Mig

The Migraine Brain

The Migraine Brain

Imaging Structure and Function

Edited by **DAVID BORSOOK, MD, PhD**
Director, Pain & Analgesia Imaging Neuroscience (P.A.I.N.) Group
McLean Hospital, Masschussetts General Hospital, and Children's Hospital
Belmont, MA

ARNE MAY, MD, PhD
Institut für Systemische Neurowissenschaften
Zentrum für Experimentelle Medizin
Universitätsklinikum Hamburg-Eppendorf
Hamburg, Germany

PETER J. GOADSBY, MD, PhD
Director, UCSF Headache Center
Department of Neurology
University of California, San Francisco
San Francisco, CA

RICHARD HARGREAVES, PhD
Vice President, Worldwide Discovery Head
Neuroscience
Merck Research Laboratories
West Point, PA and Kenilworth, NJ

OXFORD
UNIVERSITY PRESS

OXFORD
UNIVERSITY PRESS

Oxford University Press, Inc., publishes works that further
Oxford University's objective of excellence
in research, scholarship, and education.

Oxford   New York
Auckland   Cape Town   Dar es Salaam   Hong Kong   Karachi
Kuala Lumpur   Madrid   Melbourne   Mexico City   Nairobi
New Delhi   Shanghai   Taipei   Toronto

With offices in
Argentina   Austria   Brazil   Chile   Czech Republic   France   Greece
Guatemala   Hungary   Italy   Japan   Poland   Portugal   Singapore
South Korea   Switzerland   Thailand   Turkey   Ukraine   Vietnam

Copyright © 2012 by Oxford University Press, Inc.

Published by Oxford University Press, Inc.
198 Madison Avenue, New York, New York 10016
www.oup.com

Oxford is a registered trademark of Oxford University Press

Library of Congress Cataloging-in-Publication Data

The migraine brain: imaging structure and function/[edited by] David Borsook . . . [et al.].
p.; cm.
Includes bibliographical references and index.
ISBN 978–0–19–975456-4
I. Borsook, David.
[DNLM: 1. Migraine Disorders—diagnosis. 2. Migraine Disorders—physiopathology.
3. Brain—physiopathology. WL 344]
616.8'4912—dc23   2011036770

9 8 7 6 5 4 3 2 1

Printed in China on acid-free paper

FOREWORD

High-resolution imaging of the nervous system is the most useful and compelling approach to interrogate the living human brain. Without exception, neuroimaging has impacted the way we think about nearly every disorder of the human nervous system, providing a unique signature and sometimes disease-specific information of pathophysiological significance. It often provides the most relevant biomarkers for disease circa 2012. Still, these methodologies have hardly reached their potential as higher field strength magnets and more sophisticated computational and other analytical approaches improve the power, efficiency, and resolution of functional imaging. On the research side, imaging has been useful to examine the dynamics of brain connectivity during rest and after noxious stimulation, and can help to unravel the correlates of psychophysical or behavioral stimulation to brain activation and its central modulation. It also has been useful to explore the structural and functional consequences of chronic pain. Particularly relevant to the theme of this book, neuroimaging approaches have informed us about cerebral blood flow regulation and the coupling that exists between flow, metabolism, and neurophysiological activity in disorders of neurovascular regulation. Although admittedly at an early stage of investigation, these methods both alone and in combination (multimodal imaging) are now being exploited to unravel the biological underpinnings of migraine headache, among the most complex problems in contemporary neurology. There is no more compelling application of these tools than to study the migraine brain.

On the clinical side, migraine headaches are among the most common and economically burdensome neurological conditions. Affecting females more than males, the headaches are often one-sided and sometimes accompanied by nausea, vomiting, and sensitivity to light, sound, and smell. Originally considered a disorder primarily of blood vessels, the preponderance of recent data implicate the brain, its trigeminovascular system, neurovascular dysfunction, and the role of genetics and hormones as well as a host of susceptibility factors. Organized temporally into prodrome, aura, headache, and resolution, it remains uncertain in what way these phases represent the hyperexcitable state reflecting neuronal network excitability; or relate to cortical spreading depression, the putative biological event underlying migraine aura; or both. It has become increasingly recognized that the migraine brain between attacks may differ from so-called normals. Headache, although not invariate, is often the most troublesome symptom that brings patients to medical attention, along with allodynia, an underappreciated accompaniment in some migraineurs with implications for the timing of treatment and for the modulation of pain. Of considerable importance are the unexplained brain and vascular changes found in migraineurs by imaging techniques, including small infarcts within the posterior circulation, small demyelinating foci, and iron accumulation within the upper midbrain.

These and many other contemporary matters are considered in *The Migraine Brain*. Beginning with a description of the history and neurobiological issues of relevance today, the book continues with a description of its principal clinical conundrums (e.g., transition from acute to chronic pain) as it builds toward a description of studies that utilize a wide range of functional imaging tools. Chapters consider changes in white matter and connectivity, blood flow and meningeal vessel caliber, central correlates of headache and aura, and meningeal vessel caliber and their metabolic consequences. This book underscores the innumerable ways in which imaging can be used to decipher the phases of migraine described above and the interictal migraine brain. Arguably, there is no better way to conduct a functional postmortem examination (either during the interictal state or during an attack), not only in the service of nosology and a biologically based headache classification system, but also as an approach to understanding the hyperexcitable brain, its rewired state, and relevant pharmacological mechanisms essential for next-generation therapeutics. Indeed, the subject and book are timely, the tools are increasingly powerful (and getting more so), and the future of functional imaging in diagnosis and treatment of migraine looks bright.

Michael A. Moskowitz, MD
Professor of Neurology
Harvard Medical School
Affiliate, Harvard-MIT Division of
Health Sciences and Technology

PREFACE

The field of migraine has undergone advances in a number of scientific domains. Yet, treatment modalities, as is the case with many disorders affecting the central nervous system, are not optimal. Pharmacological and biobehavioral approaches for the most part do not eliminate migraine attacks. Recent advances in neuroimaging have provided unparalleled opportunities to noninvasively evaluate brain changes in migraine patients, both during the ictal and interictal phases. These approaches have included electroencephalography, magnetoencephalography, functional magnetic resonance imaging, and transcranial magnetic stimulation. In this book we have attempted to bring together the current state of the field in imaging and modulation of the brain in the migraine patient. Experts from around the world have enthusiastically come together to define the current state of these modalities. We believe that these initial steps in evaluating brain systems biology are a new beginning that will integrate with other domains of the science (including genetics, translational research, pharmacotherapy, and behavioral research) to further improve the lot of those who suffer from migraine.

This book was instigated through Elizabeth Loder, who approached us to see if we would be willing to undertake the process of recruiting authors for the project. We would like to thank all the authors for their participation and Dr. Michael Moskowitz for his willingness to write the Foreword to the book. We would also like to thank Jeanette Cohan for managing the process with those at Oxford University Press, and both Craig Panner and Kathryn Winder, whose help was invaluable. Finally, we dedicate this book to migraine sufferers including those who have participated in clinical research, without whom novel insights would not be possible. It is the promise of new therapies through research, of which imaging is now a major part, that we move forward into the future. Hopefully, it is a future where new insights translate into decreasing or curing the burden of migraine.

David Borsook, MD, PhD
Arne May, MD, PhD
Peter Goadsby, MD
Richard Hargreaves, PhD

CONTENTS

CONTRIBUTORS

M. Sohail Asghar, MD, PhD
Danish Headache Center
Department of Neurology
Glostrup Hospital
Faculty of Health Sciences
University of Copenhagen
Copenhagen, Denmark

Messoud Ashina, MD, PhD
Associate Professor
Danish Headache Center
Department of Neurology
Glostrup Hospital
Faculty of Health Sciences
University of Copenhagen
Copenhagen, Denmark

Sheena K. Aurora, MD
Director
Swedish Pain and Headache Center
Seattle, WA

Lino Becerra, PhD
Associate Professor of Psychiatry
Harvard Medical School; and
    Associate Biophysicist
McLean Hospital
Boston, MA

Marcelo E. Bigal, MD, PhD
Associate Clinical Professor
Headache Division
Saul R. Korey Department of Neurology
Albert Einstein College of Medicine
Bronx, NY

David Borsook, MD, PhD
Director, Pain & Analgesia Imaging
    Neuroscience (P.A.I.N.) Group
McLean Hospital, Massachusetts
    General Hospital, and Children's Hospital
Belmont, MA

Susan M. Bowyer, PhD
MEG Physicist
Department of Neurology
Henry Ford Hospital
Detroit, MI

Rami Burstein, PhD
Associate Professor
Anesthesia, Critical Care & Pain Medicine
Harvard University
Boston, MA

Sabina Cevoli, MD, PhD
Department of Neurological Sciences
University of Bologna Medical School
Bologna, Italy

Gianluca Coppola, MD, PhD
Department of Medico-Surgical Sciences and
    Biotechnologies
"Sapienza" University of Rome Polo Pontino; and
G.B. Bietti Eye Foundation-IRCCS
Department of Neurophysiology of Vision and
    Neuroophtalmology
Rome, Italy

Pietro Cortelli, MD
Department of Neurological Sciences
University of Bologna Medical School
Bologna, Italy

Geneviève Demarquay, MD, PhD
Neurology Unit
Hôpital Croix-Rousse
Hospices Civils de Lyon
Lyon, France

Marie Denuelle, MD
Department of Neurology
University Hospital of Toulouse
Toulouse, France

Boukje de Vries, MSc
Department of Human Genetics
Leiden University Medical Center
Leiden, The Netherlands

Hans-Christoph Diener, MD
Professor of Neurology and
    Chairman
Department of Neurology
University Duisburg-Essen
Essen, Germany

David W. Dodick, MD
Professor of Neurology
Mayo Clinic in Arizona
Scottsdale, AZ

Peter D. Drummond, PhD
Professor of Psychology
School of Psychology
Murdoch University
Perth, Australia

Mervyn J. Eadie, MD, PhD, FRACP
Emeritus Professor of Clinical Neurology and
    Neuropharmacology
Honorary Research Consultant
University of Queensland
Brisbane, Australia

Randolph W. Evans, MD
Clinical Professor of Neurology
Baylor College of Medicine
Houston, TX

Nelly Fabre, MD
Department of Neurology
University Hospital of Toulouse
Toulouse, France

Michel D. Ferrari, MD, PhD
Professor of Neurology
Leiden University Medical Center
Leiden, The Netherlands

Massimo Filippi, MD
Neuroimaging Research Unit
Institute of Experimental Neurology
Division of Neuroscience
San Raffaele Scientific Institute and Vita-Salute
    San Raffaele University
Milan, Italy

Felipe Fregni, MD, PhD
Laboratory of Neuromodulation
Department of Physical Medicine & Rehabilitation
Spaulding Rehabilitation Hospital and Massachusetts
    General Hospital
Harvard Medical School
Boston, MA

Andreas R. Gantenbein, MD
Department of Neurology
University Hospital Zurich
Zurich, Switzerland

Gilles Géraud, MD
Department of Neurology
University Hospital of Toulouse
Toulouse, France

Peter J. Goadsby, MD, PhD
Director, UCSF Headache Center
Department of Neurology
University of California, San Francisco
San Francisco, CA

Cristina Granziera, MD, PhD
Department of Clinical Neurosciences Centre
    Hospitalier Universitaire Vaudois and Advanced
    Clinical Imaging Technology Group, Centre
    d'imagerie biomédical
Ecole Polytechnique Fédéral de Lausanne
Lausanne, Switzerland

Joost Haan, MD, PhD
Department of Neurology
Leiden University Medical Center
Leiden, The Netherlands

Nouchine Hadjikhani, MD, PhD
Associate Professor of Radiology
A. A. Martinos Center for Biomedical Imaging
Harvard Medical School
Boston, MA

Richard Hargreaves, PhD
Vice President, Worldwide Discovery Head
Neuroscience
Merck Research Laboratories
West Point, PA and Kenilworth, NJ

Mark C. Kruit, MD, PhD
Department of Radiology
Leiden University Medical Center
Leiden, The Netherlands

Richard B. Lipton, MD
Professor of Neurology, Psychiatry & Behavioral
    Medicine, and Epidemiology and Population Health
Albert Einstein College of Medicine
Bronx, NY

Raffaele Lodi, MD
Functional MR Unit
Department of Biomedical and NeuroMotor Sciences
University of Bologna
Bologna, Italy

Nasim Maleki, PhD
Research Fellow in Radiology
Children's Hospital Boston
Boston, MA

Farooq H. Maniyar, MD
UCSF Headache Center
University of California, San Francisco
San Francisco, CA

François Mauguière, MD, PhD
Neurology Unit
Neurological hospital
Hospices Civils de Lyon
University Lyon1
Lyon, France

Arne May, MD, PhD
Institut für Systemische Neurowissenschaften
Zentrum für Experimentelle Medizin
Universitätsklinikum Hamburg-Eppendorf
Hamburg, Germany

Panayiotis D. Mitsias, MD, PhD
Professor of Neurology
Director, Stroke and Neurovascular Center
Neurosciences Institute
Henry Ford Health System
Detroit, MI

Eric A. Moulton, PhD
Pain/Analgesia Imaging Neuroscience Group
Department of Psychiatry, Harvard Medical School
Brain Imaging Center, McLean Hospital
Belmont, MA

Jes Olesen, MD, DMSc, DHonC
Professor of Neurology
Department of Neurology
University of Copenhagen
Glostrup Hospital
Copenhagen, Denmark

Inge H. Palm-Meinders, MD
Department of Radiology
Leiden University Medical Center
Leiden, The Netherlands

Pierre Payoux, MD, PhD
Department of Nuclear Medicine
University Hospital of Toulouse
Toulouse, France

Giulia Pierangeli, MD, PhD
Department of Neurological Sciences
University of Bologna Medical School
Bologna, Italy

Franz Riederer, MD
Department of Neurology
University Hospital Zurich
Zurich, Switzerland

Maria A. Rocca, MD
Neuroimaging Research Unit
Institute of Experimental Neurology
Division of Neuroscience
San Raffaele Scientific Institute and Vita-Salute
    San Raffaele University
Milan, Italy

Sidra Saeed
Swedish Pain and Headache Center
Seattle, WA

Peter S. Sándor, MD
Senior Physician of Head, Headaches,
    and Pain Clinic
Department of Neurology
University Hospital Zurich
Zurich, Switzerland

Jean Schoenen, MD, PhD
Professor of Neurology
Headache Research Unit
University Department of Neurology
University of Liège
Liège, Belgium

Todd J. Schwedt, MD
Director, Washington University
    Headache Center
Department of Neurology
Washington University School of Medicine
St. Louis, MO

Christian L. Seifert, MD
Klinikum rechts der Isar
Neurologische Klinik und Poliklinik
Technische Universität München
Munich, Germany

Christos Sidiropoulos, MD
Movement Disorders Fellow
Henry Ford Health System
Detroit, MI

Stephen D. Silberstein, MD
Professor of Neurology
Department of Neurology
Director, Jefferson Headache Center
Thomas Jefferson University
Philadelphia, PA

Till Sprenger, MD
Department of Neurology
Universitätsspital Basel
Basel, Switzerland

Anne Stankewitz, PhD
Professor of Neuroscience
Department of Systems Neuroscience
University Medical Center Hamburg-Eppendorf
Hamburg, Germany

Gisela M. Terwindt, MD
Department of Neurology
Leiden University Medical Center
Leiden, The Netherlands

Peer Tfelt-Hansen, MD, DMS
Danish Headache Center
Department of Neurology
University of Copenhagen
Glostrup Hospital
Glostrup, Denmark

Caterina Tonon, MD
Functional MR Unit
Department of Biomedical and NeuroMotor Sciences
University of Bologna
Bologna, Italy

Arn M.J.M. van den Maagdenberg, PhD
Department of Human Genetics
Leiden University Medical Center
Leiden, The Netherlands

Maurice B. Vincent, MD, PhD
Department of Neurology
Hospital Universitário Clementino Fraga Filho
Universidade Federal do Rio de Janeiro
Rio de Janeiro, Brazil

Magdalena Sarah Volz
Laboratory of Neuromodulation
Department of Physical Medicine & Rehabilitation
Spaulding Rehabilitation Hospital and Massachusetts
    General Hospital
Harvard Medical School
Boston, MA

Claudia M. Weller, MD
Department of Human Genetics
Leiden University Medical Center
Leiden, The Netherlands

Part 1

Migraine: History

1 A History of Migraine

MERVYN J. EADIE

INTRODUCTION

The true beginnings of the story of migraine have been lost in the obscurity of prehistory. This review selects a number of vignettes that have been recorded over time to illustrate the evolution in the history of migraine.

Antiquity

The oldest record of human headache may date from about 6,000 years ago. Thompson (1903), after translating some late-8th-century BCE Babylonian cuneiform tablets that included material on headache, concluded from internal and other evidence that their original versions were prepared around 4000 BCE. The details in his translation do not permit identification of the type or types of headache mentioned. Headache was also recorded in various Egyptian papyri (Karenberg & Leitz, 2001) dating from around 1550 BCE, but the types of headache cannot be determined. Chapter 4 of the Old Testament Second Book of Kings (circa 7th century BCE) contains the story of a boy who one morning went to his father in the fields and then cried out, "My head, my head!" The boy was taken to his mother, sat on her knees till noon, and then died. The mother sent for the prophet Elisha, who found the child had "neither voice nor hearing." Elisha then seems to have breathed into the boy's mouth and the child became warm and, after an interval, opened his eyes again. At that point the account ended. Clearly, the story could have more than one explanation in terms of pathology, but could it be accounted for by an episode of childhood migraine culminating in deep sleep, with full recovery by the time of waking?

This interpretation of this ancient biblical tale raises the question of how migraine may be recognized in writings from a bygone day when the entity itself was not defined. The word *migraine*, of French origin, is a corruption of the late Latin *hemicrania* ("half a head"), which itself is derived from the Greek ἡμικρανία. It has been customary to take the word *hemicrania* in earlier writings to refer to what would now be accepted as migraine. This may often be correct, because migraine is such a frequent type of headache. However, the ancients thought of *hemicrania* in its literal sense of a one-sided head pain, and such pain may have causes other than migraine, for example, the various hemicranial pains described in the *Observationes* of Wepfer (1727) and Sauvages' (1772) list of 10 varieties of *hemicrania* (the ocular, dental, sinus, hemorrhoidal, purulent, and infective types; those associated with coryza, kidney disease, and the phase of the moon; and *clavus hystericus*). For at least two centuries, it has been increasingly realized that the headache of migraine is not necessarily strictly one sided (Labarraque, 1837). Therefore, the *hemicrania* of the past can be assumed to include today's migraine, but disorders other than migraine may be included; however, instances of nonunilateral migraine will be excluded. Indeed, to be reasonably sure that an earlier account of headache has dealt with the modern entity of migraine, there probably should be at least a history of either otherwise unexplained recurrent reasonably similar headache attacks occurring over a period of months or longer, or headache attacks associated with typical migraine aura phenomena. Ancient medical writing often does not seem to have been particularly concerned with the long-term course of illness. Therefore, the recorded occurrence of an aura in older descriptions of headache has great importance in recognizing migraine. If this point is accepted, the earliest known account of reasonably unequivocal migraine is present in the later writings of the Hippocratic school (circa 200 BCE), though not in what are often considered the genuine works of Hippocrates. In the words of Smith's translation of one of the two very similar passages present in the original version (Hippocrates, 1994, p. 207):

> Phoenix's problem: he seemed to see flashes like lightning in his eye, mostly the right. And when he had suffered that a short time, a terrible pain developed toward his right temple and then around his whole head and on to the part of the neck where the head is attached behind the vertebrae. And there was tension and hardening around the tendons. If he tried to move his head or opened his teeth, he could not, as being violently stretched. Vomits, whenever they occurred, averted the pains I have described, or made them gentler.

The accompanying text contained no interpretation of the cause or mechanism of production of this headache.

Early Christian Era Greco-Roman Medicine

Early Greek medical authors appear to have subdivided headache on the basis of its time course into short-lived varieties (*cephalalgia*) and persistent or recurrent types (*cephalaea*). Aretaeus the Cappadocian (probably early 2nd century CE) wrote about *cephalalgia* in a part of his work that has been lost. In the surviving portions (Adams, 1856), he dealt with *cephalaea* (i.e., chronic or recurrent headache). This could involve the whole head or part of it. Aretaeus considered it due to coldness with dryness. When such headache was strictly localized to one half of the head, he called it (*h*)*eterocrania*. This pain could begin suddenly with:

> unseemly and dreadful symptoms; spasm and distortion of the countenance takes place; the eyes either fixed intently like horns, or they are rolled inwardly to this side or that; vertigo, deep-seated pain of the eyes as far as the meninges; irresistible sweat; sudden pain of the tendons, as of one striking with a club; nausea; vomiting of bilious matter; collapse of the patient; but, if the affection be protracted, the patient will die, or, if more slight and not deadly, it becomes chronic; there is much torpor, heaviness of the head, anxiety, and *ennui*. For they flee the light; the darkness soothes their disease; nor can they bear readily to look upon or hear anything agreeable. (Adams, 1856, pp. 294–295)

Some such instances could be accounted for by migraine; others obviously could not.

Aretaeus recommended treating worsening *cephalaea* by bleeding from a vein at the elbow followed by the use of purgatives. Further bleeding from a forehead vein could be carried out, and the shaved head at the vertex or the interscapular area cupped. Excision of part of the superficial temporal or postauricular arteries could also be considered to be necessary. Phlegm was to be removed from the body via the alimentary tract (employing clysters or sialogogues) or by inducing sneezing (using sternutatories, e.g., pepper powder, beaver's testicle). He mentioned that *heterocrania* was treated similarly to *cephalaea*, except that any locally acting remedies were applied at the headache site.

Galen of Pergamon (121 to circa 200 CE), probably a little later in the 2nd century CE than Aretaeus, dealt with the subject of headache in a number of places in his voluminous surviving writings. The different accounts are not entirely consistent, possibly reflecting different times of composition. Galen usually used the word *hemicrania* instead of *heterocrania*, but he occasionally employed the latter. Book II of Volume 12 of the Kühn edition of Galen's *Opera omnia* (1821–1833) contains individual chapters on the treatment of head pain (*dolor capitis,* seemingly equivalent to *cephalalgia*), *cephalaea,* and *hemicrania.* This arrangement suggests that Galen might have been the first to define the latter as a separate headache entity, though the later Byzantine commentator Alexander of Tralles (6th century CE) is usually credited for this classification.

James's *Medical Dictionary* (1745, p. 207) stated that Galen "beautifully described" *cephalea* (in what could pass as an account of an attack of migraine without aura):

> A Cephalea is a lasting Pain of the whole Head, which is with Difficulty remov'd, and which, by the slightest Accidents, is so increased, that the Patient can neither endure any Noise, any loud Voice, the Splendor of the Light, or any Motion, but seeks Retirement from Noise, and a dark Chamber, on account of the intense Pain: For some imagine, that they are beaten with a Mallet, others that their Heads left contus'd and distended, and in some few the Pain reaches to the Roots of the Eyes, so that, in this Species of Pain, we have no Reason to doubt but the whole Membrane of the Head is severely affected.

Galen at different places in his writings indicated that either yellow bile or a hot vaporous pneuma, which had accumulated in the stomach, could rise to the head to produce headache. The pain itself originated in the meninges and pericranium. He also cited an observation from the now lost writings of Archigenes (circa 100 CE) that suggested that cranial blood vessels, particularly arteries, were involved in headache causation. In the words of Siegel's (1976, p. 52) translation of Galen's *De locis affectis* (Kühn, Vol. 8): "If blood vessels which are not inflamed are strongly compressed, the headaches [Kephalgias] are stopped as if the influx [of humours] is prevented." This observation had to wait more than 1,500 years to be recorded in medical literature again.

It seems likely that Galen would have followed Archigenes and applied such ideas to the interpretation of headaches which would fit into the category of present-day migraine. Galen listed a large array of therapeutic approaches that might afford headache relief, including the use of phlegm-removing apophlegmatics (taken by mouth or inserted into the nostrils), clysters, and cataplasms (plasters or poultices); local applications of sternutatories (to induce sneezing); and even wearing amulets.

The later Byzantine commentators (e.g., Caelius Aurelianus, Oribasius, Alexander of Tralles, Paul of Aegina) added little that was original and conceptually important to the knowledge of their predecessors regarding the origin and classification of headache. However, the range of therapeutic material that they advocated became more extensive, and Caelius Aurelianus (1950), in particular, provided considerable lifestyle-type advice.

Arabic and Medieval European Medicine

The Arabic medical writers of the 11th to 13th centuries (Haly Abbas, Rhases, Avicenna) largely reiterated the ideas of the early Greco-Roman physicians concerning headache, its causes, and its treatment. They named recurrent unilateral headache *shaqhiqheh* (Gorji & Ghadiri, 2002). Conceptually, in relation to the emergence of the modern entity of migraine, there was, however, little real advance.

Singer (2005) considered that several of the visions described and illustrated by the medieval mystical philosopher Hildegard of Bingen (1098–1179), abbess of a Benedictine convent in the Rhineland, suggest that she may have experienced the visual aura of migraine. For instance, part of one of her illustrations showed falling sparks in a pattern that a migraine sufferer might describe, while the remainder of the illustration included a reasonably well-executed sketch of a humanlike figure. This illustration was explained as follows:

> I saw a great star most splendid and beautiful, and with it an exceeding multitude of falling sparks which the star followed southward. And they examined Him upon His throne almost as something hostile, and turning from Him they sought rather the north. And suddenly they were all annihilated, being turned into black coals. (p. 78)

If Singer's interpretation is correct, a probable medieval migraine sufferer has been identified. Knowledge about the disorder was not otherwise advanced.

The Parisian physician Jean Fernel (1497–1558) continued to deal with headache under the conventional triad of headache types. The French translation of his *Pathologie* (Fernel, 1655) contained the idea that the ordinary headache, which was often suffered over many years and occurred on the slightest occasion, was either *cephalaea* or "migraine." The latter was one sided, usually commenced with beating or throbbing in the temple, and sometimes was due to sympathy with the abdominal viscera. The sympathy was mediated by a sharp bilious humor from the stomach, which impacted on the meninges. As Fernel elsewhere in his account had already considered head pain due to organic disease, it seems fairly clear that he was referring to what would pass as present-day migraine. His account really adds no important new insights to existing concepts of migraine pathogenesis, though he provided an explanation for the mechanism of the "sympathy" that he postulated.

The 17th Century

During the 17th century, medical reports in which migraine was recognizable increased in number and new ideas concerning its pathogenesis began to appear.

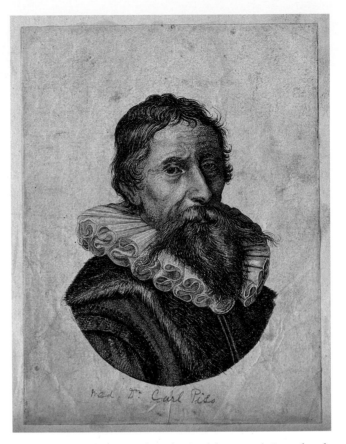

FIGURE 1–1 *Charles Le Pois (Carolus Piso) (1563–1635). Reproduced with permission of the Wellcome Library, London.*

Charles Le Pois (*Carolus Piso*, 1563–1635; Fig. 1–1), professor of medicine at the University of Pont-à-Mousson in northern France, described the course of his own recurrent headache with vomiting of bile. He had suffered from this since he had been a student in Paris in his youth (Le Pois, 1618). He also described the instance of a 12-year-old girl who developed a sensation of formication, which began in the little finger of the left hand and spread over the hand to the forearm, upper arm, and neck, while severe headache occurred in the front part of the left side of her head. The episode ended with vomiting of bile. No disturbance of vision was mentioned. Milder recurrences occurred. This may be the first report of what was later somewhat loosely called "hemiplegic migraine." Le Pois ascribed the headache of what obviously was migraine to an acrid bilious humor from the stomach that boiled up and flowed over the head, causing distension of the membranes of the brain, thus producing headache. This explanation owed something to ancient humoral pathology but also contained an element of Paracelsian iatrochemistry and included a mechanism through which the irritated meninges might cause pain. Le Pois reasoned that vomiting during the attacks was a result of the headache and not of a primary gastric disturbance, writing (in the words of Liveing's [1873] translation, p. 239):

> Since the headache invariably precedes the abdominal pains and spasms, as I have experienced in my own case and that of others, and as will appear from the following narrative, it may be hence inferred that the head suffers idiopathically, but the stomach and bowels by sympathy with the head.

In 1666 Van der Linden drew attention to the relation between the menstrual cycle and migraine when he described the consistent association between the two in the then 31-year-old Marchioness of Brandenberg (*hemicrania menstrua*). Thomas Sydenham (1624–1689), when discussing "the affection called hysteria in women; and hypochondriasis in men," mentioned a new entity of *clavus hystericus*: "a racking pain in the head, so limited as to be covered by your thumb, accompanied by the vomiting-up of green matter like rancid bile" (Sydenham, 1848, p. 231).

The term *clavus* continued to appear in the literature in relation to such localized headache for some two centuries afterward. Campbell (1894) considered that it was merely a variant of migraine.

Thomas Willis (1621–1675; Fig. 1–2) in his *De Anima Brutorum* (1672) wrote on "headach" in general rather

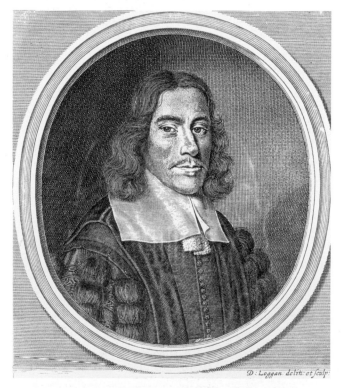

FIGURE 1–2 *Thomas Willis (1621–1675). The frontispiece of the remaining medical works of that famous and renowned physician Dr Thomas Willis. London. Dring, Harper, Leigh and Martyn. 1681.*

than on migraine specifically. He proposed a mechanism to explain *hemicrania*, which Pordage translated as "meagrim":

> Secondly, The other kind of Headach, to wit, within the skull, is more frequent, and much more cruel, because the Membranes, cloathing the Brain, are very sensible, and the Blood is poured upon them by a manifold passage, and by many and greater Arteries. Further, because the Blood or its Serum, sometimes passing thorow all the Arteries at once, both the *Carotides* and the *Vertebrals*, and sometimes apart, thorow these or those, on the one side or the opposite, bring hurt to the Meninges, hence the pain is caused that is interior; which is either universal, infesting the whole Head or its greatest part, or particular, which is limited to some private region; and sometimes produces a Meagrim on the side, sometimes in the forepart, and sometimes in the hinder part of the Head. (Willis, 1683, p. 106)

Thus, Willis related the headache of migraine to increased localized or more widespread cranial artery blood flow. Elsewhere in his account he wrote of the meninges being distended or pulled on, so that the irritated meningeal nerves produced head pain. Willis was an iatrochemist and in his explanations for the most part eschewed the humoral misbehaviors that had dominated concepts of the pathogenesis of migraine for centuries. Instead, he invoked the existence of (imaginary) chemical entities and unprovable intellectual creations such as the animal spirits and the vital spirits. Conceptually, his major insight was to postulate a vascular basis with a secondary neural component in the pathogenesis of migraine. His lists of treatments contained some novel components as compared with earlier writers, but clearly he and his contemporaries knew of no invariably effective remedy, as he confessed when writing of the treatment of the migraine of Anne, Countess of Conway (Willis, 1672, p.122):

> there was no kind of Medicines both *Cephalicks, Antiscorbutics, Hystericals,* all famous *Specificks,* which she took not, both from the Learned and the unlearned, from quacks, and old Women; and yet notwithstanding, she professed, that she had received from no Remedy, or method of Curing, any thing of Cure or Ease, but that the contumacious and rebellious Disease, refused to be tamed, being deaf to the charms of every Medicine.

Willis's great Swiss contemporary Johann Jakob Wepfer (1620–1695; Fig. 1–3), in his posthumously published (1727) *Observationes medico-practicae de affectibus capitis,* provided a number of accounts of *cephalaea* and *hemicrania.* The exact allocation of some of these to modern headache categories is arguable, but Wepfer's Observation

54 described the course of a headache that was very probably migraine with a visual aura (blurred vision beginning on the right side with moving flies being seen). This occurred in a 23-year-old woman ill with a urinary tract infection. According to Isler (1985), Wepfer took the view that the "headache of emicrania was of vascular origin, and that the vascular disturbance was due to postulated defective serum, or overfilled vessels" and that brain disturbance accounted for the migraine aura and vomiting in the attacks. Isler (1987) also considered Wepfer's Observation 108 and thought it likely that here he described so-called basilar artery migraine. However, the existence of previous probable cerebrovascular events in this case makes that interpretation questionable. Interestingly, Wepfer did not offer any overall hypothesis concerning the pathogenesis of *hemicrania*. Rather, he preferred to interpret the headache mechanisms in his cases individually and did not go into the mechanism of the headache in the commentary accompanying what probably was his most convincing instance of migraine (Observation 54, outlined above).

The 18th Century

In the mid-18th century, a monograph reviewing *hemicrania* appeared (Fordyce, 1758), containing the suggestion that hemicranial pain could originate in the temporal muscles and the falx cerebri. The latter is a part of the dura not specifically mentioned previously as a site of origin of head pain.

In the 1770s, Samuel Tissot's (Fig. 1–4) influential *Traité des nerfs*, dealing with both psychological and neurological illness, appeared in stages. One chapter dealt with migraine under that designation (Tissot, 1780). The text has never been published in English translation, but Tissot's description of the clinical features of the disorder is detailed and thorough and contains most of what one would expect in a modern-day account. He recognized that every unilateral headache was not necessarily migraine and mentioned that there were instances of headache that resembled migraine in all respects except that the pain was not restricted to one side of the head.

Tissot rejected the idea of Le Pois, Wepfer, and others that migraine was due to the accumulation of an acid

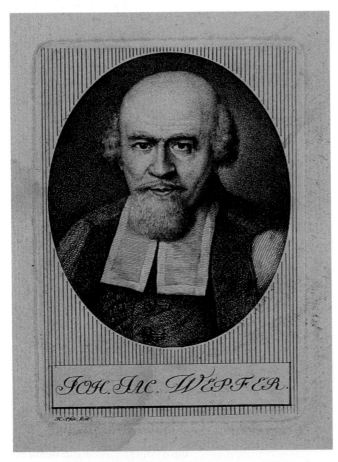

FIGURE 1–3 *Johann Jakob Wepfer (1620–1695). Reproduced with permission of the Wellcome Library, London.*

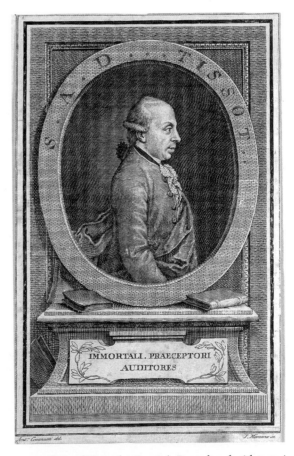

FIGURE 1–4 *Samuel Tissot (1728–1787). Reproduced with permission of the Wellcome Library, London.*

serosity. In contrast, he believed that the stomach was the usual primary source of migraine and that the head symptoms resulted from a process of sympathy with the stomach. The mechanism mediating the sympathy was that the effect of the stomach abnormality was transmitted by nerves (presumably the vagus) to branches of the trigeminal nerves, especially the supraorbital ones. Therefore, the headache site usually corresponded to the territory of distribution of the latter nerves. However, the pain could be present more extensively in areas innervated by the trigeminal nerves. Spread of the neural activity to other parts of the central nervous system accounted, for instance, for vomiting in migraine attacks. Tissot's interpretation led him to advocate the use of milk as a treatment for migraine and in general to recommend less vigorous therapies than his predecessors.

Tissot's writings had important consequences. They were intended to reach and educate the medical profession in Western Europe. On the whole they did so, making physicians more aware of migraine and its frequency. Tissot abandoned any lingering notions about a humoral pathogenesis of migraine and introduced a neurally mediated hypothesis instead, ignoring the vascular-based type of hypothesis found in Willis's writings. As well, Tissot's ideas discouraged overly vigorous therapy for the disorder. They probably played a very significant role in initiating the veritable torrent of French language publications and theses concerning migraine that appeared during the 19th century. Before discussing some of this French output, three late-18th-century British contributions warrant mention.

John Fothergill of London, in 1778, tried to emphasize to English readers the frequency of so-called "sick headach," that is, migraine. In doing this, he attributed the disorder to "inattention to diet" but did not explain how this would produce headache. He noted that symptoms of alimentary tract disturbance usually appeared after the headache began. Hence, he probably would have disagreed with Tissot's interpretation of migraine pathogenesis, had he known of it.

Whether or not he knew of Tissot's writings, William Heberden (1802) held that migraine usually originated from the stomach, the headache being brought about through the effects of "sympathy," though he allowed the possibility that the head could be affected primarily in migraine.

Probably without knowing that it had been observed in the 1st century CE, Caleb Hillier Parry of Bristol (1792) reported that unilateral carotid compression on the headache-affected side temporarily relieved *hemicrania* and bilious headache. Thereafter, this observation continued to be relevant to the interpretation of the pathogenesis of

migraine. Parry later described scintillating scotoma in migraine (Parry, 1825).

The 19th Century

Remarkably little was published on the aura of migraine between its description in the later Hippocratic school's writings and the early 19th century, though instances of aura documented in the works of Charles Le Pois and Wepfer were referred to by Tissot (1780), who added his own examples of migraine with aura. In the 1830s, Pierre-Adolphe Piorry (1831; Fig. 1–5) described the visual aura of the disorder in considerable detail and proposed a novel and wide-ranging hypothesis to account for it and the ensuing headache. He suggested that an exciting cause, probably ambient light, acted on the retina and the iris to cause pupil constriction. Local neural activity then resulted in an oscillation of the iris. When contracted, the iris produced an image of a small luminous circle with irregular margins—the so-called fortification spectra. This grew larger whenever the iris dilated. If the local neural disturbance spread into nearby trigeminal branches, particularly the supraorbital nerve, pain occurred in the nerve's territory of supply. The neural disturbance might extend to the sympathetic nervous system and the vagus via anastomotic neural communications, causing nausea and vomiting. Piorry considered that migraine with aura was an iridial or ciliary neuralgia, an "irisalgia." Forty-four years later his interpretation remained unchanged (Piorry, 1875). Indeed, the idea that migraine was a neuralgia was present previously in the literature, for example, to an extent in the writings of Willis (1672) and Whytt (1768), and this concept held for some time in that migraine was thought to be a neuralgia of trigeminal nerve branches (e.g., Garrett Anderson, 1870; Romberg, 1853; Symonds, 1858; Woakes, 1868).

Over the next few decades numerous publications on migraine continued to appear in the French language. Calmeil (1839) thought that migraine was a trigeminal neuralgia but considered that the visual aura symptoms were cerebral in origin. He recognized that most of the factors that precipitated migraine attacks must act through neural pathways in the brain to involve the trigeminal innervation of the head. Calmeil also noted that there sometimes was evidence of increased local blood flow in the painful area and increased arterial pulsation during migraine attacks. He thought that these phenomena probably were of neural origin but could not explain them further.

Auzias Turenne (1849), again in Paris, produced a reasonably comprehensive hypothesis of migraine pathogenesis based on the concept of intracranial venous distension. He proposed that distended venous sinuses near the base

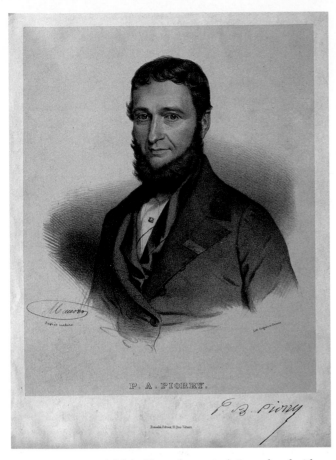

FIGURE 1–5 *Pierre-Adolphe Piorry (1792–1879). Reproduced with permission of the Wellcome Library, London.*

of the skull compressed the trigeminal nerve, particularly its first division, in the cavernous sinus. The compression could be mainly one sided, thus explaining unilateral headache. Pulsation of the carotid artery within the sinus made the nerve compression, and therefore the pain, pulsatile in character. If venous blood in the foramen lacerum or the distended jugular vein within the carotid sheath in the neck compressed the vagus nerve, nausea and vomiting could result. Congestion of the ophthalmic vein possibly caused blurred vision. Turenne's idea perished for want of evidence of the proposed mechanism. A similar fate befell the related but less developed notion that Marshall Hall (1849), in Britain, put forward in the same year as Turenne. Hall invoked the reflex arc mechanism he had earlier discovered to suggest that irritation of the afferent limb of the arc caused reflex neck muscle spasm, which obstructed the jugular veins. The resulting cranial venous congestion (Hall's *phlebismus*) brought about migraine.

These vascular-based ideas of migraine pathogenesis, which had appeared in parallel with the neuralgia-type hypotheses, were given a stronger scientific basis by the Berlin physiologist Emil Du Bois-Reymond (1861).

He attempted to interpret the mechanism of his own migraine, stressing (though it proved of little avail) that he was not attempting to explain the mechanism of all migraines. Since he was 20 years old he had experienced attacks of moderately severe headache in his right temple. The pain increased with each pulsation of the superficial temporal artery, which in the attacks felt like a hard cord compared with its left-sided counterpart. His face was pale and his right eye a little injected during the attacks. As an attack was passing off, his right ear became red and his skin warmer. During an attack, he had seen in a mirror that his right pupil was dilated. He interpreted the phenomena in terms of overaction of his right cervical sympathetic trunk causing painful spasm of the muscle coat of the arteries in the painful part of his head. He assumed that the ophthalmic, internal carotid, and vertebral arteries were also contracted during his attacks. Cerebral blood pressure fluctuations caused his nausea. Decreased blood pressure in the visual apparatus explained the visual aura phenomena that others might experience in their attacks. Ultimately, the spasm of the arterial walls would pass off due to smooth muscle fatigue so that his facial skin became warmer. Du Bois-Reymond thought that the sympathetic nervous system overaction that underlay his migraine (a *hemicrania sympathotonica*) originated in the upper thoracic portion of his spinal cord (the ciliospinal region).

Brown-Séquard (1861), then in London, promptly rejected the idea that arterial wall muscle spasm was painful, on the basis of his animal experimental work stimulating the cervical sympathetic trunk. He also commented that there were signs of cervical sympathetic paralysis, rather than overaction, during the headaches in most of the cases of migraine that he had seen. Du Bois-Reymond's fellow Berliner Möllendorf (1867) reinforced the latter point and claimed that there was ophthalmoscopic evidence of increased retinal blood flow in the eye on the affected side during migraine attacks. Möllendorf also pointed out that, while carotid compression on the side of the headache was maintained, the headache was relieved. He concluded, in the words of Liveing's (1873, page 307) translation:

> Hemicrania is a partly typical partly a-typical one-sided loss of power in the vaso-motor nerves governing the carotid artery, whereby a relaxation of the artery and a flow of arterial blood towards the brain are established.

Very probably in ignorance of Möllendorf's paper, in 1869 Samuel Wilks, a great Victorian-era English scientific clinician, proposed a similar interpretation of the mechanism of migraine headache. Later Wilks (1878, p. 427) expressed the idea thus:

The fact is, that in this distended throbbing carotid and its branches lies the source of the trouble. The vasomotor nerve on one side seems for the time paralysed, the vessels of the head dilate, more blood is sent to it, hence the increased heat, throbbing, and pain which the patient must suffer till the tone of the nerve is restored.

Albert Eulenburg (1877), then of the University of Greifswald, recognized that neither Du Bois-Reymond's idea nor Möllendorf's *hemicrania neuro-paralytica* explained the phenotype of migraine sufferers who had no detectable vasomotor disturbance during their headaches. Eulenburg suggested that any rapid-onset change in cranial arterial diameter might irritate nearby trigeminal nerve endings and so produce the pain of migraine. Thus, he neatly accommodated most features of the two earlier sympathetic nervous system–based hypotheses:

> Probably, in migraine, the local anomalies of circulation, without regard to their special mode of origin, are to be regarded as the essential and universal causal condition, while, on the other hand, tetanus or relaxation of the muscles of the vessels exercises rather an indirect influence, confined to single cases, and acting through the local anaemia or hyperaemia of which it is an important cause. (Eulenburg, 1877, pp. 21–22)

In fact, this type of sympathetic neurovascular interpretation had been anticipated in print in a slightly different way by Jaccoud (1869), who thought that the discrepancy between Du Bois-Reymond's and Möllendorf's interpretations might have resulted from observations having been made at different stages in migraine attacks, and suggested that in migraine an initial phase of sympathetic excitation was followed by a phase of sympathetic paralysis.

The British astronomer royal Sir George Biddell Airy (1865), in a response to a paper "On Hemianopsy" written by Sir David Brewster, principal of Edinburgh University, in the *Philosophical Magazine*, described and illustrated his own typically migrainous visual illusions, which occurred without accompanying headache. Airy's son Hubert (Airy, 1870), then a medical graduate, published a detailed account of the visual aura (for which he coined the term *teichopsia*, i.e., "town-wall vision") that preceded his own attacks of headache. Airy's colored illustration of the evolution of his visual changes has often been republished. Airy's (1870) paper was enhanced by its account of similar visual illusions that occurred in contemporary scientific notables and which he probably knew about through his father's connections with the Royal Society. Airy offered no explanation for the mechanism of the aura

but raised pertinent questions about it and the ensuing headaches. Was the aura due to a temporary suspension of brain function? Was the headache due to spread of the initial disturbance in the brain? Obviously he was thinking along the lines that migraine was a neural and not a vascular disorder, and that the neural element was cerebral and not located peripherally.

P. W. Latham attempted to answer Airy's questions, and so did another Cambridge medical graduate, Edward Liveing. Latham (1872, 1873) reasoned that circumstances that favored the onset of migraine (e.g., fatigue, anxiety, or other depressing causes) would decrease the brain's capacity to restrain the sympathetic nervous system. The resulting cervical sympathetic overactivity would cause cerebral artery constriction. Decreased cerebral arterial blood flow then caused the aura. When the sympathetic nervous system became exhausted from its overactivity, a state of sympathetic underactivity ensued. Cranial artery dilatation and headache would then occur. Latham's concept was a mixture of Du Bois-Reymond's and Wilks's ideas and had been anticipated by Jaccoud (1869). The concept was very similar to the interpretation of the mechanism of migraine that was to reappear and hold sway in the middle decades of the 20th century, though by then Jaccoud's and Latham's role as its originators had, by many, long been forgotten.

Almost simultaneously with Latham, Edward Liveing (1872, 1873) published a paper on migraine and also what became the classical monograph *On Megrim, Sick Headache and Some Allied Disorders* (Fig. 1–6). Liveing proposed that migraine was the result of a "nerve storm." He was working at a time when John Hughlings Jackson thought that epileptic seizures were produced by sudden bursts of localized cerebral cortical overactivity. Liveing's nerve storm seems to have been envisaged as an inherited tendency to irregular accumulation and subsequent discharge of nerve force, a "neurosal seizure." This event could occur anywhere along a line of brain structures extending from the optic thalamus to the vagal nucleus in the lower brainstem. The thalamic disturbance accounted for the visual aura—the course of the visual pathway beyond the thalamus had not been established at that time. Vagal nuclear disturbance accounted for the nausea and vomiting of migraine. Disturbance in between these anatomical extremes somehow accounted for the headache. Liveing's concept was an ingenious application of Jackson's then novel ideas concerning epileptogenesis and localization of function in the brain. His location of the site of origin of migraine headache appears prescient in light of quite recent knowledge.

The remaining years of the 19th century saw no major advances in the understanding of migraine. There was

ON MEGRIM, SICK-HEADACHE,

AND

SOME ALLIED DISORDERS:

A CONTRIBUTION

TO THE PATHOLOGY OF NERVE-STORMS.

BY

EDWARD LIVEING, M.D. Cantab.

HONORARY FELLOW OF KING'S COLLEGE, LONDON;
FORMERLY ASSISTANT PHYSICIAN TO KING'S COLLEGE HOSPITAL;
EXAMINER IN MEDICINE, UNIVERSITY OF CAMBRIDGE, 1870–71.

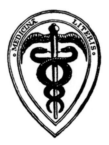

LONDON:
J. AND A. CHURCHILL, NEW BURLINGTON STREET.
1873.

FIGURE 1–6 *Title page of Edward Liveing's classical monograph on migraine (1873).*

some refinement of ideas, and an ergot alkaloid, the first specific agent against the headache, was used therapeutically without its significance then being realized.

John Hughlings Jackson (1835–1911) began to speculate on the range of intermittent disorders that might be accounted for by his "discharging lesion" idea, and included migraine among them (Jackson 1876, 1879). He wrote (Jackson, 1879, p. 278):

scientifically migraine is, I think, to be classed with the epilepsies, provisionally, as being dependent on a "discharging lesion" of some part of the cerebral cortex – probably of some part of Ferrier's sensory region.

His idea was taken up by others, and even half a century later can be found in a paper by Collier (1928). The persistence of his theory may reflect both Jackson's enormous medical reputation and the absence of completely satisfactory theories of the genesis of migraine.

William Gowers (1845–1915), in Volume 2 of his *Manual of Diseases of the Nervous System* (1888), often considered the greatest of all neurology single-authored texts, expressed the view that a cerebral cortical disturbance explained both the aura and the pain of migraine. He was cautious concerning the nature of the process in the cortex, possibly because he knew that his University College London colleague Sidney Ringer (1877) had suggested that migraine was not caused by release of excess nervous system energy (i.e., Liveing's "nerve storms"). Instead, it resulted from loss of "resistance," more or less tantamount to inhibition, in the "nucleus of the supraorbital nerve." This postulated loss of resistance might spread to other brain areas to explain, for instance, the nausea and vomiting of the migraine attack.

Moebius (1894) suggested that an initial brain disturbance in the migraine attack might affect cervical sympathetic tone. The resulting change in cranial blood flow produced the headache. Thus, he linked a cerebral origin to a vascular element via the sympathetic nervous system to explain the mechanism of the migraine attack.

Overall, by the end of the 19th century, the dominant view seems to have been that migraine resulted from a cerebral disturbance, though some, for instance, Wilfred Harris (1907), continued to favor Latham's vascular-based concept.

Over the preceding centuries an enormous array of substances were used therapeutically in attempts to relieve migraine. None proved consistently useful. Then, in August 1868, Edward Woakes (1837–1912), a medical practitioner from Luton in England, reported the use of liquid extract of ergot of rye in seven patients (four with sciatica). The extract proved effective in two young women with probable migraine (though diagnosed by Woakes as having *tic douloureux*) and in a 35-year-old man with *hemicrania*. Woakes's account marks the beginning of the use of ergot derivatives in migraine, a story that belongs to the 20th century.

The French librarian Louis Hyacinthe Thomas (1887) published a competent monograph on migraine in which he divided the topic into *migraine vulgaire* (common migraine, i.e., migraine without aura) and *migraine ophthalmique* (more or less equivalent to migraine with aura, the so-called classical migraine). This distinction has continued in use ever since.

The 20th Century

During much of the first half of the 20th century, the absence of satisfactory hypotheses that explained all aspects of migraine pathogenesis, the lack of adequate investigational methods applicable to humans, and the disruption of medical research produced by two world wars and their aftermaths probably account for the failure to develop major new ideas about migraine, though there were therapeutic advances. A good deal of attention was paid to migraine causes, as distinct from migraine mechanisms.

MIGRAINE TREATMENT

As mentioned above, Woakes had used ergot of rye in 1868 and others tried various ergot-derived preparations with some success in the late 19th century. The Swiss chemist Stoll (1918) isolated pure ergotamine from the mix of alkaloids in ergot. The pure substance, given parenterally and later by mouth, proved efficacious in relieving migraine attacks in small numbers of sufferers (Maier, 1926; Rothlin, 1955) and came into increasing therapeutic use despite growing awareness of the long record of ergot's toxicity, as described, for instance, by Barger (1931). Synthetic analgesics (e.g., aspirin), as they became available, also were employed. Perhaps surprisingly, Osler (1892) observed that "*cannabis indica* is probably the most satisfactory remedy," although this has not subsequently been proven to be so.

Over the centuries a great variety of physical activities, or occasionally inactivity, had been recommended to be therapeutic for preventing migraine, and vast numbers of substances were used as preventative treatments without any single agent proving satisfactory. Careful and critical thinkers such as Gowers had their personal favorites (e.g., bromide, glyceryl trinitrate). However, during the 20th century, therapeutic trials and statistical methodology gradually established that certain agents (e.g., methysergide, certain antihistamines with antiserotonin properties, and β-adrenergic blocking agents) did possess genuine, though decidedly modest, migraine-preventing actions. More recently anticonvulsants such as valproate and topiramate and toxins such as onabotulinum toxin have been approved for prevention. Unfortunately, there has been a paucity of research directed to the discovery of migraine prophylaxis drugs in recent years.

THE UNDERSTANDING OF MIGRAINE

In the earlier part of the 20th century, allergy was considered a major precipitating cause of migraine, mainly on the basis of anecdotal and circumstantial evidence. However, reasonably adequately designed experiments failed to substantiate the association (Loveless, 1950). Hurst (1924), and numerous others, made claims for the causal role of vision defects or refractive errors, though the idea was soon rejected by Bramwell (1926). Nonetheless, it lingered much longer in popular awareness.

Sigmund Freud put forward a psychodynamic interpretation of the origin of the disorder (Karwautz, Wober-Bingol, & Wober, 1996). Some new, either unprovable or demonstrably unsatisfactory, hypotheses of the mechanism of the migraine attack were proposed. For instance, Spitzer (1901) suggested that part of the choroid plexus of one lateral ventricle might herniate temporarily into an already congenitally narrow foramen of Munro. This would block cerebrospinal fluid (CSF) outflow and produce painful distension of one lateral ventricle. No pathological evidence to confirm the possibility ever became available. Timme (1926) and Thompson (1932) suggested that episodic pituitary swelling could cause the headache. If the gland herniated upward, it might touch the optic chiasm and produce the visual disturbance of the migraine aura. If it protruded laterally into the cavernous sinus, it might involve trigeminal nerve branches and so produce headache and also the cranial nerve palsies that occasionally complicate migraine attacks. Pituitary tumors may behave in these ways as they grow, but no evidence exists that the pituitary may swell episodically to a sufficient extent to explain migraine.

From the early 1940s onward the interpretation of migraine began to be based on human and animal experimental data as well as clinical observation. Harold Wolff (1898–1962) in New York undertook a program of studies into headache mechanisms that culminated in the publication of the first two editions of his book *Headache and Other Head Pain*. The major outcome of his studies was encapsulated in the following statement concerning the pathogenesis of the migraine attack (Wolff, 1963, p. 682).

> . . . an initial local vasoconstriction of cerebral arteries produces visual and other non-painful, sensory, preheadache phenomena. As the vasoconstrictor preheadache phenomena recede, vasodilator headache manifestations begin. . . . In most patients the headache arises in one or another of the distended branches of the external carotid arteries, although any or all of the major cranial arteries may be involved at one time or another in headache of the migraine type. . . . Vasodilatation sustained during several hours leads to a thickening or edema of the affected artery wall and often to edema of the adjacent tissues. Because of transient thickening of their walls, the soft, readily collapsible arteries become rigid and pipe-like. Further, the pulsating pain becomes a steady ache, and the artery itself becomes tender on palpation.
>
> Secondary to such prolonged pain in distension of cranial arteries, skeletal muscles of the head and neck contract. Prolonged muscle contraction in

itself becomes painful, and adds a component to the migraine headache which may outlast the vascular pain.

Much of this interpretation is similar to those of Jaccoud, Latham, and Eulenburg more than eight decades before, but Wolff's views were derived from sound experimental data as well as clinical observation. Further, they included the recognition of a later-stage tension-type headache mechanism in the migraine attack that had escaped the notice of his predecessors.

There was a great deal more original observation in Wolff's work that cannot be dealt with here because of limitations of space. His ideas proved very influential, both at the time they appeared and subsequently. They seemed to finally establish the vascular nature of migraine. Yet even as the second (posthumous) edition of Wolff's book (1963) became available, two observations had been made that opened new directions in the understanding of the pathogenesis and treatment of the disorder. Evidence became available that serotonin (5-hydroxytryptamine [5-HT]) could play a role in the migraine mechanism, and the phenomenon of cortical spreading depression was first recognized.

SEROTONIN

Several lines of evidence from human clinical physiology and pharmacology (e.g., Curran, Hinterberger, & Lance, 1965; Sicuteri, 1976; Sicuteri, Testi, & Anselmi, 1961) suggested a role for serotonin in migraine pathogenesis and therapy (Humphrey, 2007). In the 1980s and 1990s, molecules with serotoninlike structures but selectivity for intracranial and trigeminal 5-HT receptors were synthesized in the hope that they would relieve migraine symptoms. On the whole this hope was realized, and a series of triptan derivatives (Humphrey, 2007) became available for treating the attacks. Also, the old migraine-specific agent ergotamine was shown to be a very potent serotonin agonist. The role of serotonin agonism in migraine pathogenesis as compared to treatment remains poorly understood, and emphasis has shifted from its vascular role to its role in brainstem pain modulation.

Evidence that one biological molecule played a role in migraine inevitably led to a search for others that might. From this search quite strong evidence emerged that at least calcitonin gene–related peptide (CGRP) was involved in the mechanism of the attacks (Doods, Arndt, Rudolf, & Just, 2007). CGRP, a very potent vasodilator, possesses pain-producing properties and occurs in trigeminal nerve terminals near blood vessels in the pia and dura and also in trigeminal afferent terminals in the descending spinal nucleus of the nerve. CGRP antagonists have been shown effective in clinical trials in treating migraine attacks (e.g., Olesen et al., 2004).

CORTICAL SPREADING DEPRESSION

Aristides Leão, in the 1943–1944 period, while investigating experimental epileptogenesis, observed that local stimulation of the cerebral cortex of anesthetized rabbits caused a spreading wave of decreased electrical activity in the cortex. The wave moved at an approximate rate of 2 to 3 mm per minute and was accompanied by a spreading dilatation of the local pial arteries. Later it was noticed that there was an initial phase of spreading excitation that preceded the depression (Leão, 1944a, 1944b, 1947). Leão and Morison (1945) suggested that the phenomenon could account for the aura of migraine. They were apparently unaware that Lashley (1941) had mapped the course of his own migraine visual aura and calculated that it could be explained by a disturbance of function of his visual cortex that spread at the rate of about 3 mm per minute. After some delay, it has been increasingly accepted that cortical spreading depression is the basis of the migraine aura, and the phenomenon has become the 20th-century version of Liveing's "nerve storms."

MIGRAINE GENETICS

It has been known for a very long time that a tendency to have migraines is often inherited. Willis (1672, p. 107) wrote of headache that "the Disease is often delivered from the Parents to the Children," and Gowers (1888, p. 777) stated: "Migraine is strongly hereditary; in more than half the cases, inheritance can be traced, and it is usually direct, *i.e.* other members of the family (very often a parent) suffer from paroxysmal headache."

It has been assumed that the usually encountered forms of migraine have a multigenic basis (Wessman, Terwindt, Kaunisto, Palotie, & Ophoff, 2007). The specific genes responsible for the migraine tendency remained elusive until very recently (Chasman et al., 2011), except in the case of the rare variants with extreme phenotypes such as familial hemiplegic migraine (Ducros, Tournier-Lasserve, & Bousser, 2002).

By the end of the 20th century a great deal of information about migraine and its mechanism had been accumulated. Aspects of the pathogenesis of the disorder (e.g., the headache and the aura) could be explained by what appears to be high-quality evidence. However, there still remains difficulty in incorporating the susceptibility, pathogenesis, and pain of the disorder into one comprehensive interpretation, though attempts have been made (e.g., Iadecola [2002], Moskowitz [2007]).

Obviously, the long saga of the human encounter with migraine is not near its end. In historically modern times,

hypotheses of its cause and mechanism have come and gone, with their dominant emphasis shifting between predominantly vascular and predominantly neural factors, but usually involving an admixture of the two. The neural elements have at different times involved the trigeminal nerve, the cervical sympathetic trunk, and the neuraxis at sites between the brainstem and the cortex. The present-day simplification that migraine is a trigeminovascular disorder has a long and rather varied ancestry, while the treatment of the disorder, though enhanced by recent scientific advances, continues to fall short of what is desirable.

REFERENCES

Adams, F (Ed.). (1856). *The extant works of Aretaeus, the Cappadocian.* London: New Sydenham Society.

Airy, G. B. (1865). The Astronomer Royal on hemianopsy. *Philosophical Magazine, 30*, 19–21.

Airy, H. (1870). On a distinct form of transient hemiopsia. *Philosophical Transactions, 159*, 247–264.

Barger, G. (1931). *Ergot and ergotism.* London: Gurney & Jackson.

Bramwell, E. (1926). Discussion on migraine. *British Medical Journal, ii*, 765–769.

Brown-Séquard, C. E. (1861). Remarques sur le travail precedent. *Journal de la physiologie de l'homme er des animaux, 4*, 137–139.

Caelius Aurelianus. (1950). *On acute diseases and on chronic diseases.* (I. E. Drabkin, Trans.). Chicago: University of Chicago Press.

Calmeil, L-F. (1839). Migraine. In: B. Béclard (Ed.), *Adelon's Dictionnaire de médicine ou répetoirre* (2nd ed., Vol. 20, pp. 3–10.). Paris: Béchet & Labé.

Campbell, H. (1894). *Headache and other morbid cephalic sensations.* London: Lewis.

Chasman, D. I., Schürks, M., Anttila, V., de Vries, B., Schmink, U., Launer, L. J., et al. (2011). Genome-wide association study reveals three susceptibility loci for common migraine in the general population. *Nature Genetics. 43*, 695–698.

Collier, J. (1928). Lumleian lectures on epilepsy. *Lancet, 221*, 587–591, 642–647.

Curran, D. A., Hinterberger, H., & Lance, J. W. (1965). Total plasma serotonin, 5-hydroxyindoleacetic acid excretion in normal and migrainous subjects. *Brain, 88*, 997–1010.

Doods, H., Arndt, K., Rudolf, K., & Just, S. (2007). CGRP antagonists: Unravelling the role of CGRP in migraine. *Trends in Pharmacological Science, 28*, 580–587.

Du Bois-Reymond, E. H. (1861). De l'hémicrânie ou migraine. *Journal de la physiologie de l'homme er des animaux, 4*, 130–137.

Ducros, A., Tournier-Lasserve, E., & Bousser, M-G. (2002). The genetics of migraine. *Lancet Neurology, 1*, 285–293.

Eulenburg, A. (1877). Vasomotor and trophic neuroses. Hemicrania (migraine). In: H. van Ziemssen (Ed.), *Cyclopedia of the practice of medicine* (Vol. 14, pp. 3–30). New York: Wood.

Fernel, J. (1655). *La pathologie ou discours des maladies.* (J. Guingard, Trans.). Paris: Faret & Guingard.

Fordyce, J. (1758). *De hemicrania.* Durham: Wilson.

Fothergill, J. (1778). Remarks on that complaint commonly known under the name of sick headach. *Medical Observations and Inquiries*, 103–137.

Garrett Anderson, E. (1870). *Sur la migraine* (Thesis). Paris: Bibliotheque Interuniversitaire de Medecine et d'Odontologie.

Gorji, A., & Ghadiri, M. K. (2002). History of headache in medieval Persian medicine. *Lancet Neurology, 1,* 510–515.

Gowers, W. R. (1888). *A manual of the diseases of the nervous system* (Vol. 2). London: J & A Churchill.

Hall, M. (1849). The neck as a medical region. *Lancet, 53,* 174–176, 285–287, 394–395, 506–508, 687–688; 54, 66–69, 75–77.

Harris, W. (1907). The causation and treatment of some headaches. *Lancet, 169,* 276–278.

Heberden, W. (1802). *Commentaries on the history and cure of diseases.* London: Payne.

H*ippocrates.* (1994). (W. D. Smith, Ed. & Trans.). Cambridge, MA: Harvard University Press.

Humphrey, P. P. A. (2007). The discovery of a new drug class for the acute treatment of migraine. *Headache, 47*(Suppl. 1), S10–S19.

Hurst, A. F. (1924). The Savill lecture on migraine. *Lancet, 204,* 1–6.

Iadecola, C. (2002). From CSD to headache: A long and winding road. *Nature Medicine, 8,* 110–112.

Isler. H. (1985). Johann Jakob Wepfer (1620–1695): Discoveries in headache. *Cephalalgia, 5*(Suppl. 3), 423–425.

Isler, H. (1987). Retrospect: The history of thought about migraine from Aretaeus to 1920. In: J. N. Blau (Ed.), *Migraine. Clinical and research aspects* (pp. 659–674). Baltimore: Johns Hopkins Press.

Jaccoud, S. F. (1869). *Migraine—hémicrânie. Traité de pathologie interne* (Vol. 1, book 3, pp. 452–456). Paris: Delahaye.

Jackson, J. H. (1876). On epilepsies and on the after-effects of epileptic discharges (Todd and Robertson's hypothesis). *West Riding Asylum Medical Reports, 6,* 266–309. (Reprinted in *Selected writings of John Hughlings Jackson,* pp. 135–161, by J. Taylor, Ed., 1958, London: Staples Press)

Jackson, J. H. (1879). Lectures on the diagnosis of epilepsy. *Medical Times and Gazette, i,* 29–33, 85–88, 141–143, 223–226. (Reprinted in *Selected writings of John Hughlings Jackson,* pp. 276–307, by J. Taylor, Ed., 1958, London: Staples Press)

James, T. (1745). Cephalalgia, cephalaea. In: *A medical dictionary* (7 pages, unnumbered). London: Roberts.

Karenberg, A., & Leitz, C. (2001). Headache in magical and medical papyri of ancient Egypt. *Cephalalgia, 21,* 911–916.

Karwautz, A., Wober-Bingol, C., & Wober, C. (1996). Freud and migraine: The beginnings of a psychodynamically oriented view of headache a hundred years ago. *Cephalalgia, 16,* 22–26.

Kühn, K. G. E. (Ed.). (1821–1833). *Galen's Omnia opera* (Vols. 1–20). Leipzig: Cnoblochii.

Labarraque, H. (1837). *Essai sur la céphalalgie et la migraine* (Thesis). Paris: Bibliotheque Interuniversitaire de Medecine et d'Odontologie.

Lashley, K. S. (1941). Patterns of cerebral integration indicated by the scotomas of migraine. *Archives of Neurology and Psychiatry, 49,* 331–339.

Latham, P. W. (1872). Nervous or sick headache. *British Medical Journal, i,* 305–306, 336–337.

Latham, P. W. (1873). *On nervous or sick headache, its varieties and treatment.* Cambridge: Deighton, Bull & Co.

Le Pois, C. (1618). *Selectiorum observationum et consiliorum de praetevisis hactenus morbis affectibusque praeter naturam.* Pont-à-Mausson: Carolum Mercatorem.

Leão A. A. P. (1944a). Pial circulation and spreading depression of activity in the cerebral cortex. *Journal of Neurophysiology, 7,* 391–396.

Leão, A. A. P. (1944b). Spreading depression of activity in the cerebral cortex. *Journal of Neurophysiology, 7,* 359–390.

Leão, A. A. P. (1947). Further observations on the spreading depression of activity in the cerebral cortex. *Journal of Neurophysiology, 10,* 409–414.

Leão, A. A. P., & Morison, R. S. (1945). Propagation of spreading cortical depression. *Journal of Neurophysiology, 8,* 33–46.

Liveing, E. (1872). Observations on megrim or sick-headache. *British Medical Journal, 1,* 364–366.

Liveing, E. (1873). *On megrim, sick-headache, and some allied disorders: A contribution to the pathology of nerve-storms.* London: Churchill.

Loveless, M. (1950). Milk allergy: A survey of its incidence: Experiments with a masked ingestion test; allergy for corn and its derivatives: Experiments with a masked ingestion test for its diagnosis. *Journal of Allergy, 21,* 489–499.

Maier, H-W. (1926). L'ergotamine, inhibiteur du sympathetique étudié en clinique, comme moyen d'exploration et comme agent thérapeutique. *Revue Neurologique Paris, 33,* 1104–1108.

Moebius, P. J. (1894). Die migraine. In: H. Nothnagel (Ed.), *Specielle Pathologie und Therapie.* (Cited by Schiller, F. [1975]. The migraine tradition. *Bulletin of the History of Medicine, 49,* 1–19).

Moskowitz, M. A. (2007). Pathophysiology of headache—past and present. *Headache, 47*(Suppl. 1), S58–S63.

Möllendorf, F. W. (1867). Ueber Hemikranie. *Archiv fur pathologische Anatomie und Physiologie, 47,* 385–395.

Olesen, J., Diener, H. C., Husstedt, I. W., Goadsby, P. J., Hall, D., Meier, U., et al. (2004). Calcitonin gene-related peptide receptor antagonist BIBN 4096 BS for the acute treatment of migraine. *New England Journal of Medicine, 350,* 1104–1110.

Osler, W. (1892). *The principles and practice of medicine.* New York: Appleton & Co.

Parry, C. H. (1792). On the effect of compression of the arteries in various diseases and particularly in those of the head: With hints towards a new mode of treating nervous disorders. *Memoirs of the Medical Society of London, 3,* 77–113.

Parry, C. H. (1825). Scintillating scotoma. In: W. E.Parry (Ed.), *Collections from the unpublished medical writings of Caleb Hillier Parry* (Vol. 1, p. 557). London: Underwoods.

Piorry, P-A. (1831). *Mémoire sur la migraine.* Paris: Ballière.

Piorry, P. A. (1875). Mémoire sur le vertige. *Bulletin de l'Acadamie de Médecine, 66,* 1–12.

Ringer, S. (1877). A suggestion concerning the condition of the nervous centres in migraine, epilepsy, and other explosive neuroses. *Lancet, 111,* 228–229.

Romberg, M. H. (1853). *A manual of the nervous diseases of man.* (E. H. Sieveking, Trans.). London: New Sydenham Society.

Rothlin, E. (1955). Historical development of the ergot therapy of migraine. *International Archives of Allergy and Immunology, 7,* 205–209.

Sauvages, F. B. de. (1772). *Nosologie méthodolique* (Vol. 16). Lyon: Gouvion.

Sicuteri, F. (1976). Hypothesis: Migraine, a central biochemical dysnocioception. *Headache, 16,* 145–159.

Sicuteri, F., Testi, A., & Anselmi, B. (1961). Biochemical investigations in headache: Increase in the hydroxyindoleacetic acid excretion during migraine attacks. *International Archives of Allergy and Applied Immunology, 19,* 55–58.

Siegel, R. E. (1976). *Galen on the affected parts.* Basel: Karger.

Singer, C. (2005). The visions of Hildegard of Bingen. *Yale Journal of Biology and Medicine, 78,* 57–82. (Reprint of 1917 paper)

Spitzer, J. (1901). *Uber migräne.* Jena: Fischer.

Stoll, A. (1918). Zur Kenntnis der Mutterkornalkaloide. *Varhandlungen der Schweizerischen Naturforschungsgesellschaft, 101,* 190–191.

Sydenham, T. (1848). On the affection called hysteria in women; and hypochondriasis in men. In: *The works of Thomas Sydenham MD* (Vol. 2, pp. 231–235). London: Sydenham Society.

Symonds, J. A. (1858). Gulstonian lectures for 1858. On headache. *Medical Times and Gazette, 37,* 285–288, 393–396, 419–422.

Thomas, L. H. (1887). *La migraine.* Paris: Delahaye & Lecrosnier.

Thompson, A. P. (1932). A contribution to the study of intermittent headache. *Lancet, 220,* 229–235.

Thompson, R. (1903). *The devils and evil spirits of Babylonia.* London: Luzac & Co.

Timme, W. (1926). General discussion. *British Medical Journal, ii,* 771–772.

Tissot, S. A. (1780). *Traité des nerfs et de leurs maladies* (Vol. 3). Paris: Didot.

Turenne, A. (1849). Theory on the production of hemicrania. *Lancet, 53,* 177–179.

Van der Linden, J. A. (1666). *De hemicrania menstrua. Historia et consilium Lugundum Batavorum.* London. Elsevirum.

Wepfer, J. J. (1727). *Observationes medico-practicae de affectibus capitis.* Schaffenhausen: Ziegler.

Wessman, M., Terwindt, G. M., Kaunisto, M. A., Palotie, A., & Ophoff, R. A. (2007). Migraine: A complex genetic disorder. *Lancet Neurology, 6,* 521–532.

Whytt, R. (1768). *The works of Robert Whytt.* Edinburgh: Becket & DeHondt; Balfour.

Wilks, S. (1869). Lectures on diseases of the nervous system. Hemicrania or sick-headache. *Medical Times and Gazette 1,* 1–2.

Wilks, S. (1878). *Lectures on diseases of the nervous system.* London: J & A Churchill.

Willis, T. (1672). *De anima brutorum quae hominis vitalis ac sensitiva est, exercitationes duae.* Oxford: Davis.

Willis, T. (1672). Two discourses concerning the soul of brutes *[De anima brutorum quae hominis vitalis ac sensitiva est, exercitationes duae].* (S. Pordage, Trans.). London: Dring, Harper & Leigh.

Woakes, E. (1868). On ergot of rye in the treatment of neuralgia. *British Medical Journal, 2,* 350–361.

Wolff, H. G. (1963). *Headache and other head pain* (2nd ed.). New York: Oxford University Press.

Part 2

Neurobiology of the
Migraine Brain

2 Migraine—Some Theories and Controversies

FAROOQ H. MANIYAR AND PETER J. GOADSBY

INTRODUCTION

Migraine is a disabling disorder characterized by unilateral, throbbing headache associated with nausea and hypersensitivity to a variety of external stimuli. We have largely moved away from the *vascular* theory of migraine; vasodilatation is an epiphenomenon neither necessary nor sufficient for the symptoms (Rahmann, Wienecke et al., 2008). There are still many unanswered questions concerning migraine that lead to controversial issues needing clarification to make progress. One might consider the neural versus vascular basis of the disorder primary among these, since without an answer we cannot know the primary organ system involved and thus, how will truly novel therapeutics be developed? Our view is that migraine is, primarily, a brain disorder. Moreover, neuroimaging studies have concentrated on the headache phase, although clearly the migraine process begins before the headache as patients commonly experience one or more symptoms during the premonitory phase. What structures drive the premonitory symptoms that lead to the headache? Does the hypothalamus play a significant role in this? If it does, how important is the role of the orexins, neuropeptides only recently implicated in migraine? What role does the pons play in migraine? Functional neuroimaging studies have consistently shown activation of the dorsal pons during migraine headache (Afridi, Matharu et al., 2005; Weiller, May et al., 1995), an area that may play a key role in the sensory hypersensitivity that patients commonly experience. Lastly, do antimigraine drugs have access to the brain areas important in migraine, and what is the status of the blood-brain barrier during migraine? We address these issues as examples of crucial questions that neuroimaging may answer for clinicians and for the greater good of patients.

PREMONITORY SYMPTOMS IN MIGRAINE: WHEN DOES AN ATTACK REALLY START?

Between 7% and 88% of patients with migraine have one or more symptoms during the period before the onset of headache (Drummond & Lance, 1984; Rasmussen & Olesen, 1992; Russell, Rasmussen et al., 1996; Waelkens, 1985). This phase has been called the premonitory phase. These studies were retrospective and hence subject to recall bias. Two studies have prospectively studied premonitory symptoms (Giffin, Ruggiero et al., 2003; Quintela, Castillo et al., 2006). Giffin and colleagues used electronic diaries wherein patients were asked to register entries daily that could not be changed once entered. This, along with the prospective nature of the study, makes it an interesting approach to study premonitory symptoms. Migraine was correctly predicted to occur within 72 hours by 72% of entries. The most common symptoms were tiredness, present in two thirds of patients, and difficulty concentrating and stiff neck, present in half the patients. However, these were not the most predictive for a migraine attack as can be estimated by the lack of specificity and common occurrence of these symptoms in the population. The symptoms with the highest predictive value were yawning, difficulties in speech and reading, and emotional disturbance, correctly predicting a migraine headache in more than two thirds of patients. Yawning and increased energy and hunger/cravings were the only symptoms that became less common with the occurrence of headache. Other symptoms were common during and after the headache. The study mentioned that mild pain was frequently mentioned by patients in the premonitory phase in the form of neck discomfort, dull pain behind the eyes, or pain around the ears. However, the percentage of patients with this symptom was not mentioned. This is in keeping with the clinical observation of mild pain frequently present along with other symptoms in the premonitory phase.

Quintela and colleagues (2006) studied 100 patients with migraine. Symptoms present during headache-free days in the interictal period were discounted. Patients visited the research office 2 to 5 days after a migraine attack started and were asked to fill out a questionnaire regarding the occurrence of premonitory symptoms present 24 hours before the start of the headache. Thus, patient ascertainment was prospective, although data collection was not. Of these patients, 84% had one or more premonitory symptoms, and the average number was seven for each patient. Anxiety, phonophobia, irritability, unhappiness, yawning, photophobia, asthenia, and concentration difficulties were the most frequent, present in around 40% patients. About two thirds of symptoms were present in at least two out of three attacks and more than half were present in three out of three attacks, indicating these were highly consistent. The constellation of symptoms in the premonitory phase clearly indicates that the origin of the problem is in the brain. The events leading to these symptoms occur before the aura and before the events causing pain. Exploring the premonitory phase will help us understand where migraine starts, and indeed if it starts in the brain.

Dopamine and Migraine

Yawning is one of the most predictive premonitory symptoms. Yawning is a phylogenetically old, stereotyped event occurring alone or associated with stretching and/or penile erection in humans and other mammalians, thought to be associated with the release of several neurotransmitters including dopamine (Argiolas & Melis, 1998). Apomorphine induces yawning, penile erection, genital grooming, and reduced motility in rats. Hypophysectomy prevented the yawning, penile erection, and genital grooming but not the effect on locomotion in response to apomorphine in a study (Serra, Collu et al., 1983), suggesting a role for the hypothalamus–pituitary connection driven by dopamine receptors. We have encountered patients with sexual ideas during spontaneous and nitroglycerin-induced migraines in the premonitory phase. Hypothalamus and midbrain substantia nigra are the main sources of dopamine in the brain, and it is possible—indeed, based on clinical observation, likely—that these areas are involved in the premonitory phase. It is interesting that a recent diffusion tensor imaging study has shown strong connections between the hypothalamus and the prefrontal cortex (Lemaire, Frew et al., 2011).

Domperidone, a dopamine D_2 receptor antagonist, was able to prevent 63% of migraine attacks at a dose of 40 mg when taken in the premonitory phase (Waelkens, 1984). Thus, there is some evidence for the involvement of dopamine in the premonitory phase, the source of which could be either the hypothalamus or the brainstem. Dopamine can mediate other symptoms, such as nausea, that are also common in the premonitory phase, and it is common practice to use antidopaminergic drugs to treat nausea and vomiting during headache, although most medicines used have complex pharmacology. One of the questions often raised is if antidopaminergic agents can prevent or treat migraine, why is migraine more common in dopamine deficiency states such as restless legs syndrome? Though there is no clear answer to this at the moment, it is likely to be related to the timing of dopamine

release. The A11 region of the hypothalamus has an inhibitory effect on nociception transmission in the trigeminal complex, which is mediated through dopamine (Charbit, Akerman et al., 2009). Lack of dopamine may remove this inhibition, making the trigeminal complex more "ready" for transmission of pain, and dopamine substitution or dopamine agonists may restore the balance. A recent functional neuroimaging study showed increased trigeminal activation in response to noxious stimulation in the trigeminal distribution up to 72 hours before a migraine attack as compared to the interictal and attack phases (Stankewitz, Aderjan et al., 2011). This could result from inhibition of the normal descending inhibitory influence over the trigeminal complex, a situation that will be exacerbated by lack of dopamine. On exposure to a trigger, dopamine release from the brainstem or hypothalamus would engage a cascade; dopamine blockers at this stage would be useful in arresting the progression of events. In addition to yawning, other symptoms, such as thirst and frequent urination, can be explained by hypothalamic involvement possibly related to the release of vasopressin (Krowicki & Kapusta, 2011). During nitroglycerin-induced migraine, we have observed cranial parasympathetic symptoms of lacrimation and conjunctival injection in the premonitory phase along with hypothalamic symptoms of thirst, yawning, and frequent urination in the absence of trigeminal pain. We propose that the hypothalamus directly stimulates the cranial parasympathetic outflow to cause cranial autonomic symptoms in the premonitory phase.

Photophobia, Phonophobia, and Neuroimaging

It was interesting to find symptoms such as photophobia and phonophobia during the premonitory phase. A recent positron emission tomography (PET) study showed that the visual cortex is hyperexcitable during migraine attacks and this persists after treatment of pain with sumatriptan (Denuelle, Boulloche et al., 2011), suggesting that the cortical hyperactivity is not just a reaction to pain. It is not known if this is a de novo cortical process or cortical modulation by subcortical structures. Thalamic neurons responding to both light and trigeminal pain projecting to the visual cortex can modulate the visual cortex (Noseda & Burstein, 2011). Similarly, brainstem areas such as the dorsal pons, which includes the locus coeruleus, and dorsal midbrain, which includes the dorsal raphe nucleus, are active during migraine, and this persists after pain is treated with sumatriptan (Weiller et al., 1995). It is not known if these thalamic and brainstem areas, which could potentially modulate and increase cortical excitability, are active during the premonitory phase, though serotonergic mechanisms are probably involved as suggested by the serotonin 5-HT$_{1B/1D}$ agonist naratriptan, 2.5 mg, preventing 60% of migraine headaches when taken in the premonitory phase (Luciani, Carter et al., 2000).

Electrophysiological Changes and the Premonitory Phase

Electrophysiological studies also suggest a biological change during the period before the headache in migraine. Kropp and Gerber (1998) measured contingent negative variations (CNVs), a slow cortical potential employing a two-stimulus paradigm. The CNV was more negative in migraine patients than controls. There was a significant difference between the day before and the day after a migraine attack, with more negative CNVs on the day before. These findings indicated cortical hyperexcitability and lack of cortical habituation in patients with migraine as compared to controls and also that the cortex was particularly hyperexcitable just before the onset of migraine headache. Evers and colleagues (1999) studied reaction times, latency, and amplitude of event-related potentials (ERPs) to visual stimuli along with 5-HT levels in platelets in patients with episodic migraine. The findings showed that the ERPs increased continuously throughout the interictal period, suggestive of lack of cortical habituation, with the maximum increase occurring a few days before the migraine attack. During the migraine attack, there was abrupt normalization of habituation on the first day. Findings suggested slowed cerebral processing during the migraine attack, which correlated with reduced 5-HT platelet levels. These findings confirmed that cortical hyperexcitability is at its maximum just before the onset of the migraine headache. More recently Sand and colleagues (2008) found that the N2 component of the visual evoked potential was increased in the 72 hours before an attack as compared to the interictal period, suggesting cortical hyperresponsiveness particularly of the extrastriate region of the visual cortex. These electrophysiological data clearly show brain function is altered in the period before the headache starts, a time when the majority of patients have one or more symptoms. A better understanding of this phase and the generation of the migraine attack is pivotal in our effort to develop better preventive approaches.

MIGRAINE AND THE HYPOTHALAMUS

The hypothalamus has been linked to migraine for many years. Daro and colleagues (1964) successfully treated migraine patients with posterior pituitary extract. Pearce (1969) suggested that the hypothalamus could account for the periodicity in migraine and connections with the limbic system could explain the emotional changes in migraine. The hypothalamus is a small structure at the base of the brain weighing 4 to 5 g and measuring 4 cm³ in volume (Amionff et al., 2004). It can be arbitrarily divided into a medial and lateral part, with the medial part further divided into anterior, middle (tuberal), and posterior parts (Young & Stanton, 1994). The posteriormost part of the lateral region along with the mamillary bodies constitutes the posterior region of the hypothalamus. The boundaries of this region are not distinct and merge with the ventral tegmental area of the midbrain. The anterior part contains the supraoptic and paraventricular nuclei, which contain the hormones oxytocin and vasopressin. The paraventricular nucleus plays an important role in control of the autonomic   system. The suprachiasmatic nucleus, also present in the anterior part, controls the circadian rhythm. Although the anterior part is thought to control the sympathetic and the posterior part the parasympathetic system, this division of function may not be strictly true (Holstege, 1987). The hypothalamus controls the endocrine system; the tuberal part contains the luteinizing hormone–releasing hormone (LHRH) generator, which controls the menstrual cycle. Thus, the hypothalamus plays an important role in maintaining homeostasis via control over the endocrine and autonomic systems and has a role in pain modulation.

Observations Suggesting Hypothalamic Involvement in Migraine

1. *Premonitory symptoms*: Many of the premonitory symptoms suggest a hypothalamic origin (e.g., thirst, yawning, tiredness, frequent urination, and food cravings). This is further described in the premonitory symptoms section.
2. *Sexual dimorphism in migraine*: Migraine is equally common in boys and girls until puberty (Waters & O'Connor, 1971), after which it becomes three times more common in females than males (Lipton, Stewart et al., 2001). Menstrual migraine is more likely to occur 2 days before and on the first 2 days of the menstrual period (Stewart, Lipton et al., 2000); hormonal changes are likely to be contributory, though it may not be just estrogen withdrawal (Almen-Christensson, Hammar et al., 2011). Migraine often becomes troublesome during perimenopause before becoming less common (MacGregor, 2006). Up to 90% of women experience a decrease in the frequency of migraine during pregnancy (Goadsby, Goldberg et al., 2008).

A sexually dimorphic nucleus has been identi-fied in the preoptic area of the hypothalamus, and the hormonal-related changes in migraine are likely to be related to LHRH secretion (Facchinetti, Sgarbi et al., 2000).

3. *Antinociceptive effect of the hypothalamus—relevance in migraine:* Evidence suggests that the hypothalamus can modulate nociception. It has ascending and descending connections with the dorsal horns of the spinal cord (Giesler, Katter, et al. 1994; Millan, 1999). Direct orexinergic projections terminate in the spinal and trigeminal dorsal horns (Van den Pol, 1999). Though these connections are mostly excitatory, orexinergic neurons also synapse with spinal inhibitory interneurons (Siegel, 2004) and have been shown to produce antinociceptive effects at the level of the spinal cord (Yamamoto, Saito et al., 2003). The trigeminovascular neurons project to the hypothalamus through the trigeminohypothalamic tract (Malick, Strassman et al., 2000). Various hypothalamic nuclei are connected to structures such as periaqueductal gray matter, nucleus tractus solitarius (NTS), rostroventromedial medulla, and nucleus raphe magnus, as well as corticolimbic structures involved in the cognitive and affective aspects of pain (Millan, 1999). Deep brain stimulation of the medial and lateral hypothalamic nuclei has an antinociceptive effect on rat dorsal horn (Carstens, 1986). The A11 region of the posterior hypothalamus has an inhibitory effect on nociceptive transmission in the trigeminal complex, and this is predominantly dopamine D_2 receptor mediated (Charbit et al., 2009). Destruction of the ventromedial posterior hypothalamus caused transient hyperalgesia, indicating this area helps to maintain a basal antinociceptive action (Millan, Przewlocki et al., 1983). Pretreatment of rats with anandamide, a cannabinoid, reduced nitroglycerin-induced activity in the trigeminal nucleus caudalis (TNC) and increased c-Fos in the paraventricular and supraoptic nuclei of the hypothalamus (Greco, Mangione et al., 2011). Thus, the predominant effect of hypothalamic stimulation with regard to pain is antinociceptive. The antinociceptive action of the hypothalamus could be mediated by several peptides such as endogenous opioids, vasopressin, somatostatin, angiotensin II, calcitonin (Amionff et al., 2004), oxytocin (Lund, Ge et al., 2002), and ghrelin, among others.

A recent PET study within 4 hours of migraine onset showed hypothalamic activations that persisted after treatment of pain with sumatriptan (Denuelle, Fabre et al., 2007). It is not known when the hypothalamic activation starts and if it is present in the premonitory state. Hypothalamic activation was shown during dobutamine-induced cardiac stress in patients with overt angina as compared to baseline but not in patients with silent angina as compared to baseline (there was no difference with direct comparison between overt angina and silent angina), suggesting, again, that hypothalamic activation occurs if pain is perceived (Rosen, Paulesu et al., 1996). This does not, however, exclude a more fundamental role for the hypothalamus in migraine. Hypothalamic dysfunction in the form of either inhibition or stimulation of areas different from those involved in antinociception could have a pronociceptive effect on the trigeminal complex leading to the pain phase.

4. *Hypothalamus and autonomic symptoms in migraine:* The hypothalamus controls the autonomic system, and the paraventricular nucleus has been termed as the *master control*. Various nuclei in the anterior and posterior hypothalamus are linked with autonomic functions. Afferent information from the periphery reaches the autonomic ganglia and brainstem nuclei, which then relay it to the hypothalamus and limbic system. The limbic system and hypothalamus are connected to the NTS and brainstem nuclei. The trigeminal pathway connects with the cranial parasympathetic pathways, forming the trigeminal-autonomic reflex that is thought to account for cranial autonomic symptoms such as lacrimation, conjunctival injection, nasal congestion, rhinorrhea, and others commonly seen in trigeminal autonomic cephalalgias (Goadsby, 2005a, 2005b; Goadsby & Lipton, 1997). Cranial autonomic symptoms are also common in migraine, occurring in up to half of the cases, and are frequently bilateral (Lai, Fuh et al., 2009). During nitroglycerin-induced migraine, we have observed cranial autonomic symptoms along with hypothalamic symptoms of thirst, yawning, and frequent urination during the premonitory phase in the absence of trigeminal pain. This is likely to be a hypothalamic influence on the efferent arc of the trigeminal-autonomic reflex as the afferent arc has not been recruited yet. Alternatively, disinhibition of the hypothalamic control would

lead to hyperactivity of the reflex, causing cranial autonomic symptoms.

The sympathetic system is also involved and may contribute to symptoms of presyncope and syncope seen in migraine. In the interictal period, norepinephrine (NE) levels are lower in the supine and upright positions. Response to α-adrenoceptor agonists is prolonged in migraineurs as compare to controls, more so in migraine patients with syncope, suggestive of receptor supersensitivity. Similarly, systolic and diastolic blood pressures are lower in the upright position, and there is a lesser increase in the diastolic blood pressure on isometric exercise and a reduced blood pressure response on Valsalva maneuver in migraine patients as compared to controls. It is interesting that prolonged stimulation of the cervical sympathetic ganglion led to a decrease of NE but an increase in the dopamine levels in the salivary glands. Lower NE levels were associated with increased levels of dopamine, adenosine triphosphate, and adenosine at various levels of activation (Peroutka, 2004). Thus, after exposure to a triggerlike stress, hypothalamic involvement may lead to sympathetic stimulation and eventually decreased NE and increased dopamine levels, unfolding a cascade of events leading to the premonitory phase followed by the headache.

5. *Hypothalamus and circadian rhythm*: Periodicity is well known in migraine, and in some patients, attacks tend to recur in a particular season, time of the month, week, or day, pointing toward the involvement of the suprachiasmatic nucleus, the master clock of circadian rhythm (Alstadhaug, 2006). Many patients get their attacks upon first waking up from sleep, and migraine attacks were found to peak around the middle of the day (Alstadhaug, Salvesen et al., 2008). The tuberomammillary complex is thought to be involved in the process of waking up, mediated by histamine (Burstein & Jakubowski, 2005), although antihistaminergic drugs are not useful in migraine. Most studies indicate a strong protective effect of sleep (Alstadhaug et al., 2008). Rarely patients get attacks during sleep, and an association with rapid eye movement (REM) sleep has been shown (Dexter & Weitzman, 1970). The circadian occurrence and relation to sleep suggest a role for the hypothalamus.

6. *Hypothalamus and orexins*: Also referred to as hypocretins, orexins are neuropeptides and exist in two forms: orexin A and orexin B. Orexin A has both the N-terminal pyroglutamyl cyclization and C-terminal amidation, whereas orexin B has the C-terminal amidation only after translation (Lee, Bang et al., 1999). Orexin A structure is homologous in various mammalian species, but orexin B differs (Dyer, Touchette et al., 1999; Shibahara, Sakurai et al., 1999). Orexins bind to two G-protein-coupled receptors: 1 and 2. Orexin A has equal affinity to both receptors, whereas orexin B has 10 times more affinity to the orexin 2 receptor. Both receptors upon stimulation lead to release of intracellular calcium, which stimulates the action of phospholipase C. Orexinergic neurons are mainly located in the lateral/perifornical, posterior, and paraventricular parts of the hypothalamus. Through connections to various parts of the brain, orexins are thought to be involved in maintenance of cycles such as sleep, feeding, thermoregulation, and neuroendocrine, autonomic, and nociceptive functions (Ferguson & Samson, 2003; Samson, Taylor et al., 2005; Siegel, 2004).

Orexinergic system involvement in migraine is suggested by the epidemiological finding that migraine is significantly overrepresented in patients with narcolepsy compared to the normal population (Dahmen, Querings et al., 1999). Loss of orexinergic neurons is thought to be central to the pathogenesis of narcolepsy. Activation of orexin 1 receptors in the posterior hypothalamus was found to be antinociceptive to trigeminal stimulation, whereas activation of orexin 2 receptors was pronociceptive (Bartsch, Levy et al., 2004). Direct orexinergic descending pathways to the spinal dorsal horn and trigeminal nucleus are present. Although the predominant action of orexins is stimulation, at higher concentration orexins stimulate the inhibitory neurons (Siegel, 2004). As an example, at low concentration, orexins stimulate the serotonergic dorsal raphe nucleus neurons, but at higher concentration, they also stimulate GABAergic neurons, which would inhibit the release of serotonin (Liu, van den Pol et al., 2002). This dual functional ability renders flexibility in the control of nociceptive transmission. Along with pain, the hypothalamic orexinergic system is likely involved in other disturbances with migraine, such as sleep, appetite, cravings, circadian nature of attacks, and autonomic abnormalities. Clearly orexin receptors may be therapeutic targets in migraine.

7. *Obesity, hypothalamus, and migraine*: Both migraine and obesity are common disorders.

Although the prevalence of obesity is not increased in episodic migraineurs, the frequency of migraine attacks is increased in obese people as compared to normal-weighted people and directly varies with the degree of obesity (Bigal, Tsang et al., 2007). Obesity was a risk factor for chronic daily headache, much more strongly related to chronic migraine than chronic tension-type headache (Bigal & Lipton, 2006). Obesity increases several mediators such as interleukins and calcitonin gene–related peptide, which are important in migraine and may increase the frequency, severity, and duration of migraine (Bigal, Lipton et al., 2007). As mentioned above, orexins can modulate pain as well as feeding behaviors; hypothalamic orexinergic dysfunction may be the link between primary headaches and comorbidities such as obesity.

8. *Neuroimaging studies in migraine*: Despite the strong pointers for the involvement of the hypothalamus in migraine, neuroimaging studies, except one (Denuelle et al., 2007), have not shown changes suggestive of its involvement in migraine. These include studies in spontaneous as well as nitroglycerin-induced migraine (Afridi, Giffin, et al., 2005; Afridi, Matharu, et al., 2005; Weiller, May et al., 1995). The study by Denuelle and colleagues was the only one to show hypothalamic activation, mainly in the anterior region. They scanned their patients within 4 hours of headache onset, whereas in all other studies patients were scanned later. It is therefore possible that hypothalamic activation occurs early in migraine and then turns off. Having said that, we cannot be sure if this activation is a response to pain or to the various autonomic and endocrine changes that pain induces, if it is an antinociceptive response, or if it helps generate the pain. Hypothalamic activation during pain is not specific to migraine. A PET study in dobutamine-induced cardiac stress showed hypothalamic activation during clinically overt angina compared to baseline but not during silent angina compared to baseline (there was no difference with direct comparison between clinical and silent angina), though both groups had similar levels of cardiac stress (Rosen, Paulesu et al., 1996).

BLOOD-BRAIN BARRIER

The blood-brain barrier (BBB) is formed by nonfenestrated endothelial cells and tight junctions between them strengthened by foot processes of pericytes. The tight junctions make it necessary for substances to pass through the endothelial cells (i.e., transcellular rather than paracellular transport). Small gaseous molecules, such as O_2 and CO_2, and lipophilic drugs, such as barbiturates and ethanol, can freely pass through the lipid membranes. The presence of active transport systems on both the luminal and abluminal surfaces regulates passage of small hydrophilic substances across the BBB. Intracellular and extracellular enzymes metabolize harmful and neuroactive substances, preventing their entry. Large hydrophilic compounds such as peptides and proteins are generally excluded unless there are specific mechanisms for their transport (Abbott, Ronnback et al., 2006). This arrangement maintains a stable environment that is very important for normal functioning of the brain.

The question of where antimigraine drugs act has been heavily debated (Humphrey & Goadsby, 1994). Peripheral as well as central sites have been proposed. If it is a predominantly central action, treatments need to cross the BBB to be effective.

Sumatriptan was the first triptan to be introduced into routine clinical practice in 1991 in Australia, New Zealand, and Europe. It has been widely used successfully in migraine. The initial mechanism for its anti-nociceptive action was thought to be through cerebral vasoconstriction (Humphrey & Goadsby, 1994; Humphrey, Feniuk et al., 1990). Later on sumatriptan was thought to act on peripheral trigeminovascular neurons (Humphrey & Goadsby, 1994). However, vascular changes were shown to be unrelated to the pain phase; cranial blood flow can be normal or reduced during pain (Olesen, Friberg et al., 1990). There was no change in the diameter of intracranial arteries in the migraine phase compared to baseline in nitroglycerin-induced migraine (Schoonman, van der Grond et al., 2008), although the situation is less clear in spontaneous attacks (Asghar, Hansen et al., 2011). Vasodilators such as nitroglycerin (Sances, Tassorelli et al., 2004) and pituitary adenylate cyclase activating peptide (PACAP-38) (Schytz, Birk et al., 2009) could trigger delayed migraine-like headache. However, another vasodilator, vasoactive intestinal polypeptide—like PACAP, a member of the secretin/glucagon peptide family—could not trigger delayed headache in migraineurs (Rahmann et al., 2008). Taken together, the available data suggest vasodilation is an epiphenomenon neither sufficient nor necessary for migraine. It has been suggested that some part of migraine headache is due to dural plasma protein extravasation and sterile neurogenic inflammation (Moskowitz, 1990). Sumatriptan can block the release of plasma proteins induced by electrical stimulation of the trigeminal ganglion (Buzzi & Moskowitz, 1990). However, other substances such as substance P- neurokinin 1 receptor antagonists (Goldstein, Offen et al., 2001; May & Goadsby, 2001) are not useful in migraine, suggesting blocking of neurogenic inflammation is not the mechanism of action for pain relief for sumatriptan.

So where do triptans act in migraine? Sumatriptan reduced Fos protein expression in the TNC after irritation of the dura with autologous blood (Nozaki, Moskowitz et al., 1992). Sumatriptan reduced Fos protein expression in the TNC in response to dilatation of the superior sagittal sinus (Hoskin, Kaube et al., 1996a). Both these experiments indicate that sumatriptan when given systemically can inhibit activity in the TNC in response to peripheral trigeminal stimulation; the experiments do not tell us about the site of action, which may be peripheral on the trigeminovascular neurons or centrally in the brain. In another experiment sumatriptan was able to prevent sensitization in central but not peripheral trigeminal neurons when given intravenously after application of inflammatory soup over the meninges in rats. After peripheral and central sensitization was established, sumatriptan was not able to reverse these. The authors concluded this is due to agonist activity of sumatriptan on $5HT_{1B/1D}$ receptors on the presynaptic trigeminal terminals in the dorsal horn, though one may argue this may also be a more central site, if sumatriptan is able to cross the BBB (Levy, Jakubowski et al., 2004). Kaube et al. found that sumatriptan given intravenously was not able to alter the electrical activity of central trigeminal neurons in response to electrical stimulation of the superior sagittal sinus but was able to do so when the BBB had been opened up with mannitol (Kaube, Hoskin et al., 1993). Shepheard et al. (1995) also found that intravenous sumatriptan did not alter c-Fos mRNA in the TNC after stimulation of the trigeminal ganglion but was able to decrease this after the BBB had been altered with hyperosmolar mannitol. These two experiments seem to suggest a central site of action on trigeminal neurons, and considering that sumatriptan is a highly effective drug, it is tempting to conceive that a similar change in BBB occurs during migraine. Alternatively, only small amounts of sumatriptan are able to enter the brain with an intact BBB (Humphrey et al., 1990) in keeping with its low lipophilicity.

Magnetic resonance imaging (MRI) scans during migraine do not show vasogenic edema except in some cases of status migrainosus (Gentile, Rainero et al., 2009) and familial hemiplegic migraine (Dreier, Jurkat-Rott et al., 2005). Therefore, if the BBB does not change, then it would indicate that the small amount of sumatriptan entering the brain is enough for its therapeutic activity.

Things are clearer with reference to other drugs used in migraine. In a cat model radioactive dihydroergotamine

($[^3H$-DHE]) binding was seen in the dorsal horn of the cervical spinal cord: in the medulla, associated with the nucleus of the tractus solitarius area postrema and descending spinal trigeminal nucleus, and in the mesencephalon and the cerebral cortex. The highest density was found in the dorsal and medial raphe nuclei of the midbrain, suggesting DHE can cross the BBB and may act centrally at these sites in migraine (Goadsby & Gundlach, 1991). Stimulation of the superior sagittal sinus by hook electrodes, which stimulate the trigeminal neurons only without stimulating the nerve–vessel interface, thus avoiding peripheral $5-HT_{1B/1D}$ receptors, led to accumulation of Fos protein and increased electrical activity in the TNC. This was blocked by intravenous DHE, indicating it can cross the BBB and bind to $5-HT_{1B/1D}$ receptors in the TNC since these receptors are not present in the trigeminal nerve axons or the trigeminal ganglion (Hoskin, Kaube et al., 1996b).

Other more lipophilic triptans, such as eletriptan and zolmitriptan, can more easily cross the BBB as suggested by similar serotonergic agonist activity after intravenous and intracerebral administration (Johnson, Rollema et al., 2001). In humans the best evidence about antimigraine drugs crossing the BBB comes from the study by Bergstrom et al. (2006), who showed that intravenous ^{11}C-zolmitriptan entered the brain within 5 minutes, with brain tissue concentration reaching about 25% of the plasma concentration.

To conclude, the status of the BBB in acute migraine is unclear. Most antimigraine drugs are able to cross the BBB to some extent. Either the BBB opens up, allowing greater access to these drugs, or the amounts that enter the brain with an intact BBB are enough for their therapeutic action. Migraine is a disease of the brain and it is likely that these drugs act centrally within the brain tissue.

So How Will Neuroimaging Help Solve These Questions?

Functional neuroimaging with PET and functional MRI allows us to measure changes in cerebral blood flow as a marker of synaptic activity. Though these tests do not tell us if the synaptic activity is excitatory or inhibitory, they have the potential of showing which areas are functionally active during various stages of migraine, for example, for the premonitory phase. Similarly, ligand PET studies can show brain areas to which the ligand binds during migraine, indicating the site and possible mechanism of action of these drugs. This is an exciting era and functional neuroimaging is likely to help us make key inroads in the understanding of migraine, a common and disabling disorder.

REFERENCES

Abbott, N. J., Ronnback, L., & Hansson, E. (2006). Astrocyte-endothelial interactions at the blood-brain barrier. *Nature Reviews Neuroscience, 7*(1), 41–53.

Afridi, S. K., Giffin, N. J., Kaube, H., Friston, K. J., Ward, N. S., Frackowiak, R. S., et al. (2005). A positron emission tomographic study in spontaneous migraine. *Archives of Neurology, 62*(8), 1270–1275.

Afridi, S. K., Matharu, M. S., Lee, L., Kaube, H., Friston, K. J., Frackowiak, R. S., et al. (2005). A PET study exploring the laterality of brainstem activation in migraine using glyceryl trinitrate. *Brain, 128*(Pt 4), 932–939.

Almen-Christensson, A., Hammar, M., Lindh-Åstrand, L., Landtblom, A. M., Brynhildsen, J. (2011). Prevention of menstrual migraine with perimenstrual transdermal 17-beta-estradiol: A randomized, placebo-controlled, double-blind crossover study. *Fertility and Sterility, 96*(2), 498–500.

Alstadhaug, K. B. (2006). Periodicity of migraine. *Headache, 46*(3), 532–533.

Alstadhaug, K., Salvesen, R., & Bekkelund, S. (2008). 24-hour distribution of migraine attacks. *Headache, 48*(1), 95–100.

Amionff, M. J., Boller, F., & Swaab, D. F. (2004). *The human hypothalamus: Basic and clinical aspects* (Part II, Vol. 80). Amsterdam, London: Elsevier.

Argiolas, A., & Melis, M. R. (1998). The neuropharmacology of yawning. *European Journal of Pharmacology, 343*(1), 1–16.

Asghar, M. S., Hansen, A. E., et al. (2011). Evidence for a vascular factor in migraine. *Annals of Neurology, 69*(4), 635–645.

Bartsch, T., Levy, M. J., et al. (2004). Differential modulation of nociceptive dural input to [hypocretin] orexin A and B receptor activation in the posterior hypothalamic area. *Pain, 109*(3), 367–378.

Bergstrom, M., Yates, R., Wall, A., Kågedal, M., Syvänen, S., & Långström, B. (2006). Blood-brain barrier penetration of zolmitriptan—modelling of positron emission tomography data. *Journal of Pharmacokinetics and Pharmacodynamics, 33*(1), 75–91.

Bigal, M. E., & Lipton, R. B. (2006). Obesity is a risk factor for transformed migraine but not chronic tension-type headache. *Neurology, 67*(2), 252–257.

Bigal, M. E., Lipton, R. B., Holland, P. R., & Goadsby, P. J. (2007). Obesity, migraine, and chronic migraine: Possible mechanisms of interaction. *Neurology, 68*(21), 1851–1861.

Bigal, M. E., Tsang, A., Loder, E., Serrano, D., Reed, M. L., & Lipton, R. B. (2007). Body mass index and episodic headaches: A population-based study. *Archives of Internal Medicine, 167*(18), 1964–1970.

Burstein, R., & Jakubowski, M. (2005). Unitary hypothesis for multiple triggers of the pain and strain of migraine. *Journal of Comparative Neurology, 493*(1), 9–14.

Buzzi, M. G., & Moskowitz, M. A. (1990). The antimigraine drug, sumatriptan (GR43175), selectively blocks neurogenic plasma extravasation from blood vessels in dura mater. *British Journal of Pharmacology, 99*(1), 202–206.

Carstens, E. (1986). Hypothalamic inhibition of rat dorsal horn neuronal responses to noxious skin heating. *Pain, 25*(1), 95–107.

Charbit, A. R., Akerman, S., Holland, P. R., & Goadsby, P. J. (2009). Neurons of the dopaminergic/calcitonin gene-related peptide A11 cell group modulate neuronal firing in the trigeminocervical complex: An electrophysiological and immunohistochemical study. *Journal of Neuroscience, 29*(40), 12532–12541.

Dahmen, N., Querings, K., Grün, B., & Bierbrauer, J. (1999). Increased frequency of migraine in narcoleptic patients. *Neurology, 52*(6), 1291–1293.

Daro, A. F., Gollin, H. A., & Samos, F. H. (1964). The tranquilizing effect of posterior pituitary extract. *Journal of the International College of Surgeons, 41*, 297–300.

Denuelle, M., Boulloche, N., Payoux, P., Fabre, N., Trotter, Y., & Géraud, G. (2011). A PET study of photophobia during spontaneous migraine attacks. *Neurology, 76*(3), 213–218.

Denuelle, M., Fabre, N., Payoux, P., Chollet, F., & Geraud, G. (2007). Hypothalamic activation in spontaneous migraine attacks. *Headache, 47*(10), 1418–1426.

Dexter, J. D., & Weitzman, E. D. (1970). The relationship of nocturnal headaches to sleep stage patterns. *Neurology, 20*(5), 513–518.

Dreier, J. P., Jurkat-Rott, K., Petzold, G. C., Tomkins, O., Klingebiel, R., & Kopp, U. A. (2005). Opening of the blood-brain barrier preceding cortical edema in a severe attack of FHM type II. *Neurology, 64*(12), 2145–2147.

Drummond, P. D., & Lance, J. W. (1984). Neurovascular disturbances in headache patients. *Clinical and Experimental Neurology, 20*, 93–99.

Dyer, C. J., Touchette, K. J., Carroll, J. A., Allee, G. L., & Matteri, R. L. (1999). Cloning of porcine prepro-orexin cDNA and effects of an intramuscular injection of synthetic porcine orexin-B on feed intake in young pigs. *Domestic Animal Endocrinology, 16*(3), 145–148.

Evers, S., Quibeldey, F., Grotemeyer, K. H., Suhr, B., & Husstedt, I. W. (1999). Dynamic changes of cognitive habituation and serotonin metabolism during the migraine interval. *Cephalalgia, 19*(5), 485–491.

Facchinetti, F., Sgarbi, L., & Piccinini, F. (2000). Hypothalamic resetting at puberty and the sexual dimorphism of migraine. *Functional Neurology, 15*(Suppl 3), 137–142.

Ferguson, A. V., & Samson, W. K. (2003). The orexin/hypocretin system: A critical regulator of neuroendocrine and autonomic function. *Frontiers in Neuroendocrinology, 24*(3), 141–150.

Gentile, S., Rainero, I., Daniele, D., Binello, E., Valfrè, W., & Pinessi, L. (2009). Reversible MRI abnormalities in a patient with recurrent status migrainosus. *Cephalalgia, 29*(6), 687–690.

Giesler, G. J., Jr., Katter, J. T., & Dado, R. J. (1994). Direct spinal pathways to the limbic system for nociceptive information. *Trends in Neuroscience, 17*(6), 244–250.

Giffin, N. J., Ruggiero, L., Lipton, R. B., Silberstein, S. D., Tvedskov, J. F., & Olesen, J. (2003). Premonitory symptoms in migraine: An electronic diary study. *Neurology, 60*(6), 935–940.

Goadsby, P. J. (2005a). Trigeminal autonomic cephalalgias: Fancy term or constructive change to the IHS classification? *Journal of Neurology, Neurosurgery, and Psychiatry, 76*(3), 301–305.

Goadsby, P. J. (2005b). Trigeminal autonomic cephalalgias. Pathophysiology and classification. *Review Neurologique (Paris), 161*(6–7), 692–695.

Goadsby, P. J., Goldberg, J., & Silberstein, S. D. (2008). Migraine in pregnancy. *BMJ, 336*(7659), 1502–1504.

Goadsby, P. J., & Gundlach, A. L. (1991). Localization of 3H-dihydroergotamine-binding sites in the cat central nervous system: Relevance to migraine. *Annals of Neurology, 29*(1), 91–94.

Goadsby, P. J., & Lipton, R. B. (1997). A review of paroxysmal hemicranias, SUNCT syndrome and other short-lasting headaches with autonomic features, including new cases. *Brain, 120*(Pt 1), 193–209.

Goldstein, D. J., Offen, W. W., Klein, E. G., Phebus, L. A., Hipskind, P., & Johnson, K. W. (2001). Lanepitant, an NK-1 antagonist, in migraine prevention. *Cephalalgia, 21*(2), 102–106.

Greco, R., Mangione, A. S., Sandrini, G., Maccarrone, M., Nappi, G., & Tassorelli, C. (2011). Effects of anandamide in migraine: Data from an animal model. *Journal of Headache and Pain, 12*(2), 177–183.

Holstege, G. (1987). Some anatomical observations on the projections from the hypothalamus to brainstem and spinal cord: An HRP and autoradiographic tracing study in the cat. *Journal of Comparative Neurology, 260*(1), 98–126.

Hoskin, K. L., Kaube, H., & Goadsby, P. J. (1996a). Sumatriptan can inhibit trigeminal afferents by an exclusively neural mechanism. *Brain, 119*(Pt 5), 1419–1428.

Hoskin, K. L., Kaube, H., & Goadsby, P. J. (1996b). Central activation of the trigeminovascular pathway in the cat is inhibited by dihydroergotamine. A c-Fos and electrophysiological study. *Brain, 119*(Pt 1), 249–256.

Humphrey, P. P., Feniuk, W., Perren, M. J., Beresford, I. J., Skingle, M., & Whalley, E. T. (1990). Serotonin and migraine. *Annals of the New York Academy of Sciences, 600*, 587–598; discussion 598–600.

Humphrey, P. P., & Goadsby, P. J. (1994). The mode of action of sumatriptan is vascular? A debate. *Cephalalgia, 14*(6), 401–410; discussion 393.

Johnson, D. E., Rollema, H., Schmidt, A. W., & McHarg, A. D. (2001). Serotonergic effects and extracellular brain levels of eletriptan, zolmitriptan and sumatriptan in rat brain. *European Journal of Pharmacology, 425*(3), 203–210.

Kaube, H., Hoskin, K. L., & Goadsby, P. J. (1993). Inhibition by sumatriptan of central trigeminal neurons only after blood-brain barrier disruption. *British Journal of Pharmacology, 109*(3), 788–792.

Kropp, P., & Gerber, W. D. (1998). Prediction of migraine attacks using a slow cortical potential, the contingent negative variation. *Neuroscience Letters, 257*(2), 73–76.

Krowicki, Z. K., & Kapusta, D. R. (2011). Microinjection of glycine into the hypothalamic paraventricular nucleus produces diuresis, natriuresis, and inhibition of central sympathetic outflow. *Journal of Pharmacology and Experimental Therapeutics, 337*(1), 247–255.

Lai, T. H., Fuh, J. L., & Wang, S. J. (2009). Cranial autonomic symptoms in migraine: Characteristics and comparison with cluster headache. *Journal of Neurology, Neurosurgery, and Psychiatry, 80*(10), 1116–1119.

Lee, J. H., Bang, E., Chae, K. J., Kim, J. Y., Lee, D. W., & Lee, W. (1999). Solution structure of a new hypothalamic neuropeptide, human hypocretin-2/orexin-B. *European Journal of Biochemistry, 266*(3), 831–839.

Lemaire, J. J., Frew, A. J., McArthur, D., Gorgulho, A. A., Alger, J. R., & Salomon, N. (2011). White matter connectivity of human hypothalamus. *Brain Research, 1371*, 43–64.

Levy, D., Jakubowski, M., & Burstein, R. (2004). Disruption of communication between peripheral and central trigeminovascular neurons mediates the antimigraine action of 5HT 1B/1D receptor agonists. *Proceedings of the National Academy of Sciences of the United States of America, 101*(12), 4274–4279.

Lipton, R. B., Stewart, W. F., Diamond, S., Diamond, M. L., & Reed, M. (2001). Prevalence and burden of migraine in the United States: Data from the American Migraine Study II. *Headache, 41*(7), 646–657.

Liu, R. J., van den Pol, A. N., & Aghajanian, G. K. (2002). Hypocretins (orexins) regulate serotonin neurons in the dorsal raphe nucleus by excitatory direct and inhibitory indirect actions. *Journal of Neuroscience, 22*(21), 9453–9464.

Luciani, R., Carter, D., Mannix, L., Hemphill, M., Diamond, M., & Cady, R. (2000). Prevention of migraine during prodrome with naratriptan. *Cephalalgia, 20*(2), 122–126.

Lund, I., Ge, Y., Yu, L. C., Uvnas-Moberg, K., Wang, J., & Yu, C. (2002). Repeated massage-like stimulation induces long-term effects on nociception: Contribution of oxytocinergic mechanisms. *European Journal of Neuroscience, 16*(2), 330–338.

MacGregor, E. A. (2006). Migraine and the menopause. *Journal of the British Menopause Society, 12*(3), 104–108.

Malick, A., Strassman, R. M., & Burstein, R. (2000). Trigemino-hypothalamic and reticulohypothalamic tract neurons in the upper cervical spinal cord and caudal medulla of the rat. *Journal of Neurophysiology, 84*(4), 2078–2112.

May, A., & Goadsby, P. J. (2001). Substance P receptor antagonists in the therapy of migraine. *Expert Opinion on Investigational Drugs, 10*(4), 673–678.

Millan, M. J. (1999). The induction of pain: An integrative review. *Progress in Neurobiology, 57*(1), 1–164.

Millan, M. J., Przewlocki, R., Millan, M. H., & Herz, A. (1983). Evidence for a role of the ventro-medial posterior hypothalamus in nociceptive processes in the rat. *Pharmacology, Biochemistry, and Behavior, 18*(6), 901–907.

Moskowitz, M. A. (1990). Basic mechanisms in vascular headache. *Neurology Clinics, 8*(4), 801–815.

Noseda, R., & Burstein, R. (2011). Advances in understanding the mechanisms of migraine-type photophobia. *Current Opinion in Neurology, 24*(3), 197–202.

Nozaki, K., Moskowitz, M. A., & Boccalini, P. (1992). CP-93, 129, sumatriptan, dihydroergotamine block c-fos expression within rat trigeminal nucleus caudalis caused by chemical stimulation of the meninges. *British Journal of Pharmacology, 106*(2), 409–415.

Olesen, J., Friberg, L., Olsen, T. S., Iversen, H. K., Lassen, N. A., Andersen, A. R., et al. (1990). Timing and topography of cerebral blood flow, aura, and headache during migraine attacks. *Annals of Neurology, 28*(6), 791–798.

Pearce, J. (1969). *Migraine: Clinical features, mechanisms and management.* Springfield, IL: Charles C. Thomas.

Peroutka, S. J. (2004). Migraine: A chronic sympathetic nervous system disorder. *Headache, 44*(1), 53–64.

Quintela, E., Castillo, J., Muñoz, P., & Pascual, J. (2006). Premonitory and resolution symptoms in migraine: A prospective study in 100 unselected patients. *Cephalalgia, 26*(9), 1051–1060.

Rahmann, A., Wienecke, T., Hansen, J. M., Fahrenkrug, J., Olesen, J., & Ashina, M. (2008). Vasoactive intestinal peptide causes marked cephalic vasodilation, but does not induce migraine. *Cephalalgia, 28*(3), 226–236.

Rasmussen, B. K., & Olesen, J. (1992). Migraine with aura and migraine without aura: An epidemiological study. *Cephalalgia, 12*(4), 221–228; discussion 186.

Rosen, S. D., Paulesu, E., Nihoyannopoulos, P., Tousoulis, D., Frackowiak, R. S., Frith, C. D., et al. (1996). Silent ischemia as a central problem: Regional brain activation compared in silent and painful myocardial ischemia. *Annals of Internal Medicine, 124*(11), 939–949.

Russell, M. B., Rasmussen, B. K., Fenger, K., & Olesen, J. (1996). Migraine without aura and migraine with aura are distinct clinical entities: A study of four hundred and eighty-four male and female migraineurs from the general population. *Cephalalgia, 16*(4), 239–245.

Samson, W. K., Taylor, M. M., & Ferguson, A. V. (2005). Non-sleep effects of hypocretin/orexin. *Sleep Medicine Reviews, 9*(4), 243–252.

Sances, G., Tassorelli, C., Pucci, E., Ghiotto, N., Sandrini, G., & Nappi, G. (2004). Reliability of the nitroglycerin provocative test in the diagnosis of neurovascular headaches. *Cephalalgia, 24*(2), 110–119.

Sand, T., Zhitniy, N., White, L. R., & Stovner, L. J. (2008). Visual evoked potential latency, amplitude and habituation in migraine: A longitudinal study. *Clinical Neurophysiology, 119*(5), 1020–1027.

Schoonman, G. G., van der Grond, J., Kortmann, C., van der Geest, R. J., Terwindt, G. M., & Ferrari, M. D. (2008). Migraine headache is not associated with cerebral or meningeal vasodilatation—a 3T magnetic resonance angiography study. *Brain, 131*(Pt 8), 2192–2200.

Schytz, H. W., Birk, S., Wienecke, T., Kruuse, C., Olesen, J., & Ashina, M. (2009). PACAP38 induces migraine-like attacks in patients with migraine without aura. *Brain, 132*(Pt 1), 16–25.

Serra, G., Collu, M., Loddo, S., Celasco, G., & Gessa, G. L. (1983). Hypophysectomy prevents yawning and penile erection but not hypomotility induced by apomorphine. *Pharmacology, Biochemistry, and Behavior, 19*(16), 917–919.

Shepheard, S. L., Williamson, D. J., Williams, J., Hill, R. G., & Hargreaves, R. J. (1995). Comparison of the effects of sumatriptan and the NK1 antagonist CP-99,994 on plasma extravasation in Dura mater and c-fos mRNA expression in trigeminal nucleus caudalis of rats. *Neuropharmacology, 34*(3), 255–61.

Shibahara, M., Sakurai, T., Nambu, T., Takenouchi, T., Iwaasa, H., & Egashira, S. I. (1999). Structure, tissue distribution, and pharmacological characterization of Xenopus orexins. *Peptides, 20*(10), 1169–1176.

Siegel, J. M. (2004). Hypocretin (orexin): Role in normal behavior and neuropathology. *Annual Review of Psychology, 55*, 125–148.

Stankewitz, A., Aderjan, D., Eippert, F., & May, A. (2011). Trigeminal nociceptive transmission in migraineurs predicts migraine attacks. *Journal of Neuroscience, 31*(6), 1937–1943.

Stewart, W. F., Lipton, R. B., Chee, E., Sawyer, J., & Silberstein, S. D. (2000). Menstrual cycle and headache in a population sample of migraineurs. *Neurology, 55*(10), 1517–1523.

Van den Pol, A. N. (1999). Hypothalamic hypocretin (orexin): Robust innervation of the spinal cord. *Journal of Neuroscience, 19*(8), 3171–3182.

Waelkens, J. (1984). Dopamine blockade with domperidone: Bridge between prophylactic and abortive treatment of migraine? A dose-finding study. *Cephalalgia, 4*(2), 85–90.

Waelkens, J. (1985). Warning symptoms in migraine: Characteristics and therapeutic implications. *Cephalalgia, 5*(4), 223–228.

Waters, W. E., & O'Connor, P. J. (1971). Epidemiology of headache and migraine in women. *Journal of Neurology, Neurosurgery, and Psychiatry, 34*(2), 148–153.

Weiller, C., May, A., Limmroth, V., Jüptner, M., Kaube, H., Schayck, R. V. (1995). Brain stem activation in spontaneous human migraine attacks. *Nature Medicine, 1*(7), 658–660.

Yamamoto, T., Saito, O., Shono, K., & Hirasawa, S. (2003). Activation of spinal orexin-1 receptor produces anti-allodynic effect in the rat carrageenan test. *European Journal of Pharmacology, 481*(2–3), 175–180.

Young, J. K., & Stanton, G. B. (1994). A three-dimensional reconstruction of the human hypothalamus. *Brain Research Bulletin, 35*(4), 323–327.

3 Neural System Changes in Migraine

PETER D. DRUMMOND

INTRODUCTION

Migraine is complex—attacks are often heralded by premonitory and prodromal disturbances and may be associated with heightened sensitivity to light, noise, and smells; with allodynia and hyperalgesia that spread from the head and neck to other parts of the body; and with dizziness, vertigo, and gastrointestinal complaints. Many of these symptoms persist subclinically between episodes of headache and may increase susceptibility to recurrent attacks and to comorbid conditions such as motion sickness (Cuomo-Granston & Drummond, 2010).

Elucidating this complexity is a challenging task. The approach taken in this chapter is to review neural mechanisms that might underlie some of the major symptoms of migraine—premonitory and prodromal changes, headache, sensory hypersensitivity, gastrointestinal disturbances, and vestibular instability. How these symptoms might interact during attacks of migraine is then discussed.

PREMONITORY AND PRODROMAL CHANGES

Premonitory Symptoms

In a clinical survey of 893 migraine sufferers who attended a tertiary care center for treatment of headache, approximately 30% of patients reported that premonitory symptoms such as fatigue, mood change, or gastrointestinal disturbances preceded their headache by several hours (Kelman, 2004a). These premonitory symptoms appear to be associated more frequently with symptoms of migraine (unilateral pain, gastrointestinal disturbances, and focal neurological symptoms) than with tension-type headache (Drummond & Lance, 1984a). Premonitory symptoms were studied prospectively in a recent electronic diary study of 97 patients who recorded symptoms before, during, and after attacks of migraine (Giffin et al., 2003). The most common premonitory symptoms were tiredness, difficulty concentrating and having a stiff neck, but some of these symptoms were also common at other times. Gastrointestinal disturbances and sensitivity to light and noise frequently preceded and sometimes

outlasted the headache, suggesting that these symptoms might contribute to the evolution of headache. Symptoms that most accurately predicted headache within the next 72 hours included yawning; difficulty with reading, writing, or speech; and increased emotionality. Using quantitative electroencephalography (EEG), Bjørk, Stovner, Hagen, and Sand (2011) identified slow and asymmetric EEG activity interictally, and reported an association between depressed responses to photic stimuli up to 36 hours before the onset of migraine and the severity of photophobia during attacks. Thus, a decrease in cortical excitability may be important in attack initiation.

The nature of certain premonitory symptoms (such as changes in mood, appetite, and fatigue) suggests that they are driven by a hypothalamic disturbance (Blau, 1980). The hypothalamus has multiple functions. Its key roles include regulating the endocrine system, coordinating circadian rhythms and states of arousal, synchronizing activity within the sympathetic and parasympathetic nervous systems, regulating appetitive drives, and modulating pain. It is also an important component of limbic circuits that regulate emotion. Involvement of the hypothalamus in migraine might account for links between the menstrual cycle and migraine and for circadian patterns in the timing of early-morning attacks (Alstadhaug, 2009).

The first direct evidence of hypothalamic activation during spontaneous attacks of migraine was presented in a positron emission study of seven patients studied within 4 hours of attack onset (Denuelle et al., 2007). In addition to activation at other sites in the cerebral cortex, midbrain, and pons, hypothalamic activation was detected both during headache and following headache relief with sumatriptan. Whether an activated hypothalamus is the source of migraine, generates attacks via projections to a vulnerable cerebral cortex or excitable brainstem nuclei, or reflects the activation of an antinociceptive mechanism remains unclear.

The Migraine Prodrome

The migraine aura typically begins within 30 minutes of an attack and is associated with neurological disturbances likened to the effects of a slow wave of cortical activation followed by prolonged depression of activity in the previously activated neurons. The close temporal relationship between the migraine aura and headache suggests that the aura triggers the headache, perhaps due to painful ischemia or perivascular inflammation. However, the aura is neither necessary nor sufficient for migraine, as only some attacks are preceded by an aura and some patients report auras without migraine. Lambert and Zagami (2009) suggested that activation of cortical neurons during the migraine aura inhibits midbrain neurons involved in pain modulation, leading to withdrawal of descending inhibition. That is, the migraine aura could act as a migraine trigger in much the same way that migraine might be provoked by strong sensory stimulation or intense emotional experiences.

Much evidence from divergent sources points toward an abnormal excitability of cortical and subcortical regions during the interictal period in migraine sufferers with or without aura (Aurora & Wilkinson, 2007). For example, visual evoked potential and neuromagnetic studies show that cortical excitability increases from a low base with repeated stimulation in migraine sufferers, whereas responses habituate in headache-free controls (Chen et al., 2011; Schoenen et al., 2003). A deficit in habituation has also been noted in auditory and somatosensory evoked potentials, laser evoked potentials, and trigeminal nociceptive blink reflexes (reviewed comprehensively by Coppola et al., 2009).

Psychophysical studies also demonstrate an abnormal excitability of the visual cortex in migraine sufferers during the interictal period. For example, migraine sufferers are particularly sensitive to striped patterns with a spatial frequency of around one to three cycles per degree, not only in regard to visual discomfort and distortions, but also in terms of visual cortical activation measured with blood oxygenation level–dependent functional magnetic resonance imaging (fMRI) (Huang et al., 2003; Shepherd, 2000). The effect of individually-prescribed precision ophthalmic tinted lenses on visual discomfort and fMRI visual cortical activation was investigated recently by Huang et al. (2011). Under control conditions, stressful striped patterns induced greater visual cortical activation in patients than controls. However, the precision ophthalmic tinted lenses alleviated visual discomfort and suppressed cortical activation in extra-striate areas. This normalization of cortical activity might account for the therapeutic benefits of the lenses.

HEADACHE

Source of Pain in Migraine

Despite many years of investigation, the source of pain in migraine remains unclear (Olesen et al., 2009). The most likely candidates are the cranial vessels and dura mater as noxious chemical, mechanical, and electrical stimulation of these structures evokes headache in a migrainelike distribution (Wolff, 1963). However, it has also been suggested that headache represents the failure of pain modulation processes to inhibit sensations arising from normal sensory traffic (Lambert, 2010). That is, the source of pain in migraine may be more to do with the "abnormal perception of the normal" than the activation of nociceptive pathways in the usual way that pain is generated (Goadsby, 2001). Each of these possibilities is discussed below.

Trigeminovascular System

Cells in the trigeminal ganglion that project to the large cranial vessels and meninges supply pathways for the transmission of pain signals from these structures and also provide a framework for neurovascular control (Borsook et al., 2006). This may take two forms: a trigeminal-parasympathetic vasodilator reflex and a neurogenic inflammatory process that involves release of neuropeptides such as calcitonin gene–related peptide from trigeminovascular nerve terminals (Goadsby et al., 1986; Lambert et al., 1984). An interaction between these processes could establish a vicious circle of vasodilatation, inflammation, and pain, driven by trigeminal nociceptive discharge.

An increase in inflammatory mediators in the external jugular vein (Sarchielli, Alberti, et al., 2006) and the peripheral bloodstream (Perini et al., 2005) during attacks of migraine has provided support for the view that meningeal inflammation is a source of pain. Whether this inflammatory response is associated with trigeminal activation is uncertain, as neuropeptide levels in the external jugular vein appear to remain unchanged in most patients during migraine attacks (Tfelt-Hansen & Le, 2009; Tvedskov et al., 2005). However, it is worth noting that levels of calcitonin gene–related peptide in the external jugular vein during attacks of migraine were greater in patients who responded to rizatriptan than nonresponsive patients, and that levels fell in the responsive patients after administration of rizatriptan (Sarchielli, Pini, et al., 2006). In addition, the generation of migrainelike headache after intravenous administration of calcitonin gene–related peptide (Lassen et al., 2002) and the beneficial effects of calcitonin gene–related peptide antagonists in migraine (Ho et al., 2008; Olesen et al., 2004) suggest that trigeminal activation and associated neurogenic vasodilatation is a source of pain.

Neurophysiological observations are also consistent with trigeminal activation during attacks of migraine. Kaube et al. (2002) reported a shortening in the latency of blink reflexes evoked from a concentric stimulating electrode on the ipsilateral side during attacks of unilateral migraine, together with an increase in the strength of the blink reflex. Unlike standard electrodes, the concentric electrode appears to preferentially evoke activity in superficial nociceptive afferent fibers rather than deeper fibers activated by innocuous electrical stimuli (Kaube et al., 2000). Thus, the findings suggest that the excitability of trigeminal nociceptive pathways increases on the headache-affected side during attacks of unilateral migraine.

Headache Mechanisms

Trigeminal activation may initiate two opposing processes within the brainstem. The first involves sensitization of second-order neurons in the medullary dorsal horn that receive convergent inputs from the meninges and the facial skin (Burstein et al., 1998). This central sensitization may result in the scalp tenderness that accompanies most attacks of migraine, outlasting the headache by up to a week (Drummond, 1987). Hyperalgesia often extends from the scalp to encompass the limbs as the attack progresses, possibly due to the rostral spread of sensitization in nociceptive pathways (Burstein, Cutrer, et al., 2000; Burstein, Yarnitsky, et al., 2000).

In addition to central sensitization, trigeminal nerve discharge may initiate a second opposing process that involves heightened activity in pain modulation pathways that originate in the periaqueductal gray and rostroventral medulla. Higher subcortical and cortical centers such as the amygdala and anterior cingulate cortex, which process the unpleasant and distressing aspects of pain and modulate attention to pain, communicate with the midbrain periaqueductal gray, which, in turn, projects downstream to the serotonergic raphe nuclei and brainstem adrenergic nuclei (Bajic & Proudfit, 1999). Inhibitory pain control pathways descend from these brainstem nuclei to the trigeminal nucleus caudalis and dorsal horn of the spinal cord (Bajic & Proudfit, 1999; Basbaum & Fields, 1978). The dorsolateral periaqueductal gray contains "command modules" that activate the cardiovascular system and trigger nonopioid analgesia in threatening circumstances (Bandler & Shipley, 1994). Microinjections of the synaptic excitant d,l-homocysteic acid into the pretentorial part of the lateral periaqueductal gray of decerebrate cats evokes extracranial vasodilatation, whereas more caudal injections evoke hind-limb vasodilatation (Carrive & Bandler, 1991). A second major command module in the ventrolateral periaqueductal gray initiates opioid analgesia and inhibits cardiovascular activity, locomotion, and responsiveness to the environment during periods of inescapable pain and stress (the "defeat" response). Both of these command modules may be overactive in migraine

sufferers, first in association with extracranial vasodilatation during stressful encounters and then in association with pain modulation during migraine headache. From a teleological perspective, some attacks of migraine might represent forced withdrawal from engagement with environmental or physiological stressors, followed by a period of recuperation.

Increases in activity in midbrain and brainstem regions during attacks of migraine and following headache relief with sumatriptan (Afridi, Giffin, et al., 2005; Afridi, Matharu, et al., 2005; Denuelle et al., 2007; Weiller et al., 1995) may reflect increased activity in these pain modulation circuits. Alternatively, increased brainstem activity could represent a failure of pain modulation processes to inhibit neural discharge in circuits that generate headache and symptoms associated with migraine. These pain modulation processes appear to work less efficiently in migraine sufferers than controls. In particular, the nociceptive RIII flexion reflex was found to increase in migraine sufferers during concurrent pain but to decrease in controls (consistent with normal inhibitory pain modulation via "diffuse noxious inhibitory controls") (Sandrini et al., 2006). Failure of inhibitory control might result in the rapid sensitization of central nociceptive pathways during attacks of migraine.

Welch et al. (2001) provided neuroanatomical evidence of disturbed function of the periaqueductal gray in migraine sufferers. Iron levels increased in proportion to the number of years with migraine, suggesting that iron may accumulate in the periaqueductal gray during repeated attacks. Welch et al. suggested that neurons with high iron content may be particularly vulnerable to iron-catalyzed free radical damage, which, in turn, could compromise descending inhibitory pain control.

The cranial nociceptive system appears to be more excitable in migraine sufferers during the headache-free interval than in controls. For example, the prevalence of "ice-cream headache" and stabbing, ice pick–like pains is elevated in migraine sufferers (Drummond & Lance, 1984a; Fuh et al., 2003; Raskin & Knittle, 1976; Raskin & Schwartz, 1980; Selekler & Budak, 2004). Migraine sufferers were found to be more sensitive to painful stimulation of the temple with ice than controls, and more readily developed headache (Drummond & Granston, 2005). In addition, temporal summation to painful stimulation of the forehead with a firm bristle was found to be greater in migraine sufferers than controls, consistent with induction of wind-up in second-order trigeminal nociceptive neurons (Weissman-Fogel et al., 2003). Moreover, the threshold of the electrically elicited corneal reflex was lower and the trigeminal nociceptive blink reflex habituated more slowly in migraine sufferers than controls

(Katsarava et al., 2003; Sandrini et al., 2002). In patients with strictly unilateral migraine, pressure-pain thresholds were found to be lower and pericranial tenderness greater on the symptomatic than nonsymptomatic side during the headache-free interval, and pressure-pain thresholds were lower on both sides than in controls (Fernandez-de-las-Penas et al., 2008). In addition, pain to palpation over the supraorbital nerve was greater on the symptomatic than nonsymptomatic side of the forehead in patients with strictly unilateral migraine (Fernandez-de-las-Penas et al., 2009). Conversely, the frequency and intensity of migrainous attacks decreased following local anesthetic blockade of the distal emergence points of tender supraorbital and greater occipital nerves (Caputi & Firetto, 1997). Together, these findings suggest that nociceptive discharge in hyperexcitable cranial nerves may increase susceptibility to headache in migraine sufferers.

By and large, migraine sufferers tolerate pain to the same extent as headache-free controls (Drummond, 1987). Nevertheless, migraine sufferers generally appear to be more sensitive to pain than people who rarely or never suffer from headaches. For example, pressure-pain thresholds were found to be lower in migraine sufferers than in controls not only over the supraorbital nerves but also over peripheral nerve trunks in the upper extremities during the headache-free interval (Fernandaz-de-las-Penas et al., 2009). Similarly, migraine sufferers reported more intense and diffuse limb pain during cold pressor tests than controls (Drummond & Granston, 2003), and limb pain evoked by mechanical stimulation increased in migraine sufferers but not controls during motion sickness (Drummond, 2002). These findings suggest that nociceptive networks may become more readily sensitized in migraine sufferers than controls, possibly due to failure of pain modulation processes (Sandrini et al., 2006).

Vascular Disturbances
Dilatation of pain-sensitized cranial arteries is a source of pain in migraine (Iversen et al., 1990; Olesen et al., 2009; Wolff, 1963), but this may vary from one attack to another or even across different stages of the same attack (Drummond & Lance, 1983, 1984b). Headache associated with signs of extracranial vasodilatation can usually be alleviated temporarily by digital compression of the superficial temporal artery, and intracranial vessels may be an alternate source of pain in another subgroup of cases (Drummond & Lance, 1983). However, in the majority of patients, headache persists despite occlusion of flow through the common carotid artery, implying that headache arises from a nonvascular source (e.g., tender scalp muscles, inflamed meningeal tissues, or a sensitized

trigeminal nociceptive network) (Drummond & Lance, 1984b).

To investigate the vascular changes associated with migraine, Asghar et al. (2011) employed high-resolution magnetic resonance arteriography to measure the circumference of the extracranial middle meningeal artery and the intracranial middle cerebral artery during attacks provoked by infusion of calcitonin gene-related peptide. They detected arterial dilatation of 9 to 12% on the painful side but no change on the pain-free side during attacks, and constriction of the middle meningeal artery (but not the middle cerebral artery) when the headache was alleviated by sumatriptan. These findings contrast with those reported by Schoonman et al. (2008) in a study of vascular changes associated with nitroglycerin-induced headache, possibly because Ashgar et al. were able to measure arterial changes more precisely. The vascular changes of migraine might induce—or be induced by—activation of sensitized peri-vascular nociceptors (Levy & Burstein, 2011).

During the headache-free period, extracranial vasodilator responses to pain and other forms of physical and emotional discomfort appear to be greater in migraine sufferers than controls. For example, increases in extracranial blood flow were greater in migraine sufferers than controls in anticipation of and response to facial pain (Drummond, 1997; Drummond & Granston, 2005), immersing the foot in painfully cold water (Drummond & Granston, 2003), motion sickness provocation (Drummond & Granston, 2004), and psychological stress (Drummond, 1982, 1985), and were greater on the habitually affected than headache-free side during exercise in patients with unilateral attacks (Drummond & Lance, 1981). Thus, it seems plausible that stress-evoked dilatation of pain-sensitized cranial vessels aggravates the throbbing component of pain during attacks of migraine.

Pain Arising within the Brain
In the absence of definitive peripheral pathology, it has been suggested that migraine headache might originate in the brain (Lambert, 2010). In particular, withdrawal of descending inhibition could facilitate the discharge of trigeminal nociceptive afferents, evoke trigeminal-parasympathetic vasodilator reflexes and neurogenic inflammation, and set the wheels of migraine in motion.

This view requires confirmation that spontaneous traffic in trigeminal nociceptive afferents or second-order neurons is great enough to evoke headache and trigeminovascular responses when freed from the constraints of descending inhibitory control (Olesen et al., 2009). Nevertheless, parallels have been drawn between migraine and other forms of central pain (e.g., deafferentation pain, poststroke pain, or phantom limb pain) (Sicuteri, 1987; Sicuteri & Nicolodi, 1986). In particular, Sicuteri et al. (1979) noted similarities between migraine and opiate withdrawal syndrome (headache, autonomic disturbances, emotional distress, and supersensitivity of venous smooth muscle to monoamines). Sicuteri (1987) postulated that a central supersensitivity to monoamines, due to a chronically deficient opioid system, could mediate many of the symptoms of migraine.

SENSITIVITY TO LIGHT, NOISE, AND SMELLS

Sensitivity to light, noise, and/or smells accompanies most attacks of migraine and often persists to some extent between attacks. This sensitivity of the special senses may increase during the migraine prodrome (Giffin et al., 2003), and intense sensory stimuli (e.g., bright or flickering lights or odors such as perfumes or wet paint) may trigger some attacks. Heightened sensitivity in one sensory modality (e.g., light) is associated with heightened sensitivity in other modalities (e.g., noise or smells) (De Carlo et al., 2010; Demarquay et al., 2006), suggesting the involvement of a common mechanism.

Photophobia

Photophobia consists of two components: a sense of heightened glare and an experience of light-induced pain (Lebensohn, 1934). In a study in our laboratory, both components were found to be greater in migraine sufferers during the interictal period than in controls, and light-induced pain increased further during attacks (Drummond, 1986). Light-induced pain generally was greater on the side of headache than on the headache-free side in patients with unilateral attacks. Subsequent studies confirmed that thresholds for light-induced discomfort and pain were lower in migraine sufferers than controls, both during and outside of attacks (Vanagaite et al., 1997). However, light-induced pain was similar on both sides in patients with unilateral headache, possibly because each eye was tested sequentially rather than simultaneously (Vanagaite et al., 1997). Martin et al. (2011) recently employed fMRI to investigate the cortical response to differing light intensities. They found that photophobia and reactivity of the occipital cortex to low- and medium-low luminance levels were greater in migraine sufferers than controls. Surprisingly, however, there was no association between the intensity of photophobia and the extent of cortical activation, implying independent mechanisms.

Wolff (1963) reported that injection of sodium chloride into the frontalis muscle above the supraorbital margin increased the rate of winking (a sign of photophobia), and

concluded that irritation anywhere within the region supplied by the ophthalmic division of the trigeminal nerve could facilitate photophobia. He postulated that the motor components of photophobia, such as blinking, conjunctival vasodilatation and lacrimation, involved spread of excitatory influences in the brainstem from trigeminal and optic nerve nuclei to the facial nerve, while higher centers were responsible for the intensification of photophobia in bright light. Drummond and Woodhouse (1993) investigated whether painful stimulation within the distribution of the ophthalmic nerve increased the subjective sensation of photophobia to the same extent in migraine sufferers and headache-free controls. To induce pain, ice was applied to the midforehead while the discomfort threshold to an increasingly intense light was assessed. Tolerance to bright light decreased during cold-induced pain in migraine sufferers but not in headache-free controls, suggesting that the mechanism responsible for photophobia was more responsive to trigeminal input in migraine sufferers than controls. Similarly, ratings of glare and light-induced pain increased during painful stimulation of various facial sites in migraine sufferers but remained steady in headache-free controls (Drummond, 1997). Together, these findings suggest that the mechanism responsible for photophobia is more responsive to trigeminal input in migraine sufferers than controls.

The cortical correlates of photophobia were investigated recently during migraine attacks using positron emission tomography (Boulloche et al., 2010; Denuelle et al., 2011). Cortical responses to static visual stimulation of the whole visual field were examined during eight attacks of migraine and after headache relief by sumatriptan. During migraine, visual stimulation at an intensity that evoked photophobia (an increase of 2 points on a 0 to 10 headache intensity scale) evoked activity in the primary visual cortex. This response decreased but was still present to some extent after sumatriptan was administered. However, the same level of visual stimulation evoked no change in activity in the primary visual cortex during the headache-free interval. Cortical responses to three static luminous intensities were also compared in seven migraine sufferers and seven headache-free controls with and without noxious heating of the forehead (Boulloche et al., 2010). In migraine sufferers, visual stimulation increased activity in the primary and secondary visual cortex and the adjacent posterior cingulate cortex in proportion to the intensity of stimulation, and pain potentiated the response. In contrast, visual stimulation evoked cortical activity only in the presence of pain in controls. Together, these findings suggest that photophobia in migraine is linked with cortical excitability, and that this is facilitated by trigeminal nociception.

Noseda et al. (2010) reported recently that migraine sufferers without image-forming vision but with a preserved sense of light still experienced photophobia during attacks of migraine, whereas patients without a preserved sense of light did not. Noseda et al. identified light-sensitive neurons in the posterior thalamus of rats that also were sensitive to stimulation of the dura mater. The thalamic neurons received information from intrinsically photosensitive retinal ganglion cells that entrain the biological clock to the dark–light cycle, form the afferent pathway of the pupillary light reflex, and suppress melatonin release by light. Nerve fibers were found to project widely from the posterior thalamus to the somatosensory cortex and to regions involved in cognitive, motor, and visual functions. Thus, the thalamus may form a point of convergence between the trigeminal nociceptive signals that mediate headache and the visual inputs that underlie photophobia.

Phonophobia

During attacks of migraine, patients often retreat into a quiet room to wait out the attack. A heightened sensitivity to sound, likened to "hearing the sound of a pin drop in the next room," appears to be a common experience. Quantitative measures of sound aversion thresholds have confirmed that phonophobia strengthens during attacks of migraine but persists to some extent during the headache-free interval (Ashkenazi et al., 2009; Vanagaite Vingen et al., 1998). Woodhouse and Drummond (1993) measured the hearing threshold and the auditory discomfort threshold to an 8,000-Hz tone during the headache-free interval and again during attacks in 16 migraine sufferers. The auditory discomfort threshold decreased during attacks (consistent with phonophobia), and the hearing threshold increased (three patients) or decreased significantly (three patients) compared with normal variation in headache-free controls, indicating that multiple mechanisms may contribute to phonophobia.

Kayan and Hood (1984) suggested that phonophobia in migraine might be due to a cochlear disturbance that evokes loudness recruitment (an abnormally rapid increase in loudness with increase in intensity of sound, associated with unilateral cochlear hearing loss). Cochlear function in migraine sufferers was examined recently by testing otoacoustic emissions (Bolay et al., 2008), which are produced by movements of the eardrum in response to vibrations generated by outer hair cells within the cochlea. Otoacoustic emissions can be measured from the external ear canal and can be suppressed by auditory stimulation of the contralateral ear, an effect mediated by neurons in the medial superior olivary complex in the brainstem. During the headache-free interval, otoacoustic emissions were similar in migraine sufferers and controls. However,

suppression of otoacoustic emissions by contralateral sound stimulation was impaired in migraine sufferers, implying decreased activation of neurons in the medial olivary complex or reduced synaptic transmission between olivocochlear nerve fibers and outer hair cells in the cochlea. Similarly, Hamed, Youssef, and Elattar (2011) reported that nearly two-thirds of patients with migraine had one or more abnormalities in electrophysiological tests of otoacoustic emissions and auditory brainstem reflexes. Whether these peripheral and central auditory disturbances contribute to phonophobia in migraine is unknown.

Cochlear disturbances that provoke loudness recruitment might account for partial hearing loss during attacks of migraine, but do not account for increases in auditory acuity. Although additional mechanisms that contribute to phonophobia in migraine are unknown, possibilities might include disruption to pain modulation processes mediated by disturbances in noradrenergic or serotonergic pathways that modulate transfer of sensory information to the cerebral cortex (Vanagaite Vingen et al., 1998). An association between phonophobia and cutaneous allodynia during attacks of migraine supports the view that a central integrative mechanism mediates aversion to multiple sensory modalities in migraine (Ashkenazi et al., 2010).

Olfactory Discomfort

Many patients with migraine describe an aversion to odors normally perceived as innocuous (osmophobia) or, less commonly, a heightened acuity to certain odors. These symptoms are more frequently associated with migraine than tension-type headache, both in adults (Kelman, 2004b; Zanchin et al., 2007) and children (Corletto et al., 2008; De Carlo et al., 2010). Olfactory discomfort persists in some patients during the interictal period, and certain odors (e.g., perfume, car exhaust fumes, or cigarette smoke) may trigger attacks (Demarquay et al., 2006; Sjostrand et al., 2010).

Despite the clear association between migraine and olfactory discomfort in clinical surveys, the characteristics of olfactory disturbances in migraine remain unclear. For example, in olfactory tests with pyridine, 12 of 67 migraine sufferers (18%) had elevated thresholds, compared with the prevalence of hyposmia or anosmia of only 1% in the general population of the United States (Hirsh, 1992). In contrast, the olfactory threshold for vanillin (a pure olfactory stimulus) was found to be lower in migraine sufferers than controls during the interictal period (Snyder & Drummond, 1997). In addition, migraine sufferers who reported olfactory hypersensitivity during attacks were able to detect the odor of acetone (a mixed olfactory–trigeminal stimulus) at a lower concentration than most other patients. In a more recent study, neither the identification accuracy to a range of odors nor the odor detection threshold to *n*-butanol differed between migraine sufferers and controls (Grosser et al., 2000). However, the N1 amplitude of the event-related potential to short pulses of carbon dioxide (a pure trigeminal stimulus) was greater in migraine sufferers than controls, whereas the peak-to-peak amplitude of the P1N1 wave to hydrogen sulfide (an olfactory stimulus) was smaller in migraine sufferers than controls.

Neural networks that might mediate olfactory discomfort in migraine sufferers were explored recently using positron emission tomography in 11 patients who were vulnerable to odor-triggered attacks (Demarquay et al., 2008). During olfactory stimulation, activation of the left inferior frontal gyrus, left and right middle frontal gyri, left and right angular gyri, right posterosuperior temporal gyrus, posterior cingulate gyrus, and right locus coeruleus was smaller in migraine sufferers than controls. As many of these cortical regions respond directly to olfactory stimulation, the findings suggest that processing of olfactory stimuli differs between migraine sufferers and controls. This might be due to deficiencies in cortical activation in migraine sufferers, or could reflect inhibitory processes that aim to suppress olfactory discomfort. Further studies that compare patients with and without olfactory discomfort may be required to clarify these results. In addition to these findings, activation of the left temporal pole (which is involved in olfactory emotional processing) was greater in migraine sufferers than controls (Demarquay et al., 2008), perhaps reflecting greater olfactory discomfort in migraine sufferers.

Cortical and subcortical fMRI responses to a pure olfactory stimulus (rose odor) were recently investigated between and during attacks of migraine by Stankewitz and May (2011). Intensity ratings were similar in patients and controls and did not change during attacks, possibly due to the small sample size. Nevertheless, activation was greater in the amygdala, insular cortex, temporal pole, superior temporal gyrus, rostral pons, and cerebellum during than outside attacks. These findings are consistent with greater sensitivity to olfactory stimuli in a cortical network of olfactory-related brain areas during attacks. In addition, olfactory activation of the rostral pons (the so-called "migraine generator") during migraine implies a link with trigeminal sensory processing, perhaps explaining the aversive quality of odors during attacks.

VESTIBULAR AND GASTROINTESTINAL DISTURBANCES

Vestibular Symptoms

Dysfunction in peripheral or central vestibular pathways seems to be characteristic of migraine. The vestibular evoked myogenic potential is induced less readily in migrainous patients than in controls, even in patients with no other features of vestibular migraine (Boldingh, Ljostad, Mygland, & Monstad, 2011; Hong, Kim, Park, & Lee, 2011). Vestibular disturbances such as vertigo and related symptoms such as nonspecific dizziness often develop before or during attacks of migraine and frequently recur during the headache-free interval (Calhoun, Ford, Pruitt, & Fisher, 2011; Cha et al., 2009; Kuritzky et al., 1981; Lempert et al., 2009). Migraine is also associated with vestibular disturbances such as benign paroxysmal positional vertigo and Ménière disease (Neuhauser & Lempert, 2009).

Various explanations have been put forward to account for these associations. When linked with other symptoms of the migraine aura, vertigo may represent a manifestation of "cortical spreading depression" involving the parieto-insular vestibular cortex. Alternatively, vertigo and other cochlear symptoms associated with migraine could be due to periodic vasospasm of the internal auditory artery or the vertebrobasilar artery when accompanied by other symptoms of brainstem ischemia, or might more broadly reflect aberrant regulation of activity in brainstem nuclei linked with the trigeminovascular system.

Evidence of a functional relationship between the vestibular and trigeminal systems in migraine sufferers was presented in a study that involved measuring eye movements during supraorbital electrical stimulation at pain threshold intensity (Marano et al., 2005). Supraorbital stimulation evoked or modified nystagmus in 8 of 10 migraine sufferers but had no effect on spontaneous eye movements in controls. In another 10 patients, supraorbital stimulation again evoked or modified nystagmus, whereas median nerve stimulation altered nystagmus in only 1 case. The nystagmus appeared to be of peripheral origin as it could be suppressed by eye fixation; in addition, the velocity of the slow phase of eye movement was linear rather than exponential, which supports a peripheral rather than central mechanism. Marano et al. (2005) postulated that supraorbital electrical stimulation evoked an axon reflex in trigeminal neurons with collateral projections to the supraorbital skin and cochlea, thereby modifying vestibular function. Alternatively, the trigeminal–vestibular interaction might involve communication between trigeminal sensory afferents or second-order trigeminal neurons and vestibular neurons in the brainstem (Buisseret-Delmas et al., 1999; Marfurt & Rajchert, 1991).

From early childhood, migraine sufferers appear to be vulnerable not only to vertigo but also to nausea and other abdominal complaints (Barabas et al., 1983; Li et al., 1999). A history of motion sickness is predictive of childhood migraine (Jan, 1998), and a history of motion sickness, migraine, or family history of migraine predicts vomiting after mild head injury (Jan et al., 1997). Motion sickness arises due to a mismatch between vestibular and visual or proprioceptive cues of movement during passive locomotion (e.g., riding in a car or boat) or when stationary while the visual surround is in motion (e.g., watching three-dimensional movies). It is associated with many of the symptoms of migraine (primarily nausea and vomiting, but also dizziness, headache, and facial pallor). Migraine sufferers appear to be vulnerable both to movement-induced and visually induced motion sickness (Drummond, 2002, 2005b; Drummond & Granston, 2004; Grunfeld & Gresty, 1998; Grunfeld et al., 1998), suggesting the involvement not only of the peripheral vestibular system but also of central vestibular nuclei. Evidence both of peripheral and central vestibular disturbances in migraine was obtained recently in patients with an array of vestibular symptoms (Jeong et al., 2010; Teggi et al., 2009).

Effects of motion sickness provocation may be greater in migraine sufferers than controls not only for symptoms of motion sickness but also in terms of photophobia and heightened sensitivity to pain (Drummond, 2002). Consistent with this possibility, pain evoked by a sharp probe applied to the fingertips increased after motion sickness induction in migraine sufferers but did not change in controls (Drummond, 2002). It would be interesting to determine whether motion sickness disrupts pain-modulating processes such as diffuse noxious inhibitory controls or stress-induced analgesia and, if so, whether the disruptive effects of motion sickness are greater in migraine sufferers than controls.

Gastrointestinal Disturbances

Nausea is generally described as an unpleasant wave-like sensation in the throat, epigastrium, or abdomen that often precedes but does not always culminate in vomiting. The physiological basis of nausea is uncertain, but may involve communication between afferent pathways involved in vomiting (e.g., the chemoreceptor trigger zone, gastrointestinal visceral afferents, and/or the labyrinth) (Takeda et al., 1993) and forebrain regions that integrate this sensory input with past experiences and concurrent sensory-motor and emotional activity (Horn et al., 2007). Nausea might also arise from preparatory activation of motor pathways in the nucleus tractus solitarius and the dorsal motor nucleus of the vagus—the so-called vomiting or emetic center (Dahlof & Hargreaves, 1998; Mitchelson, 1992; Takeda et al., 2001).

In addition to regulating cardiovascular, respiratory, and gastrointestinal functions, the nucleus tractus

solitarius receives convergent visceral, spinal, and trigeminal nociceptive inputs that could mediate gastrointestinal disturbances in migraine (Benarroch, 2006; Knight, 2005; Ruggiero et al., 2000). In support of this possibility, periodic head pain (evoked by applying an ice block to the temple for 30 seconds) was found to provoke nausea in migraine sufferers but not controls (Drummond & Granston, 2005). This effect was particularly striking during and after motion sickness provocation, presumably reflecting excitability within emetic or trigeminal nociceptive circuits (Drummond & Granston, 2004, 2005). In addition, application of ice to the temple aggravated headache during motion sickness provocation (Drummond & Granston, 2004). Conversely, scalp tenderness increased in the most nauseated participants after motion sickness provocation (Drummond, 2002). Thus, it seems plausible that nausea and headache reinforce each other in a vicious circle (Fig. 3–1).

This possibility was investigated in migraine sufferers who attended our laboratory on three occasions spread over several months to participate in experiments that involved exposure to optokinetic stimulation (to provoke symptoms of motion sickness), together with painful stimulation of the temple or hand (Granston & Drummond, 2005). The daily incidence of migrainelike attacks (headache associated with nausea) averaged 8% throughout the monitoring period. This increased only slightly after sessions that involved painful stimulation of the hand but jumped to 44% after sessions that involved painful stimulation of the temple (Fig. 3–2). As the development of nausea and headache during optokinetic stimulation increased the likelihood of migrainelike attacks afterward, head pain and nausea appeared to interact synergistically to provoke these attacks.

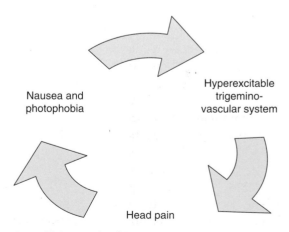

FIGURE 3–1 *Vicious circle of symptoms in migraine.*

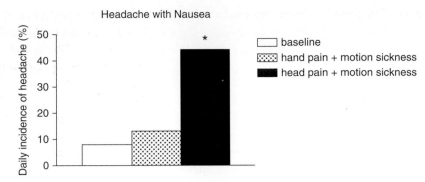

FIGURE 3–2 *Daily incidence of headaches associated with nausea throughout the monitoring period (baseline), after sessions involving motion sickness provocation and hand pain (immersing one hand in ice water), and after sessions involving motion sickness provocation and head pain (applying an ice block to the temple) in a study by Granston and Drummond (2005). The incidence of migrainelike headaches was greater after sessions involving motion sickness provocation and head pain than after sessions that involved motion sickness provocation and hand pain (*p < .05).*

SYMPTOM INTERACTION IN MIGRAINE

As noted above, multiple sources of evidence point to subclinical disturbances that persist interictally and that might increase vulnerability to migraine. This includes signs of altered cortical excitability, heightened sensitivity to light and noise, vestibular disturbances, compromised pain control, and increased reactivity of extracranial blood vessels. Heightened sensitivity to head pain, aggravated by gastrointestinal disturbances, vestibular instability, and stimulation of the special senses, is consistent with the notion of an underlying disturbance to pain modulation processes that might increase vulnerability to recurrent attacks. Neurogenic inflammation and dilatation of intracranial and extracranial vessels appear to be the most likely sources of pain in migraine, although spontaneous activity in a disinhibited trigeminal nociceptive system could also contribute to headache. Reciprocal interaction between headache and symptoms such as photophobia, nausea, and vertigo may create a vicious circle of symptoms and pain.

The neural mechanisms that might underlie susceptibility to recurrent attacks of migraine are illustrated in Figure 3–3. In particular, disturbances in the trigeminal nucleus caudalis, nucleus tractus solitarius, and vestibular nuclei may respectively mediate headache, nausea, and dizziness. Trigeminovascular reflexes and neurogenic inflammation could develop in response to, then aggravate, the brainstem disturbances responsible for symptoms of migraine. This may establish a vicious circle akin to a neural "wind-up" phenomenon. Disruption of pain modulation processes that normally inhibit discomfort to light, noise, and head pain might result in the sensitization of trigeminal nociceptive neurons and their rostral projections. Sensory stimulation then intensifies activity in, and promotes sensitization of, these neural circuits.

The sequence illustrated in Figure 3–3 does not address one of the cardinal features of migraine—more often than not the headache is limited to one side of the head. Thus, it may be necessary to postulate asymmetric activation of the trigeminovascular system and brainstem nuclei. Afridi, Giffin, et al. (2005) reported that the thalamus contralateral to the side of pain was activated during spontaneous attacks of migraine, as might be expected on anatomical grounds. They also detected left-sided activation of the dorsolateral pons, irrespective of whether the headache was left or right sided. In attacks provoked by glyceryl trinitrate, activation in the dorsolateral pons was ipsilateral to the side of pain in patients with unilateral headache, and bilateral with a left-sided preponderance in patients with bilateral headache (Afridi, Matharu, et al., 2005). This left-sided tendency might account for the left-sided preponderance of activation in the dorsolateral pons during spontaneous attacks of migraine.

By definition, the axon reflexes that mediate neurogenic inflammation are limited to the receptive field of the activated nerve (i.e., in a unilateral distribution); in addition, trigeminal-parasympathetic vasodilator reflexes are predominantly ipsilateral to the site of stimulation (Drummond, 1992; Lambert et al., 1984). Persistent deficits in sympathetic vasoconstrictor tone in extracranial vessels (Drummond, 1991) could increase extracranial vasodilatation during attacks of migraine and aggravate pain. Curiously, nociceptive stimulation of the limbs also dilates ipsilateral extracranial blood vessels due to release of sympathetic vasoconstrictor tone (Drummond, 2006a) (Fig. 3–4), but whether this response is relevant to migraine is uncertain. In any case, mechanisms within the brainstem and trigeminovascular system that could initiate unilateral episodes of headache clearly exist.

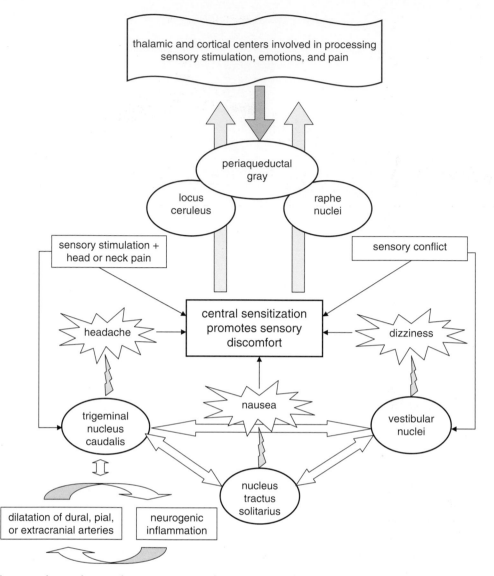

FIGURE 3–3 *Neural systems that might contribute to symptoms of migraine. Within the brainstem, headache, nausea, and dizziness may be mediated respectively by activity in the trigeminal nucleus caudalis, nucleus tractus solitarius, and vestibular nuclei. Simultaneous discharge within these nuclei could intensify symptoms via "reverberating circuits" (positive loops). Trigeminal nociceptive discharge may be associated with neurogenic inflammation and dilatation of dural, pial, or extracranial arteries; this could intensify pain and promote rostral spread of central sensitization within nociceptive circuits. In the posterior thalamus, convergence between trigeminal nociceptive signals and input from the special senses may result in photophobia and phonophobia. Ascending nociceptive discharge and activity in cortical centers that process sensory stimulation, emotions, and pain mobilize pain modulation processes in the periaqueductal gray that project to the locus coeruleus and raphe nuclei. Failure of these pain modulation processes to inhibit pain could escalate symptoms of migraine.*

At least some of the interactions among symptoms of migraine may be mediated by serotonin. This was investigated in our laboratory by administering an amino acid drink that omitted l-tryptophan (the precursor to serotonin) before motion sickness provocation (Drummond, 2005a). This procedure (called tryptophan depletion) rapidly reduces brain serotonin synthesis. In headache-free controls, tryptophan depletion enhanced dizziness, nausea, and the illusion of movement to levels that approached those reported by migraine sufferers. In addition, tryptophan depletion augmented headache in migraine sufferers and enhanced ratings of glare, light-induced pain, and nausea both in migraine sufferers and controls (Drummond, 2006b). These findings suggest that migrainous symptoms intensify following a rapid reduction in brain synthesis of serotonin.

Migraine is associated with chronically low concentrations of plasma serotonin and a heightened sensitivity to

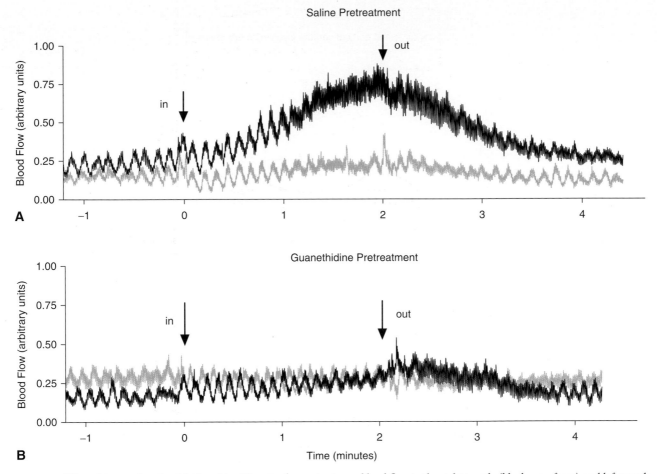

Saline Pretreatment

Guanethidine Pretreatment

Time (minutes)

FIGURE 3–4 *Effect of immersing the right hand in 2°C water for 2 minutes on blood flow in the right temple (black waveform) and left temple (gray waveform) after bilateral saline pretreatment (A) and after guanethidine pretreatment to the right temple (to block adrenergic vasoconstriction) and saline pretreatment to the left temple (B). The right hand was immersed in the water at the arrow marked "in" and removed from the water at the arrow marked "out." The guanethidine pretreatment inhibited increases in blood flow in the right temple during the cold pressor test, indicating that the vasodilator response was mediated by release of adrenergic vasoconstrictor tone. Pulse amplitude (indicated by the thickness of the blood flow signal) also increased in the right temple after saline pretreatment, and this response was inhibited by guanethidine pretreatment. Reprinted with permission from Drummond, P. D. (2006). Immersion of the hand in ice water releases adrenergic vasoconstrictor tone in the ipsilateral temple.* Autonomic Neuroscience, 128, 70–75.

serotonin agonists (Ferrari & Saxena, 1993; Panconesi & Sicuteri, 1997). Disruption of serotonergic neurotransmission within the central nervous system might compromise endogenous pain control and information processing, thereby increasing vulnerability to triggers of migraine (Coppola et al., 2009). Against this background, symptoms could escalate quickly once attacks are under way.

disturbances, and vestibular instability—are complex. Many of these symptoms persist subclinically between episodes of headache and may increase susceptibility to recurrent attacks and to comorbid conditions. Understanding the neural basis of migraine-associated symptoms can provide a unique view of the changes in central nervous system function that characterize migraineurs and their vulnerability to migraine headache attacks.

CONCLUSIONS

The neural mechanisms that underlie some of the major symptoms of migraine—premonitory and prodromal changes, headache, sensory hypersensitivity, gastrointestinal

REFERENCES

Afridi, S. K., Giffin, N. J., Kaube, H., Friston, K. J., Ward, N. S., Frackowiak, R. S., et al. (2005). A positron emission tomographic study in spontaneous migraine. *Archives of Neurology, 62*, 1270–1275.

Afridi, S. K., Matharu, M. S., Lee, L., Kaube, H., Friston, K. J., Frackowiak, R. S., et al. (2005). A PET study exploring the laterality of brainstem activation in migraine using glyceryl trinitrate. *Brain, 128*, 932–939.

Alstadhaug, K. B. (2009). Migraine and the hypothalamus. *Cephalalgia, 29*, 809–817.

Asghar, M. S., Hansen, A. E., Amin, F. M., van der Geest, R. J., Koning, P., Larsson, H. B., Olesen, J., & Ashina, M. (2011). Evidence for a vascular factor in migraine. *Annals of Neurology, 69*, 635–645.

Ashkenazi, A., Mushtaq, A., Yang, I., & Oshinsky, M. L. (2009). Ictal and interictal phonophobia in migraine-a quantitative controlled study. *Cephalalgia, 29*, 1042–1048.

Ashkenazi, A., Yang, I., Mushtaq, A., & Oshinsky, M. L. (2010). Is phonophobia associated with cutaneous allodynia in migraine? *Journal of Neurology, Neurosurgery, and Psychiatry, 81*, 1256–1260.

Aurora, S. K., & Wilkinson, F. (2007). The brain is hyperexcitable in migraine. *Cephalalgia, 27*, 1442–1453.

Bajic, D., & Proudfit, H. K. (1999). Projections of neurons in the periaqueductal gray to pontine and medullary catecholamine cell groups involved in the modulation of nociception. *Journal of Comparative Neurology, 405*, 359–379.

Bandler, R., & Shipley, M. T. (1994). Columnar organization in the midbrain periaqueductal gray: Modules for emotional expression? *Trends in Neuroscience, 17*, 379–389.

Barabas, G., Matthews, W. S., & Ferrari, M. (1983). Childhood migraine and motion sickness. *Pediatrics, 72*, 188–190.

Basbaum, A. I., & Fields, H. L. (1978). Endogenous pain control mechanisms: Review and hypothesis. *Annals of Neurology, 4*, 451–462.

Benarroch, E. E. (2006). Pain-autonomic interactions. *Neurological Sciences, 27*(Suppl 2), S130–S133.

Bjørk, M., Stovner, L. J., Hagen, K., & Sand, T. (2011). What initiates a migraine attack? Conclusions from four longitudinal studies of quantitative EEG and steady-state visual-evoked potentials in migraineurs. *Acta Neurologica Scandinavica Supplement*, 56–63.

Blau, J. N. (1980). Migraine prodromes separated from the aura: Complete migraine. *BMJ, 281*, 658–660.

Bolay, H., Bayazit, Y. A., Gunduz, B., Ugur, A. K., Akcali, D., Altunyay, S., et al. (2008). Subclinical dysfunction of cochlea and cochlear efferents in migraine: An otoacoustic emission study. *Cephalalgia, 28*, 309–317.

Boldingh, M. I., Ljostad, U., Mygland, A., & Monstad, P. (2011). Vestibular sensitivity in vestibular migraine: VEMPs and motion sickness susceptibility. *Cephalalgia, 31*, 1211–1219.

Borsook, D., Burstein, R., Moulton, E., & Becerra, L. (2006). Functional imaging of the trigeminal system: Applications to migraine pathophysiology. *Headache, 46*(Suppl 1), S32–S38.

Boulloche, N., Denuelle, M., Payoux, P., Fabre, N., Trotter, Y., & Geraud, G. (2010). Photophobia in migraine: An interictal PET study of cortical hyperexcitability and its modulation by pain. *Journal of Neurology, Neurosurgery, and Psychiatry, 81*, 978–984.

Buisseret-Delmas, C., Compoint, C., Delfini, C., & Buisseret, P. (1999). Organisation of reciprocal connections between trigeminal and vestibular nuclei in the rat. *Journal of Comparative Neurology, 409*, 153–168.

Burstein, R., Cutrer, M. F., & Yarnitsky, D. (2000). The development of cutaneous allodynia during a migraine attack clinical evidence for the sequential recruitment of spinal and supraspinal nociceptive neurons in migraine. *Brain, 123*(Pt 8), 1703–1709.

Burstein, R., Yamamura, H., Malick, A., & Strassman, A. M. (1998). Chemical stimulation of the intracranial dura induces enhanced responses to facial stimulation in brain stem trigeminal neurons. *Journal of Neurophysiology, 79*, 964–982.

Burstein, R., Yarnitsky, D., Goor-Aryeh, I., Ransil, B. J., & Bajwa, Z. H. (2000). An association between migraine and cutaneous allodynia. *Annals of Neurology, 47*, 614–624.

Calhoun, A. H., Ford, S., Pruitt, A. P., & Fisher, K. G. (2011). The point prevalence of dizziness or vertigo in migraine—and factors that influence presentation. *Headache, 51*(9), 1388–1392.

Caputi, C. A., & Firetto, V. (1997). Therapeutic blockade of greater occipital and supraorbital nerves in migraine patients. *Headache, 37*, 174–179.

Carrive, P., & Bandler, R. (1991). Control of extracranial and hindlimb blood flow by the midbrain periaqueductal grey of the cat. *Experimental Brain Research, 84*, 599–606.

Cha, Y. H., Lee, H., Santell, L. S., & Baloh, R. W. (2009). Association of benign recurrent vertigo and migraine in 208 patients. *Cephalalgia, 29*, 550–555.

Chen, W. T., Wang, S. J., Fuh, J. L., Lin, C. P., Ko, Y. C., & Lin, Y. Y. (2011). Persistent ictal-like visual cortical excitability in chronic migraine. *Pain, 152*, 254–258.

Coppola, G., Pierelli, F., & Schoenen, J. (2009). Habituation and migraine. *Neurobiology of Learning and Memory, 92*, 249–259.

Corletto, E., Dal Zotto, L., Resos, A., Tripoli, E., Zanchin, G., Bulfoni, C., et al. (2008). Osmophobia in juvenile primary headaches. *Cephalalgia, 28*, 825–831.

Cuomo-Granston, A., & Drummond, P. D. (2010). Migraine and motion sickness: What is the link? *Progress in Neurobiology, 91*, 300–312.

Dahlof, C. G., & Hargreaves, R. J. (1998). Pathophysiology and pharmacology of migraine. Is there a place for antiemetics in future treatment strategies? *Cephalalgia, 18*, 593–604.

De Carlo, D., Dal Zotto, L., Perissinotto, E., Gallo, L., Gatta, M., Balottin, U., et al. (2010). Osmophobia in migraine classification: A multicentre study in juvenile patients. *Cephalalgia, 30*, 1486–1494.

Demarquay, G., Royet, J. P., Giraud, P., Chazot, G., Valade, D., & Ryvlin, P. (2006). Rating of olfactory judgements in migraine patients. *Cephalalgia, 26*, 1123–1130.

Demarquay, G., Royet, J. P., Mick, G., & Ryvlin, P. (2008). Olfactory hypersensitivity in Migraineurs: A H(2)(15)O-PET study. *Cephalalgia, 28*, 1069–1080.

Denuelle, M., Boulloche, N., Payoux, P., Fabre, N., Trotter, Y., & Geraud, G. (2011). A PET study of photophobia during spontaneous migraine attacks. *Neurology, 76*, 213–218.

Denuelle, M., Fabre, N., Payoux, P., Chollet, F., & Geraud, G. Hypothalamic activation in spontaneous migraine attacks. *Headache, 47*, 1418–1426.

Drummond, P. D. (1982). Extracranial and cardiovascular reactivity in migrainous subjects. *Journal of Psychosomatic Research, 26*, 317–331.

Drummond, P. D. (1985). Vascular responses in headache-prone subjects during stress. *Biological Psychology, 21*, 11–25.

Drummond, P. D. (1986). A quantitative assessment of photophobia in migraine and tension headache. *Headache, 26*, 465–469.

Drummond, P. D. (1987). Scalp tenderness and sensitivity to pain in migraine and tension headache. *Headache, 27*, 45–50.

Drummond, P. D. (1991). Effects of body heating and mental arithmetic on facial sweating and blood flow in unilateral migraine headache. *Psychophysiology, 28*, 172–176.

Drummond, P. D. (1992). The mechanism of facial sweating and cutaneous vascular responses to painful stimulation of the eye. *Brain, 115*(Pt 5), 1417–1428.

Drummond, P. D. (1997). Photophobia and autonomic responses to facial pain in migraine. *Brain, 120*(Pt 10), 1857–1864.

Drummond, P. D. (2002). Motion sickness and migraine: Optokinetic stimulation increases scalp tenderness, pain sensitivity in the fingers and photophobia. *Cephalalgia, 22*, 117–124.

Drummond, P. D. (2005a). Effect of tryptophan depletion on symptoms of motion sickness in migraineurs. *Neurology, 65*, 620–622.

Drummond, P. D. (2005b). Triggers of motion sickness in migraine sufferers. *Headache, 45*, 653–656.

Drummond, P. D. (2006a). Immersion of the hand in ice water releases adrenergic vasoconstrictor tone in the ipsilateral temple. *Autonomic Neuroscience, 128*, 70–75.

Drummond, P. D. (2006b). Tryptophan depletion increases nausea, headache and photophobia in migraine sufferers. *Cephalalgia, 26*, 1225–1233.

Drummond, P. D., & Granston, A. (2003). Facilitation of extracranial vasodilatation to limb pain in migraine sufferers. *Neurology, 61*, 60–63.

Drummond, P. D., & Granston, A. (2004). Facial pain increases nausea and headache during motion sickness in migraine sufferers. *Brain, 127*, 526–534.

Drummond, P. D., & Granston, A. (2005). Painful stimulation of the temple induces nausea, headache and extracranial vasodilation in migraine sufferers. *Cephalalgia, 25*, 16–22.

Drummond, P. D., & Lance, J. W. (1981). Extracranial vascular reactivity in migraine and tension headache. *Cephalalgia, 1*, 149–155.

Drummond, P. D., & Lance, J. W. (1983). Extracranial vascular changes and the source of pain in migraine headache. *Annals of Neurology, 13*, 32–37.

Drummond, P. D., & Lance, J. W. (1984a). Neurovascular disturbances in headache patients. *Clinical and Experimental Neurology, 20*, 93–99.

Drummond, P. D., & Lance, J. W. (1984b). Facial temperature in migraine, tension-vascular and tension headache. *Cephalalgia, 4*, 149–158.

Drummond, P. D., & Woodhouse, A. (1993). Painful stimulation of the forehead increases photophobia in migraine sufferers. *Cephalalgia, 13*, 321–324.

Fernandez-de-las-Penas, C., Arendt-Nielsen, L., Cuadrado, M. L., & Pareja, J. A. (2009). Generalized mechanical pain sensitivity over nerve tissues in patients with strictly unilateral migraine. *Clinical Journal of Pain, 25*, 401–406.

Fernandez-de-las-Penas, C., Cuadrado, M. L., Arendt-Nielsen, L., & Pareja, J. A. (2008). Side-to-side differences in pressure pain thresholds and pericranial muscle tenderness in strictly unilateral migraine. *European Journal of Neurology, 15*, 162–168.

Ferrari, M. D., & Saxena, P. R. (1993). On serotonin and migraine: A clinical and pharmacological review. *Cephalalgia, 13*, 151–165.

Fuh, J. L., Wang, S. J., Lu, S. R., & Juang, K. D. (2003). Ice-cream headache—a large survey of 8359 adolescents. *Cephalalgia, 23*, 977–981.

Giffin, N. J., Ruggiero, L., Lipton, R. B., Silberstein, S. D., Tvedskov, J. F., Olesen, J., et al. (2003). Premonitory symptoms in migraine: An electronic diary study. *Neurology, 60*, 935–940.

Goadsby, P. J. (2001). Migraine, aura, and cortical spreading depression: Why are we still talking about it? *Annals of Neurology, 49*, 4–6.

Goadsby, P. J., Lambert, G. A., & Lance, J. W. (1986). Stimulation of the trigeminal ganglion increases flow in the extracerebral but not the cerebral circulation of the monkey. *Brain Research, 381*, 63–67.

Granston, A., & Drummond, P. D. (2005). Painful stimulation of the temple during optokinetic stimulation triggers migraine-like attacks in migraine sufferers. *Cephalalgia, 25*, 219–224.

Grosser, K., Oelkers, R., Hummel, T., Geisslinger, G., Brune, K., Kobal, G., et al. (2000). Olfactory and trigeminal event-related potentials in migraine. *Cephalalgia, 20*, 621–631.

Grunfeld, E., & Gresty, M. A. (1998). Relationship between motion sickness, migraine and menstruation in crew members of a "round the world" yacht race. *Brain Research Bulletin, 47*, 433–436.

Grunfeld, E. A., Price, C., Goadsby, P. J., & Gresty, M. A. (1998). Motion sickness, migraine, and menstruation in mariners. *Lancet, 351*, 1106.

Hamed, S. A., Youssef, A. H., & Elattar, A. M. (2011). Assessment of cochlear and auditory pathways in patients with migraine. *American Journal of Otolaryngology*, in press.

Hirsch, A. R. (1992). Olfaction in migraineurs. *Headache, 32*, 233–236.

Ho, T. W., Ferrari, M. D., Dodick, D. W., Galet, V., Kost, J., Fan, X., et al. (2008). Efficacy and tolerability of MK-0974 (telcagepant), a new oral antagonist of calcitonin gene-related peptide receptor, compared with zolmitriptan for acute migraine: A randomised, placebo-controlled, parallel-treatment trial. *Lancet, 372*, 2115–2123.

Hong, S. M., Kim, S. K., Park, C. H., & Lee, J. H. (2011). Vestibular-evoked myogenic potentials in migrainous vertigo. *Otolaryngology–Head and Neck Surgery, 144*, 284–287.

Horn, C. C., Ciucci, M., & Chaudhury, A. (2007). Brain Fos expression during 48 h after cisplatin treatment: Neural pathways for acute and delayed visceral sickness. *Autonomic Neuroscience, 132*, 44–51.

Huang, J., Cooper, T. G., Satana, B., Kaufman, D. I., & Cao, Y. (2003). Visual distortion provoked by a stimulus in migraine associated with hyperneuronal activity. *Headache, 43*, 664–671.

Huang, J., Zong, X., Wilkins, A., Jenkins, B., Bozoki, A., & Cao, Y. (2011). fMRI evidence that precision ophthalmic tints reduce cortical hyperactivation in migraine. *Cephalalgia, 31*, 925–936.

Iversen, H. K., Nielsen, T. H., Olesen, J., Tfelt-Hansen, P. (1990). Arterial responses during migraine headache. *Lancet, 336*, 837–839.

Jan, M. M. (1998). History of motion sickness is predictive of childhood migraine. *Journal of Paediatrics and Child Health, 34*, 483–484.

Jan, M. M., Camfield, P. R., Gordon, K., & Camfield, C. S. (1997). Vomiting after mild head injury is related to migraine. *Journal of Pediatrics, 130*, 134–137.

Jeong, S. H., Oh, S. Y., Kim, H. J., Koo, J. W., & Kim, J. S. (2010). Vestibular dysfunction in migraine: Effects of associated vertigo and motion sickness. *Journal of Neurology, 257*, 905–912.

Katsarava, Z., Giffin, N., Diener, H. C., & Kaube, H. (2003). Abnormal habituation of "nociceptive" blink reflex in migraine—evidence for increased excitability of trigeminal nociception. *Cephalalgia, 23*, 814–819.

Kaube, H., Katsarava, Z., Kaufer, T., Diener, H., & Ellrich, J. (2000). A new method to increase nociception specificity of the human blink reflex. *Clinical of Neurophysiology, 111*, 413–416.

Kaube, H., Katsarava, Z., Przywara, S., Drepper, J., Ellrich, J., & Diener, H. C. (2002). Acute migraine headache: Possible sensitization of neurons in the spinal trigeminal nucleus? *Neurology, 58*, 1234–1238.

Kayan, A., & Hood, J. D. (1984). Neuro-otological manifestations of migraine. *Brain, 107*(Pt 4), 1123–1142.

Kelman, L. (2004a). The premonitory symptoms (prodrome): A tertiary care study of 893 migraineurs. *Headache, 44*, 865–872.

Kelman, L. (2004b). The place of osmophobia and taste abnormalities in migraine classification: A tertiary care study of 1237 patients. *Cephalalgia, 24*, 940–946.

Knight, Y. E., Classey, J. D., Lasalandra, M. P., Akerman, S., Kowacs, F., Hoskin, K. L., et al. (2005). Patterns of fos expression in the rostral medulla and caudal pons evoked by noxious craniovascular stimulation and periaqueductal gray stimulation in the cat. *Brain Research, 1045*, 1–11.

Kuritzky, A., Toglia, U. J., & Thomas, D. (1981). Vestibular function in migraine. *Headache, 21*, 110–112.

Lambert, G. A. (2010). The lack of peripheral pathology in migraine headache. *Headache, 50*, 895–908.

Lambert, G. A., Bogduk, N., Goadsby, P. J., Duckworth, J. W., & Lance, J. W. (1984). Decreased carotid arterial resistance in cats in response to trigeminal stimulation. *Journal of Neurosurgery, 61*, 307–315.

Lambert, G. A., & Zagami, A. S. (2009). The mode of action of migraine triggers: A hypothesis. *Headache, 49*, 253–275.

Lassen, L. H., Haderslev, P. A., Jacobsen, V. B., Iversen, H. K., Sperling, B., & Olesen, J. (2002). CGRP may play a causative role in migraine. *Cephalalgia, 22*, 54–61.

Lebensohn, J. E. (1934). The nature of photophobia. *Archives of Ophthalmology, 12*, 380–390.

Lempert, T., Neuhauser, H., & Daroff, R. B. (2009). Vertigo as a symptom of migraine. *Annals of the New York Academy of Sciences, 1164*, 242–251.

Levy, D., & Burstein, R. (2011). The vascular theory of migraine: leave it or love it? *Annals of Neurology, 69*, 600–601.

Li, B. U., Murray, R. D., Heitlinger, L. A., Robbins, J. L., & Hayes, J. R. (1999). Is cyclic vomiting syndrome related to migraine? *Journal of Pediatrics, 134*, 567–572.

Marano, E., Marcelli, V., Di Stasio, E., Bonuso, S., Vacca, G., Manganelli, F., et al. (2005). Trigeminal stimulation elicits a peripheral vestibular imbalance in migraine patients. *Headache, 45*, 325–331.

Marfurt, C. F., & Rajchert, D. M. (1991). Trigeminal primary afferent projections to "non-trigeminal" areas of the rat central nervous system. *Journal of Comparative Neurology, 303*, 489–511.

Martin, H., Del Rio, M. S., de Silanes, C. L., Alvarez-Linera, J., Hernandez, J. A., & Pareja, J. A. (2011). Photoreactivity of the Occipital Cortex Measured by Functional Magnetic Resonance Imaging-Blood Oxygenation Level Dependent in Migraine Patients and Healthy Volunteers: Pathophysiological Implications. *Headache, 51*, 1520–1528.

Mitchelson, F. (1992). Pharmacological agents affecting emesis. A review (Part I). *Drugs, 43*, 295–315.

Neuhauser, H., & Lempert, T. (2009). Vestibular migraine. *Neurology Clinics, 27*, 379–391.

Noseda, R., Kainz, V., Jakubowski, M., Gooley, J. J., Saper, C. B., Digre, K., et al. (2010). A neural mechanism for exacerbation of headache by light. *Nature Neuroscience, 13*, 239–245.

Olesen, J., Burstein, R., Ashina, M., Tfelt-Hansen, P. (2009). Origin of pain in migraine: Evidence for peripheral sensitisation. *Lancet Neurology, 8*, 679–690.

Olesen, J., Diener, H. C., Husstedt, I. W., Goadsby, P. J., Hall, D., Meier, U., et al. (2004). Calcitonin gene-related peptide receptor antagonist BIBN 4096 BS for the acute treatment of migraine. *New England Journal of Medicine, 350*, 1104–1110.

Panconesi, A., & Sicuteri, R. (1997). Headache induced by serotonergic agonists—a key to the interpretation of migraine pathogenesis? *Cephalalgia, 17*, 3–14.

Perini, F., D'Andrea, G., Galloni, E., Pignatelli, F., Billo, G., Alba, S., et al. (2005). Plasma cytokine levels in migraineurs and controls. *Headache, 45*, 926–931.

Raskin, N. H., & Knittle, S. C. (1976). Ice cream headache and orthostatic symptoms in patients with migraine. *Headache, 16*, 222–225.

Raskin, N. H., & Schwartz, R. K. (1980). Icepick-like pain. *Neurology, 30*, 203–205.

Ruggiero, D. A., Underwood, M. D., Mann, J. J., Anwar, M., & Arango, V. (2000). The human nucleus of the solitary tract: Visceral pathways revealed with an "in vitro" postmortem tracing method. *Journal of the Autonomic Nervous System, 79*, 181–190.

Sandrini, G., Proietti Cecchini, A., Milanov, I., Tassorelli, C., Buzzi, M. G., & Nappi, G. (2002). Electrophysiological evidence for trigeminal neuron sensitization in patients with migraine. *Neuroscience Letters, 317*, 135–138.

Sandrini, G., Rossi, P., Milanov, I., Serrao, M., Cecchini, A. P., & Nappi, G. (2006). Abnormal modulatory influence of diffuse noxious inhibitory controls in migraine and chronic tension-type headache patients. *Cephalalgia, 26*, 782–789.

Sarchielli, P., Alberti, A., Baldi, A., Coppola, F., Rossi, C., Pierguidi, L., et al. (2006). Proinflammatory cytokines, adhesion molecules, and lymphocyte integrin expression in the internal jugular blood of migraine patients without aura assessed ictally. *Headache, 46*, 200–207.

Sarchielli, P., Pini, L. A., Zanchin, G., Alberti, A., Maggioni, F., Rossi, C., et al. (2006). Clinical-biochemical correlates of migraine attacks in rizatriptan responders and non-responders. *Cephalalgia, 26*, 257–265.

Schoenen, J., Ambrosini, A., Sandor, P. S., & Maertens de Noordhout, A. (2003). Evoked potentials and transcranial magnetic stimulation in migraine: Published data and viewpoint on their pathophysiologic significance. *Clinical Neurophysiology, 114*, 955–972.

Schoonman, G. G., van der Grond, J., Kortmann, C., van der Geest, R. J., Terwindt, G. M., & Ferrari, M. D. (2008). Migraine headache is not associated with cerebral or meningeal vasodilatation—a 3T magnetic resonance angiography study. *Brain, 131*, 2192–2200.

Selekler, H. M., & Budak, F. (2004). Idiopathic stabbing headache and experimental ice cream headache (short-lived headaches). *European Neurology, 51*, 6–9.

Shepherd, A. J. (2000). Visual contrast processing in migraine. *Cephalalgia, 20*, 865–880.

Sicuteri, F. (1987). Quasi-phantom head pain from functional deafferentation. *Clinical Journal of Pain, 3*, 63–80.

Sicuteri, F., Del Bianco, P. L., & Anselmi, B. (1979). Morphine abstinence and serotonin supersensitivity in man: Analogies with the mechanism of migraine? *Psychopharmacology (Berlin), 65*, 205–209.

Sicuteri, F., & Nicolodi, M. (1986). Electroencephalographic alterations in migraine as an expression of "self-deafferentation": A hypothesis. *Functional Neurology, 1,* 455–460.

Sjostrand, C., Savic, I., Laudon-Meyer, E., Hillert, L., Lodin, K., & Waldenlind, E. (2010). Migraine and olfactory stimuli. *Current Pain and Headache Reports, 14,* 244–251.

Snyder, R. D., & Drummond, P. D. (1997). Olfaction in migraine. *Cephalalgia, 17,* 729–732.

Stankewitz, A., & May, A. (2011). Increased limbic and brainstem activity during migraine attacks following olfactory stimulation. *Neurology, 77*(5), 476–482.

Takeda, N., Morita, M., Hasegawa, S., Horii, A., Kubo, T., & Matsunaga, T. (1993). Neuropharmacology of motion sickness and emesis. A review. *Acta Otolaryngologica Supplementum, 501,* 10–15.

Takeda, N., Morita, M., Horii, A., Nishiike, S., Kitahara, T., & Uno, A. (2001). Neural mechanisms of motion sickness. *Journal of Medical Investigation, 48,* 44–59.

Teggi, R., Colombo, B., Bernasconi, L., Bellini, C., Comi, G., & Bussi, M. (2009). Migrainous vertigo: Results of caloric testing and stabilometric findings. *Headache, 49,* 435–444.

Tfelt-Hansen, P., & Le, H. (2009). Calcitonin gene-related peptide in blood: Is it increased in the external jugular vein during migraine and cluster headache? A review. *Journal of Headache and Pain, 10,* 137–143.

Tvedskov, J. F., Lipka, K., Ashina, M., Iversen, H. K., Schifter, S., & Olesen, J. (2005). No increase of calcitonin gene-related peptide in jugular blood during migraine. *Annals of Neurology, 58,* 561–568.

Vanagaite, J., Pareja, J. A., Storen, O., White, L. R., Sand, T., & Stovner, L. J. (1997). Light-induced discomfort and pain in migraine. *Cephalalgia, 17,* 733–741.

Vanagaite Vingen, J., Pareja, J. A., Storen, O., White, L. R., & Stovner, L. J. (1998). Phonophobia in migraine. *Cephalalgia, 18,* 243–249.

Weiller, C., May, A., Limmroth, V., Juptner, M., Kaube, H., Schayck, R. V., et al. (1995). Brain stem activation in spontaneous human migraine attacks. *Nature Medicine, 1,* 658–660.

Weissman-Fogel, I., Sprecher, E., Granovsky, Y., & Yarnitsky, D. (2003). Repeated noxious stimulation of the skin enhances cutaneous pain perception of migraine patients in-between attacks: Clinical evidence for continuous sub-threshold increase in membrane excitability of central trigeminovascular neurons. *Pain, 104,* 693–700.

Welch, K. M., Nagesh, V., Aurora, S. K., & Gelman, N. (2001). Periaqueductal gray matter dysfunction in migraine: Cause or the burden of illness? *Headache, 41,* 629–637.

Wolff, H. G. (1963). *Headache and other head pain.* New York: Oxford University Press.

Woodhouse, A., & Drummond, P. D. (1993). Mechanisms of increased sensitivity to noise and light in migraine headache. *Cephalalgia, 13,* 417–421.

Zanchin, G., Dainese, F., Trucco, M., Mainardi, F., Mampreso, E., & Maggioni, F. (2007). Osmophobia in migraine and tension-type headache and its clinical features in patients with migraine. *Cephalalgia, 27,* 1061–1068.

4 Sensitization of Trigeminovascular Pathway
Implications to Migraine Pathophysiology

RAMI BURSTEIN AND DAVID BORSOOK

INTRODUCTION

Migraine is a neurological disorder of recurring, unilateral, throbbing headache, associated with variable incidence of aura, nausea and vomiting, photophobia and phonophobia, fatigue, and irritability. We have shown that migraine headache is also associated with cephalic and extracephalic allodynia. Patients exhibiting signs of cephalic allodynia testify that during migraine their facial skin hurts in response to otherwise innocuous activities such as combing their hair, shaving, letting water run over their face in the shower, or wearing glasses or earrings. Patient exhibiting signs of extracephalic allodynia testify that during migraine their bodily skin is hypersensitive and that wearing tight clothes, bracelets, rings, necklaces, and socks or using a heavy blanket can be uncomfortable and/or painful.

Here, we will present evidence to support the view that the development of throbbing in the initial phase of migraine is mediated by sensitization of peripheral trigeminovascular neurons that innervate the meninges, that the development of cephalic allodynia is propelled by sensitization of second-order trigeminovascular neurons in the spinal trigeminal nucleus that receive converging sensory input from the meninges as well as from the scalp and facial skin, and that the development of extracephalic allodynia is mediated by sensitization of third-order trigeminovascular neurons in the posterior thalamic nuclei that receive converging sensory input from the meninges and facial and body skin.

SENSITIZATION OF FIRST-ORDER TRIGEMINOVASCULAR NEURONS

In 1996, we reported that mechanically insensitive meningeal nociceptors (i.e., peripheral trigeminovascular neurons) in the trigeminal ganglion became mechanically sensitive several minutes after chemical stimulation of

their dural receptive fields and as a result, began to respond to dural indentation (Strassman et al., 1996). Since the slightest mechanical pressure (producing no visible indentation of the dura) was sufficient to induce activity in the sensitized neurons (Fig. 4–1), we concluded that when meningeal nociceptors become sensitized, they become responsive to otherwise unperceived rhythmic fluctuation in intracranial pressure (i.e., throbbing) produced by normal arterial pulsation. Based on this conclusion, we proposed that during migraine, such mechanical hypersensitivity could mediate the throbbing of the headache and its worsening during coughing, bending, or other physical activities that increase intracranial pressure (Blau & Dexter, 1981).

SENSITIZATION OF SECOND-ORDER TRIGEMINOVASCULAR NEURONS

In 1998, we reported that chemical irritation of the dura with inflammatory agents activates and sensitizes central trigeminovascular neurons in the spinal trigeminal nucleus for up to 10 hours (Burstein et al., 1998). The sensitized neurons in the medullary dorsal horn showed increased responsiveness to mechanical indentation of dural receptive fields and to mechanical and thermal stimulation of cutaneous receptive fields; their response thresholds decreased and their response magnitudes increased (Fig. 4–2). Since their response to innocuous skin stimulation after induction of sensitization was greater than their responses to noxious stimulation before induction of sensitization, we proposed that during migraine, sensitization of these second-order trigeminovascular neurons could mediate scalp (Liveing, 1873; Selby & Lance, 1960; Wolff et al., 1953) and muscle (Tfelt-Hansen et al., 1981) tenderness, as well as facial allodynia.

In 2000, we used a more scientific approach to characterize cutaneous allodynia using repeated measurements of mechanical and thermal pain thresholds of facial skin

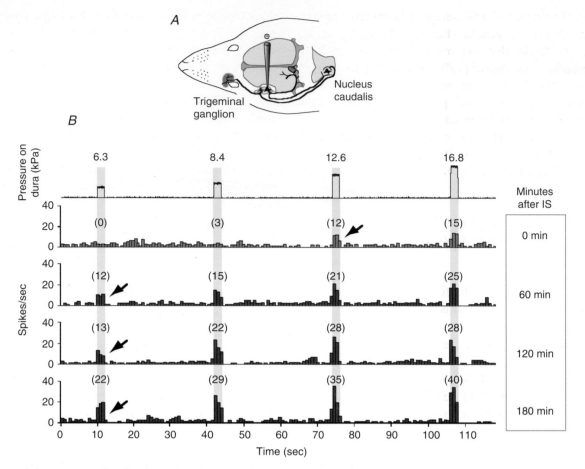

FIGURE 4–1 *(A) Exposure to dura for electrophysiolical recordings. (B) Sensitization of meningeal nociceptor to mechanical stimulation of the dura. Recording location in the trigeminal ganglion. IS (inflammatory soup).*

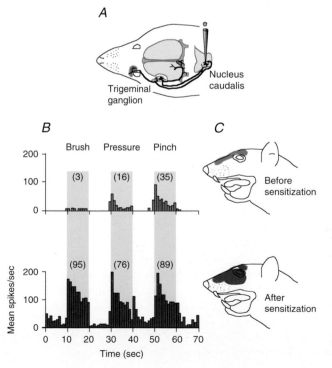

FIGURE 4–2 *Sensitization of a second-order trigeminovascular neuron reflected by enhanced responses to innocuous (nonpainful) stimulation of the facial skin. Recording location in lamina V of the spinal trigeminal nucleus. (A) Exposure of dura for application of inflammatory soup with recording in the nucleus caudalis. (B) Sensitization of trigeminal neurons (lamina V) to brush, pressure and pinch before (green) and after (red) inflammatory soup applied to the dura. (C) Expansion of area facial sensitivity to non-painful stimuli that activates lamina V neurons that correlates with changes observed in B.*

areas in the absence of, and during (4 hours from onset), unilateral migraine attacks (Burstein, Yarnitsky, et al., 2000). We found that the mean cold pain threshold decreased by an average of 12.7°C (from 16.3°C to 29.0°C), heat pain threshold decreased by 7.4°C (from 44.3°C to 36.9°C), and mechanical pain threshold decreased by 7.1 VFH numbers (from above 100 g to <10 g force) (Fig. 4–3A). The prevalence of cutaneous allodynia among migraine patients has been estimated at 65% to 70% (Bigal et al., 2008; Lipton et al., 2008).

SENSITIZATION OF THIRD-ORDER TRIGEMINOVASCULAR NEURONS

In the course of studying cephalic allodynia during migraine, we unexpectedly found clear evidence for allodynia in remote skin areas outside the innervation territory of the trigeminal nerve (Fig. 4–3B) (Burstein, Yarnitsky, et al., 2000). In the discussion of that study, we proposed that ipsilateral cephalic allodynia is mediated by sensitization of dura-sensitive neurons in the medullary dorsal horn because their cutaneous receptive field is confined to innervation territory of the ipsilateral

trigeminal nerve (Burstein et al., 1998; Craig & Dostrovsky, 1991; Davis & Dostrovsky, 1988; Ebersberger et al., 1997; Strassman et al., 1994; Yamamura et al., 1999) and that extracephalic allodynia must be mediated by neurons that process sensory information they receive from all levels of the spinal and medullary dorsal horn. Our search of such neurons focused on the thalamus since an extensive axonal mapping of sensitized trigeminovascular neurons in the spinal trigeminal nucleus revealed distinguish projections to the posterior (PO), the ventral posteromedial (VPM), and the sub-parafascicular (PF) nuclei.

In 2010, we reported that topical administration of inflammatory molecules to the dura sensitized thalamic trigeminovascular neurons that process sensory information from the cranial meninges and cephalic and extracephalic skin (Burstein et al., 2010). Sensitized thalamic neurons developed ongoing firing and exhibited hyperresponsiveness (increased response magnitude) and hypersensitivity (lower response threshold) to mechanical and thermal stimulation of extracephalic skin areas (Fig. 4–4). Relevant to migraine pathophysiology was the finding that in such neurons, innocuous extracephalic skin stimuli that did not induce neuronal firing before sensitization

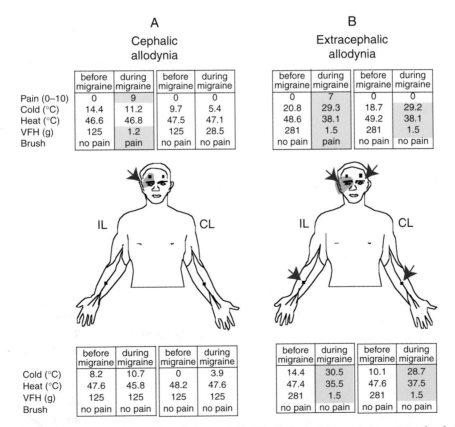

FIGURE 4–3 *Quantitative measurements of cephalic (A) and extracephalic (B) allodynia during migraine. Pain thresholds to cold, heat, and mechanical skin stimulation were determined when patients were pain-free (left columns) and during migraine (right columns).*

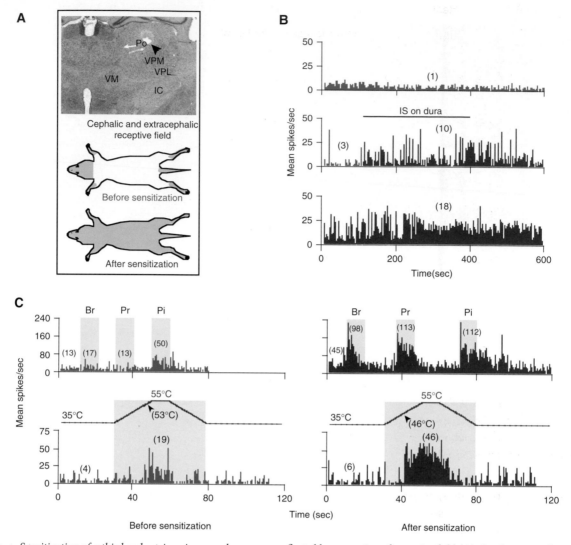

FIGURE 4–4 *Sensitization of a third-order trigeminovascular neuron reflected by expansion of receptive field (A), development of spontaneous activity (B), and enhanced responses to innocuous and noxious mechanical and heat stimulation of the hind paw (C). Recording location in the dorsal region of the posterior thalamic nucleus. Key: Po = posterior nucleus; VPM = ventroposteromedial nuclues; VPL = ventroposterolateral nucleus; VM = ventromedial nuclues; IC = internal capsule.*

(e.g., brush) became as effective as noxious stimuli (e.g., pinch) in triggering large bouts of activity after sensitization was established.

To understand better the transformation of migraine headache into widespread, cephalic and extracephalic allodynia, we also studied the effects of extracephalic brush and heat stimuli on thalamic activation registered by functional magnetic resonance imaging (fMRI) during migraine in patients with whole-body allodynia (Burstein et al., 2010). Functional assessment of blood oxygenation level–dependent (BOLD) signals showed that brush and heat stimulation at the skin of the dorsum of the hand produced larger BOLD responses in the posterior thalamus of subjects undergoing a migraine attack with extracephalic allodynia than the corresponding responses

registered when the same patients were free of migraine and allodynia (Fig. 4–5).

TEMPORAL ASPECTS OF SENSITIZATION DURING MIGRAINE

There are remarkable similarities between the temporal changes in the development of peripheral and central sensitization in the rat and their corresponding clinical manifestations during the course of migraine. The induction of peripheral sensitization in the rat occurs rapidly within 5 to 20 minutes after applying inflammatory soup (IS) onto the dura, whereas sensitization of trigeminovascular neurons in the dorsal horn and thalamus develops over 20

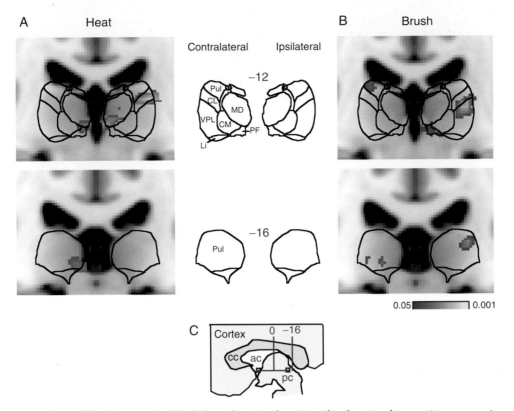

FIGURE 4–5 *Contrast analysis of blood oxygenation level–dependent signals registered in functional magnetic resonance imaging scans of the human posterior thalamus following innocuous (B) and noxious (A) skin stimuli during migraine attacks that were associated with extracephalic allodynia. Note evidence for enhanced activation in the pulvinar (C) shows a diagram of the location of the images within a coronal section of the brain (0 to [-16]).*

to 60 and 60 to 240 minutes, respectively. Similarly in patients, throbbing transpires some 5 to 20 minutes after the onset of headache, whereas cutaneous allodynia starts between 20 and 120 minutes and becomes firmly established only 120 to 240 minutes after the onset of headache (Burstein, Cutrer, et al., 2000). According to this scenario, meningeal nociceptors become sensitized a few minutes after their initial activation, resulting in throbbing headache and its exacerbation by bending over. The continued barrage of impulses arriving from sensitized meningeal nociceptors gradually stimulates the development of central sensitization in spinal trigeminovascular neurons, resulting in cutaneous allodynia in the same area as the referred head pain. Eventually, the ongoing bombardment of thalamic trigeminovascular neurons by sensitized second-order neurons renders the third-order neurons sensitized.

REFERENCES

Bigal, M. E., Ashina, S., Burstein, R., Reed, M. L., Buse, D., Serrano, D., et al. (2008). Prevalence and characteristics of allodynia in headache sufferers: A population study. *Neurology, 70*(17), 1525–1533.

Blau, J. N., & Dexter, S. L. (1981). The site of pain origin during migraine attacks. *Cephalalgia, 1*(3), 143–147.

Burstein, R., Cutrer, F. M., & Yarnitsky, D. (2000). The development of cutaneous allodynia during a migraine attack: Clinical evidence for the sequential recruitment of spinal and supraspinal nociceptive neurons in migraine. *Brain, 123*, 1703–1709.

Burstein, R., Jakubowski, M., Garcia-Nicas, E., Kainz, V., Bajwa, Z., Hargreaves, R., et al. (2010). Thalamic sensitization transforms localized pain into widespread allodynia. *Annals of Neurology, 68*(1), 81–91.

Burstein, R., Yamamura, H., Malick, A., & Strassman, A. M. (1998). Chemical stimulation of the intracranial dura induces enhanced responses to facial stimulation in brain stem trigeminal neurons. *Journal of Neurophysiology, 79*(2), 964–982.

Burstein, R., Yarnitsky, D., Goor-Aryeh, I., Ransil, B. J., & Bajwa, Z. H. (2000). An association between migraine and cutaneous allodynia. *Annals of Neurology, 47*, 614–624.

Craig, A. D., & Dostrovsky, J. O. (1991). Thermoreceptive lamina I trigeminothalamic neurons project to the nucleus submedius in the cat. *Experimental Brain Research, 85*(2), 470–474.

Davis, K. D., & Dostrovsky, J. O. (1988). Responses of feline trigeminal spinal tract nucleus neurons to stimulation of the middle meningeal artery and sagittal sinus. *Journal of Neurophysiology, 59*(2), 648–666.

Ebersberger, A., Ringkamp, M., Reeh, P. W., & Handwerker, H. O. (1997). Recordings from brain stem neurons responding to chemical stimulation of the subarachnoid space. *Journal of Neurophysiology, 77*(6), 3122–3133.

Lipton, R. B., Bigal, M. E., Ashina, S., Burstein, R., Silberstein, S., Reed, M. L., et al. (2008). Cutaneous allodynia in the migraine population. *Annals of Neurology, 63*(2), 148–158.

Living, E. (1873). *On megrim, sick headache*. Nijmegen: Arts & Boeve Publishers.

Selby, G., & Lance, J. W. (1960). Observations on 500 cases of migraine and allied vascular headache. *Journal of Neurology, Neurosurgery, and Psychiatry*, 23–32.

Strassman, A. M., Potrebic, S., & Maciewicz, R. J. (1994). Anatomical properties of brainstem trigeminal neurons that respond to electrical stimulation of dural blood vessels. *Journal of Comparative Neurology, 346*(3), 349–365.

Strassman, A. M., Raymond, S. A., & Burstein, R. (1996). Sensitization of meningeal sensory neurons and the origin of headaches. *Nature, 384*(6609), 560–564.

Tfelt-Hansen, P., Lous, I., & Olesen, J. (1981). Prevalence and significance of muscle tenderness during common migraine attacks. *Headache, 21*(2), 49–54.

Wolff, H. G., Tunis, M. M., & Goodell, H. (1953). Studies on migraine. *Archives of Internal Medicine, 92*, 478–484.

Yamamura, H., Malick, A., Chamberlin, N. L., & Burstein, R. (1999). Cardiovascular and neuronal responses to head stimulation reflect central sensitization and cutaneous allodynia in a rat model of migraine. *Journal of Neurophysiology, 81*(2), 479–493.

5 Brain Measures of the Interictal Migraine Brain State

NASIM MALEKI, LINO BECERRA, RAMI BURSTEIN, AND DAVID BORSOOK

INTRODUCTION

Given that repeated migraine events occur in episodic migraine and that some patients not only have an increased frequency of migraine but also may go on to develop chronic daily headache, the notion of an altered brain state even in the interictal period has begun to attract more attention in clinical research. The definition of the interictal migraine state is not clear since prodromes and pre-migraine attacks may be subtle and take the form of altered behavior or mood changes such as tiredness or irritability. Here we define the interictal migraine brain state (IMBS) as that period outside of migraine when there are no premonitory symptoms 72 hours prior to or 72 hours after a migraine.

IBMS has been the focus of studies ranging across research spectrums, including clinical, electrophysiological, and imaging studies that suggest that an altered brain state, compared to healthy controls, may exist. Such evidence has come from studies reporting the following: consistent lack of habituation to repetitive stimulation (Afra, 2005; Ozkul & Uckardes, 2002; Schoenen, 2006) as well as a reduced capacity for diffuse noxious inhibitory control (DNIC) to modulate pain (de Tommaso et al., 2007); increased sensitivity to noise (phonophobia) in the interictal period (Ashkenazi et al., 2009); increased sensitivity to smell (Demarquay et al., 2008) and sensory input (Boulloche et al., 2010; Lang et al., 2004); diminished modulatory tone (Moulton et al., 2011) and dysfunction of brainstem structures (e.g., the periaqueductal gray [PAG] and dorsal rostral pons) (Aurora et al., 2007; Coppola, Pierelli, et al., 2007; Welch et al., 2001); and altered excitatory neurotransmitters in brain regions in migraine patients (Prescot et al., 2009). Other evidence that points to an altered brain state includes altered brain morphology (Geuze et al., 2008; May, 2009), changes in brain blood flow (Bartolini et al., 2005; Dora & Balkan, 2002; Shinoura & Yamada, 2005), and changes in interictal cognitive functioning (Mulder et al., 1999). Such data strongly support the hypothesis of an altered brain state with migraine playing a key role in the pathogenesis of migraine.

The implications of a better understanding of the interictal migraine state relate to issues of chronification and medication resistance, and thus developing and having measures of efficacy for novel medications. Chronification of migraine is a significant process affecting relatively few individuals but resulting in a huge economic burden. Whether the cause or effect of migraine, the simple alteration in the form of either increased migraine frequency or progression to chronic daily headache must underlie some alteration in brain processing.

In this chapter we review the literature for evidence on morphometric, functional, and metabolic brain alterations in migraine patients during their interictal state. We focus on imaging findings that also support findings from neurophysiological techniques such as evoked potentials (EPs), transcranial magnetic stimulation (TMS), and transcranial direct current stimulation, which have also been important contributors to understanding migraine brain pathophysiology.

STRUCTURAL ALTERATIONS

A number of studies have reported alteration in brain structure in migraine patients (Kruit et al., 2004, 2005; Rocca et al., 2006). The largest of these studies is the Dutch-based CAMERA study, which has reported increased white matter lesions, interpreted by the authors as subclinical infarcts in the posterior circulation and brain iron accumulation (Kruit et al., 2010). Attack frequency and disease burden correlate with measures of brain alterations in migraine (Schmitz, Admiraal-Behloul, et al., 2008).

High-resolution anatomical scans of the human brain with structural magnetic resonance imaging (SMRI) or

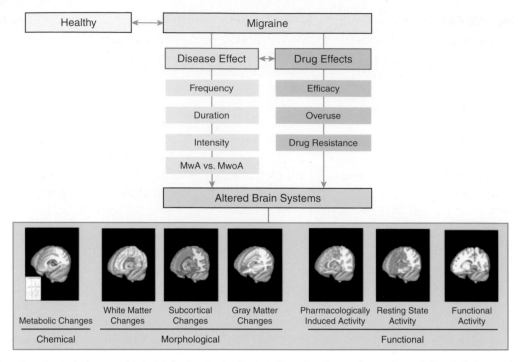

FIGURE 5–1 *Neuroimaging techniques and interictal migraine brain state. Functional, morphometric, and chemical changes in the brain can be assessed using an array of information obtainable from neuroimaging techniques. The data can be correlated with different aspects of migraine disease or drug effects interictally or ictally. MwA, migraine with aura; MwoA, migraine without aura.*

computed tomography (CT) combined with recent sophisticated semiautomatic or automatic image processing techniques provide the means for characterization of brain neuroanatomy in health and disease. Most typically these methods are used to assess changes in the gray matter. The most common methods for this purpose include volumetric comparisons of neuroanatomical regions of interest (ROI), whole-brain voxel-based morphometric comparisons, and surface-based cortical thickness comparisons.

Multiple studies report morphological abnormalities in patients with migraine (DaSilva, Granziera, Snyder, et al., 2007; DaSilva, Granziera, Tuch et al., 2007; Rocca et al., 2003), although the findings are not consistent among all of the studies. Decreased gray matter in pain-transmitting areas such as the anterior cingulate cortex (Kim et al., 2008; Schmidt-Wilcke et al., 2008; Valfre et al., 2008) and insula (Kim et al., 2008; Valfre et al., 2008) in migraine patients has been reported. Significant correlation between progressive gray matter reduction in these structures and frequency or duration of migraine attacks has also been reported (Kim et al., 2008; Valfre et al., 2008). Increased density of brainstem structures in migraine patients in the periaqueductal gray matter has been reported. Structural abnormalities in migraineurs

have also been reported in the frontal and parietal lobes (Schmitz, Admiraal-Behloul, et al., 2008; Schmitz, Arkink, et al., 2008), basal ganglia, and cerebellum (Schmitz, Admiraal-Behloul, et al., 2008). Changes in cortical gray matter volume have also been reported in other conditions such as neuropathic pain in a rat model (Seminowicz et al., 2009), in which there is an association of increased hyperalgesia with decreased volume in the anterior cingulate cortex and insula and the changes coincide with the onset of anxiety-like behaviors. In patients with chronic tension-type headache, a significant decrease of gray matter has been reported, observed only in cortical areas involved in pain processing (Kim et al., 2008; Schmidt-Wilcke et al., 2008; Valfre et al., 2008). These findings may suggest that volume reduction might be due to a central sensitization generated by prolonged nociceptive input, although there is not enough evidence to determine whether these changes are the cause or the consequence of chronic pain.

Thickening in the somatosensory cortex of patients with migraine has been reported (DaSilva, Granziera, Snyder, et al., 2007). This area is involved in noxious somatosensory processing, especially in the trigeminal area, which includes the head and face (DaSilva, Granziera, Snyder, et al., 2007). Thickening in the somatosensory cortex is in line with diffusional abnormalities observed in the subcortical trigeminal somatosensory pathway (DaSilva, Granziera, Tuch et al., 2007). Areas involved in motion processing in the visual cortex of migraineurs with or without aura show increased cortical thickness in areas MT + and V3A compared to healthy subjects (Granziera et al., 2006). This finding specifically relates to the findings of a separate study where the source of the cortical spreading depression (CSD) during migraine aura had also been identified to be in the V3A area of the cortex (DaSilva, Granziera, Snyder, et al., 2007). Cortical thickening may relate to increased afferent input to these regions in a manner analogous to activation-dependent thickening following motor training (Anderson et al., 2002) or musical training (Lappe et al., 2008).

FUNCTIONAL ALTERATIONS

Functional magnetic resonance imaging (fMRI) has contributed a lot to understanding abnormal cortical and subcortical processing due to migraine. fMRI has been used extensively to study the migraine brain during migraine attacks and interictally and to study the effect of medication/treatment. Positron emission tomography (PET) imaging studies have also contributed a lot to understanding the functional changes in the brain interictally. Most of the findings have been repeatedly replicated by several groups, which has led to a new understanding of the pathophysiology of migraine and specifically of the central role of the brain, which will be described in the following.

There are multiple reports on alterations in sensory, emotional, and autonomic function during the interictal period, including altered visual evoked responses (Afra et al., 2000; Backer et al., 2001; Coppola, Ambrosini, et al., 2007) and altered auditory evoked responses (Afra et al., 2000; Ambrosini et al., 2003; Wang et al., 1996). Enhanced excitability of somatosensory (Lang et al., 2004) and motor (Afra et al., 1998) evoked responses in the interictal migraine brain have also been reported. There is also evidence for altered nociceptive processing in migraineurs interictally (Moulton et al., 2011).

One of the major focuses in studying the interictal functional changes in migraine has been on the role of PAG. The PAG modulates trigeminovascular nociceptive input, and its main role has been described in terms of pain facilitation and inhibition. The damaged PAG does not filter or block pain as effectively as in the intact state, and whatever peripheral activators of migraine may be (e.g., circulating cytokines, stress, hormonal changes), the activations are not modulated (inhibited) at the PAG level

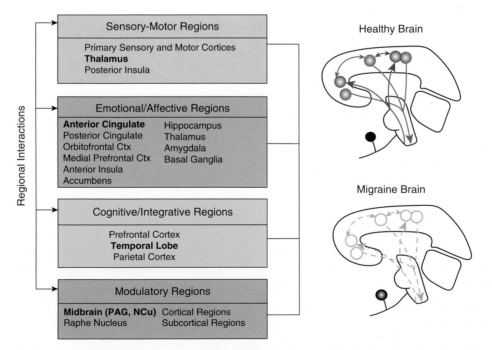

FIGURE 5–2 *Schematic of anatomical sites and pathways that show changes in migraine. Migraine involves alterations in sensory/motor, emotional/affective, cognitive/integrative, and modulatory regions that are involved in the complex processing of pain and are altered interictally. Ctx, cortext; PAG, periaqueductal gray; NCu, nucleus cuneiformis.*

(Aurora et al., 2007; Coppola, Pierelli, et al., 2007; Welch et al., 2001).

Abnormalities in the PAG in migraine patients are supported by a number of imaging studies assessing abnormalities in this region (Rocca et al., 2006; Tortorella et al., 2006), including abnormal iron homeostasis (Welch et al., 2001) in patients both with episodic and with episodic and chronic migraines and altered endogenous modulation (Moulton et al., 2008). In prior fMRI studies both increased and decreased blood oxygenation level–dependent (BOLD) activation in the PAG to noxious stimulation (Becerra et al., 2001) and diminished activation in the PAG with analgesics such as morphine (Becerra et al., 2006) have been reported.

Given the structural changes in the IMBS, it is perhaps not surprising that functional imaging studies would demonstrate altered brain function in migraine patients during their interictal state when they are migraine free. Some studies have shown that changes in the gray matter in areas related to pain transmission or pain processing are accompanied by functional activity or functional connectivity changes in these areas, suggesting that these changes might be the consequence of frequent nociceptive input. For example, changes in the functional activity and connectivity of the brainstem (specifically in the PAG) with the cortex may imply inhibitory deficiency in migraineurs (Becerra et al., 2001). In fact, axonal tracing studies along with immunohistochemistry have shown central termination of nociceptive afferent terminals in the trigeminal brainstem nuclear complex (TNBC). Tract tracing studies also have demonstrated that trigeminal afferent and TNBC projections trace to a number of other brainstem nuclei (Hayashi, 1985; Henry et al., 1996; Liu et al., 2004; Panneton & Burton, 1981).

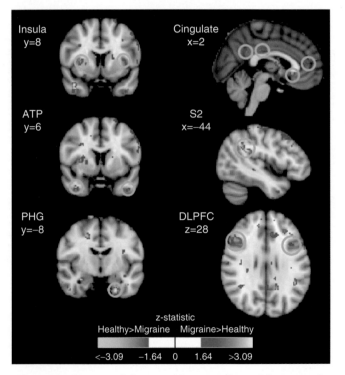

FIGURE 5–3 *Functional changes: Contrast analysis of the interictal migraine versus a gender- and age-matched control group in response to noxious heat (pain threshold + 1C) of the face shows significant differences in several regions including increased activation in migraine patients in the contralateral anterior temporal pole (ATP) and within the ipsilateral parahippocampal gyrus (PHG) and secondary somatosensory cortex (S2), along with decreases in the insula and the dorsolateral prefrontal cortex (DLPFC). From Moulton, E. A., Becerra, L., Maleki, N., Pendse, G., Tully, S., Hargreaves, R., et al. (2011). Painful heat reveals hyperexcitability of the temporal pole in interictal and ictal migraine States. Cerebral Cortex, 21, 435–448.*

WHITE MATTER ALTERATIONS

Multiple studies have reported the presence of white matter abnormalities in the brain of migraine patients in the form of focal hyperintense lesions using magnetic resonance imaging (Cooney et al., 1996; Fazekas et al., 1992; Robbins & Friedman, 1992; Rocca et al., 2000). These white matter abnormalities may be the result of ischemic damages that are secondary to the repeated regional blood flow reductions known to occur during headache attacks. However, these signal abnormalities are most often nonspecific (Fazekas et al., 1992) and do not correlate with age, sex, disease duration, or frequency of attacks (Pavese et al., 1994), and the frequency of their occurrence does not correlate to the subtype of migraine (Cooney et al., 1996).

Migraine patients with white matter lesions display a significantly higher frequency of antineuronal antibodies than migraine patients without white matter lesions (Turkoglu et al., 2011), implying the involvement of inflammation in migraine pathogenesis, which is reflected in the form of white matter lesions detectable with MRI. The inflammatory reaction predominantly involves the cerebellum, consistent with the reduction of fractional anisotropy (FA) in that area (Turkoglu et al., 2011). Multiple sclerosis patients or healthy subjects do not show similar antineuronal antibodies.

Diffusion is a natural physical property in the tissues, which describes the microscopic random motion of water molecules as a result of their internal thermal energy. Diffusivity of water depends primarily on the presence of microscopic structural barriers in tissues, and thus diffusion measures provide information on the tissue structure. Diffusion-weighted MR imaging (DWI) has been used to study the white matter anatomy and integrity in the brain. DWI is a one-dimensional technique to measure the projection of all molecular displacements along one direction at a time. Diffusion tensor imaging (DTI) is another approach that is used to provide information on diffusion directionality from which fiber tracts can be tracked and brain connectivity can be studied. MR diffusion imaging is a technique that allows early detection of white matter damage, sometimes even in regions that appear normal on conventional anatomical images.

Alterations in the postcentral gyrus white matter in migraineurs has been reported using DTI (Whitcher et al., 2007), which traverses the length of the gyrus, consistent with the expected geometry of the fiber pathway originating from the ventral posterolateral (VPL) nucleus of the thalamus and targeting primary somatosensory cortex (SI) via the internal capsule and corona radiata. This finding is consistent with other evidence from magnetoencephalographic (Lang et al., 2004) and fMRI (Rocca et al., 2003) studies supporting the involvement of the somatosensory cortex in migraine pathophysiology.

Fiber tracking using the DTI/MRI can be used to determine the structural connectivity basis for the observed functional changes in migraineurs. For instance, in migraine patients, during their interictal phase, there is a significant change in the temporal pole in response to noxious heat (Moulton et al., 2011). Using DTI, it has been shown that there is a potential trigeminothalamic pathway through the pulvinar nucleus that may send nociceptive information to the temporal pole. This structural connectivity between the temporal pole and the pulvinar nucleus suggests the presence of an afferent pathway that could provide the substrate for functional changes in the temporal pole in migraine patients (Moulton et al., 2011).

DTI also shows changes in diffusion properties of the optic radiation in migraine patients with aura (Rocca et al., 2008), which shows reduced FA. Decline in FA is often used as an index of decreasing white matter integrity. These migraineurs also show areas of lower FA along the ventral trigeminothalamic white matter tract (DaSilva, Granziera, Tuch, et al., 2007). Migraineurs without aura have lower FA in the ventrolateral periaqueductal gray matter. Migraineurs with or without aura show areas of lower FA along the thalamocortical tract compared to healthy controls (DaSilva, Granziera, Tuch, et al., 2007). These findings may represent phenotypic biomarkers of the disease and emphasize the effect of migraine on the trigeminal somatosensory and modulatory pain systems.

CHEMICAL ALTERATIONS

Neurochemical evidence suggests that interictal migraine patients have altered levels of neurotransmitters (Prescot et al., 2009), which may be linked to the increased cortical excitability that has been well documented in migraine patients, particularly those with migraine aura. One imaging approach for assessing neurochemical changes in the brain is magnetic resonance spectroscopy (MRS). MRS is a noninvasive method for investigating tissue metabolism. MRS is based on the chemical shifts that occur when the resonance frequency of a nucleus is modified by its surrounding chemical environment. Changes in brain metabolites due to activation in response to a particular stimulus or potential mechanisms of action of medications can also readily be assessed using MRS. MRS can be used to measure the concentrations or synthesis rates of neurotransmitters such as glutamate, glycine, and γ-aminobutyric acid (GABA) by measuring the distribution of chemical shifts from a single volume or region of interest in vivo. The most common nuclei studied in vivo include ^{31}P, ^{1}H, ^{13}C, and ^{19}F. These nuclei are nonradioactive and occur naturally, although often in small physiologic concentrations.

Studies have reported that increased platelet levels of neuroexcitatory amino acids including aspartate (Asp), glutamate (Glu), glutamine (Gln), and glycine (Gly) exist in migraine patients compared with healthy control subjects (Alam et al., 1998; Cananzi et al., 1995; D'Andrea et al., 1991). Cerebrospinal fluid (CSF) Gln, Gly, and taurine (Tau) concentrations are elevated in migraineurs (Rothrock et al., 1995), which strongly implicates increased activity in glutamatergic systems in the migraine brain. Increased synaptic concentrations of excitatory amino acid neurotransmitters may lead to excessive activity at the N-methyl-d-aspartate (NMDA) Glu receptor subtype, which in turn may amplify and reinforce pain transmission in migraine and other types of headache. Low-affinity NMDA receptor (NMDAr) antagonists, such as memantine, have been shown to reduce the frequency of migraine and tension-type headaches (Krusz, 2002). One other potential mechanism for neuronal excitability includes an abnormality of the presynaptic release of excitatory amino acid neurotransmitters.

The aura aspect of migraine headaches has been particularly studied with respect to chemical changes in the brain. As aura duration in migraine patients increases with certain aura phenotypes, phosphocreatine/phosphate ratios in gray matter seem to decrease (Boska et al., 2002). During the migraine interictal period, increased levels of lactate (Watanabe et al., 1996), decreased levels of choline (Macri et al., 2003), and reduced levels of

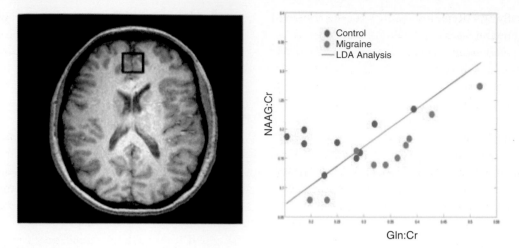

FIGURE 5–4 *Chemical alterations: (Left Panel) Axial high-resolution T1-weighted fluid-attenuated inversion recovery magnetic resonance images recorded from a 42-year-old male migraine patient showing an 8-cm³ spectroscopy voxel (black box) positioned within the ACC. (Right Panel) This figure depicts two metabolite ratios (e.g., NAAG:Cr and Glu:Cr) that separate controls from migraineurs through the black line in the cingulate using linear discriminant analysis (LDA). From Prescot, A., Becerra, L., Pendse, G., Tully, S., Jensen, E., Hargreaves, R., et al. (2009). Excitatory neurotransmitters in brain regions in interictal migraine patients.* Molecular Pain, 5, 34.

naphthalic acetic acid (NAA) (Dichgans et al., 2005; Sarchielli et al., 2005) have been reported.

Chemical changes have been difficult to interpret in terms of increased excitability as a result of enhanced inhibitory systems (e.g., GABA, glycine). Various amino acid neurotransmitters have been found to have effects in migraine sufferers; however, these observed changes are not always good measures or indicators of changes in the brain.

CEREBROVASCULAR HEMODYNAMICS

Identification of structural alterations in the cerebral vasculature of migraine patients may have important pathophysiological and clinical implications. Reversible vessel and perfusion abnormalities may be observed in patients with visual symptoms and headache (Beccia et al., 2009). There are several studies looking at the association between migraine and cerebrovascular hemodynamic abnormalities. The findings, however, are not conclusive. While impaired adaptive cerebral hemodynamic mechanisms in the posterior circulation (Silvestrini et al., 2004) and repressed pressure-related vasoreactivity in the right hemisphere of migraineurs during the interictal period have been reported (Silvestrini et al., 2004), there are other reports of no significant water diffusion or cerebral perfusion changes in the brains of migraine patients with aura (Jager et al., 2005).

PATHOPHYSIOLOGY OF THE INTERICTAL BRAIN

So far we have discussed some of the potential processes that contribute to the altered interictal brain. However, there remains a very important and most obvious question of which comes first: Are the brains of migraineurs different to begin with and their condition exacerbates the process, or does the process of the migraine alter the brain? Support for each of these scenarios is provided below.

Migraine Itself Produces Brain Changes

1. *Pain and central sensitization:* The phenomenon of central sensitization may occur with each migraine attack. Central sensitization, as it occurs in migraine, represents the augmentation of central neuronal responses (see Woolf, 2011) to stimuli as a result of the afferent barrage resulting from nociceptor activation in the trigeminovascular system in migraineurs (Burstein et al., 2000). While the peripheral manifestations such as tactile allodynia, secondary hyperalgesia, and enhanced temporal summation may be observed as hypersensitivity even outside the region innervated by the trigeminal nerve (Burstein et al., 2005), the phenomenon represents enhanced synaptic efficacy of neurons in the brain's

pain pathways. Repetitive central sensitization and altered neural function may thus contribute to activity-dependent plasticity of brain structure and function, including processes underlying chronification in migraine (Buchgreitz et al., 2006).

2. *Repeated drug use*: The use of medications in migraine patients may contribute to brain changes. While this has been observed in other conditions (e.g., prescription opioid abuse [Upadhyay et al., 2010]), little data are available on the main classes of drugs used in episodic migraine (nonsteroidal anti-inflammatory drugs, triptans). Opioid resistance has been reported in migraine patients (Biondi, 2003; Saper & Lake, 2008). Medication overuse headaches have been associated with barbiturate-containing analgesics or caffeine-containing analgesics but may also be associated with triptan overuse (Cupini & Calabresi, 2005). Overuse of triptans has been reported to alter the brain and increase the brain's sensitivity to migraine triggers in a rodent model of migraine (De Felice, Ossipov, Wang, Dussor, et al., 2010; De Felice, Ossipov, Wang, Lai, et al., 2010). Here, the data suggest that triptans produce a pronociceptive adaptation and enhanced responses to normal migraine triggers.

3. *Repeated stress*: Acute stressors may produce chronic changes and thus disease (see Eggers, 2007). Such stressors have been shown to alter structure and cell function in brain regions in the rat (Alfarez et al., 2003; Joels et al., 2004). As such, brain changes observed in migraine patients may result through the same mechanisms which leads to changes that have been noted in animal studies, particularly in hippocampal regions as has been defined in animal models (McEwen, 2001).

4. *Cytokines and neurotrophic factors*: Increases in some of these chemicals including brain-derived neurotrophic factor (BDNF) (Tanure et al., 2010), interleukin-5 (IL-5), and IL-4 (Bockowski et al., 2010; Munno et al., 1998) have been reported in migraine. Some cytokines are proinflammatory (e.g., IL-1) and others are anti-inflammatory (e.g., IL-4, IL-10) (Munno et al., 1998). Cytokines may alter neuroplasticity via a number of mechanisms, including via glutamatergic synapses (Fourgeaud & Boulanger, 2010). Cytokines may thus act as neuromodulators that can be induced through astrocytes (Fellin, 2009) and have been implicated in a number of central nervous system diseases including depression (Miller et al., 2009).

Brain Changes Produce Migraine

1. *Altered modulatory processes in the brainstem*: Changes in the functional activity and connectivity of the brainstem (specifically in the PAG) with the cortex may, on the other hand, imply inhibitory deficiency in migraineurs.

2. *Trauma*: Headaches are relatively common following head trauma, including concussion (Elkind, 1989; Packard, 1999). Following concussion, some 37% of soldiers reported headaches, of which some 58% were determined to

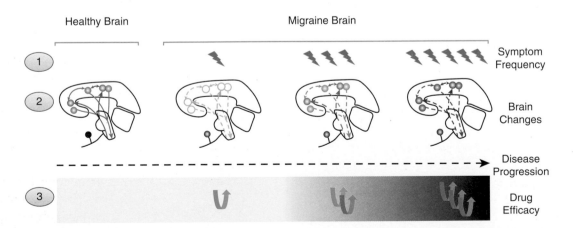

FIGURE 5–5 *Migraine chronification. (1) The frequency, duration, and intensity of migraine attacks may increase gradually over the years in some patients. (2) There are brain alterations associated with changes in the number and severity of migraine attacks. (3) The drug resistance or drug modification of the brain may also happen in patients. In fact, there is usually concomitant use of medication with increased frequency of migraine attacks. The changes in the brain may reflect alterations that may be indicators of migraine chronification/ transformation.*

be migraine headaches (Theeler et al., 2010). Similar data have been found in the civilian population (Lew et al., 2006). The former group is associated with a higher frequency of headache attacks and an increased prevalence of chronic daily headache (Theeler et al., 2010). Alterations in brain microstructural change (Maruta et al., 2010) and function (Ptito et al., 2007) may occur following concussion.

3. *Familial/genetic*: Genetics of migraine has focused on a rare subtype (familial hemiplegic migraine [FHM]) that has as its basis alterations in coding of ion transporters (Stam et al., 2008; Van Den Maagdenberg et al., 2010). Patients with FHM exhibit brain changes including alterations in cerebrocerebellar circuits that may be a basis for cognitive deficits (Karner et al., 2010). However, although currently the focus of a number of laboratories, a gene for the more common forms of migraine is still not defined.

4. *Comorbid conditions*: This topic has been reviewed elsewhere (Guidetti et al., 2010; Scher et al., 2005), and these conditions include psychiatric (anxiety disorders, depression, and eating disorders) (Baskin & Smitherman, 2009; Keck et al., 1994), neurological (epilepsy, brain trauma), and medical (congenital heart defects). With respect to brain changes, there are some important considerations. In the pain field, chronic pain is associated with depression (Antonaci et al., 2011) and primary depression may result in a generalized pain disorder in a significant number of individuals (Lepine & Briley, 2004). This is less clear-cut in the migraine field. However, recent epidemiological data suggest that comorbidity plays a significant role (Louter et al., 2010; Ortiz et al., 2010; Peterlin et al., 2011), which, along with shared genetics between migraine and some of the comorbid diseases (Haan et al., 2008; Ligthart et al., 2010), further implicates alterations in brain structure and function in migraine disorders.

CONCLUSIONS

The independent studies that were reviewed in this chapter have one particular common finding, which is the central and fundamental role of the brain in migraine pathophysiology. These studies collectively suggest that migraine brain, even in the migraine-free state, is structurally and functionally altered and "functions" abnormally.

Despite all these findings, however, no reliable biomarker exists for what appears to be an abnormal brain state. Having such a biomarker would allow for (a) a better understanding of the disease; (b) objective measures of the interictal state and an index of transition from acute migraine to chronic daily headache; and (c) the ability to monitor potential benefits of therapeutic interventions, including clinical trials, where beneficial changes may take longer to be elucidated. Moreover, a better understanding of the specific abnormalities in the interictal migraine brain may provide a unique signature for the underlying dysfunction. Therefore, these specificities may provide a better understanding of the disease in terms of what are the detrimental effects of the frequency and duration of repeated migraine headaches on the brain, and may help discover what the potential underlying mechanisms are that trigger the progression of the disease to more severe or chronic stages. The acquirement of this knowledge could eventually help with the development of better therapeutic or preventive interventions.

ACKNOWLEDGMENTS

The work was supported by grants from NIH (K24 NS064050 [NINDS] and R01 NS056195 [NINDS] to D.B.).

REFERENCES

Afra, J. (2005). Intensity dependence of auditory evoked cortical potentials in migraine. Changes in the peri-ictal period. *Functional Neurology, 20*, 199–200.

Afra, J., Mascia, A., Gerard, P., Maertens de Noordhout, A., & Schoenen, J. (1998). Interictal cortical excitability in migraine: A study using transcranial magnetic stimulation of motor and visual cortices. *Annals of Neurology, 44*, 209–215.

Afra, J., Proietti Cecchini, A., Sandor, P. S., & Schoenen, J. (2000). Comparison of visual and auditory evoked cortical potentials in migraine patients between attacks. *Clinical Neurophysiology, 111*, 1124–1129.

Alam, Z., Coombes, N., Waring, R. H., Williams, A. C., & Steventon, G. B. (1998). Plasma levels of neuroexcitatory amino acids in patients with migraine or tension headache. *Journal of the Neurological Sciences, 156*, 102–106.

Alfarez, D. N., Joels, M., & Krugers, H. J. (2003). Chronic unpredictable stress impairs long-term potentiation in rat hippocampal CA1 area and dentate gyrus in vitro. *European Journal of Neuroscience, 17*, 1928–1934.

Ambrosini, A., Rossi, P., De Pasqua, V., Pierelli, F., & Schoenen, J. (2003). Lack of habituation causes high intensity dependence of auditory evoked cortical potentials in migraine. *Brain, 126*, 2009–2015.

Anderson, B. J., Eckburg, P. B., & Relucio, K. I. (2002). Alterations in the thickness of motor cortical subregions after motor-skill learning and exercise. *Learning and Memory, 9*, 1–9.

Antonaci, F., Nappi, G., Galli, F., Manzoni, G. C., Calabresi, P., & Costa, A. (2011). Migraine and psychiatric comorbidity: A review of clinical findings. *Journal of Headache and Pain, 12*(2):115–125.

Ashkenazi, A., Mushtaq, A., Yang, I., & Oshinsky, M. L. (2009). Ictal and interictal phonophobia in migraine-a quantitative controlled study. *Cephalalgia, 29,* 1042–1048.

Aurora, S. K., Barrodale, P. M., Tipton, R. L., & Khodavirdi, A. (2007). Brainstem dysfunction in chronic migraine as evidenced by neurophysiological and positron emission tomography studies. *Headache, 47,* 996–1003; discussion 1004–1007.

Backer, M., Sander, D., Hammes, M. G., Funke, D., Deppe, M., Conrad, B., et al. (2001). Altered cerebrovascular response pattern in interictal migraine during visual stimulation. *Cephalalgia, 21,* 611–616.

Bartolini, M., Baruffaldi, R., Paolino, I., & Silvestrini, M. (2005). Cerebral blood flow changes in the different phases of migraine. *Functional Neurology, 20,* 209–211.

Baskin, S. M., & Smitherman, T. A. (2009). Migraine and psychiatric disorders: comorbidities, mechanisms, and clinical applications. *Neurological Sciences, 30*(Suppl 1), S61–S65.

Beccia, M., Ceschin, V., Bozzao, A., Romano, A., Biraschi, F., Fantozzi, L. M., et al. (2009). Headache and visual symptoms in two patients with MRI alterations in posterior cerebral artery territory. La *Clinica Terapeutica, 160,* 125–127.

Becerra, L., Breiter, H. C., Wise, R., Gonzalez, R. G., & Borsook, D. (2001). Reward circuitry activation by noxious thermal stimuli. *Neuron, 32,* 927–946.

Becerra, L., Harter, K., Gonzalez, R. G., & Borsook, D. (2006). Functional magnetic resonance imaging measures of the effects of morphine on central nervous system circuitry in opioid-naive healthy volunteers. *Anesthesia and Analgesia, 103,* 208–216, table of contents.

Biondi, D. M. (2003). Opioid resistance in chronic daily headache: A synthesis of ideas from the bench and bedside. *Current Pain Headache Reports, 7,* 67–75.

Bockowski, L., Smigielska-Kuzia, J., Sobaniec, W., Zelazowska-Rutkowska, B., Kulak, W., & Sendrowski, K. (2010). Anti-inflammatory plasma cytokines in children and adolescents with migraine headaches. *Pharmacology Reports, 62,* 287–291.

Boska, M. D., Welch, K. M., Barker, P. B., Nelson, J. A., & Schultz, L. (2002). Contrasts in cortical magnesium, phospholipid and energy metabolism between migraine syndromes. *Neurology, 58,* 1227–1233.

Boulloche, N., Denuelle, M., Payoux, P., Fabre, N., Trotter, Y., & Geraud, G. (2010). Photophobia in migraine: An interictal PET study of cortical hyperexcitability and its modulation by pain. *Journal of Neurology, Neurosurgery, and Psychiatry, 81,* 978–984.

Buchgreitz, L., Lyngberg, A. C., Bendtsen, L., & Jensen, R. (2006). Frequency of headache is related to sensitization: A population study. *Pain, 123,* 19–27.

Burstein, R., Cutrer, M. F., & Yarnitsky, D. (2000). The development of cutaneous allodynia during a migraine attack clinical evidence for the sequential recruitment of spinal and supraspinal nociceptive neurons in migraine. *Brain, 123*(Pt 8), 1703–1709.

Burstein, R., Levy, D., & Jakubowski, M. (2005). Effects of sensitization of trigeminovascular neurons to triptan therapy during migraine. *Review Neurologique (Paris), 161,* 658–660.

Cananzi, A. R., D'Andrea, G., Perini, F., Zamberlan, F., & Welch, K. M. (1995). Platelet and plasma levels of glutamate and glutamine in migraine with and without aura. *Cephalalgia, 15,* 132–135.

Cooney, B. S., Grossman, R. I., Farber, R. E., Goin, J. E., & Galetta, S. L. (1996). Frequency of magnetic resonance imaging abnormalities in patients with migraine. *Headache, 36,* 616–621.

Coppola, G., Ambrosini, A., Di Clemente, L., Magis, D., Fumal, A., Gerard, P., et al. (2007). Interictal abnormalities of gamma band activity in visual evoked responses in migraine: An indication of thalamocortical dysrhythmia? *Cephalalgia, 27,* 1360–1367.

Coppola, G., Pierelli, F., Schoenen, J. (2007). Is the cerebral cortex hyperexcitable or hyperresponsive in migraine? *Cephalalgia, 27,* 1427–1439.

Cupini, L. M., & Calabresi, P. (2005). Medication-overuse headache: Pathophysiological insights. *Journal of Headache and Pain, 6,* 199–202.

D'Andrea, G., Cananzi, A. R., Joseph, R., Morra, M., Zamberlan, F., Ferro Milone, F., et al. (1991). Platelet glycine, glutamate and aspartate in primary headache. *Cephalalgia, 11,* 197–200.

DaSilva, A. F., Granziera, C., Snyder, J., & Hadjikhani, N. (2007). Thickening in the somatosensory cortex of patients with migraine. *Neurology, 69,* 1990–1995.

DaSilva, A. F., Granziera, C., Tuch, D. S., Snyder, J., Vincent, M., & Hadjikhani, N. (2007). Interictal alterations of the trigeminal somatosensory pathway and periaqueductal gray matter in migraine. *Neuroreport, 18,* 301–305.

De Felice, M., Ossipov, M. H., Wang, R., Dussor, G., Lai, J., Meng, I. D., et al. (2010). Triptan-induced enhancement of neuronal nitric oxide synthase in trigeminal ganglion dural afferents underlies increased responsiveness to potential migraine triggers. *Brain, 133,* 2475–2488.

De Felice, M., Ossipov, M. H., Wang, R., Lai, J., Chichorro, J., Meng, I., et al. (2010). Triptan-induced latent sensitization: A possible basis for medication overuse headache. *Annals of Neurology, 67,* 325–337.

Demarquay, G., Royet, J. P., Mick, G., & Ryvlin, P. (2008). Olfactory hypersensitivity in migraineurs: A H(2)(15)O-PET study. *Cephalalgia, 28,* 1069–1080.

de Tommaso, M., Difruscolo, O., Sardaro, M., Libro, G., Pecoraro, C., Serpino, C., et al. (2007). Effects of remote cutaneous pain on trigeminal laser-evoked potentials in migraine patients. *Journal of Headache and Pain, 8,* 167–174.

Dichgans, M., Herzog, J., Freilinger, T., Wilke, M., & Auer, D. P. (2005). 1H-MRS alterations in the cerebellum of patients with familial hemiplegic migraine type 1. *Neurology, 64,* 608–613.

Dora, B., & Balkan, S. (2002). Exaggerated interictal cerebrovascular reactivity but normal blood flow velocities in migraine without aura. *Cephalalgia, 22,* 288–290.

Eggers, A. E. (2007). Redrawing Papez' circuit: A theory about how acute stress becomes chronic and causes disease. *Medical Hypotheses, 69,* 852–857.

Elkind, A. H. (1989). Headache and head trauma. *Clinical Journal of Pain, 5,* 77–87.

Fazekas, F., Koch, M., Schmidt, R., Offenbacher, H., Payer, F., Freidl, W., et al. (1992). The prevalence of cerebral damage varies with migraine type: A MRI study. *Headache, 32,* 287–291.

Fellin, T. (2009). Communication between neurons and astrocytes: Relevance to the modulation of synaptic and network activity. *Journal of Neurochemistry, 108,* 533–544.

Fourgeaud, L., & Boulanger, L. M. (2010). Role of immune molecules in the establishment and plasticity of glutamatergic synapses. *European Journal of Neuroscience, 32,* 207–217.

Geuze, E., Westenberg, H. G., Heinecke, A., de Kloet, C. S., Goebel, R., & Vermetten, E. (2008). Thinner prefrontal cortex in veterans with posttraumatic stress disorder. *Neuroimage, 41,* 675–681.

Granziera, C., DaSilva, A. F., Snyder, J., Tuch, D. S., & Hadjikhani, N. (2006). Anatomical alterations of the visual motion processing network in migraine with and without aura. *PLoS Medicine, 3*, e402.

Guidetti, V., Galli, F., & Sheftell, F. (2010). Headache attributed to psychiatric disorders. *Handbook of Clinical Neurology, 97*, 657–662.

Haan, J., van den Maagdenberg, A. M., Brouwer, O. F., & Ferrari, M. D. (2008). Migraine and epilepsy: Genetically linked? *Expert Reviews in Neurotherapy, 8*, 1307–1311.

Hayashi, H. (1985). Morphology of central terminations of intra-axonally stained, large, myelinated primary afferent fibers from facial skin in the rat. *Journal of Comparative Neurology, 237*, 195–215.

Henry, M. A., Johnson, L. R., Nousek-Goebl, N., & Westrum, L. E. (1996). Light microscopic localization of calcitonin gene-related peptide in the normal feline trigeminal system and following retrogasserian rhizotomy. *Journal of Comparative Neurology, 365*, 526–540.

Jager, H. R., Giffin, N. J., & Goadsby, P. J. (2005). Diffusion- and perfusion-weighted MR imaging in persistent migrainous visual disturbances. *Cephalalgia, 25*, 323–332.

Joels, M., Karst, H., Alfarez, D., Heine, V. M., Qin, Y., van Riel, E., et al. (2004). Effects of chronic stress on structure and cell function in rat hippocampus and hypothalamus. *Stress, 7*, 221–231.

Karner, E., Delazer, M., Benke, T., & Bosch, S. (2010). Cognitive functions, emotional behavior, and quality of life in familial hemiplegic migraine. *Cognitive and Behavioral Neurology, 23*, 106–111.

Keck, P. E., Jr., Merikangas, K. R., McElroy, S. L., & Strakowski, S. M. (1994). Diagnostic and treatment implications of psychiatric comorbidity with migraine. *Annals of Clinical Psychiatry, 6*, 165–171.

Kim, J. H., Suh, S. I., Seol, H. Y., Oh, K., Seo, W. K., Yu, S. W., et al. (2008). Regional grey matter changes in patients with migraine: A voxel-based morphometry study. *Cephalalgia, 28*, 598–604.

Kruit, M. C., Launer, L. J., van Buchem, M. A., Terwindt, G. M., & Ferrari, M. D. (2005). MRI findings in migraine. *Review Neurologique (Paris), 161*, 661–665.

Kruit, M. C., van Buchem, M. A., Hofman, P. A., Bakkers, J. T., Terwindt, G. M., Ferrari, M. D., et al. (2004). Migraine as a risk factor for subclinical brain lesions. *Journal of the American Medical Association, 291*, 427–434.

Kruit, M. C., van Buchem, M. A., Launer, L. J., Terwindt, G. M., & Ferrari, M. D. (2010). Migraine is associated with an increased risk of deep white matter lesions, subclinical posterior circulation infarcts and brain iron accumulation: The population-based MRI CAMERA study. *Cephalalgia, 30*, 129–136.

Krusz, J. C. (2002). Prophylaxis for chronic daily headache and chronic migraine with neuronal stabilizing agents. *Current Pain and Headache Reports, 6*, 480–485.

Lang, E., Kaltenhauser, M., Neundorfer, B., & Seidler, S. (2004). Hyperexcitability of the primary somatosensory cortex in migraine——a magnetoencephalographic study. *Brain, 127*, 2459–2469.

Lappe, C., Herholz, S. C., Trainor, L. J., & Pantev, C. (2008). Cortical plasticity induced by short-term unimodal and multimodal musical training. *Journal of Neuroscience, 28*, 9632–9639.

Lepine, J. P., & Briley, M. (2004). The epidemiology of pain in depression. *Human Psychopharmacology, 19*(Suppl 1), S3–S7.

Lew, H. L., Lin, P. H., Fuh, J. L., Wang, S. J., Clark, D. J., & Walker, W. C. (2006). Characteristics and treatment of headache after traumatic brain injury: A focused review. *American Journal of Physical Medicine and Rehabilitation, 85*, 619–627.

Ligthart, L., Nyholt, D. R., Penninx, B. W., & Boomsma, D. I. (2010). The shared genetics of migraine and anxious depression. *Headache, 50*, 1549–1560.

Liu, Y., Broman, J., & Edvinsson, L. (2004). Central projections of sensory innervation of the rat superior sagittal sinus. *Neuroscience, 129*, 431–437.

Louter, M. A., Veen, G., Ferrari, M. D., Zitman, F. G., & Terwindt, G. M. (2010). [Migraine and depression should be treated concurrently]. *Nederlands tijdschrift voor geneeskunde, 154*, A1044.

Macri, M. A., Garreffa, G., Giove, F., Ambrosini, A., Guardati, M., Pierelli, F., et al. (2003). Cerebellar metabolite alterations detected in vivo by proton MR spectroscopy. *Magnetic Resonance Imaging, 21*, 1201–1206.

Maruta, J., Lee, S. W., Jacobs, E. F., & Ghajar, J. (2010). A unified science of concussion. *Annals of the New York Academy of Sciences, 1208*, 58–66.

May, A. (2009). New insights into headache: An update on functional and structural imaging findings. *Nature Reviews Neurology, 5*, 199–209.

McEwen, B. S. (2001). Plasticity of the hippocampus: Adaptation to chronic stress and allostatic load. *Annals of the New York Academy of Sciences, 933*, 265–277.

Miller, A. H., Maletic, V., & Raison, C. L. (2009). Inflammation and its discontents: The role of cytokines in the pathophysiology of major depression. *Biological Psychiatry, 65*, 732–741.

Moulton, E. A., Becerra, L., Maleki, N., Pendse, G., Tully, S., Hargreaves, R., et al. (2011). Painful heat reveals hyperexcitability of the temporal pole in interictal and ictal migraine States. *Cerebral Cortex, 21*, 435–448.

Moulton, E. A., Burstein, R., Tully, S., Hargreaves, R., Becerra, L., & Borsook, D. (2008). Interictal dysfunction of a brainstem descending modulatory center in migraine patients. *PLoS ONE, 3*, e3799.

Mulder, E. J., Linssen, W. H., Passchier, J., Orlebeke, J. F., & de Geus, E. J. (1999). Interictal and postictal cognitive changes in migraine. *Cephalalgia, 19*, 557–565; discussion 541.

Munno, I., Centonze, V., Marinaro, M., Bassi, A., Lacedra, G., Causarano, V., et al. (1998). Cytokines and migraine: Increase of IL-5 and IL-4 plasma levels. *Headache, 38*, 465–467.

Ortiz, A., Cervantes, P., Zlotnik, G., van de Velde, C., Slaney, C., Garnham, J., et al. (2010). Cross-prevalence of migraine and bipolar disorder. *Bipolar Disorder, 12*, 397–403.

Ozkul, Y., & Uckardes, A. (2002). Median nerve somatosensory evoked potentials in migraine. *European Journal of Neurology, 9*, 227–232.

Packard, R. C. (1999). Epidemiology and pathogenesis of post-traumatic headache. *Journal of Head Trauma Rehabilitation, 14*, 9–21.

Panneton, W. M., & Burton, H. (1981). Corneal and periocular representation within the trigeminal sensory complex in the cat studied with transganglionic transport of horseradish peroxidase. *Journal of Comparative Neurology, 199*, 327–344.

Pavese, N., Canapicchi, R., Nuti, A., Bibbiani, F., Lucetti, C., Collavoli, P., et al. (1994). White matter MRI hyperintensities in a hundred and twenty-nine consecutive migraine patients. *Cephalalgia, 14*, 342–345.

Peterlin, B. L., Rosso, A. L., Sheftell, F. D., Libon, D. J., Mossey, J. M., & Merikangas, K. R. (2011). Post-traumatic stress disorder, drug abuse and migraine: New findings from the National Comorbidity Survey Replication (NCS-R). *Cephalalgia, 31*, 235–244.

Prescot, A., Becerra, L., Pendse, G., Tully, S., Jensen, E., Hargreaves, R., et al. (2009). Excitatory neurotransmitters in brain regions in interictal migraine patients. *Molecular Pain, 5*, 34.

Ptito, A., Chen, J. K., & Johnston, K. M. (2007). Contributions of functional magnetic resonance imaging (fMRI) to sport concussion evaluation. *NeuroRehabilitation, 22*, 217–227.

Robbins, L., & Friedman, H. (1992). MRI in migraineurs. *Headache, 32*, 507–508.

Rocca, M. A., Ceccarelli, A., Falini, A., Colombo, B., Tortorella, P., Bernasconi, L., et al. (2006). Brain gray matter changes in migraine patients with T2-visible lesions: A 3-T MRI study. *Stroke, 37*, 1765–1770.

Rocca, M. A., Colombo, B., Pagani, E., Falini, A., Codella, M., Scotti, G., et al. (2003). Evidence for cortical functional changes in patients with migraine and white matter abnormalities on conventional and diffusion tensor magnetic resonance imaging. *Stroke, 34*, 665–670.

Rocca, M. A., Colombo, B., Pratesi, A., Comi, G., & Filippi, M. (2000). A magnetization transfer imaging study of the brain in patients with migraine. *Neurology, 54*, 507–509.

Rocca, M. A., Pagani, E., Colombo, B., Tortorella, P., Falini, A., Comi, G., et al. (2008). Selective diffusion changes of the visual pathways in patients with migraine: A 3-T tractography study. *Cephalalgia, 28*, 1061–1068.

Rothrock, J. F., Mar, K. R., Yaksh, T. L., Golbeck, A., & Moore, A. C. (1995). Cerebrospinal fluid analyses in migraine patients and controls. *Cephalalgia, 15*, 489–493.

Saper, J. R., & Lake, A. E., 3rd. (2008). Continuous opioid therapy (COT) is rarely advisable for refractory chronic daily headache: Limited efficacy, risks, and proposed guidelines. *Headache, 48*, 838–849.

Sarchielli, P., Pedini, M., Alberti, A., Rossi, C., Baldi, A., Corbelli, I., et al. (2005). Application of ICHD 2nd edition criteria for primary headaches with the aid of a computerised, structured medical record for the specialist. *Journal of Headache and Pain, 6*, 205–210.

Scher, A. I., Bigal, M. E., & Lipton, R. B. (2005). Comorbidity of migraine. *Current Opinion in Neurology, 18*, 305–310.

Schmidt-Wilcke, T., Ganssbauer, S., Neuner, T., Bogdahn, U., & May, A. (2008). Subtle grey matter changes between migraine patients and healthy controls. *Cephalalgia, 28*, 1–4.

Schmitz, N., Admiraal-Behloul, F., Arkink, EB., Kruit, M. C., Schoonman, G. G., Ferrari, M. D., et al. (2008). Attack frequency and disease duration as indicators for brain damage in migraine. *Headache, 48*, 1044–1055.

Schmitz, N., Arkink, E. B., Mulder, M., Rubia, K., Admiraal-Behloul, F., Schoonman, G. G., et al. (2008). Frontal lobe structure and executive function in migraine patients. *Neuroscience Letters, 440*, 92–96.

Schoenen, J. (2006). Neurophysiological features of the migrainous brain. *Neurological Sciences, 27*(Suppl 2), S77–81.

Seminowicz, D. A., Laferriere, A. L., Millecamps, M., Yu, J. S., Coderre, T. J., & Bushnell, M. C. (2009). MRI structural brain changes associated with sensory and emotional function in a rat model of long-term neuropathic pain. *Neuroimage, 47*, 1007–1014.

Shinoura, N., & Yamada, R. (2005). Decreased vasoreactivity to right cerebral hemisphere pressure in migraine without aura: A near-infrared spectroscopy study. *Clinical Neurophysiology, 116*, 1280–1285.

Silvestrini, M., Baruffaldi, R., Bartolini, M., Vernieri, F., Lanciotti, C., Matteis, M., et al. (2004). Basilar and middle cerebral artery reactivity in patients with migraine. *Headache, 44*, 29–34.

Stam, A. H., van den Maagdenberg, A. M., Haan, J., Terwindt, G. M., & Ferrari, M. D. (2008). Genetics of migraine: An update with special attention to genetic comorbidity. *Current Opinion in Neurology, 21*, 288–293.

Tanure, M. T., Gomez, R. S., Hurtado, R. C., Teixeira, A. L., & Domingues, R. B. (2010). Increased serum levels of brain-derived neurotropic factor during migraine attacks: A pilot study. *Journal of Headache and Pain, 11*, 427–430.

Theeler, B. J., Flynn, F. G., & Erickson, J. C. (2010). Headaches after concussion in US soldiers returning from Iraq or Afghanistan. *Headache, 50*, 1262–1272.

Tortorella, P., Rocca, M. A., Colombo, B., Annovazzi, P., Comi, G., & Filippi, M. (2006). Assessment of MRI abnormalities of the brainstem from patients with migraine and multiple sclerosis. *Journal of the Neurological Sciences, 244*, 137–141.

Turkoglu, R., Tuzun, E., Icoz, S., Birisik, O., Erdag, E., Kurtuncu, M., et al. (2011). Antineuronal antibodies in migraine patients with white matter lesions. *International Journal of Neuroscience, 121*, 33–36.

Upadhyay, J., Maleki, N., Potter, J., Elman, I., Rudrauf, D., Knudsen, J., et al. (2010) Alterations in brain structure and functional connectivity in prescription opioid-dependent patients. *Brain 133*, 2098–2114.

Valfre, W., Rainero, I., Bergui, M., & Pinessi, L. (2008). Voxel-based morphometry reveals gray matter abnormalities in migraine. *Headache, 48*, 109–117.

Van Den Maagdenberg, A. M., Terwindt, G. M., Haan, J., Frants, R. R., & Ferrari, M. D. (2010). Genetics of headaches. *Handbook of Clinical Neurology, 97*, 85–97.

Wang, W., Timsit-Berthier, M., & Schoenen, J. (1996). Intensity dependence of auditory evoked potentials is pronounced in migraine: An indication of cortical potentiation and low serotonergic neurotransmission? *Neurology, 46*, 1404–1409.

Watanabe, H., Kuwabara, T., Ohkubo, M., Tsuji, S., & Yuasa, T. (1996). Elevation of cerebral lactate detected by localized 1H-magnetic resonance spectroscopy in migraine during the interictal period. *Neurology, 47*, 1093–1095.

Welch, K. M., Nagesh, V., Aurora, S. K., & Gelman, N. (2001). Periaqueductal gray matter dysfunction in migraine: Cause or the burden of illness? *Headache, 41*, 629–637.

Whitcher, B., Wisco, J. J., Hadjikhani, N., & Tuch, D. S. (2007). Statistical group comparison of diffusion tensors via multivariate hypothesis testing. *Magnetic Resonance in Medicine, 57*, 1065–1074.

Woolf, C. J. (2011). Central sensitization: Implications for the diagnosis and treatment of pain. *Pain, 152*, S2–S15.

6 From Episodic to Chronic Migraine

RICHARD B. LIPTON AND MARCELO E. BIGAL

INTRODUCTION

Over the past decade, our understanding of the migraine brain has evolved in many ways (Dodick, 2006). Once viewed as a purely episodic pain disorder, migraine is now understood as a chronic disorder with episodic attacks (CDEA) (Haut et al., 2006). It has features in common with both episodic and chronic pain disorders. Like purely episodic pain disorders (postoperative or posttraumatic pain), migraine attacks are acute, self-limited episodes of intense pain. Like chronic pain disorders (osteoarthritis or painful neuropathy), episodic migraine (EM) sufferers experience recurrent attacks of pain that vary in frequency. In addition, persons with migraine have an enduring predisposition to attacks marked by interictal brain sensitivity or hyperexcitability (Coppolla et al., 2005; Di Clemente et al., 2007), as well as impaired health-related quality of life (Lipton et al., 2000; Terwindt et al., 2000). Finally, both clinic-based and epidemiological studies show that a substantial minority of persons with episodic migraine progress to chronic migraine (CM). Available data suggest that 2.5% of persons with EM develop CM annually (Bigal, Serrano, et al., 2008).

The conceptual definition of CM focuses on the process of accelerating headache frequency (Manack et al., 2009). The several operational definitions of CM require headache on 15 or more days per month and a link to migraine (Manack et al., 2009). The definitions vary in the nature of that required link. In addition, some definitions use medication overuse to modify the diagnosis of CM, while others consider it an exclusion. The issues of case definition have been discussed in detail elsewhere (Manack et al., 2009; Olesen et al., 2006).

Epidemiological studies have revealed a number of environmental risk factors and comorbidities that play a role in the progression of EM to CM (Manack et al., 2011). Familial and genetic factors also seem to play a role. In this chapter, we begin with a description of our emerging understanding of the natural history of migraine as a sometimes progressive disorder. We then discuss the risk factors for migraine progression including sociodemographic factors, headache features, and comorbidities. We close with a brief discussion of the clinical implications of these data.

THE NATURAL HISTORY OF MIGRAINE

Longitudinal population studies as well as clinic-based observational studies have improved our understanding of the natural history and the prognosis of migraine (Bigal & Lipton, 2008a, 2008b; Manack et al., 2011). We distinguish four partially overlapping outcomes in persons with episodic migraine. These outcomes include complete remission, partial remission, persistence, and progression (see Fig. 6–1) (Buzzi et al., 2005; Kelman, 2007; Lipton & Bigal, 2005; Nachit-Ouinekh et al., 2005; Pryse-Phillips et al., 2006). Insights into the progression of migraine have emerged from several studies, including the American Migraine Prevalence and Prevention (AMPP) study. The AMPP study includes a longitudinal population-based assessment of migraine and other severe headache sufferers in the United States. Most migraine sufferers have persistent episodic headache (83.9%) (Buzzi et al., 2005; Kelman, 2007; Lipton & Bigal, 2005; Nachit-Ouinekh et al., 2005; Pryse-Phillips et al., 2006). Some lucky migraine sufferers remit completely (3.3%) and remain symptom free for long periods of time (*clinical remission*) (Bigal & Lipton, 2008a, 2008b; Buzzi et al., 2005; Kelman, 2007; Lipton & Bigal, 2005; Nachit-Ouinekh et al., 2005; Pryse-Phillips et al., 2006). Others have a partial remission (9.9%), continuing to have attacks with fewer migraine features (*partial remission*). Some patients with partial remission have occasional full-blown migraine attacks. Finally, in some, migraine attack frequency and disability may increase over time (*progression*) (Lipton & Bigal, 2005).

Typically, progression refers to increases in attack frequency over time leading to CM (*clinical progression*) (Bigal & Lipton, 2008a). Clinical progression is often

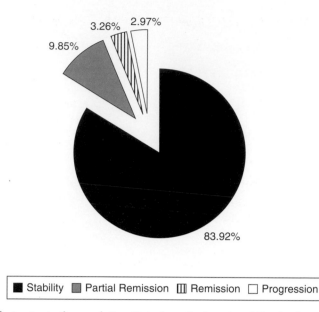

9.85% 3.26% 2.97%

83.92%

■ Stability   ■ Partial Remission   ⊞ Remission   □ Progression

FIGURE 6–1 *One-year prognosis of migraine in the population. Data from the American Migraine Prevalence and Prevention study.*

associated with emergence of cutaneous allodynia due to sensitization at various levels of the trigeminal pathway. Allodynia due to sensitization in the trigeminocervical complex, the thalamus, and perhaps the sensory cortex represents a form of *physiological progression* (Bigal & Lipton, 2008a). In addition, there may be anatomic correlates of attack frequency including stroke and deep white matter lesions (Kruit et al., 2004), as well as alteration in the volume of specific brain regions, a phenomenon we call anatomic progression (Bigal & Lipton, 2008a; May, 2009).

The population prevalence of CM is 1% to 2% (Manack et al., 2011), much lower than the 12% population prevalence of migraine. Studies show that CM develops in 2.5% of EM sufferers annually and that the remission rate of CM is high (Bigal, Serrano, et al., 2008).

SOCIODEMOGRAPHIC RISK FACTORS FOR CHRONIC MIGRAINE

The sociodemographic profile of EM is well known (Table 6–1). EM is most common between the ages of 25 and 55, shows a 3:1 gender prevalence ratio favoring women, and is inversely associated with income and education. Recent data have shown that the epidemiologic profile of CM differs from that of EM (Buse et al., 2010). Persons with CM are older and have marginally higher body mass indexes (BMIs). There is no gender predilection, but African Americans are underrepresented in the CM population. Household incomes are lower and persons with CM are less likely to be employed full time and more likely to be disabled (Table 6–1).

GENETIC AND PERINATAL RISK FACTORS FOR CHRONIC MIGRAINE

Since only a subset of episodic migraine sufferers progress to chronic migraine in any given year, progression may occur as a function of risk factors (Bigal & Lipton, 2008a; Lipton & Bigal, 2005; Manack et al., 2011). Understanding the risk factors that differentiate migraine sufferers who progress to chronic migraine from those who do not may provide insights into the mechanisms, prevention, and treatment of chronic migraine. In this section, we first consider biological predisposition and then environmental risk factors.

Genetic Factors in the Development of Chronic Migraine

Twin studies and family studies suggest that genetic factors account for about half of the risk for developing episodic migraine (Russell & Olesen, 1996; Stewart et al., 1997, 2006; Ulrich et al., 1999). The influences of genetic factors on the progression of episodic migraine to CM are not well understood. There is emerging evidence that CM aggregates within families (Lemos et al., 2009; Rueda-Sanchez & Diaz-Martinez, 2008). The prevalence of CM is elevated in first-degree relatives of probands with CM. This finding is best explained by a heritable biological predisposition, though other explanations are possible (Lemos et al., 2009; Rueda-Sanchez & Diaz-Martinez, 2008). Family aggregation also increases with illness severity as measured by pain intensity or degree of headache-related disability (Stewart et al., 1997, 2006).

TABLE 6–1 *Sociodemographic Profiles of Chronic (CM) and Episodic Migraineurs (EM)*

Variables		CM $N = 655$[a] Mean (SD)	EM $N = 11{,}249$[a] Mean (SD)	p value
Age		47.7 (14.0)	46.0 (13.8)	0.03
BMI		29.8 (8.3)	29.2 (7.9)	0.06
Gender	Female	515 (78.6)	8,469 (80.0)	0.46
Race	Caucasian	594 (90.7)	9,263 (87.3)	0.01
	African American	26 (4.0)	759 (7.2)	
	Other/no answer	35 (5.3)	587 (5.5)	
Highest level of education[b]	8 grades or less	14 (2.3)	122 (1.1)	0.35
	Some HS	28 (4.3)	506 (4.6)	
	HS graduate or GED	163 (25.3)	2,672 (24.0)	
	Some college or technical school	264 (40.8)	4,309 (38.7)	
	College graduate	124 (19.8)	2,281 (20.5)	
	Graduate degree	54 (8.4)	1,252 (11.2)	
Household income[c]	<$22,500 (Reference)	196 (29.9)	2,798 (24.9)	0.02
	$22,500–$39,999	140 (21.4)	2,249 (20.0)	
	$40,000–$59,999	106 (16.2)	2,120 (18.9)	
	$60,000–$89,999	121 (18.5)	2,078 (18.5)	
	$90,000+	92 (14.1)	2,004 (17.8)	
Employment status[c]	Employed full time	242 (37.8)	5,772 (52.3)	<0.001
	Employed part time	72 (11.3)	1,435 (13.1)	0.26
	Unemployed	48 (7.5)	811 (7.4)	0.76
	Retired	95 (14.8)	1,385 (12.6)	0.54
	Student	20 (3.1)	414 (3.8)	0.63
	Homemaker	124 (19.4)	1,781 (16.14)	0.04
	Disabled	128 (20.0)	1,225 (11.10)	<0.001
	Volunteer	20 (3.1)	253 (2.29)	0.25
Marital status[c]	Single	126 (19.4)	2,286 (20.6)	0.04
	Married	384 (59.3)	6,763 (60.8)	
	Divorced	112 (17.3)	1,502 (13.5)	
	Widowed	26 (4.0)	571 (5.1)	

[a] Ns vary as a function of response/nonresponse (missing data) to each individual item.

[b] Statistical test used was ordered logistic regression, in which odds ratio indicates how contrasted groups differ in probability of higher response category.

[c] Effects of income were adjusted for age and gender, while the effects of education, employment, and marital statuses were adjusted for age, gender, and income.

Numbers may sum to more than 100% because respondents were instructed to endorse all response options that applied to them.

From Buse, D. C., Manack, A., Serrano, D., Turkel, C., Lipton, R. B., et al. (2010). Sociodemographic and comorbidity profiles of chronic migraine and episodic migraine sufferers. *Journal of Neurology, Neurosurgery, and Psychiatry, 81*, 428–432.

The Attention Brazil Project (ABP) investigated the influence of parental headache history on headaches in offspring. In this study, using offspring of parents with a negative lifetime family history of headache, offspring of parents with any headache history were at increased risk of both episode headache (odds ratio [OR] = 1.6; 95% confidence interval [CI]: 1.3–1.8) and chronic daily headache (CDH) (OR = 6.6, 95% CI: 1.4–28.4) (Arruda et al., 2010). Frequency of headaches in the mother predicted frequency of headaches in the children. When mother had low-frequency headaches, children had an increased chance to have low or intermediate headache frequency (relative risk = 1.4, 1.2–1.6), but not chronic daily headaches. When the mother had CDH, risk of CDH was increased by almost 13-fold, but not the risk of infrequent headaches. In multivariate models, frequency of headaches in the children was independently predicted by frequency of headaches in the mother after adjustments, suggesting that headache frequency (not only headache status) aggregates in the family (Arruda et al., 2010).

We have hypothesized that the genetic factors for migraine progression and the genetic factors that contribute to migraine onset may be distinct (Bigal & Lipton, 2008a; Lipton & Bigal, 2005). Specific genetic variations may increase the risk of incident chronic pain in individuals with episodic pain (Diatchenko et al., 2006; Max et al., 2006; Nackley et al., 2007). A number of genes associated with chronic pain have been identified, though their role in migraine progression remains to be determined (Diatchenko et al., 2006; Max et al., 2006; Nackley et al., 2007). In particular, functional variants in the genes that code for enzymes involved in catecholamine metabolism have been implicated in chronic pain. These enzymes include catechol-O-methyl transferase (COMT) and dopamine β-hydroxylase (DBH), among others (Diatchenko et al., 2006; Max et al., 2006; Nackley et al., 2007).

The genetics of addiction has been better studied than the genetics of pain progression. Genetic factors may modify vulnerability to opioid addiction, for example (Goldman et al., 2005). For opioid addiction, genes associated with the serotonin transporter (SLC6A4) gene, the dopamine D_2 and D_4 receptor (DRD$_2$ and DRD$_4$) genes, the COMT gene, the monoamine oxidase A (MAOA) gene, and the opioid receptor mu-1 (OPRM1) gene are of interest (Uhl, 2006). These catecholamine pathways have also been implicated in the pathophysiology of migraine and the predisposition to pain progression (Hagen et al., 2002).

For barbiturate addiction, quantitative trait locus mapping suggests that relevant genes directly or indirectly affect γ-aminobutyric acid A (GABA$_A$) receptor-mediated transmission, which has been implicated in some of the actions of alcohol and other drugs. These include a cluster of GABA$_A$ receptor genes and genes encoding the enzymes steroid 5α-reductase-1 (involved in biosynthesis of the neuroactive steroid allopregnanolone) and glutamic acid decarboxylase-1 (involved in GABA biosynthesis) (Buck & Finn, 2001).

Accordingly, we recommend that studies of the genetics of pain progression focus on candidates from the following categories: (a) genes potentially linked to migraine or pain progression, (b) genes potentially linked to medication overuse (addiction), and (c) other genes relevant to neuronal hyperexcitability.

Prenatal Risk Factors

Among the prenatal exposures, tobacco and alcohol are of particular interest for the development of chronic pain based on both empirical data and biological plausibility (Arruda et al., 2011; Brent et al., 2004; Handmaker et al., 2006; Shumilla et al., 2004; Slotkin et al., 1998). In a large population study (Attention Brazil Project), mothers were asked about active or passive exposure to nicotine during pregnancy, as well as alcohol consumption (Table 6–2). The children of these mothers were directly interviewed in elementary school to assess headache status (Arruda et al., 2011). Odds of CDH were significantly higher when maternal tobacco use was reported. For active *and* passive smoking the OR for CDH was elevated in the offspring of exposed mothers (OR = 2.29; 95% CI: 1.6 vs. 3.6). For the offspring of mothers who actively smoked, the OR for CDH was even higher (OR = 4.2; 95% CI: 2.1–8.5). Alcohol use in pregnancy more than doubled the risk of CDH in the offspring, from 11% in unexposed individuals to 24% in the exposed (OR = 2.3; 95% CI: 1.2–4.7). The risk remained significantly elevated after adjusting for family income, parental headache status, medical care during pregnancy, hypertension during pregnancy, and use of illegal drugs (Table 6–2). The study illustrates the enormous susceptibility of the pain pathways during early development.

Preclinical studies, using primarily rodent models, have shown acetylcholine to have a critical role in brain maturation via activation of nicotinic acetylcholine receptors (nAChRs) (Brent et al., 2004). Nicotine exposure due to maternal smoking may lead to alterations in cell proliferation and differentiation in the fetal brain. There is evidence of consequent shortfalls in neuronal number as well as altered synaptic density (Brent et al., 2004; Slotkin, 1998). For ethanol, early exposure may alter the maturation of somatosensory pathways and hence alter nociceptive responses at later time points (Shumilla et al., 2004). Alterations in fetal biometric measurements were reported in those with consistent exposure to alcohol during pregnancy (Arruda et al., 2011).

TABLE 6–2 *Headache Status as a Function of Tobacco Exposure During Pregnancy in Unadjusted Analyses*

	No Headache	Episodic Headaches		CDH	
	2>N (%)	N (%)	OR (95% CI)	N (%)	**OR (95% CI)**
Overall					
Neither active nor passive tabagism	146 (41.2%)	253 (38.4%)	Reference	4 (16%)	Reference
Active + passive	66 (18.6%)	142 (21.5%)	1.15 (0.9–1.46)	10 (40%)	*2.29 (1.6–3.6)*
Active only	22 (6.2%)	30 (4.5%)	0.81 (0.48–1.36)	5 (20%)	*4.2 (2.1–8.5)*
Passive only	120 (33.9%)	233 (35.4%)	1.1 (0.9–1.2)	6 (24%)	1.33 (0.88–2.25)
Active or passive	142 (40.1%)	263 (39.9%)	1.13 (0.96–1.32)	11 (44%)	*1.55 (1.1–2.1)*
Boys					
Neither active nor passive tabagism	123 (30.5%)	118 (34.2%)	Reference	2 (18.2%)	Reference
Active + passive	109 (27.0%)	88 (25.5%)	0.90 (0.7–1.1)	4 (36.3%)	1.4 (0.9–2.5)
Active only	28 (6.9%)	19 (5.5%)	0.73 (0.4–1.2)	2 (18.2%)	2.7 (0.95–7.6)
Passive only	143 (35.5%)	120 (34.8%)	0.93 (0.8–1.1)	3 (27.3%)	0.8 (0.4–2.3)
Active or passive	171 (42.4%)	138 (40.1%)	0.91 (0.8–1.1)	5 (45.4%)	1.2 (0.7–1.9)
Girls					
Neither active nor passive tabagism	146 (41.2%)	145 (43.1%)	Reference	2 (14.3%)	Reference
Active + passive	66 (18.7%)	54 (17.2%)	0.87 (0.6–1.2)	6 (42.9%)	*2.40 (1.5–3.8)*
Active only	22 (6.1%)	11 (3.5%)	0.54 (0.3–1.1)	2 (14.3%)	*3.82 (1.3–10.9)*
Passive only	120 (33.9%)	113 (36.1%)	0.97 (0.9–1.2)	4 (28.6%)	1.48 (0.8–2.6)
Active or passive	142 (40.1%)	124 (39.7%)	0.93 (0.8–1.1)	8 (57.1%)	*1.62 (1.2–.2)*

Notes: CDH = chronic daily headaches (15 or more days of headache per month); OR (95% CI) = odds ratio and 95% confidence interval of the odds ratio.

When the CI does not include the number 1, the difference is significant and is illustrated by in italics.

In unadjusted analyses the two-sided chi-squared test was used.

From Arruda, M. A., Guidetti, V., Galli, F., Albuquerque, R. C., and Bigal, M. E. (2011). Prenatal exposure to tobacco and alcohol are associated with chronic daily headaches at childhood: A population-based study. *Arquivos de neuro-psiquiatria, 69*, 27–33.

CURRENT HEADACHE PAIN FEATURES AND ALLODYNIA AS RISK FACTORS FOR PROGRESSION

In both clinic and population studies, number of headache days at baseline is one of the most important risk factors for progression from EM into CM (Bigal, Serrano, et al., 2008; Castillo et al., 1999; Katsarava et al., 2004; Scher, Stewart, et al., 2003). Furthermore, the risk increases in a nonlinear manner with baseline headache frequency (Castillo et al., 1999; Scher, Stewart, et al., 2003). In the Frequent Headache Epidemiological Study, the risk of transformation in individuals that had a baseline frequency of less than 3 headache days per month was uniformly low but then rapidly increased for higher baseline frequencies (Scher, Stewart, et al., 2003). In clinic-based studies the risk of new-onset CM also increased rapidly with attack frequency (Katsarava et al., 2004). In the AMPP study, among persons with episodic migraine, baseline headache frequency was an important risk factor for progression to CM (Bigal, Serrano, et al., 2008).

There are several possible explanations for the longitudinal influence of headache frequency on the transition from EM to CM. Headache frequency may be a marker of headache evolution, that is, a consequence of a biological process and not the cause of the process that leads to CM. Alternatively, repetitive episodes of pain may lead to central sensitization and alteration in synaptic connectivity in areas or pathways that mediate or modulate pain. Repeated attacks may increase synaptic strength in the primary pain pathways or damage pain-modulating pathways, perhaps through the generation of free radicals (Welch et al., 2001). Lastly, as described in the section below, increased headache frequency may reflect an inherent predisposition to pain.

In this context, the role of cutaneous allodynia (CA) is of great interest. CA refers to the perception of pain after ordinarily nonpainful stimuli. Migraine patients with cutaneous allodynia report pain in response to innocuous stimuli including wearing a hat, earrings, or a necklace; taking a shower; or hair brushing. CA is a clinical marker of sensitization of the trigeminal pathways. Sensitization in the trigeminocervical complex produces allodynia in the distribution of the trigeminal nerve (Burstein & Jakubowski, 2004; Burstein et al., 2004). Extracephalic allodynia likely arises from sensitization of thalamic neurons (Burstein et al., 2010).

Clinic- and population-based studies show that about two thirds of migraine sufferers develop CA (Bigal, Ashina, et al., 2008; Burstein et al., 2000; Lipton et al., 2008; Selby & Lance, 1960). In the AMPP study, the population prevalence of CA was significantly higher in CM (68.3%) than in EM (63.2%; $p < .01$), and higher in both of these groups compared to persons with other headaches (Bigal, Ashina, et al., 2008; Lipton et al., 2008). The prevalence of severe CA followed the same pattern.

There are a number of risk factors for CA (Bigal, Ashina, et al., 2008). Nonmodifiable risk factors include male gender (prevalence ratio [PR] = 1.7, 95% CI: 1.55–1.82), African American race (PR = 1.14, 95% CI: 1.04–1.25), and decreased level of educational achievement (graduated vs. less than high school) (PR = 0.68, 95% CI: 0.55–0.83). Risk of CA increases with headache features including attack frequency, pain intensity, and headache-related disability. In addition, obesity and depression are also risk factors for allodynia (Bigal, Ashina, et al., 2008).

Increasing severity of allodynia, as measured by the Allodynia Symptom Checklist, is also associated with an increased risk of progression (Bigal, Ashina, et al., 2008; Lipton et al., 2008). Finally, in episodic migraine, allodynia is a phenomenon of the ictal state. In chronic migraine, allodynia may persist between attacks. In aggregate, these findings suggest that recurrent severe headaches lead to persistent sensitization and other alterations in nociceptive pathways. According to this hypothesis, repeated attacks of persistent pain may alter the threshold for activation of pain pathways (both primary pain pathways and modulatory pathways), potentially leading to a pain-prone state marked by cutaneous allodynia and sensitization.

SELECTED COMORBIDITIES AND CONCOMITANT ILLNESSES

Obesity

The link between obesity and the frequency of primary headaches has been demonstrated by several population studies. In the Frequent Headache Epidemiology Study, Scher et al. found that relative odds of CDH were five times higher in individuals with a BMI greater than 30 than in the normal weighted. Overweight individuals (BMI ranging from 25 to 29) had a threefold increased risk (Scher, Stewart, et al., 2003).

In the Baltimore County Migraine Study, BMI was associated with the frequency of headache attacks in migraineurs (Bigal et al., 2006). In the normal-weighted group, just 4.4% of migraine sufferers had 10 to 14 headache days per month. This increased to 5.8% of the overweight group (BMI: 25 to 29; OR = 1.3, 95% CI: 0.6–2.8), 13.6% of the obese (BMI: 30 to 34; OR = 2.9, 95% CI: 1.9–4.4), and 20.7% of the severely obese (BMI: 35+; OR = 5.7, 95% CI: 3.6–8.8). Obesity was not a risk factor for chronic tension-type headache; this specificity of association suggests a biological link between CM and obesity and not a general link to all headaches (Bigal & Lipton, 2006c). For CM, the prevalence ranged from 0.9% of the normal weighted (reference group) to 2.5% of the severely obese (OR = 2.2, 95% CI: 1.5–3.2) (Bigal & Lipton, 2006c). More recently, as part of the AMPP study, obesity was shown to be an exacerbating factor for migraine and not for headaches overall (Bigal, Tsang, et al., 2007).

Putative biological mechanisms that account for the obesity–migraine progression link have been proposed elsewhere (Bigal & Lipton, 2008c; Bigal, Lipton, et al., 2007). Briefly, several inflammatory mediators that are elevated in obese individuals are thought to be important in the pathophysiology of migraine. Migraine and obesity are prothrombotic states. Substances that are important in metabolic control (e.g., adiponectin) are nociceptive at lower levels. Hypothalamic dysfunction in the orexin pathways seems to be a risk factor for both conditions. Finally, metabolic syndrome and autonomic dysfunction may also participate in the obesity–migraine progression relationship (Bigal & Lipton, 2008c).

Snoring and Sleep Apnea

The relationship between headache progression and snoring has been studied. In a large, cross-sectional study of 3,323 Danish men, snoring was associated with any form of headache (Jennum & Sjol, 1992). The authors reported that this association was independent of weight, age, gender, hypertension, and other sleep disturbances, including secondary to caffeine consumption (Jennum & Sjol, 1992). In a separate population-based case-control study, CDH sufferers were more likely to be habitual or daily snorers than controls (Scher, Lipton, et al., 2003). Snoring remained a predictor of CDH after adjusting for obesity.

The mechanistic relationship of snoring and sleep apnea to headache progression is uncertain. Increased intracranial and arterial pressure fluctuations during snoring may contribute to pain progression. Alternatively, hypoxia, hypercapnia, sleep fragmentation, or increased muscle activity during awakenings could play a role.

Psychiatric Comorbidity and Stressful Life Events

In cross-sectional studies, the prevalence of depression and anxiety is higher in persons with migraine than in the general population (Breslau & Andreski, 1995). The prevalence of depression and anxiety is higher still in population studies of persons with chronic migraine than in persons with episodic migraine (Blumenfeld et al., 2011; Buse et al., 2010). In a cross-sectional study, persons with CM were more likely to have symptoms of depression (70% vs. 59%, $p = .062$) and anxiety (43% vs. 25%, $p = .005$) than persons with chronic tension-type headache (Karakurum et al., 2004; Zwart et al., 2003b).

The increased cross-sectional risk of depression and anxiety in persons with CM could arise in several ways. First, depression or anxiety could emerge as a consequence of increasing headache frequency. Second, depression or anxiety could be risk factors for migraine progression. Third, depression or anxiety could be associated with some other factor that drives the increased risk of CM (confounding). As a first step toward disentangling these possibilities, Ashina et al. analyzed data from the AMPP study and examined persons with EM who did and did not develop CM at follow-up (Ashina et al., 2011). They found that both depression and anxiety were risk factors for the progression of EM to CM and that increasing depression severity was associated with increased risk of new-onset CM after adjusting for many covariates (see Table 6–4). Because depression preceded the onset of CM and had a dose-dependent effect, after adjusting for confounders the authors suggested that depression is likely a risk factor for the onset of CM (Ashina et al., 2011).

The Frequent Headache Epidemiology Study assessed the role of major life events as risk factors for the new onset of CDH using a case-control design (Scher et al., 2008). Major life changes included change of residence, employment status, and marital status; changes related to their children; deaths of relatives or close friends; and "extremely stressful," ongoing situations. CDH cases were asked about events during the same year or the year before CDH onset. Controls were asked about the same events in an equivalent time period in the past. Events reported after the onset of CDH were considered subsequent events. Compared with episodic headache controls, CDH cases had more major life changes in the year before or same year. After adjusting for age, gender, headache type, and year of event, the odds of frequent headaches

increased additionally with each antecedent event (OR = 1.20, 95% CI: 1.1–1.3), but not with subsequent events (OR = 0.94, 95% CI: 0.8–1.1) (Scher et al., 2008). The specificity of association for events preceding but not following the onset of CDH supports a causal relationship.

Temporomandibular Disorders

The links between migraine and temporomandibular disorders (TMDs) have received recent attention (Bevilaqua-Grossi, Lipton, & Bigal, 2009). The term TMD includes a range of disorders characterized by alterations or dysfunction of the masticatory muscles, the temporomandibular joint (TMJ), and structures associated with it (Dworkin & LeResche, 1992). Because TMD produces both headache and face pain, this association is difficult to study.

Population studies show that headache is more common in persons with TMD than in persons free of TMD ($p = .000$). Treating the no-headache group as the reference, incremental TMD symptoms yielded increased relative odds of all other headaches (Table 6–3). When one and two symptoms of TMD were present, the magnitude of increase was higher in the CDH group, intermediate for migraine, and nonsignificant for episodic tension type headache (ETTH); when more than three symptoms were present, odds were significantly increased for all headache groups and numerically higher for migraine than for CDH, although the confidence intervals were broad. Medication overuse and magnitude of exposure increased chance of transitioning (Table 6–3).

In clinic-based studies, TMD is associated with allodynia (Bevilaqua-Grossi, Lipton, Napchan, et al., 2009). Rates and severity of allodynia were compared in individuals with episodic migraine and TMD, as assessed by research diagnostic criteria, and individuals with episodic migraine but not TMD. Allodynia was assessed in the two groups using the Allodynia Symptom Checklist (ASC-12). Individuals with TMD were more likely to have moderate or severe CA associated with their headaches. Interictally (quantitative sensory testing), thresholds for heat and mechanical nociception were significantly lower in individuals with TMD. TMDs were also associated with change in extracephalic pain thresholds. In logistical regression, TMD remained associated with CA after adjusting for aura, gender, and age (Bevilaqua-Grossi, Lipton, Napchan, 2009).

These findings are of interest, because CA is an important risk factor for migraine progression. As a proallodynic comorbidity, TMD is a candidate risk factor for the onset of CM in persons with EM.

TABLE 6–3 *Relative Risk of Headache Types as a Function of Number of Symptoms Suggestive of Temporomandibular Disorder*

Headache Type	No TMD	1 TMD Symptom N (%, OR [95% CI])	2 TMD Symptoms N (%, OR [95% CI])	≥ 3 TMD Symptoms N (%, OR [95% CI])
No Headache	489 (72.3%) Reference	120 (17.8%) Reference	39 (5.8%) Reference	28 (4.1%) Reference
Episodic tension-type headache	118 (59.0%, OR = 0.81 [0.77–0.92])	44 (22.0%, OR = 1.23 [0.9–1.7])	17 (8.5%, OR = 1.67 [0.95–1.98])	21 (10.5%, OR = 2.5 [1.4–4.3])
Migraine	100 (41.5%, OR = 0.57 [0.49–0.67])	61 (25.3%, OR = 1.192 [1.49–2.04])	27 (11.2%, OR = 2.8 [1.8–4.5])	51 (22.0%, OR = 6.2 [4.1–9.5])
Chronic daily headaches	11 (19.2%, OR = 0.26 [0.12–0.58])	13 (42.4%, OR = 2.38 [1.47–3.84])	6 (19.2%, OR = 4.8 [2.3–9.7])	3 (19.2%, OR = 4.0 [1.4–11.5])

Notes. TMD = temporomandibular disorder; OR = odds ratio; CI = confidence interval.
From Bevilaqua-Grossi, D., Lipton, R. B., & Bigal, M. E. (2009). Temporomandibular disorders and migraine chronification. *Current Pain and Headache Reports, 13*, 314–318.

OTHER RISK FACTORS

Excessive Symptomatic Medication Use

Symptomatic medication overuse (SMO) has long been associated with poor outcomes in persons with migraine (Goadsby, 2006). Several clinic-based studies suggest that medication overuse is a risk factor for headache transformation (Bahra et al., 2003; Katsarava et al., 2004; Paemeleire et al., 2008; Wilkinson et al., 2001; Williams et al., 2008). These studies suggest excessive use of analgesics for any reason (headache relief, relief of nonheadache pain, to control bowel movements) is associated with an increased risk for developing CM. In persons free of migraine, CDH rarely develops despite daily use of analgesics. These studies suggest a diathesis-stress model for the onset of CDH. Developing CDH is most likely in persons with a migraine diathesis exposed to the "stress" of medication overuse.

Several population studies also demonstrated that SMO is a risk factor for the new onset of CM in persons with EM (Table 6–3) (Bigal, Serrano, et al., 2008; Scher, Stewart, et al., 2003; Zwart et al., 2003a, 2004). As part of the American Migraine Prevalence and Prevention study, we studied factors that predict the new onset of CM after 1 year of follow-up in persons with EM (Bigal, Serrano, et al., 2008).

Persons with EM in 2005 who took barbiturate- or opioid-containing analgesics were twice as likely to develop CM in 2006 as persons who do not use these treatments (barbiturates OR = 2.06, 95% CI: 1.3–3.1; opiates OR = 1.98, 95% CI: 1.4–2.8) (Bigal, Serrano, et al., 2008). The other classes of medications did not significantly alter the odds of transformation.

Though barbiturates and opiates are used more commonly in persons who develop CM, that does not necessarily imply a causal effect. Perhaps these classes of medications are given to patients with severe disease and the use of drugs is an epiphenomenon. To address this issue, we ran a series of adjusted models including monthly headache days, preventive medication use, and headache severity and disability in the entire sample and in gender-defined subgroups. In these adjusted analyses, barbiturates (OR = 1.73, 95% CI: 1.1–2.7) and opiates (OR = 1.4, 95% CI: 1.1–2.1) remained significant predictors of the new onset of CM at follow-up. For both opiates and barbiturates a dose–response curve was demonstrated indicating that increasing days of use were associated with increased risk of CM onset (Goadsby, 2006). In the entire study population, those using triptans (OR = 1.05, 95% CI: 0.8–1.6) or nonsteroidal anti-inflammatory drugs (OR = 0.97, 95% CI: 0.7–1.34) were not at increased risk, though there are complex interactions with headache frequency and days of dosing. Results were similar for women and men, except that the risk of incident CM associated with use of opioids was higher in men (OR = 2.76) compared to women (OR = 1.28).

Odds of transition to CM increased with barbiturate exposure (OR = 1.25, 95% CI: 1.1–1.4), controlling for the effects of gender and monthly headache frequency. Risk seemed to increase at doses of 5 days per month and greater. The barbiturate effect was stronger in women. Findings were similar for opiates (OR = 1.44, 95% CI: 1.1–1.8). Risk seemed to increase at doses of 8 days per month or greater; opioid effects were more pronounced in men (Bigal, Serrano, et al., 2008).

Triptans did not increase the risk of CM (OR = 1.07, 95% CI: 0.89–1.29) overall, although they were associated with migraine progression in those with high frequency of migraine at baseline (10 to 14 days per month) (Bigal, Serrano, et al., 2008). Anti-inflammatory medications were protective in those with fewer than 10 days of headache at baseline and, as triptans, induced migraine progression in those with high frequency of headaches (Bigal, Serrano, et al., 2008).

Caffeine Overuse

The role of caffeine in migraine progression is potentially of great importance because caffeine is a very common dietary and medicinal exposure (Scher et al., 2004; Schonewille, 2002; Shapiro, 2008). The Frequent Headache Epidemiology Study included a case-control study of dietary and medicinal caffeine (Scher et al., 2004). In that study, individuals with episodic headache who developed chronic daily headache were more likely to be high caffeine consumers than the episodic headache sufferers who did not progress (OR = 1.50, p = .05) (Scher et al., 2004). Abrupt withdrawal of caffeine in individuals with chronic daily headaches is indeed associated with rebound headaches, further supporting the importance of this substance as a risk factor (Silverman et al., 1992).

Head and Neck Trauma

Head trauma has been linked to headaches in a number of ways. Head injury can cause de novo posttraumatic headache. In addition, trauma can be a migraine-exacerbating factor sometimes leading to CM. In the Frequent Headache Epidemiology Study, cases with CDH (≥180 headaches per year) and a comparison group with episodic headache (EH, 2 to 102 headaches per year) were identified from the general population. Subjects were asked about the occurrence of headache or neck injuries. Any headache or neck injury was associated with an increased risk of CDH. The attributable risk was 15%. The odds of CDH increased with the number of lifetime injuries in all groups (p < .05 trend) (Couch et al., 2007).

MULTIVARIATE MODELS AND CLINICAL IMPLICATIONS

A broad range of factors are associated with the transition from EM to CM (Ashina et al., 2011). Ashina et al. (2011) assessed the effects of risk factors in EM sufferers in 2005 for the onset of CM in 2006 as well as risk factors in 2006 that predicted migraine onset in 2007 (Ashina et al., 2011).

TABLE 6–4 *Risk Factors for the Transition from EM to CM: Results from AMPP (2005–2007)*

Predictive Factors	Model 1 OR (95% CI)	Model 2 OR (95% CI)	Model 3 OR (95% CI)	Model 4 OR (95% CI)
Age	0.99 (0.98–1.01)	1.00 (0.98–1.01)	1.00 (0.99–1.01)	1.00 (0.99–1.01)
Gender	0.75 (0.37–1.51)	0.93 (0.53–1.65)	0.92 (0.65–1.28)	0.92 (0.65–1.30)
Income	0.90 (0.74–1.09)	0.85 (0.72–1.00)*	0.85 (0.77–0.94)*	0.84 (0.76–0.93)*
Insurance	0.82 (0.41–1.61)	0.95 (0.54–1.69)	0.91 (0.65–1.27)	0.96 (0.68–1.34)
BMI (linear)	0.91 (0.80–1.04)	0.91 (0.81–1.03)	0.92 (0.87–0.97)*	0.92 (0.87–0.97)*
BMI (quadratic)	1.00 (1.00–1.00)	1.00 (1.00–1.00)	1.00 (1.00–1.00)*	1.00 (1.00–1.00)*
Cutaneous allodynia		1.63 (1.04–2.55)*	1.41 (1.08–1.83)*	1.49 (1.14–1.96)*
SRPD anxiety			1.53 (1.15–2.04)*	1.52 (1.13–2.03)*
Pain intensity (4+)				3.02 (0.96–9.47)
Depression (PHQ-9)	3.22 (1.65–6.25)*	2.35 (1.32–4.22)*	2.01 (1.42–2.85)*	2.08 (1.47–2.94)*

Notes.

* Indicates that data are significant at the p < .05 level or below.

Model 1: Adjusted for age (continuous), gender (binary, reference = male), income (linear trend in cumulative categories), health insurance status (binary, reference = uninsured), and body mass index (BMI; continuous and quadratic).

Model 2: Adjusted for cutaneous allodynia (binary, diagnosis defined as score ≥3).

Model 3: Adjusted for self-report of a physician diagnosis (SRPD) of anxiety (binary, with no SRPD anxiety endorsement as reference).

Model 4: Adjusted for headache pain intensity (binary, no/mild pain [scores 0–3] vs. combination of moderate [scores 4–6], moderately severe [scores 7–8], and severe [scores 9–10]).

Model 5: Adjusted for migraine symptom severity score (MSS) (continuous) and headache frequency (headache days per month).

Depression (PHQ-9) = dichotomous definition defined by a PHQ-9 cut-score ≥15.

From Ashina, S., Serrano, D., Lipton, R. B., et al. (2011). Depression is a risk factor for the new onset of chronic migraine. (Submitted).

Table 6–4 summarizes some of those analyses in a series of nested two-stage transition models. Model 1 shows that the demographic risk factors are not associated with an increased risk of progression, while depression is a powerful predictor of new-onset CM (OR = 3.22, 95% CI: 1.65–6.25). Model 2 shows that cutaneous allodynia is a significant predictor of CM onset and that with this adjustment, increasing household income becomes protective. In Model 3, after adding self-reported medical diagnosis of anxiety, anxiety itself is a predictor of CM onset. Finally, in Model 4, income is protective, while allodynia, anxiety, and depression are independent risk factors for new-onset CM.

Risk factors can be usefully divided into those at are remediable and those that are not. Nonremediable risk factors include gender, age, race, and head trauma. Remediable risk factors include headache frequency, depression, anxiety, obesity, and the overuse of barbiturate and opiate medications (Bigal & Lipton, 2006a, 2006b). Preliminary evidence suggests that weight loss following bariatric surgery is associated with a dramatic reduction in headache frequency (Bond et al., 2011). There are a number of preventive treatment options for migraine (Silberstein, 2010). Clinical trials indicate that CM responds with a reduction in attack frequency to preventive medications such as topiramate and onabotulinum toxin A (Dodick et al., 2009; Silberstein et al., 2009). There have been efforts to prevent the onset of CM in randomized trials (Lipton et al., 2011). As of yet, there is no evidence that modifying these risk factors will reduce the rate of CM onset. Nonetheless, reducing headache frequency, treating comorbidities, encouraging weight loss, and avoiding medication overuse are beneficial for many reasons. These strategies should improve patient outcomes on a short-term basis; their ability to improve long-term outcomes should be studied. Clinicians should aspire to help patients, not just by relieving current pain and disability, but also by avoiding migraine progression.

REFERENCES

Arruda, M. A., Guidetti, V., Galli, F., Albuquerque, R. C., & Bigal, M. E. (2010). Frequency of headache in children is influenced by headache status in the mother. *Headache, 50*(6), 973–980.

Arruda, M. A., Guidetti, V., Galli, F., et al. (2011). Prenatal exposure to tobacco and alcohol are associated with chronic daily headaches at childhood: A population-based study. *Arquivos de neuro-psiquiatria, 69,* 27–33.

Ashina, S., Serrano, D., Lipton, R. B., et al. (2011). Depression is a risk factor for the new onset of chronic migraine. *Cephalalgia.*

Bahra, A., Walsh, M., Menon, S., & Goadsby, P. J. (2003). Does chronic daily headache arise de novo in association with regular use of analgesics? *Headache, 43,* 179–190.

Bevilaqua-Grossi, D., Lipton, R. B., & Bigal, M. E. (2009). Temporomandibular disorders and migraine chronification. *Current Pain and Headache Reports, 13,* 314–318.

Bevilaqua-Grossi, D., Lipton, R. B., Napchan, U., Grosberg, B., Ashina, S., & Bigal, M. E. (2009). Temporomandibular disorders and cutaneous allodynia are associated in individuals with migraine. *Cephalalgia 30*(4), 425–432.

Bigal, M. E., Ashina, S., Burstein, R., et al. (2008). Prevalence and characteristics of allodynia in headache sufferers: A population study. *Neurology, 70,* 1525–1533

Bigal, M. E., Liberman, J. N., & Lipton, R. B. (2006). Obesity and migraine: A population study. *Neurology, 66,* 545–550.

Bigal, M. E., & Lipton, R. B. (2006a). Modifiable risk factors for migraine progression. *Headache, 46,* 1334–1343.

Bigal, M. E., & Lipton, R. B. (2006b). Modifiable risk factors for migraine progression (or for chronic daily headaches)—clinical lessons. *Headache, 46*(Suppl 3), S144–S146.

Bigal, M. E., & Lipton, R. B. (2006c). Obesity is a risk factor for transformed migraine but not chronic tension-type headache. *Neurology, 67,* 252–257.

Bigal, M. E., & Lipton, R. B. (2008a). Clinical course in migraine: Conceptualizing migraine transformation. *Neurology, 71,* 848–855.

Bigal, M. E., & Lipton, R. B. (2008b). The prognosis of migraine. *Current Opinion in Neurology, 21,* 301–308.

Bigal, M. E., & Lipton, R. B. (2008c). Putative mechanisms of the relationship between obesity and migraine progression. *Current Pain and Headache Reports, 12,* 207–212.

Bigal, M. E., Lipton, R. B., Holland, P. R., & Goadsby, P. J. (2007). Obesity, migraine, and chronic migraine: Possible mechanisms of interaction. *Neurology, 68,* 1851–1861.

Bigal, M. E., Serrano, D., Buse, D., et al. (2008). Acute migraine medications and evolution from episodic to chronic migraine: A longitudinal population-based study. *Headache, 48,* 1157–1168.

Bigal, M. E., Tsang, A., Loder, E., et al. (2007). Body mass index and episodic headaches: A population-based study. *Archives of Internal Medicine, 167,* 1964–1970.

Blumenfeld, A., Varon, S., Wilcox, T. K., et al. (2011). Disability, HRQoL and resource use among chronic and episodic migraineurs: Results from the International Burden of Migraine Study (IBMS). *Cephalalgia, 31,* 301–315.

Bond, D. S., Vithiananthan, S., Nash, J., et al. (2011). Improvement of migraine headaches in severely obese patients after bariatric surgery. *Neurology, 76,* 1135–1138.

Brent, R. L., Tanski, S., & Weitzman, M. (2004). A pediatric perspective on the unique vulnerability and resilience of the embryo and the child to environmental toxicants: The importance of rigorous research concerning age and agent. *Pediatrics, 113,* 935–944.

Breslau, N., & Andreski, P. (1995). Migraine, personality, and psychiatric comorbidity. *Headache, 35,* 382–386.

Buck, K. J., & Finn, D. A. (2001). Genetic factors in addiction: QTL mapping and candidate gene studies implicate GABAergic genes in alcohol and barbiturate withdrawal in mice. *Addiction, 96,* 139–149.

Burstein, R., Collins, B., & Jakubowski, M. (2004). Defeating migraine pain with triptans: A race against the development of cutaneous allodynia. *Annals of Neurology, 55,* 19–26.

Burstein, R., & Jakubowski, M. (2004). Analgesic triptan action in an animal model of intracranial pain: A race against the development of central sensitization. *Annals of Neurology, 55,* 27–36.

Burstein, R., Jakubowski, M., Garcia-Nicas, E., et al. (2010). Thalamic sensitization transforms localized pain into widespread allodynia. *Annals of Neurology, 68,* 8191.

Burstein, R., Yarnitsky, D., & Goor-Aryeh, I., et al. (2000). An association between migraine and cutaneous allodynia. *Annals of Neurology, 47,* 614–624.

Buse, D. C., Manack, A., Serrano, D., et al. (2010). Sociodemographic and comorbidity profiles of chronic migraine and episodic migraine sufferers. *Journal of Neurology, Neurosurgery, and Psychiatry, 81,* 428–432.

Buzzi, M. G., Cologno, D., & Formisano, R. (2005). Migraine disease: Evolution and progression. *Journal of Headache and Pain, 6,* 304–306.

Castillo, J., Munoz, P., Guitera, V., & Pascual, J. (1999). Kaplan Award 1998. Epidemiology of chronic daily headache in the general population. *Headache, 39,* 190–196.

Coppola, G., Vandenheede, M., Di Clemente, L., et al. (2005). Somatosensory evoked high-frequency oscillations reflecting thalamo-cortical activity are decreased in migraine patients between attacks. *Brain, 128,* 98–103.

Couch, J. R., Lipton, R. B., Stewart, W. F., & Scher, A. I. (2007). Head or neck injury increases the risk of chronic daily headache: A population-based study. *Neurology, 69,* 1169–1177.

Diatchenko, L., Nackley, A. G., Slade, G. D., et al. (2006). Catechol-O-methyltransferase gene polymorphisms are associated with multiple pain-evoking stimuli. *Pain, 125,* 216–224.

Di Clemente, L., Coppola, G., Magis, D., et al. (2007). Interictal habituation deficit of the nociceptive blink reflex: An endophenotypic marker for presymptomatic migraine? *Brain, 130,* 765–770.

Dodick, D. W. (2006). Clinical practice. Chronic daily headache. *New England Journal of Medicine, 354,* 158–165.

Dodick, D., Turkel, C. C., DeGryse, R. E., et al. (2009). Onabotulinum toxin A for the treatment of chronic migraine. *Headache, 49,* 1153–1162.

Dworkin, S. F., & LeResche, L. (1992). Research diagnostic criteria for temporomandibular disorders: Review, criteria, examinations and specifications, critique. *Journal of Craniomandibular Disorders, 6,* 301–355.

Goadsby, P. J. (2006). Is medication-overuse headache a distinct biological entity? *Nature Clinical Practice Neurology, 2,* 401.

Goldman, D., Oroszi, G., & Ducci, F. (2005). The genetics of addictions: Uncovering the genes. *Nature Reviews Genetics, 6,* 521–532.

Hagen, K., Einarsen, C., Zwart, J. A., et al. (2002). The co-occurrence of headache and musculoskeletal symptoms amongst 51 050 adults in Norway. *European Journal of Neurology, 9,* 527–533.

Handmaker, N. S., Rayburn, W. F., Meng, C., et al. (2006). Impact of alcohol exposure after pregnancy recognition on ultrasonographic fetal growth measures. *Alcoholism, Clinical and Experimental Research, 30,* 892–898.

Haut, S. R., Bigal, M. E., & Lipton, R. B. (2006). Chronic disorders with episodic manifestations: Focus on epilepsy and migraine. *Lancet Neurology, 5,* 148–157.

Jennum, P., & Sjol, A. (1992). Epidemiology of snoring and obstructive sleep apnoea in a Danish population, age 30-60. *Journal of Sleep Research, 1,* 240–244.

Karakurum, B., Soylu, O., Karatas, M., et al. (2004). Personality, depression, and anxiety as risk factors for chronic migraine. *International Journal of Neuroscience, 114,* 1391–1399.

Katsarava, Z., Schneeweiss, S., Kurth, T., et al. (2004). Incidence and predictors for chronicity of headache in patients with episodic migraine. *Neurology, 62,* 788–790.

Kelman, L. (2007). A clinical study of migraine evolution. *Headache, 47,* 1228–1229; author reply 1229.

Kruit, M. C., van Buchem, M. A., Hofman, P. A., et al. (2004). Migraine as a risk factor for subclinical brain lesions. *Journal of the American Medical Association, 291,* 427–434.

Lemos, C., Castro, M. J., Barros, J., et al. (2009). Familial clustering of migraine: Further evidence from a Portuguese study. *Headache, 49,* 404–411.

Lipton, R. B., & Bigal, M. E. (2005). Migraine: Epidemiology, impact, and risk factors for progression. *Headache, 45*(Suppl 1), S3–S13.

Lipton, R. B., Bigal, M. E., Ashina, S., et al. (2008). Cutaneous allodynia in the migraine population. *Annals of Neurology, 63,* 148–158.

Lipton, R. B., Hemelsky, S. W., Kolodner, K. N., et al. (2000). Migraine, quality of life and depression. A population-based case-control study. *Neurology, 55,* 629–635.

Lipton, R. B., Silberstein, S. D., Dodick, D., et al. (2011). Topiramate intervention to prevent transformation of episodic migraine: The topiramate INTREPID study. *Cephalalgia, 31,* 18–30.

Manack, A. N., Buse, D. C., & Lipton, R. B. (2011). Chronic migraine: Epidemiology and disease burden. *Current Pain and Headache Reports, 15,* 70–78.

Manack, A., Turkel, C., & Silberstein, S. (2009). The evolution of chronic migraine: Classification and nomenclature. *Headache, 49,* 1206–1213.

Max, M. B., Wu, T., Atlas, S. J., et al. (2006). A clinical genetic method to identify mechanisms by which pain causes depression and anxiety. *Molecular Pain, 2,* 14.

May, A. (2009). New insights into headache: Update based on functional and structural migraine findings. *Nature Reviews Neurology, 5*(4), 199–209.

Nachit-Ouinekh, F., Dartigues, J. F., Chrysostome, V., et al. (2005). Evolution of migraine after a 10-year follow-up. *Headache, 45,* 1280–1287.

Nackley, A. G., Tan, K. S., Fecho, K., et al. (2007). Catechol-O-methyltransferase inhibition increases pain sensitivity through activation of both beta2- and beta3-adrenergic receptors. *Pain, 128,* 199–208.

Olesen, J., Bousser, M. D., Diener, H. C., et al. (2006). New appendix criteria open for a broader concept of chronic migraine. *Cephalalgia, 26,* 742–746.

Paemeleire, K., Evers, S., & Goadsby, P. J. (2008). Medication-overuse headache in patients with cluster headache. *Current Pain and Headache Reports, 12,* 122–127.

Pryse-Phillips, W., Aube, M., Bailey, P., et al. (2006). A clinical study of migraine evolution. *Headache, 46,* 1480–1486.

Rueda-Sanchez, M., & Diaz-Martinez, L. A. (2008). Prevalence and associated factors for episodic and chronic daily headache in the Colombian population. *Cephalalgia, 28,* 216–225.

Russell, M. B., & Olesen, J. (1996). Migrainous disorder and its relation to migraine without aura and migraine with aura. A genetic epidemiological study. *Cephalalgia, 16,* 431–435.

Scher, A. I., Lipton, R. B., & Stewart, W. F. (2003). Habitual snoring as a risk factor for chronic daily headache. *Neurology, 60,* 1366–1368.

Scher, A. I., Stewart, W. F., Buse, D., et al. (2008). Major life changes before and after the onset of chronic daily headache: A population-based study. *Cephalalgia, 28,* 868–876.

Scher, A. I., Stewart, W. F., & Lipton, R. B. (2004). Caffeine as a risk factor for chronic daily headache: A population-based study. *Neurology, 63,* 2022–2027.

Scher, A. I., Stewart, W. F., Ricci, J. A., & Lipton, R. B. (2003). Factors associated with the onset and remission of chronic daily headache in a population-based study. *Pain, 106*, 81–89.

Schonewille, W. J. (2002). [Chronic daily headaches caused by too much caffeine]. *Nederlands tijdschrift voor geneeskunde, 146*, 1861–1863.

Selby, G., & Lance, J. W. (1960). Observations on 500 cases of migraine and allied vascular headache. *Journal of Neurology, Neurosurgery, and Psychiatry, 23*, 23–32.

Shapiro, R. E. (2008). Caffeine and headaches. *Current Pain and Headache Reports, 12*, 311–315.

Shumilla, J. A., Sweitzer, S. M., & Kendig, J. J. (2004). Acute and chronic ethanol exacerbates formalin pain in neonatal rats. *Neuroscience Letters, 367*, 29–33.

Silberstein, S. D. (2010). Migraine preventive treatment. *Handbook of Neurology, 97*, 337–354.

Silberstein, S. D., Lipton, R. B., Dodick, D., et al. (2009). Topiramate treatment of chronic migraine. *Headache, 97*, 337–354.

Silverman, K., Evans, S. M., Strain, E. C., & Griffiths, R. R. (1992). Withdrawal syndrome after the double-blind cessation of caffeine consumption. *New England Journal of Medicine, 327*, 1109–1114.

Slotkin, T. A. (1998). Fetal nicotine or cocaine exposure: Which one is worse? *Journal of Pharmacology and Experimental Therapeutics, 285*, 931–945.

Stewart, W. F., Bigal, M. E., Kolodner, K., et al. (2006). Familial risk of migraine: Variation by proband age at onset and headache severity. *Neurology, 66*, 344–348.

Stewart, W. F., Staffa, J., Lipton, R. B., & Ottman, R. (1997). Familial risk of migraine: A population-based study. *Annals of Neurology, 41*, 166–172.

Terwindt, G. M., Ferrari, M. D., Tijhuis, M., et al. (2000). The impact of migraine on quality of life in the general population. The GEM Study. *Neurology, 55*, 624–629.

Uhl, G. R. (2006). Molecular genetics of addiction vulnerability. *NeuroRx, 3*, 295–301.

Ulrich, V., Gervil, M., Fenger, K., et al. (1999). The prevalence and characteristics of migraine in twins from the general population. *Headache, 39*, 173–180.

Welch, K. M., Nagesh, V., Aurora, S. K., & Gelman, N. (2001). Periaqueductal gray matter dysfunction in migraine: Cause or the burden of illness? *Headache, 41*, 629–637.

Wilkinson, S. M., Becker, W. J., & Heine, J. A. (2001). Opiate use to control bowel motility may induce chronic daily headache in patients with migraine. *Headache, 41*, 303–309.

Williams, L., O'Connell, K., & Tubridy, N. (2008). Headaches in a rheumatology clinic: When one pain leads to another. *European Journal of Neurology, 15*, 274–277.

Zwart, J. A., Dyb, G., Hagen, K., et al. (2003a). Analgesic use: A predictor of chronic pain and medication overuse headache: the Head-HUNT Study. *Neurology, 61*, 160–164.

Zwart, J. A., Dyb, G., Hagen, K., et al. (2003b). Depression and anxiety disorders associated with headache frequency. The Nord-Trondelag Health Study. *European Journal of Neurology, 10*, 147–152.

Zwart, J. A., Dyb, G., Hagen, K., et al. (2004). Analgesic overuse among subjects with headache, neck, and low-back pain. *Neurology, 62*, 1540–1544.

7 Concomitant Symptoms in Migraine

ARNE MAY AND ANNE STANKEWITZ

INTRODUCTION

Migraine is a complex neurological disease that manifests itself as recurrent attacks. The predominant symptom is a unilateral head pain, usually described as throbbing or pounding. And in fact, most imaging studies in migraine have investigated the headache (May, 2009b). However, a migraine attack is more than just head pain; patients are suffering from various symptoms including nausea and increased sensitivity to sensory stimuli (Kelman, 2004; Kelman & Tanis, 2006). In this chapter we focus on three sensory systems that are hyperexcitable in the migraine state: photophobia, phonophobia, and osmophobia. As such, they represent the underpinnings of a hyperexcitable state. Photophobia, phonophobia, and osmophobia occurring during attacks are so prominent in the clinical picture that they are recognized as diagnostic criteria for migraine (Headache Classification Committee of the International Headache Society, 2004). Consequently, patients usually prefer to lie in a quiet and dark room, avoiding strong sensory input during the acute attacks.

Between attacks, many patients describe themselves as being hypersensitive to sensory input, including bright or flickering light, loud sounds, and strong odors (Friedman & De ver Dye, 2009). In addition, some patients report that repetitively applied sensory stimulation (e.g., flickering light or intensive odors such as smelling perfume) is, in principle, able to trigger acute migraine attacks (Fukui et al., 2008). In sum, these symptoms point to a general alteration of sensory processing in migraine patients independently from the migraine attack. It also raises the question whether migraine-related symptoms (head pain, phobic symptoms, and other clinical phenomena including allodynia, nausea, and vomiting) occur independently or whether they are functionally linked to each other.

In the past, sensory information processing has been investigated in a large number of electrophysiological studies mainly using evoked (EPs) and event-related potentials (ERPs) and noninvasive brain stimulation techniques such as transcranial magnetic stimulation (Ambrosini et al., 2003). A loss of habituation for various sensory modalities (visual, auditory, and nociceptive stimuli) has been observed in migraineurs during their pain-free period but not during acute attacks. Just before the onset of head pain, the response pattern of migraine patients normalizes (Siniatchkin et al., 2006). By contrast, healthy control subjects showed a gradual decrease of their response pattern during the stimulation session, pointing to habituation behavior (Coppola et al., 2009). Furthermore, several studies demonstrated altered sensory thresholds in migraine patients. However, ambiguous results have been reported in the literature: Some authors described increased, others decreased thresholds for phosphenes, odors, sounds, and heat perception, whereas other authors did not find any difference between migraine patients and unaffected controls (Ambrosini et al., 2003; Antal et al., 2006; Aurora et al., 2003; Sand et al., 2008). Thus, altered sensory information processing seems to be very specific for the pathophysiology of migraine disease. The underlying neuronal mechanisms are, however, not completely understood (Stankewitz & May, 2009). There is an ongoing controversial debate about whether migraineurs' brains are hyperexcitable (Aurora et al., 1998, 2007) or hyporesponsive (Coppola et al., 2007).

Compared to electrophysiological studies, there are only a few imaging studies available in the current literature focusing on sensory pathways in migraineurs. Most of these studies focused on pain processing. Other migraine-related symptoms have been only sparsely explored (May, 2009a, 2009b).

The first imaging study exploring pathogen mechanisms of migraine disease used positron emission tomography (PET) (Weiller et al., 1995). The main finding was that a part of the brainstem showed migraine attack–specific activity. Increased regional cerebral blood flow (rCBF) was seen in the rostral pons in migraine patients during spontaneous headache attacks, persisting after pain relief reached by taking a triptan. This finding could be replicated by later PET studies (Denuelle et al., 2007) and recently, increased activity in the pons during attacks was also seen during a functional magnetic resonance imaging (fMRI) experiment applying trigeminal pain stimuli (Stankewitz et al., 2011). The rostral part of the pons has been coined the "migraine generator," and this structure has been dominantly discussed in the literature as being the main central structure involved in the pathogenesis of migraine. However, dysfunctions of other brainstem parts have also been found in migraine. Moulton et al. (2008) found decreased activity in brainstem nuclei probably involved in inhibitory circuits during pain stimulation in interictal migraineurs compared to control subjects. Furthermore, it has been recently shown that the spinal trigeminal nuclei are mainly involved in generating an acute attack during the pain-free disease interval (Stankewitz & May, 2011; Stankewitz et al., 2011).

Thus, brainstem nuclei involved in pain transmitting and in the endogenous pain control system seem to be crucially involved in the pathogenesis of migraine, a syndrome that has been traditionally seen as a vascular disorder. Following the pioneering work by the Essen group (Weiller et al., 1995), imaging studies focused their interest almost completely on brainstem findings (see Chapter 15). Significantly less attention has been paid to cortical neuronal systems. During migraine, increased rCBF was detected in several cortical regions, including the cingulate, temporal, and occipital cortices, most likely reflecting phobic symptoms to sounds and visual input during attacks (Weiller et al., 1995), but these findings were not in the focus of interest. In the last years, some studies were performed to specifically address sensory processing and phobic symptoms in migraine patients, and some studies even explored the interrelationship between sensory input and pain processing during the ictal state.

PHOTOPHOBIA

Regarding concomitant migraine symptoms, most of the available imaging studies explored the visual system in migraineurs. Especially the aura phase, occurring in one third of migraine patients before head pain starts, has been studied using imaging techniques (see Chapter 24). There are three distinct definitions of photophobia in the literature: abnormal sensitivity to light, ocular discomfort caused by light exposure, and exacerbation of headache by light (for review see Noseda & Burstein, 2010). Recently, some authors specifically focused their interest on photophobia in migraine patients. Using H_2O^{15} PET, Boulloche et al. (2010) observed increased rCBF in the occipital lobe in seven interictal migraineurs but not in control subjects during luminous stimulation. The authors used three luminance intensities—0, 600, and 1800 Cd/m²—and because the stimulations were started 30 seconds before

PET acquisitions, the activation in the visual system should have had habituated already (see Fig. 7–1). The authors showed that this indeed has happened, but only in the healthy controls and not in the migraine patients. This behavior was interpreted as a loss of habituation in the visual system of migraineurs. In a very elegant design, the authors then applied the above-mentioned light intensities both with and without concomitant trigeminal pain stimulation using a thermode and heat as a nociceptive input on the forehead. Concomitant trigeminal pain stimulation resulted in de novo visual cortex activation in the control group but potentiated the activity in the visual system in migraineurs. The authors suggested that migraineurs exhibit a lack of habituation and/or cortical hyperexcitability to light. Moreover, as the activation by light of several visual cortex areas was potentiated by trigeminal pain, they have convincingly demonstrated multisensory integration in these areas. This interaction may be specific to the ophthalmic territory of trigeminal nerve nociception and may be one interpretation to explain the photophobia in migraine headache.

The same group further observed that luminous stimulation activated the visual cortex during spontaneous migraine attacks and after the head pain was treated but not during the pain-free disease interval (Boulloche et al., 2010; Denuelle et al., 2011). Low luminous stimulation (median of 240 Cd/m²) activated the visual cortex statistically more strongly during migraine headache than after pain relief. These findings suggest that ictal photophobia is linked with a visual cortex hyperexcitability. It is quite interesting that this activation, interpreted as cortical hyperexcitability, persisted after headache relief, which means that the mechanism behind this phenomenon could not be solely explained by trigeminal nociception. Dysfunctions of brainstem nuclei responsible for cortical alterations in migraine patients have been postulated from the authors. The authors suggested that two independent systems are candidates for influencing cortical responsiveness: one in relation to the migraine attack including the preictal and postictal periods possibly modulated by brainstem nuclei, and the other dependent on trigeminal nociception (Boulloche et al., 2010; Denuelle et al., 2011). This hypothesis would in fact explain why visual cortex hyperresponsiveness is maximal during the migraine headache and why many patients describe themselves as being hypersensitive against bright or flickering lights even outside of the attack (Friedman & De ver Dye, 2009).

The possible anatomical pathway that underlies exacerbation of migraine headache by light that has been reported in a rodent model was also recently elucidated in

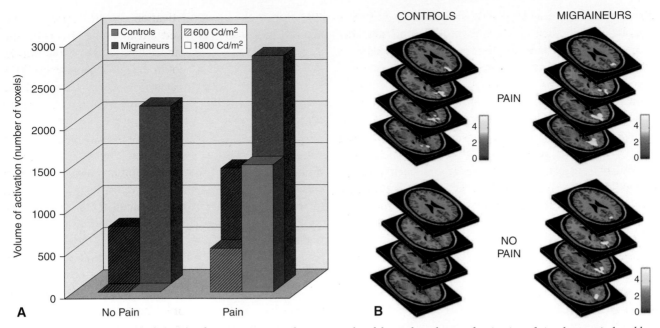

FIGURE 7–1 *(A) Activations by light. This figure summarizes the main results of the study: volumes of activation of visual cortex induced by light in both groups (purple, migraineurs; blue, controls) as a function of pain conditions (No Pain, Pain) in both light intensities (diagonal boxes, 600 Cd/m2; open boxes, 1,800 Cd/m2). (B) Activations by light at 1,800 Cd/m²: axial cross-sections at z = 0, z = 8, z = 16, and z = 24. Activations were in the cuneus, lingual gyrus, posterior cingulate cortex, and precuneus. Note that the volume of activation is greater in migraineurs. From Boulloche, N., Denuelle, M., Payoux, P., Fabre, N., Trotter, Y., & Geraud, G. (2010). Photophobia in migraine: An interictal PET study of cortical hyperexcitability and its modulation by pain. Journal of Neurology,* Neurosurgery, and Psychiatry, 81(9), 978–984.

the human brain using diffusion-weighted imaging and probabilistic tractography (Maleki et al., 2012). The authors found image-forming visual pathways from the optic nerve to the lateral geniculate and from there to the visual cortex as well as from the optic chiasm to the pulvinar, and from the pulvinar to several associative cortical brain regions. These pathways may allow photic signals to converge on a thalamic region, which was recently described to be selectively activated during migraine headache (Burstein et al., 2010). Consistent with physiological and anatomical studies in rats, the data provide an anatomical substrate for exacerbation of migraine headache by light in the human (Maleki et al., 2012). The heightened sensitivity to light during migraine may thus be mediated by convergence of nociceptive signals on visual pathways (Noseda & Burstein, 2010). This is further underlined by findings that exacerbation of migraine headache by light is prevalent among blind individuals who maintain non-image-forming photoregulation, a finding that together with animal data pointed toward the modulating effects of dura-sensitive thalamocortical nuclei in photoregulation (Noseda et al., 2011).

PHONOPHOBIA

While the visual system in migraine patients has recently been repeatedly studied, only small attention has been paid to phonophobia. Only one study described cortical activations that were interpreted as correlates of phonophobia (Weiller et al., 1995), but these findings were neither discussed in detail nor replicated in other imaging studies of migraine (May, 2009b). Several electrophysiological studies are available demonstrating cortical sensitization in response to auditory stimuli and decreased thresholds to sounds (Ambrosini et al., 2003). By contrast, not a single imaging study focused on phonophobia in migraine patients. A recent psychophysical study explored whether there is a relationship between phonophobia and aversion to the skin (cutaneous allodynia) in migraine patients (Ashkenazi et al., 2010). The data demonstrated a significant association between sound aversion thresholds and cutaneous allodynia: Allodynic patients showed lower thresholds compared to nonallodynic patients during their pain-free period. During attacks, the same pattern was observed but pronounced. Given that recently some imaging studies regarding allodynia in migraine pain have been published (Burstein et al., 2010; Moulton et al., 2011), further studies using neuroimaging methods investigating the link between allodynia and phonophobia are clearly warranted (Ashkenazi et al., 2009). If such studies are conducted, probably PET is a better choice than MRI, given the inherent noise of MRI scanners.

OSMOPHOBIA

The term *osmophobia* refers to an unpleasant or unusually intense perception of odors during an acute migraine attack that are nonaversive or even pleasurable between attacks. The olfactory system plays a pivotal role in migraine, documented by altered odor thresholds (Snyder & Drummond, 1997), hypersensitivity to odors between attacks (Demarquay et al., 2008), odor-triggered headache (Kelman, 2004), and distinct osmophobia during the headache attack (Corletto et al., 2008; Wober et al., 2007). However, perhaps due to methodological challenges, olfaction in migraine patients has received little attention so far. An early PET study investigated the activation pattern during olfactory stimulation in interictal migraine patients who reported themselves as being hypersensitive to odors during but also between migraine attacks (Demarquay et al., 2008). The authors found that migraineurs showed increased activity in the piriform cortex and the temporal gyrus as well as in the temporal pole compared to control subjects. By contrast, lower activation has been observed in frontal and temporoparietal regions, in the posterior cingulate cortex, and in the locus coeruleus. These findings have been discussed in the light of altered top-down processes in migraine patients (Demarquay et al., 2008).

Altered processing of olfactory input in migraine patients has also recently been observed using fMRI (Stankewitz & May, 2011). This study investigated cortical processes in response to event-related olfactory stimuli in migraineurs during and outside attacks using fMRI. We chose rose odor (a pure olfactory stimulus) to exclusively stimulate the olfactory nerve using a custom-built olfactometer (Stankewitz et al., 2009). We found that the piriform cortex and the amygdala were significantly activated in both groups. These structures belong to the primary olfactory cortex (Brand et al., 2001; Shipley & Ennis, 1996), receiving direct sensory input from the olfactory bulb. Increased activity was also observed bilaterally in the hippocampus in both groups. The piriform cortex, the amygdala, and the hippocampus are mainly involved in

encoding higher order representations of odor quality, identity, and familiarity and are associated with the learning and remembering of odors, as well as coordinating information between olfaction, vision, and taste (Dade et al., 2002; Gottfried et al., 2006; Howard et al., 2009). Amygdala activity has been specifically linked to intensity coding in both pleasant and unpleasant odors (Anderson et al., 2003; Royet et al., 2000; Zald & Pardo, 1997). Our data also revealed increased activity in the orbitofrontal and insular cortices (as part of the secondary olfactory cortex; Brand et al., 2001) and the caudate nucleus during olfactory processing in interictal migraine patients and controls (see Fig. 7–2). The above-named PET study (Demarquay et al., 2008) exclusively included migraine patients who reported being hypersensitive to odors at all times (i.e., interictally as well), and the findings may therefore not be migraine specific. In the fMRI study, we included migraine patients both with and without aura while ignoring any specific exclusion criteria regarding sensitivity to odors or trigger factors (Stankewitz & May, 2011). Comparing patients during the acute spontaneous headache attack with their own interictal data revealed significantly higher blood oxygenation level–dependent (BOLD) responses in the amygdala and in the insular cortex as well as in the temporal pole and the superior temporal gyrus during the attack. These findings may point to an increased sensitivity in migraineurs to odor stimuli during the headache attack compared to the interictal state. In addition to these activations in odor-specific limbic structures (Kim et al., 2010), significantly increased activity in the rostral part of the pons during the acute migraine attack compared to outside of migraine was found as well (see Fig. 7–3). The relevance of this structure for the migraine attack was demonstrated for the first time using PET during spontaneous attacks (Weiller et al., 1995) and has subsequently been replicated using both PET (Afridi et al., 2005; Denuelle et al., 2007) and fMRI (Stankewitz et al., 2011). However, it is still under debate whether this structure acts as a generator or whether other structures modulate its activity. The finding that the rostral part of the pons is activated by nociceptive (Stankewitz et al., 2011) but also by olfactory (Stankewitz & May, 2011) input suggests that this area is not exclusively "generating" migraine attacks but is at least further involved in sensory processing during attacks.

Taken together, a network of olfactory-related brain areas that are active in response to olfactory stimulation using rose odor can be identified. There appears to be no significant difference between interictal migraineurs and controls, neither in behavioral ratings of odor perception

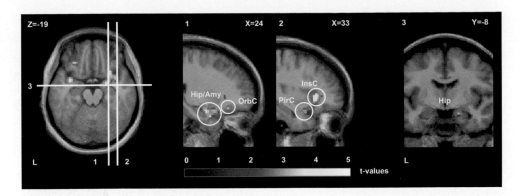

FIGURE 7–2 *Activation pattern during olfactory input in both groups. Shared activation pattern of interictal migraineurs and healthy controls (conjunction) in response to olfactory stimulation (odor > air puffs). Blood oxygenation level–dependent (BOLD) signal changes were detected in several odor-processing areas including the amygdala (Amy), the hippocampus (Hip), and the insular (InsC), piriform (PirC), and orbitofrontal cortices (OrbC). Activation maps were overlaid onto the averaged template of high-resolution structural images of healthy controls and migraine patients. For visualization purposes the threshold was set to p < .005 uncorrected; cluster size > 5 voxel; L = left side. The x, y, and z values represent the sagittal (x), coronal (y), and axial (z) level of the respective MNI coordinates. From Stankewitz, A., & May, A. (2011). Increased limbic and brainstem activity during spontaneous migraine attacks following olfactory stimulation. Neurology, 77 (5), 476–482.*

nor in imaging data. However, olfactory processing is altered during acute head pain in migraine patients, pointing to a functional link between the olfactory and trigeminal nociceptive system. As we have only assessed intensity ratings, it may well be that investigating the valence of the odor stimulus would have yielded different results. Future studies are necessary to shed light on specific neuronal connections between the olfactory and trigeminal nociceptive system.

CONCLUSIONS

It is certainly important to better understand the point of origin and role of concomitant symptoms in migraine. Despite the promising results of recent functional imaging studies, we still lack a substantial amount of knowledge regarding the underlying morphological substrate, the exact time course, and the relation of concomitant symptoms to headache in migraine. Future research faces

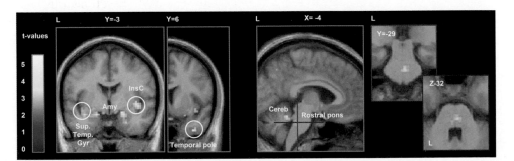

FIGURE 7–3 *Increased activation during an acute headache attack in response to olfactory stimulation. Migraine patients scanned during head pain (n = 13) showed an increased activation level in the amygdala (Amy), insular cortex (InsC), temporal pole, superior temporal gyrus (Sup. Temp. Gyr.), rostral pons, and cerebellum (Cereb) compared to their own data outside migraine attacks (n = 13). Activation maps were overlaid onto the averaged template of high-resolution structural images of healthy controls and migraine patients. For visualization threshold, the statistical threshold was set to p < .005 uncorrected; cluster size > 5 voxel; L = left side. The x, y, and z values represent the sagittal (x), coronal (y), and axial (z) level of the respective MNI coordinates. From Stankewitz, A., & May, A. (2011). Increased limbic and brainstem activity during spontaneous migraine attacks following olfactory stimulation. Neurology, 77 (5), 476–482.*

the challenge of revealing the anatomical and physiological bases of photophobia, phonophobia, and osmophobia (not to mention nausea) and adopting this knowledge for a better understanding of treatment strategies of these symptoms.

REFERENCES

Afridi, S. K., Matharu, M. S., Lee, L., Kaube, H., Friston, K. J., Frackowiak, R. S., et al. (2005). A PET study exploring the laterality of brainstem activation in migraine using glyceryl trinitrate. *Brain, 128*(Pt 4), 932–939.

Ambrosini, A., Rossi, P., De Pasqua, V., Pierelli, F., & Schoenen, J. (2003). Lack of habituation causes high intensity dependence of auditory evoked cortical potentials in migraine. *Brain, 126*(Pt 9), 2009–2015.

Anderson, A. K., Christoff, K., Stappen, I., Panitz, D., Ghahremani, D. G., Glover, G., et al. (2003). Dissociated neural representations of intensity and valence in human olfaction. *Nature Neuroscience, 6*(2), 196–202.

Antal, A., Arlt, S., Nitsche, M. A., Chadaide, Z., & Paulus, W. (2006). Higher variability of phosphene thresholds in migraineurs than in controls: A consecutive transcranial magnetic stimulation study. *Cephalalgia, 26*(7), 865–870.

Ashkenazi, A., Mushtaq, A., Yang, I., & Oshinsky, M. L. (2009). Ictal and interictal phonophobia in migraine-a quantitative controlled study. *Cephalalgia, 29*(10), 1042–1048.

Ashkenazi, A., Yang, I., Mushtaq, A., & Oshinsky, M. L. (2010). Is phonophobia associated with cutaneous allodynia in migraine? *Journal of Neurology, Neurosurgery, and Psychiatry, 81*(11), 1256–1260.

Aurora, S. K., Ahmad, B. K., Welch, K. M., Bhardhwaj, P., & Ramadan, N. M. (1998). Transcranial magnetic stimulation confirms hyperexcitability of occipital cortex in migraine. *Neurology, 50*(4), 1111–1114.

Aurora, S. K., Barrodale, P. M., Tipton, R. L., & Khodavirdi, A. (2007). Brainstem dysfunction in chronic migraine as evidenced by neurophysiological and positron emission tomography studies. *Headache, 47*(7), 996–1003; discussion 1004–1007.

Aurora, S. K., Welch, K. M., & Al-Sayed, F. (2003). The threshold for phosphenes is lower in migraine. *Cephalalgia, 23*(4), 258–263.

Boulloche, N., Denuelle, M., Payoux, P., Fabre, N., Trotter, Y., & Geraud, G. (2010). Photophobia in migraine: An interictal PET study of cortical hyperexcitability and its modulation by pain. *Journal of Neurology, Neurosurgery, and Psychiatry, 81*(9), 978–984.

Brand, G., Millot, J. L., & Henquell, D. (2001). Complexity of olfactory lateralization processes revealed by functional imaging: A review. *Neuroscience and Biobehavioral Reviews, 25*(2), 159–166.

Burstein, R., Jakubowski, M., Garcia-Nicas, E., Kainz, V., Bajwa, Z., Hargreaves, R., et al. (2010). Thalamic sensitization transforms localized pain into widespread allodynia. *Annals of Neurology, 68*(1), 81–91.

Coppola, G., Pierelli, F., & Schoenen, J. (2007). Is the cerebral cortex hyperexcitable or hyperresponsive in migraine? *Cephalalgia, 27*(12), 1427–1439.

Coppola, G., Pierelli, F., & Schoenen, J. (2009). Habituation and migraine. *Neurobiology of Learning and Memory. 92*(2), 249–259.

Corletto, E., Dal Zotto, L., Resos, A., Tripoli, E., Zanchin, G., Bulfoni, C., et al. (2008). Osmophobia in juvenile primary headaches. *Cephalalgia, 28*(8), 825–831.

Dade, L. A., Zatorre, R. J., & Jones-Gotman, M. (2002). Olfactory learning: Convergent findings from lesion and brain imaging studies in humans. *Brain, 125*(Pt 1), 86–101.

Demarquay, G., Royet, J. P., Mick, G., & Ryvlin, P. (2008). Olfactory hypersensitivity in migraineurs: A H(2)(15)O-PET study. *Cephalalgia, 28*(10), 1069–1080.

Denuelle, M., Boulloche, N., Payoux, P., Fabre, N., Trotter, Y., & Geraud, G. (2011). A PET study of photophobia during spontaneous migraine attacks. *Neurology, 76*(3), 213–218.

Denuelle, M., Fabre, N., Payoux, P., Chollet, F., & Geraud, G. (2007). Hypothalamic activation in spontaneous migraine attacks. *Headache, 47*(10), 1418–1426.

Friedman, D. I., & De ver Dye, T. (2009). Migraine and the environment. *Headache, 49*(6), 941–952.

Fukui, P. T., Goncalves, T. R., Strabelli, C. G., Lucchino, N. M., Matos, F. C., Santos, J. P., et al. (2008). Trigger factors in migraine patients. *Arquivos de neuro-psiquiatria, 66*(3A), 494–499.

Gottfried, J. A., Winston, J. S., & Dolan, R. J. (2006). Dissociable codes of odor quality and odorant structure in human piriform cortex. *Neuron, 49*(3), 467–479.

Headache Classification Committee of the International Headache Society. (2004). The international classification of headache disorders, 2nd edition. *Cephalalgia, 24*(Suppl 1), 1–160.

Howard, J. D., Plailly, J., Grueschow, M., Haynes, J. D., & Gottfried, J. A. (2009). Odor quality coding and categorization in human posterior piriform cortex. *Nature Neuroscience, 12*(7), 932–938.

Kelman, L. (2004). Osmophobia and taste abnormality in migraineurs: A tertiary care study. *Headache, 44*(10), 1019–1023.

Kelman, L., & Tanis, D. (2006). The relationship between migraine pain and other associated symptoms. *Cephalalgia, 26*, 548–553.

Kim, J. H., Kim, S., Suh, S. I., Koh, S. B., Park, K. W., & Oh, K. (2010). Interictal metabolic changes in episodic migraine: A voxel-based FDG-PET study. *Cephalalgia, 30*(1), 53–61.

Maleki, N., Becerra, L., Upadhyay, J., Burstein, R., & Borsook, D. (2012). Direct optic nerve pulvinar connections defined by diffusion MR tractography in humans: Implications for photophobia. *Human Brain Mapping, 33*(1), 75–88.

May, A. (2009a). Morphing voxels: The hype around structural imaging of headache patients. *Brain, 132*(Pt 6), 1419–1425.

May, A. (2009b). New insights into headache: An update on functional and structural imaging findings. *Nature Reviews Neurology, 5*(4), 199–209.

Moulton, E. A., Becerra, L., Maleki, N., Pendse, G., Tully, S., Hargreaves, R., et al. (2011). Painful heat reveals hyperexcitability of the temporal pole in interictal and ictal migraine states. *Cerebral Cortex, 21*(2), 435–448.

Moulton, E. A., Burstein, R., Tully, S., Hargreaves, R., Becerra, L., & Borsook, D. (2008). Interictal dysfunction of a brainstem descending modulatory center in migraine patients. *PLoS One, 3*(11), e3799.

Noseda, R., & Burstein, R. (2010). Advances in understanding the mechanisms of migraine-type photophobia. *Current Opinions in Neurology, 24*(3), 197–202.

Noseda, R., Kainz, V., Jakubowski, M., Gooley, J. J., Saper, C. B., Digre, K., et al. (2011). A neural mechanism for exacerbation of headache by light. *Nature Neuroscience, 13*(2), 239–245.

Royet, J., Zald, D. H., Versace, R., Costes, N., Lavenne, F., Koenig, O., et al. (2000). Emotional responses to pleasant and unpleasant olfactory, visual, and auditory stimuli: A positron emission tomography study. *Journal of Neuroscience, 20*(20), 7752–7759.

Sand, T., Zhitniy, N., Nilsen, K. B., Helde, G., Hagen, K., & Stovner, L. J. (2008). Thermal pain thresholds are decreased in the migraine preattack phase. *European Journal of Neurology, 15*(11), 1199–1205.

Shipley, M. T., & Ennis, M. (1996). Functional organization of olfactory system. *Journal of Neurobiology, 30*(1), 123–176.

Siniatchkin, M., Averkina, N., Andrasik, F., Stephani, U., & Gerber, W. D. (2006). Neurophysiological reactivity before a migraine attack. *Neuroscience Letters, 400*(1–2), 121–124.

Snyder, R. D., & Drummond, P. D. (1997). Olfaction in migraine. *Cephalalgia, 17*(7), 729–732.

Stankewitz, A., Aderjan, D., Eippert, F., & May, A. (2011). Trigeminal nociceptive transmission in migraineurs predicts migraine attacks. *Journal of Neuroscience, 31*(6), 1937–1943.

Stankewitz, A., & May, A. (2009). The phenomenon of changes in cortical excitability in migraine is not migraine-specific—a unifying thesis. *Pain, 145*(1–2), 14–17.

Stankewitz, A., & May, A. (2011). Increased limbic and brainstem activity during spontaneous migraine attacks following olfactory stimulation. *Neurology, 77*(5), 476–482.

Stankewitz, A., Voit, H. L., Bingel, U., Peschke, C., & May, A. (2009). A new trigemino-nociceptive stimulation model for event-related fMRI. *Cephalalgia, 30*(4), 475–485.

Weiller, C., May, A., Limmroth, V., Jüptner, M., Kaube, H., Schayck, R. V., et al. (1995). Brain stem activation in spontaneous human migraine attacks. *Nature Medicine, 1*(7), 658–660.

Wober, C., Brannath, W., Schmidt, K., Kapitan, M., Rudel, E., Wessely, P., et al. (2007). Prospective analysis of factors related to migraine attacks: The PAMINA study. *Cephalalgia, 27*(4), 304–314.

Zald, D. H., & Pardo, J. V. (1997). Emotion, olfaction, and the human amygdala: Amygdala activation during aversive olfactory stimulation. *Proceedings of National Academy of Sciences of the United States of America, 94*, 4119–4124.

Part 3

Clinical Perspective

8 Clinical Neuroimaging of Migraine

RANDOLPH W. EVANS

Most migraines can be diagnosed without diagnostic testing using the comprehensive history and neurological and focused general physical examination. In some cases, however, diagnostic testing is necessary to distinguish migraine from secondary causes that may share similar features. This chapter will review the following topics: the reasons for diagnostic testing, neuroimaging during pregnancy and lactation, incidental findings, incidence and types of pathology in adults and children, episodic and chronic migraine, and migraine mimics.

REASONS FOR DIAGNOSTIC TESTING

There are many reasons why physicians may recommend neuroimaging in migraineurs: a stubborn quest for diagnostic certainty (Kassirer, 1989), faulty cognitive reasoning (Norman & Eva, 2010), the medical decision rule where it is better to impute disease than to risk overlooking it, busy practice conditions where tests are ordered as a shortcut, patient expectations, financial incentives, professional peer pressure where recommendations for routine and esoteric tests are expected as a demonstration of competence, and medicolegal issues (Johnston, 2010; Woolf & Kamerow 1990).

Graber (2005) divides cognitive errors into the following four domains: faulty knowledge, faulty data gathering, faulty information processing, and faulty verification. Graber found that premature closure was the most common error among internists. Overconfident physicians can also make errors (Berner & Graber, 2008).

Cognitive skill errors or processing biases include the following: availability (tendency to judge diagnoses as more likely if they are more easily retrievable from memory), base rate neglect (tendency to ignore the true rate of disease and pursue rare but more exotic diagnoses), representativeness (tendency to be guided by prototypical features of disease and miss atypical variants), confirmation bias (tendency to seek data to confirm, not refute, the hypothesis), and premature closure (tendency to stop too soon and not order the critical test or gather the critical information) (Croskerry, 2003).

The attitudes and demands of patients and families and the practice of defensive medicine are especially important reasons in the case of headaches. Reliance upon guidelines alone may engender some medicolegal risk because guidelines may include studies with referral bias and a significant percentage of patients may have incidental findings (Evans & Johnston, 2011).

In the era of managed care, equally compelling reasons for not ordering diagnostic studies include economic credentialing, which is the use of economic criteria unrelated to quality of care or professional competence in determining a physician's qualifications for initial or continuing hospital medical staff membership or privileges and the use of economic data by insurance companies to determine membership in tiered provider programs and, in less common situations, to eliminate physicians from provider panels (Berry, 2010; Wong & Forese, 2010). The American Medical Association argues that cost-profiling programs by insurance companies may misclassify many patients (Stagg, 2010). In a study of specialty groups not including neurologists, the RAND Corporation concluded that physician cost profiles did not meet common thresholds of reliability (Adams et al., 2010). Information about whether current economic profiling of neurologists and headache medicine specialists is reliable is needed. Lack of funds and high deductibles continue to be barriers for appropriate diagnostic testing for many patients.

COMPUTED TOMOGRAPHY VERSUS MAGNETIC RESONANCE IMAGING

Computed tomography (CT) will detect most abnormalities that may cause headaches. CT is generally preferred over magnetic resonance imaging (MRI) for the evaluation of acute subarachnoid hemorrhage, acute head trauma, and bony abnormalities. However, there are a number of disorders that may be missed on routine CT of the head including vascular disease, neoplastic disease, cervicomedullary lesions, and infections. MRI is more sensitive than CT in the detection of posterior fossa and cervicomedullary lesions, ischemia, white matter abnormalities, cerebral venous thrombosis, subdural and epidural hematomas, neoplasms (especially in the posterior fossa), meningeal disease (such as carcinomatosis, diffuse meningeal enhancement in low cerebrospinal fluid [CSF] pressure syndrome, and sarcoid), and cerebritis and brain abscess. Pituitary pathology is more likely to be detected on a routine MRI of the brain than a routine CT.

Another concern from CT is exposure to ionizing radiation. The average radiation dose of a CT scan of the head without contrast is an effective dose of 2.0 millisieverts (mSv), which is equivalent to 100 chest radiographs (Semelka, 2007). The most common malignancies associated with radiation exposure include leukemia and breast, thyroid, lung, and stomach cancers. The latency period for solid tumors usually is long, with an average of 10 to 20 years and a persistent lifetime risk. Leukemia has an earlier latency period, with an increased risk noted 2 to 5 years after radiation exposure. The pediatric population is at increased risk due to increased radiosensitivity and more years of remaining life to potentially develop cancer. Consider the radiation exposure of some of your patients with multiple trips to the emergency department with migraine and multiple CT scans, as well as multiple CT scans of the head and sinuses in the outpatient setting as well. For a single CT scan of the head, the estimated lifetime attributable risk of death from cancer at different ages is approximately as follows: age 10 years, 0.025%; age 20 years, 0.01%; and age 50 years, 0.003%. (Brenner & Hall, 2007). Although these are relatively small numbers, were the individual studies justified? Up to 2% of all cancer deaths in the United States may be attributable to radiation exposure associated with CT use.

Berrington de González et al. (2009) estimated that approximately 29,000 future cancers could be related to CT scans performed in the United States in 2007, with 4,000 from CT scans of the head. However, there is controversy over these risk-of-future-cancer estimates as they are largely based on extrapolations from data from Japanese atomic bomb survivors; the risk may not be the same and may not necessarily be cumulative (Schenkman, 2011).

Immediate hypersensitivity reactions occur much more commonly with contrast for CT than MRI. The rate of immediate hypersensitivity reactions with low osmolal contrast material agents (LOCMs) for CT is up to 3% (with fatal reactions occurring in 1 to 3 per 100,000 administrations) (Brockow, 2009), as compared to 0.0045% (with fatal reactions occurring in <1 per million doses for most contrast agents) for gadolinium-based chelates for brain studies (Prince et al., 2011). Delayed adverse reactions with LOCMs primarily with skin exanthema may occur in 0.5% to 23%.

Patients with a serum creatinine ≥1.5 mg/dL (132 μmol/L) or an estimated glomerular filtration rate <60 mL/1.73 m², particularly in those with diabetes, are at risk of iodinated contrast–induced nephropathy. Nephrogenic systemic fibrosis (NSF) is seen only in patients with moderate to severe renal failure, particularly those on dialysis, characterized by thickening and hardening of the skin overlying the extremities and trunk and marked expansion and fibrosis of the dermis in association with CD34-positive fibrocytes, and has a mortality rate of 28% (Miskulin et al., 2011). Since the first description in 1997, over 200 cases have been reported to the international registry, with more than 95% having had recent exposure to gadolinium. The risk of developing NSF is about 2.5% to 5% after receiving gadolinium (the risk may be greatest with gadodiamide [Omniscan]) with severely impaired renal function.

Thus, MRI is generally preferred over CT for the evaluation of headaches. The yield of MRI may vary depending on the field strength of the magnetic, the use of paramagnetic contrast, the selection of acquisition sequences, and the use of magnetic resonance angiography and venography. However, MRI may be contraindicated in the presence of an aneurysm clip or pacemaker. In addition, anxiety reactions are common during MRI studies, occurring in up to 37% with reports of 0.5% to 14.5% of patients becoming claustrophobic to the point where they cannot tolerate the study (Eshed et al., 2007).

NEUROIMAGING DURING PREGNANCY AND LACTATION

When there are appropriate indications, neuroimaging should be performed during pregnancy. With the use of lead shielding, a standard CT scan of the head exposes the uterus to less than 1 mrad. The radiation dose for a typical cervical or intracranial arteriogram is less than 1 mrad. The fetus is most susceptible to the teratogenic effects of radiation between the 2nd and 20th weeks of embryonic age (de Santis et al., 2005), with a threshold radiation dose estimated between 5 and 15 rads (Berlin, 1996). Although there is no known risk of iodinated contrast use during pregnancy, contrast should be avoided without indication (American College of Radiology, 2010a).

MRI is more sensitive for rare disorders that may occur during pregnancy such as pituitary apoplexy, cerebral venous sinus thrombosis (with the addition of magnetic resonance venography), and metastatic choriocarcinoma. There is no known risk of MRI during pregnancy (Chen, 2008), but there is some controversy because the magnets induce an electric field and slightly raise the core temperature (<1 °C.). A survey of pregnant MRI workers found no adverse fetal outcome (Kanal et al., 1993), and no adverse fetal effects from MRI have been documented to date. Children exposed in utero at 1.5 Tesla were found to have no exposure-related abnormalities at 9 months of age (Clements et al, 2000) and at up to 9 years of age (Kok et al., 2004).

The 2007 American College of Radiology (ACR) Guidance Document for Safe Practices stated:

Present data have not conclusively documented any deleterious effects of MR imaging exposure on the developing fetus. Therefore, no special consideration is recommended for the first, versus any other, trimester in pregnancy. . . . Pregnant patients can be accepted to undergo MR scans at any stage of pregnancy if, in the determination of a level 2 MR personnel–designated attending radiologist, the risk–benefit ratio to the patient warrants that the study be performed. The radiologist should confer with the referring physician and document the following in the radiology report or the patient's medical record:

1. The information requested from the MR study cannot be acquired via nonionizing means (e.g., ultrasonography).
2. The data are needed to potentially affect the care of the patient or fetus *during* the pregnancy.
3. The referring physician does not feel it is prudent to wait until the patient is no longer pregnant to obtain these data.
. . . MR contrast agents should *not* be routinely provided to pregnant patients. . . . The decision to administer a gadolinium-based MR contrast agent to pregnant patients should be accompanied by a well-documented and thoughtful risk–benefit analysis. (Kanal et al., 2007, p. 1455)

The American College of Radiology (2010a) later reiterated that there is no known risk of gadolinium to the fetus.

Lactating women may be advised to discard breast milk for 24 hours after receiving intravenous iodinated contrast or gadolinium if they choose. However, only a tiny fraction of iodinated contrast or gadolinium entering the infant gut is actually absorbed. "The very small potential risk associated with absorption of contrast medium may be insufficient to warrant stopping breast-feeding for 24 hours after either iodinated or gadolinium contrast agents" (Chen et al., 2008, p.338). The American College of Radiology (2010b) concurs that the available evidence suggests that it is safe to continue breastfeeding after receiving either agent.

RISK–BENEFIT AND COST–BENEFIT OF NEUROIMAGING

The risks of neuroimaging include radiation exposure and contrast reactions as discussed above, incidental findings discussed further below, and false positives (Frishberg, 1994). Although the scan helps to relieve anxiety for many, for others the scan may produce anxiety when nonspecific abnormalities are found, such as incidental anatomical variants or white matter lesions, or the scan is misread with a false positive. I suspect that many neurologists have seen patients with isolated headaches referred by primary care physicians with a request to rule out multiple sclerosis when white matter lesions are detected.

Although the cost of finding significant pathology is quite high, the cost of neuroimaging is significantly decreasing under many managed care contracts and with Medicare/Medicaid. Cost–benefit estimates should also include the cost to the physician of malpractice suits filed when patients with significant pathology do not have neuroimaging and the cost to the patient and society of premature death and disability of undetected treatable lesions.

INCIDENTAL FINDINGS

As discussed, many MRI scans are done to reassure anxious migraineurs. Although incidental findings may not be responsible for their migraines, rarely incidental findings may be present, which raises medicolegal concerns for the physician (Evans & Johnston, 2011). In a meta-analysis of 16 studies with 19,559 participants from ages 10 to 89, the overall prevalence of incidental brain findings on MRI was 2.7, including the following: neoplasia (benign and malignant), 0.7%; vascular abnormality, 0.56% with 0.35% aneurysms; Chiari I, 0.24%; and arachnoid cysts, 0.5% (Morris et al., 2009). There was an increasing prevalence with older age. Not infrequently, MRI scans are reported as suspicious for mastoiditis, which is usually not clinical mastoiditis, or, perhaps 20% of the time, due to otitis media, Eustachian tube dysfunction, or tympanosclerosis (Polat et al., 2011).

Incidental findings are also common in strictly pediatric populations. In a retrospective study of children and adolescents ages 3 to 18 years with recurrent nonprogressive headache without abnormal physical examinations seen in a pediatric neurology clinic, 185 underwent neuroimaging, CT in 51%, MRI in 38%, and both in 11%. The scans were reported as normal in 78.4%, and 21.5% had the following incidental findings: 35%, sinus disease; 15%, Chiari I malformation; 7.5%, supratentorial parenchymal tissue; 15%, arachnoid cyst(s); 10%, brainstem or infratentorial parenchyma tissue abnormality (including one with Dandy-Walker); 5%, pineal cyst; 5%, developmental venous anomalies; 5%, Virchow-Robin spaces; and 2.5%, cavum septi pellucidi (Graf et al., 2010). These findings are similar to other pediatric studies (Gupta & Belay, 2008; Mazzotta et al., 2004; Schwedt et al., 2006; Wöber-Bingöl et al., 1996).

ABNORMALITIES IN MIGRAINEURS

Incidence of Pathology

Frishberg (1994) reviewed four CT scan studies (Cala & Mastaglia, 1976; Cuetter & Aita, 1983; Hungerford et al., 1976; Masland et al., 1978), four MRI scan studies (Igarashi et al., 1991; Jacome & Leborgne, 1990; Osborn et al., 1991; Soges et al., 1988), and one combined MRI and CT scan study (Kuhn & Sheklar, 1990) of 897 scans of patients with migraine and found any potentially treatable lesions in 0.3% on CT and 0.4% on MRI. These findings are combined with more recent reports of one CT scan study of 284 patients (Dumas et al., 1994) and six studies of MRI scans of 444 patients (Cooney et al., 1996; de Benedittis et al., 1995; Fazekas et al., 1992; Pavese et al., 1994; Robbins & Friedman, 1992; Ziegler et al., 1991) for a total of 1,625 scans of patients with various types of migraine. Other than white matter abnormalities, the studies showed no significant pathology except for four brain tumors (three of which were incidental findings) and one arteriovenous malformation (in a patient with migraine and a seizure disorder). Sempere et al. (2005) found a similarly low yield of 0.4% in migraineurs.

White Matter Abnormalities

Multiple MRI studies have investigated white matter abnormalities (WMAs) on scans of migraineurs. WMAs are foci of hyperintensity on both proton density and T2-weighted images in the deep and periventricular white matter due to either interstitial edema or perivascular demyelination. WMAs are easily detected on MRI and less well visualized on CT scan.

The percentages of WMAs for all types of migraine range from 12% (Osborn et al., 1991) to 46% (Soges et al., 1988). WMAs have been reported as both more frequent in the frontal region of the centrum semiovale (De Benedittis et al., 1995; Igarashi et al., 1991) and no more frequent (Pavese et al., 1994) than in the white matter of the parietal, temporal, and occipital lobes. Six out of the eight studies using controls found a higher incidence of WMAs in migraineurs. The incidence of WMAs in controls ranged from 0% (Rovaris et al., 2001) to 14% (Fazekas

et al., 1992). One small study reported a similar incidence of WMAs in patients with tension-type headaches, 34.3%, as those with migraine, 32.1%, and greater than the 7.4% in controls (De Benedittis et al., 1995).

Four studies found similar percentages of WMAs comparing migraine with aura to migraine without aura (Cooney et al., 1996; De Benedittis et al., 1995; Pavese et al., 1994; Prager et al., 1991), while two reported a higher percentage in migraine with aura (Fazekas et al., 1992; Igarashi et al., 1991). Three small studies of basilar migraine found WMAs in 17% (Cooney et al., 1996; Jacome & Leborgne, 1990) and 38% (Fazekas et al., 1992). WMAs are variably reported as more often present in adult migraineurs older than 40 years and younger than 60 years (Cooney et al., 1996; Prager et al., 1991) and equally present (Fazekas et al., 1992) compared to those age 40 years or younger. Cooney et al. (1996) found an increased frequency of WMAs associated with age older than 50 years and with medical risk factors (hypertension, atherosclerotic heart disease, diabetic mellitus, autoimmune disorder, or demyelinating disease) but not with gender, migraine subtype, or duration of migraine symptoms.

Migraine with aura is associated with an increased frequency of right-to-left shunts mostly due to a patent foramen ovale, which hypothetically could cause WMAs due to paradoxical microembolism of platelets or shunting of vasoactive amines that have escaped the pulmonary circulation. However, a study of 185 consecutive subjects with migraine with aura, 66% with right-to-left shunts, found no increase in white matter lesion load as compared to those without shunts (Adami et al., 2008). Periventricular WMAs were present in 19% and deep WMAs in 46%, and 11% showed coexistence of periventricular and deep lesions. Similarly, there was no increase in white matter lesions in another consecutive series of 87 migraineurs, 45% with right-to-left shunts (del Sette et al., 2008); WMAs were present in 61% of patients. In both studies, the only risk factor associated with WMAs was older age, not gender, frequency of migraines, smoking, hyperlipidemia, or oral contraceptive use.

While the cause of WMAs in migraine is not certain, various hypotheses have been advanced including increased platelet aggregability with microemboli, abnormal cerebrovascular regulation, and repeated attacks of hypoperfusion during the aura (De Benedittis et al., 1995; Igarashi et al., 1991; Kruit et al., 2004; Pavese et al., 1994). The presence of antiphospholipid antibodies might be another risk factor for WMAs in migraine (Tietjen, 1992). The reported incidence of antiphospholipid antibodies in migraine ranges from 0% (Hering et al., 1991) to 24% (Robbins, 1991). In one MRI study, however, the presence of WMAs showed no correlation with the presence of anticardiolipin antibodies (Igarashi et al., 1991). The presence of anticardiolipin antibodies is not an additional risk factor for stroke in migraineurs (Daras et al., 1995). Tietjen et al. (1998) found that, compared to control subjects, there was no increase in frequency of anticardiolipin positivity in adults younger than 60 years of age with transient focal neurological events or in those with migraine with or without aura. Additionally, antiphospholipid antibodies were not detected and antithrombin II, protein C, and protein S were normal in 102 consecutive migraineurs with WMAs (Intiso et al., 2006).

Subclinical Infarcts

Kruit et al. (2004) obtained MRI scans on a population-based sample of Dutch adults ages 30 to 60 years with migraine with aura (n = 161), migraine without aura (n = 134), and well-matched controls (n = 140). No participants reported a history of stroke or transient ischemic attack or had relevant abnormalities at standard neurological examination. There was no significant difference between patients with migraine and controls in overall infarct prevalence (8.1% vs. 5.0%). However, in the cerebellar region of the posterior circulation territory, patients with migraine had a higher prevalence of infarct than controls (5.4% vs. 0.7%). The adjusted odds ratio (OR) for posterior infarct varied by migraine subtype and attack frequency. The adjusted OR was 13.7 for patients with migraine with aura compared with controls. In patients with migraine with a frequency of attacks of one or more per month, the adjusted OR was 9.3. The highest risk was in patients with migraine with aura with one attack or more per month (OR = 15.8). Kruit et al. (2005) hypothesize that focal (possibly migraine-related) hypoperfusion rather than microembolic occlusion is responsible for most of the cerebellar infarcts.

Thirty-eight percent of the subjects in both the migraine and control groups had at least one medium-sized deep white matter lesion (DWML). Among women, the risk for high DWML load was increased in patients with migraine compared with controls (OR = 2.1); this risk increased with attack frequency (highest in those with one attack per month: OR = 2.6) but was similar in patients with migraine with or without aura. In men, controls and patients with migraine did not differ in the prevalence of DWMLs. There was no association between severity of periventricular white matter lesions (PVWMLs) and migraine, irrespective of sex or migraine frequency or subtype. There were no differences in the distributions and the mean values of grades of severity of PVWMLs between patients with migraine and controls. These results did not vary by sex, migraine subtype, and/or migraine attack frequency.

Kruit et al. (2006, 2010) further reported the brainstem and cerebellar hyperintense lesions found in their same migraine population. Infratentorial hyperintensities were identified in 13 of 295 (4.4%) migraineurs and in 1 of 140 (0.7%) controls. Migraineurs with aura had a higher prevalence of subclinical infarcts in the posterior circulation (OR = 13.7), and female migraineurs had an increased risk of WMA (OR = 2.1). Twelve cases had hyperintensities, mostly bilaterally, in the dorsal basis pontis (described for the first time in migraine). Those with infratentorial hyperintensities also had supratentorial white matter lesions more often. The cause may be small-vessel disease (arteriosclerosis), repetitive perfusion deficits, or both. It is not known whether the lesions are progressive or have relevant long-term functional correlates.

Other Causes of White Matter Abnormalities to Consider

WMAs found on MRI may at times raise concern to exclude other diseases that can be comorbid with migraine and also cause WMAs.

Migraine may be more common in persons with multiple sclerosis (MS) according to some studies (Putski & Katsarava, 2010), occurring as much as three times more in a clinic population than in controls (Kister et al., 2010). The total number of T2 lesions in migraineurs with MS does not differ from nonmigraineurs with MS (Kister et al., 2010). In a series of 16 consecutive migraineurs (14 without aura and 2 with aura), Rovaris et al. (2001) found white matter lesions in 5 (31%). The pattern of MRI lesions fulfilled diagnostic criteria suggestive of MS in four—none of the patients had any other neurological symptoms or signs. Cervical spine MRI studies were obtained in all subjects as well as in 17 age- and gender-matched controls in whom no cord lesions were detected. Primary antiphospholipid antibody syndrome can also produce a pattern of white matter abnormalities, which can be difficult to distinguish from multiple sclerosis (Stosic et al., 2010).

WMAs in migraine may be difficult to distinguish from those found in vasculitides (Schedel et al., 2010) such as neuropsychiatric systemic lupus erythematosus (SLE) (Luyendijk et al, 2011) and primary Sjögren syndrome (PSS) (Morgen et al., 2004). Confounding the distinction, migraine may be more common in both diseases, occurring in 44% of those with SLE and 35% of those with PSS (Harboe et al., 2009). In another study of 67 patients with SLE, migraine was present in 36% (13% with aura), versus 19% of controls (Harboe et al al., 2011). There was no difference in the presence of white matter hyperintensities in those patients with SLE with or without headaches.

A subgroup of migraineurs may have a genetic predisposition for white matter lesions on MRI scans.

Cerebral autosomal dominant arteriopathy with subcortical infarcts and leukoencephalopathy (CADASIL) is a familial genetic disease with migraine as a common symptom and severe WMAs on MRI as a consistent neuroimaging finding. Chabriat et al. (1995) described several members of a family with an autosomal dominant illness manifested by migraine attacks and a significant leukoencephalopathy on MRI but without other specific manifestations of CADASIL. Mourad et al. (2006) also described four patients older than the age of 60 years with typical Notch3 mutations leading to CADASIL who did not have dementia or disability but had extensive WMAs on MRI. It is possible that there is a specific gene locus for migraine with white matter changes. Variable gene penetrance could result in CADASIL at one extreme and tiny T2 hyperintense white matter foci and migraine alone at the other extreme.

Cerebral Atrophy

Diffuse cerebral atrophy with widening of the lateral ventricles and cerebral sulci is equally well detected by both MRI and CT scans (Kuhn & Shekar, 1990). The incidence of cerebral atrophy in migraineurs on CT and MRI scans has been variably reported as 4% (Cala & Mastaglia, 1976), 26% (Hungerford et al., 1976), 28% (Prager et al., 1991), 35% (Kuhn & Shekar, 1990), and 58% (du Boulay et al., 1983). The studies describe most cases of atrophy as mild to moderate. However, three subsequent studies found the incidence of atrophy in migraineurs to be no greater than in controls (De Benedittis et al., 1995; Rocca et al., 2006; Ziegler et al., 1991). The high incidence of CT changes seen in migraineurs in early studies probably reflected artifact and a failure to recognize the range of normality in the early days of imaging.

Neuroimaging in Children

Lewis and Dorbad (2000) retrospectively reviewed records of children ages 6 to 18 years with migraine and chronic daily headache with normal examinations. Of 54 patients with migraine who underwent either CT (42) or MRI (12) scans, the yield of abnormalities was 3.7%, none clinically relevant. Of 25 patients with chronic daily headache who underwent either CT (17) or MRI (8) scans, the yield of abnormalities was 16%, none clinically relevant.

Carlos et al. (2000), in a retrospective chart review, identified all pediatric migraine patients who had a CT or MRI scan to investigate their headaches. Ages ranged from 3 to 18 years. Of the 93 patients, 35 had CT, 14 had MRI, and 9 had both. Twenty-two had abnormalities, but none were felt to be related to the patients' headaches. Alehan (2002) prospectively obtained neuroimaging (49 MRI scans, 11 CT scans) in 60 out of 72 consecutive children diagnosed with migraine or tension-type headaches. Ten percent had findings related to their headache, with no neoplasms and no patients requiring surgery.

In a retrospective review of the results of brain MRI and CT of 1,562 children ages 2 to 18 years with headaches referred to nine pediatric neurology clinics, abnormal findings were present in 7% of 377 migraineurs without aura and 6% of 124 migraineurs with aura (Rho et al., 2011). Although the pathology is not provided for the migraine group (and is presumably incidental), 0.91% of all patients imaged (11 of 1,204) underwent a neurosurgical procedure.

A report of the Quality Standards Subcommittee of the American Academy of Neurology and the Practice Committee of the Child Neurology Society (Lewis et al., 2002) makes the following recommendations:

1. Obtaining a neuroimaging study on a routine basis is not indicated in children with recurrent headaches and a normal neurological examination (Level B; class II and class III evidence).
2. Neuroimaging should be considered in children with an abnormal neurological examination (e.g., focal findings, signs of increased intracranial pressure, significant alteration of consciousness), the coexistence of seizures, or both (Level B; class II and class III evidence).
3. Neuroimaging should be considered in children in whom there are historical features to suggest the recent onset of severe headache or there is change in the type of headache, or if there are associated features that suggest neurological dysfunction (Level B; class II and class III evidence).

Chronic Migraine

Wang et al. (2001) retrospectively reviewed the medical records and MRI images of 402 adult patients (286 women and 116 men) who had been evaluated by the neurology service with a primary complaint of chronic headache (a duration of 3 months or more) and no other neurological symptoms or findings. Major abnormalities (a mass, those that caused mass effect, or those believed to be the likely cause of the patient's headache) were found in 15 patients (3.7%) including a glioma, meningioma, metastases, subdural hematoma, arteriovenous malformation, hydrocephalus (three patients), and Chiari I malformations (two patients). They were found in 0.6% of patients with migraine, 1.4% of those with tension headaches, 14.1% of those with atypical headaches, and 3.8% of those with other types of headaches.

Tsushimo and Endo (2005) retrospectively reviewed the clinical data and magnetic resonance studies of 306 adult patients (136 men and 170 woman), all of whom were referred for MRI evaluation of chronic or recurrent headache with a duration of 1 month or more, no other neurological symptoms or focal findings at physical examination, and no prior head surgery, head trauma, or seizure: 55.2% had no abnormalities, 44.1% had minor abnormalities, and 0.7% (two patients) had clinically significant abnormalities (pituitary macroadenoma and subdural hematoma). Neither contrast material enhancement ($n = 195$) nor repeated MRI ($n = 23$) contributed to the diagnosis.

Sempere and colleagues (2005) reported a study of 1,876 consecutive patients (1,243 females, 633 males) aged 15 years or older, with a mean age of 38 years, with headaches that had an onset at least 4 weeks previously who were referred to two neurology clinics in Spain. One third of the headaches were new onset, and two thirds had been present for more than 1 year. Subjects had the following types: migraine (49%), tension (35.4%), cluster (1.1%), posttraumatic (3.7%), and indeterminate (10.8%). Normal neurological examinations were found in 99.2% of the patients. CT was performed in 1,432 patients and MRI in 580; 136 patients underwent both studies.

Neuroimaging studies detected significant lesions in 22 patients (1.2%), of whom 17 had a normal neurological examination. The only variable or "red flag" associated with a higher probability of intracranial abnormalities was an abnormal neurological examination, with a likelihood ratio of 42. The diagnoses in these 17 patients were pituitary adenoma ($n = 3$), large arachnoid cyst ($n = 2$), meningioma ($n = 2$), hydrocephalus ($n = 2$), and Arnold-Chiari type I malformation, ischemic stroke, cavernous angioma, arteriovenous malformation, low-grade astrocytoma, brainstem glioma, colloid cyst, posterior fossa papilloma (one of each). Of these 17 patients, 8 were treated surgically: hydrocephalus ($n = 2$) and pituitary adenoma, large arachnoid cyst, meningioma, arteriovenous malformation, colloid cyst, and papilloma (one of each).

The rate of significant intracranial abnormalities in patients with headache and normal neurological examination was 0.9%. Neuroimaging studies discovered incidental findings in 14 patients (75%): 3 pineal cysts, 3 intracranial lipomas, and 8 arachnoid cysts. The yield of neuroimaging studies was higher in the group with indeterminate headache (3.7%) than in the migraine (0.4%) or tension-type headache (0.8%) groups. The study does not provide information on white matter abnormalities in migraineurs. MRI performed in 119 patients with normal CT revealed significant lesions in 2 cases: a small meningioma and an acoustic neurinoma. No saccular aneurysms were detected; magnetic resonance angiography was not obtained.

However, the studies do not give information about the detection of paranasal sinus disease, which may be the cause of some headaches. For example, sphenoid sinusitis may cause a severe, intractable, new-onset headache that interferes with sleep and is not relieved by simple analgesics. The headache may increase in severity with no specific location. There may be associated pain or paraesthesias in the facial distribution of the fifth nerve and photophobia or eye tearing with or without fever or nasal drainage. The headache may mimic other causes such as migraine or meningitis (Silberstein, 2004).

American Academy of Neurology Practice Parameter

A report of the Quality Standards Subcommittee of the American Academy of Neurology (Silberstein, 2000) makes the following recommendation: Neuroimaging is not usually warranted in patients with migraine and a normal neurological examination (Grade B).

Although the yield is low, the following are some reasons to consider neuroimaging in migraineurs: unusual, prolonged, or persistent aura; increasing frequency, severity, or change in clinical features; first or worst migraine; basilar; confusion; hemiplegic; late-life migraine accompaniments; aura without headache; headaches always on the same side (see arteriovenous malformation discussion below); posttraumatic; and patient's or family's and friends' request.

MIGRAINE MIMICS OR SYMPTOMATIC MIGRAINE

The differential diagnosis of migraines is long (Swanson & Sakai, 2006). Some mimics will be discussed that can be diagnosed on neuroimaging. The prevalence of arteriovenous malformations (AVMs) is about 0.5% in postmortem studies (Brown et al., 1988). In contrast to saccular aneurysms, up to 50% present with symptoms or signs other than hemorrhage. Headache without distinctive features (such as frequency, duration, or severity) is the presenting symptom in up to 48% of cases (The Arteriovenous Malformation Study Group, 1999).

Migrainelike headaches with and without visual symptoms can be associated with arteriovenous malformations, especially those in the occipital lobe, which is the predominant location of about 20% of parenchymal AVMs (Frishberg, 1997; Kupersmith et al., 1996). Although headaches always occurring on the same side (side-locked) are present in 95% of those with AVMs (Bruyn, 1984), 17% of those with migraine without aura and 15% of patients with migraine with aura have side-locked headaches (Leone et al., 1993).

Migraine due to an AVM is usually atypical and rarely meets the International Headache Society criteria for migraine. In a series of 109 patients with headache and AVMs, Ghossoub et al. (2001) reported the following features: nonpulsating, 95%; nausea, vomiting, light or noise sensitivity, 4.1%; unilateral and homolateral to the AVM, 70%; duration less than 3 hours, 77%; one to two per month, 82.5%; and usually mild responding to simple analgesics. Bruyn (1984) reported the following features in patients with migrainelike symptoms and AVM: unusual associated signs (papilledema, field cut, bruit), 65%; short duration of headache attacks, 20%; brief scintillating scotoma, 10%; absent family history, 15%; atypical sequence of aura, headache, and vomiting, 10%; and seizures, 25%.

The following brainstem vascular malformations have been associated with migraine meeting International Headache Society criteria: a hemorrhagic midbrain cavernoma resulting in a contralateral headache (Goadsby, 2002); a pontine bleed from a cavernous angioma with initially ipsilateral headache, then bilateral with aura (Afridi & Goadsby 2003); pontine capillary telangiectasia with signs of residual hemorrhage with bilateral headaches initially with aura (Obermann et al., 2006); and a midbrain/upper pons hemorrhagic AVM/cavernous malformation resulting in a contralateral headache with aura (Malik & Young, 2006). These cases provide evidence for the involvement of the brainstem in the initiation of migraine.

Pituitary hemorrhage can produce a migrainelike acute headache with a normal neurological examination (Evans, 1997). Pituitary infarction, with severe headache, photophobia, and CSF pleocytosis, can initially be quite similar to aseptic meningitis or meningoencephalitis (Embil, 1997). Pituitary pathology is more likely to be detected on a routine MRI than CT scan. Acute sphenoid sinusitis can mimic migraine (also see section on chronic migraine; Silberstein, 2004).

Internal carotid artery dissection can mimic migraine with aura with a visual aura only or a march of symptoms (such as visual then sensory then dysphasia) associated with a migrainelike headache (Ramadan et al., 1991; Silverman & Wityk, 1998). In occasional cases where migraine with aura criteria are met in those with a prior history of migraine, the dissection could be incidental or could be a trigger for the migraine with aura episode(s).

Migraine or migrainelike headaches with and without aura have been reported in patients with colloid cysts of the third ventricle (Lane et al., 2010; Young & Silberstein, 1997), cerebral venous thrombosis (Agostoni, 2004), cerebral metastasis (Porta-Etessam et al., 1998), brainstem glioma (Lim et al., 2005), and pituitary tumors (Gabrielli et al., 2002; Levy, 2011). Migrainelike headaches occur in up to 15% of patients with primary and metastatic tumors (Forsyth & Posner, 1993; Schankin et al., 2007; Valentinis et al, 2010). Obstructive hydrocephalus (Lane et al., 2010) might also cause a migrainelike visual aura. Finally, rarely, with a normal scan of the brain and a white eye, subacute angle closure glaucoma can mimic migraine with and without aura, which can even recur over a period of years (Molyneux & Jordan, 2010).

REFERENCES

Adami, A., Rossato, G., Cerini, R., Thijs, V. N., Pozzi-Mucelli, R., Anzola, G. P., et al. (2008). Right-to-left shunt does not increase white matter lesion load in migraine with aura patients. *Neurology, 71,* 101–107.

Adams, J. L., Mehrotra, A., Thomas, J. W., & McGlynn, E. A. (2010). Physician cost profiling—reliability and risk of misclassification. *New England Journal of Medicine, 362*(11), 1014–1021.

Afridi, S., & Goadsby, P. J. (2003). New onset migraine with a brain stem cavernous angioma. *Journal of Neurology, Neurosurgery, and Psychiatry, 74,* 680–682.

Agostoni, E. (2004). Headache in cerebral venous thrombosis. *Neurological Sciences, 25*(Suppl 3), S206–S210.

Alehan FK. Value of neuroimaging in the evaluation of neurologically normal children with recurrent headache. J Child Neurol. 2002;17:807-809.

American College of Radiology. (2010a). Administration of contrast medium to pregnant or potentially pregnant patients. In: *Manual on contrast media* (version 7, pp. 59–60). Retrieved March 14, 2011, from http://www.acr.org/SecondaryMainMenuCategories/quality_safety/contrast_manual.asx

American College of Radiology. (2010b). Administration of contrast media to breast-feeding mothers. In: *Manual on contrast media* (version 7, pp. 61–62). Retrieved March 14, 2011, from http://www.acr.org/SecondaryMainMenuCategories/quality_safety/contrast_manual.asx

The Arteriovenous Malformation Study Group. (1999). Arteriovenous malformations of the brain in adults. *New England Journal of Medicine, 340,* 1812–1818.

Berlin, L. (1996). Radiation exposure and the pregnant patient. *AJR American Journal of Roentgenology, 167,* 1377–1379.

Berner, E. S., & Graber, M. L. (2008). Overconfidence as a cause of diagnostic error in medicine. *American Journal of Medicine, 121*(5 Suppl), S2–S23.

Berrington de González, A., Mahesh, M., Kim, K. P., Bhargavan, M., Lewis, R., Mettler, F., et al. (2009). Projected cancer risks from computed tomographic scans performed in the United States in 2007. *Archives of Internal Medicine, 169,* 2071–2077.

Berry E. (2010, October 4). Narrow networks: Will you be in or out? *American Medical News.* Retrieved from http://www.ama-assn.org/amednews/2010/10/04/bisa1004.htm

Brenner, D. J., & Hall, E. J. (2007). Computed tomography—an increasing source of radiation exposure. *New England Journal of Medicine, 357,* 2277–2284.

Brockow, K. (2009). Immediate and delayed reactions to radiocontrast media: Is there an allergic mechanism? *Immunology and Allergy Clinics of North America, 29*(3), 453–468

Brown, R. D., Wiebers, D. O., Forbes, G., O'Fallon WM, Piepgras DG, Marsh WR., et al. (1988). The natural history of unruptured intracranial arteriovenous malformations. *Journal of Neurosurgery, 68*, 352–357.

Bruyn, G. W. (1984). Intracranial arteriovenous malformation and migraine. *Cephalalgia, 4*, 191–207.

Cala, L., & Mastaglia, F. (1976). Computerized axial tomography findings in a group of patients with migrainous headaches. *Proceedings of the Australian Academy of Neurology, 13*, 35–41.

et al. (2000). Neuroimaging studies in pediatric migraine headaches. *Headache, 40*, 404.

Chabriat, H., Vahedi, K., Iba-Zizen, M. T., Joutel, A., Nibbio, A., Nagy, T. G., et al. (1995). Clinical spectrum of CADASIL: A study of 7 families. Cerebral autosomal dominant arteriopathy with subcortical infarcts and leukoencephalopathy. *Lancet, 346*, 934–939.

Chen, M. M., Coakley, F. V., Kaimal, A., Laros, R. K., Jr. (2008). Guidelines for computed tomography and magnetic resonance imaging use during pregnancy and lactation. *Obstetrics and Gynecology, 112*(2 Pt 1), 333–340.

Clements, H., Duncan, K. R., Fielding, K., Gowland, P. A., Johnson, I. R., & Baker, P. N. (2000). Infants exposed to MRI in utero have a normal paediatric assessment at 9 months of age. *British Journal of Radiology, 73*, 190–194.

Cooney, B. S., Grossman, R. I., Farber, R. E., Goin JE, Galetta SL. (1996). Frequency of magnetic resonance imaging abnormalities in patients with migraine. *Headache, 36*, 616–621.

Cuetter, A., & Aita, J. (1983). CT scanning in classic migraine [Letter]. *Headache, 23*, 195.

Daras, M., Koppel, B., Leyfermann, M., Samkoff, L., & Tuchman, A. (1995). Anticardiolipin antibodies in migraine patients: An additional risk factor for stroke? *Neurology, 45*(Suppl 4), A367–A368.

De Benedittis, G., Lorenzetti, A., Sina, C., & Bernasconi, V. (1995). Magnetic resonance imaging in migraine and tension-type headache. *Headache, 35*, 264–268.

De Santis, M., Di Gianantonio, E., Straface, G., Cavaliere, A. F., Caruso, A., Schiavon, F., et al. (2005). Ionizing radiations in pregnancy and teratogenesis: A review of literature. *Reproductive Toxicology, 20*, 323–329.

Del Sette, M., Dinia, L., Bonzano, L., Roccatagliata, L., Finocchi, C., Parodi, R. C., et al. (2008). White matter lesions in migraine and right-to-left shunt: A conventional and diffusion MRI study. *Cephalalgia, 28*, 376–382.

du Boulay, G. H., & Ruiz, J. S. (1983). CT changes associated with migraine. *AJNR American Journal of Neuroradiology, 4*, 472–473.

Dumas, M. D., Pexman, W., & Kreeft, J. H. (1994). Computed tomography evaluation of patients with chronic headache. *Canadian Medical Association Journal, 151*,1447–1452.

Embil, J. M., Kramer, M., Kinnear, S., & Light, R. B. (1997). A blinding headache. *Lancet, 349*, 182.

Eshed, I., Althoff, C. E., Hamm, B., & Hermann, K. G. (2007). Claustrophobia and premature termination of magnetic resonance imaging examinations. *Journal of Magnetic Resonance Imaging, 26*(2), 401–404.

Evans, R. W. (1997). Migrainelike headaches in pituitary apoplexy. *Headache, 37*, 455–456.

Evans, R. W., & Johnston, J. C. (2011). Migraine and medical malpractice. *Headache.* 51:434-440

Fazekas, F., Koch, M., Schmidt, R., Offenbacher H, Payer F, Freidl W et al. (1992). The prevalence of cerebral damage varies with migraine type: A MRI study. *Headache, 32*, 287–291.

Forsyth, P. A., & Posner, J. B. (1993). Headaches in patients with brain tumors: A study of 111 patients. *Neurology, 43*(9), 1678–1683.

Frishberg, B. M. (1994). The utility of neuroimaging in the evaluation of headache in patients with normal neurologic examination. *Neurology, 44*,1191–1197.

Frishberg, B. M. (1997). Neuroimaging in presumed primary headache disorders. *Seminars in Neurology, 17*, 373–382.

Gabrielli, M., Gasbarrini, A., Fiore, G., Santarelli, L., Padalino, C., De Martini, D., et al. (2002). Resolution of migraine with aura after successful treatment of a pituitary microadenoma. *Cephalalgia, 22*(2), 149–150.

Ghossoub, M., Nataf, F., Merienne, L., Devaux, B., Turak, B., & Roux, F. X. (2001). [Characteristics of headache associated with cerebral arteriovenous malformations] *Neurochirurgie, 47*(2–3 Pt 2), 177–183.

Goadsby, P. J. (2002). Neurovascular headache and a midbrain vascular malformation: Evidence for a role of the brainstem in chronic migraine. *Cephalalgia, 22*, 107–111.

Graber, M. L. (2005). Diagnostic error in internal medicine. *Archives of Internal Medicine, 165*, 1493–1499.

Graf, W. D., Kayyali, H. R., Abdelmoity, A. T., Womelduff, G. L., Williams, A. R., & Morriss, M. C. (2010). Incidental neuroimaging findings in nonacute headache. *Journal of Child Neurology, 25*, 1182–1187.

Gupta, S. N., & Belay, B. (2008). Intracranial incidental findings on brain MR images in a pediatric neurology practice: A retrospective study. *Journal of Neurological Sciences, 264*, 34–33.

Harboe, E., Gøransson, L. G., Beyer, M. K., Greve, O. J., Herigstad, A., Kvaløy, J. T., et al. (2011). Migraine is frequent in patients with systemic lupus erythematosus: A case-control study. *Cephalalgia, 31*(4), 401–408.

Harboe, E., Tjensvoll, A. B., Maroni, S., Gøransson, L. G., Greve, O. J., Beyer, M. K., et al. (2009). Neuropsychiatric syndromes in patients with systemic lupus erythematosus and primary Sjögren syndrome: A comparative population-based study. *Annals of Rheumatic Disease, 68*(10), 1541–1546.

Hering, R., Couturier, E. G. M., Steiner, T. J., Asherson, R. A., & Rose, C. F. (1991). Anticardiolipin antibodies in migraine. *Cephalalgia, 11*, 19–21.

Hungerford, G., duBoulay, G., & Zilkha, K. (1976). Computerized axial tomography in patients with severe migraine: A preliminary report. *Journal of Neurology, Neurosurgery, and Psychiatry, 39*, 990–994.

Igarashi, H., Sakai, F., Kan, S., Okada, J., & Tazaki, Y. (1991). Magnetic resonance imaging of the brain in patients with migraine. *Cephalalgia, 11*, 69–74.

Intiso, D., Di Rienzo, F., Rinaldi, G., Zarrelli, M. M., Giannatempo, G. M., Crociani, P., et al. (2006). Brain MRI white matter lesions in migraine patients: Is there a relationship with antiphospholipid antibodies and coagulation parameters? *European Journal of Neurology, 13*, 1364–1369.

Jacome, D. E., & Leborgne, J. (1990). MRI studies in basilar artery migraine. *Headache, 30*, 88–90.

Johnston, J. C. (2010). Neurological malpractice and nonmalpractice liability. *Neurologic Clinics, 28*, 441–458.

Kanal, E., Barkovich, A. J., Bell, C. (2007). ACR guidance document for safe practices: 2007. *American Journal of Roentgenology, 188*, 1447–1474.

Kanal, E., Gillen, J., Evans, J. A., et al. (1993). Survey of reproductive health among female MR workers. *Radiology, 187*, 395–399.

Kassirer, J. P. (1989). Our stubborn quest for diagnostic certainty. A cause of excessive testing. *New England Journal of Medicine, 320*, 1489–1491.

Kister, I., Caminero, A. B., Monteith, T. S., Soliman, A., Bacon, T. E., Bacon, J. H., et al. (2010). Migraine is comorbid with multiple sclerosis and associated with a more symptomatic MS course. *Journal of Headache and Pain, 11*(5), 417–425.

Kok, R. D., de Vries, M. M., Heerschap, A., van den Berg, P. P. (2004). Absence of harmful effects of magnetic resonance exposure at 1.5 T in utero during the third trimester of pregnancy: A follow-up study. *Magnetic Resonance Imaging, 22*, 851–854.

Kruit, M. C., Launer, L. J., Ferrari, M. D., & van Buchem, M. A. (2005). Infarcts in the posterior circulation territory in migraine. The population-based MRI CAMERA study. *Brain, 128*(Pt 9), 2068–2077.

Kruit, M. C., Launer, L. J., Ferrari, M. D., & van Buchem, M. A. (2006). Brain stem and cerebellar hyperintense lesions in migraine. *Stroke, 37*(4), 1109–1112.

Kruit, M. C., van Buchem, M. A., Hofman, P. A., Bakkers, J. T., Terwindt, G. M., Ferrari, M. D., et al. (2004). Migraine as a risk factor for subclinical brain lesions. *Journal of the American Medical Association, 291*, 427–434.

Kruit, M. C., van Buchem, M. A., Launer, L. J., Terwindt, G. M., Ferrari, M. D. (2010). Migraine is associated with an increased risk of deep white matter lesions, subclinical posterior circulation infarcts and brain iron accumulation: The population-based MRI CAMERA study. *Cephalalgia, 30*, 129–136.

Kuhn, M. J., & Shekar, P. C. (1990). A comparative study of magnetic resonance imaging and computed tomography in the evaluation of migraine. *Computed Medical Imaging Graphics, 14*, 149–152.

Kupersmith, M. J., Vargas, M. E., Yashar, A., Madrid, M., Nelson, K., Seton, A., et al. (1996). Occipital arteriovenous malformations: Visual disturbances and presentation. *Neurology, 46*, 953–957.

Lane, R., Jenkins, H., van Dellen, J., & Davies, P. (2010). Migraine with atypical visual aura caused by colloid cyst of the third ventricle. *Cephalalgia, 30*, 996–999.

Leone, M., D'Amico, D., Frediani, F., Torri, W., Sjaastad, O., & Bussone, G. (1993). Clinical considerations on side-locked unilaterality in long lasting primary headaches. *Headache, 33*, 381–384.

Levy, M. J. (2011). The association of pituitary tumors and headache. *Current Neurology and Neuroscience Reports, 11*(2), 164–170.

Lewis, D. W., & Dorbad, D.(2000). The utility of neuroimaging in the evaluation of children with migraine or chronic daily headache who have normal neurological examinations. *Headache, 40*, 629–632.

Lewis, D. W., Ashwal, S., Dahl, G., Dorbad, D., Hirtz, D., Prensky A., et al. (2002). Practice parameter: evaluation of children and adolescents with recurrent headaches: report of the Quality Standards Subcommittee of the American Academy of Neurology and the Practice Committee of the Child Neurology Society. *Neurology, 59*, 490–498.

Lim, E. C., Wilder-Smith, E. P., Chong, J. L., & Wong, M. C. (2005). Seeing the light: Brainstem glioma causing visual auras and migraine. *Cephalalgia, 25*(2), 154–156.

Luyendijk, J., Steens, S. C., Ouwendijk, W. J., Steup-Beekman, G. M., Bollen, E. L., van der Grond, J., et al. (2010). Neuropsychiatric SLE: Lessons learned from MRI. *Arthritis and Rheumatology*. [Epub ahead of print] 2011;63:722-732

Malik, S. N., & Young, W. B. (2006). Midbrain cavernous malformation causing migraine-like headache. *Cephalalgia, 26*, 1016–1019.

Masland, W., Friedman, A., & Buchsbaum, H. (1978). Computerized axial tomography of migraine. *Research and Clinical Studies in Headache, 6*, 136–140.

Mazzotta, G., Floridi, F., Mattioni, A., D'Angelo, R., & Gallai, B. (2004). The role of neuroimaging in the diagnosis of headache in childhood and adolescence: A multicentre study. *Neurological Sciences*, (Suppl 3), S265–S26. 25

Miskulin, D., Gul, A., Rudnick, M., & Cowper, S. (2011). Nephrogenic systemic fibrosis/nephrogenic fibrosing dermopathy in advanced renal failure. In: D. S. Basow (Ed.), *UpToDate*. Waltham, MA: UpToDate.

Molyneux, P. D., & Jordan, K. (2010). Migraine, an open and shut case? *Practical Neurology, 10*(3), 172–175.

Morgen, K., McFarland, H. F., & Pillemer, S. R. (2004). Central nervous system disease in primary Sjogrens syndrome: The role of magnetic resonance imaging. *Seminars in Arthritis and Rheumatology, 34*(3), 623–630.

Morris, Z., Whiteley, W. N., Longstreth, W. T., Jr., Weber, F., Lee, Y. C., Tsushima, Y., et al. (2009). Incidental findings on brain magnetic resonance imaging: Systematic review and meta-analysis. *BMJ, 339*, b3016.

Mourad, A., Levasseur, M., Bousser, M. G., & Chabriat, H. (2006). [CADASIL with minimal symptoms after 60 years]. *Review Neurologique* (Paris), *162*(8–9), 827–831.

Norman, G. R., & Eva, K. W. (2010). Diagnostic error and clinical reasoning. *Medical Education, 44*(1), 94–100.

Obermann, M., Gizewski, E. R., Limmroth, V., Diener, H. C., & Katsarava, Z. (2006). Symptomatic migraine and pontine vascular malformation: Evidence for a key role of the brainstem in the pathophysiology of chronic migraine. *Cephalalgia, 26*, 763–766.

Osborn, R. E., Alder, D. C., & Mitchell, C. S. (1991). MR imaging of the brain in patients with migraine headaches. *AJNR American Journal of Neuroradiology, 12*, 521–524.

Pavese, N., Canapicchi, R., Nuti, A., et al. (1994). White matter MRI hyperintensities in a hundred and twenty-nine consecutive migraine patients. *Cephalalgia, 14*, 342–345.

Polat, S., Aksoy, E., Serin, G. M., Yıldız, E., & Tanyeri, H. (2011). Incidental diagnosis of mastoiditis on MRI. *European Archives of Otorhinolaryngology*. 2011 Feb 5. [Epub ahead of print]

Porta-Etessam, J., Berbel, A., Martínez, A., & Nuñez-López, R. (1998). Cerebral metastasis presenting as Valsalva-induced migraine with aura. *Headache, 38*(10), 801.

Prager, J. M., Rosenblum, J., Mikulis, D. J., Diamond, S., & Freitag, F. G. (1991). Evaluation of headache patients by MRI. *Headache Quarterly, 2*, 192–196.

Prince, M. R., Zhang, H., Zou, Z., Staron, R. B., & Brill, P. W. (2011). Incidence of immediate gadolinium contrast media reactions. *American Journal of Roentgenology, 196*(2), W138–W143.

Putzki, N., & Katsarava, Z. (2010). Headache in multiple sclerosis. *Current Pain and Headache Reports, 14*(4), 316–320.

Ramadan, N. M., Tietjen, G. E., Levine, S. R., & Welch, K. M. A. (1991). Scintillating scotomata associated with internal carotid artery dissection: Report of three cases. *Neurology, 41*, 1084–1087.

Rho, Y. I., Chung, H. J., Suh, E. S., Lee, K. H., Eun, B. L., Nam, S. O., et al. (2011). The role of neuroimaging in children and adolescents with recurrent headaches—multicenter study. *Headache, 51*, 403–408.

Robbins, L. (1991). Migraine and anticardiolipin antibodies-case reports of 13 patients and the prevalence of antiphospholipid antibodies in migraineurs. *Headache, 31*, 537–539.

Robbins, L., & Friedman, H. (1992). MRI in migraineurs. *Headache, 32*, 507–508.

Rocca, M. A., Ceccarelli, A., Falini, A., Tortorella, P., Colombo, B., Pagani, E., et al. (2006). Diffusion tensor magnetic resonance imaging at 3.0 tesla shows subtle cerebral grey matter abnormalities in patients with migraine. *Journal of Neurology, Neurosurgery, and Psychiatry, 77,* 686–689.

Rovaris, M., Bozzali, M., Rocca, M. A., Colombo, B., & Filippi, M. (2001). An MR study of tissue damage in the cervical cord of patients with migraine. *Journal of the Neurological Sciences, 183,* 43–46.

Schankin, C. J., Ferrari, U., Reinisch, V. M., Birnbaum, T., Goldbrunner, R., & Straube, A. (2007). Characteristics of brain tumour-associated headache. *Cephalalgia, 27*(8), 904–911.

Schedel, J., Kuchenbuch, S., Schoelmerich, J., Feuerbach, S., Geissler, A., & Mueller-Ladner, U. (2010). Cerebral lesions in patients with connective tissue diseases and systemic vasculitides: Are there specific patterns? *Annals of the New York Academy of Sciences, 1193,* 167–175.

Schenkman, L. (2011). Radiology. Second thoughts about CT imaging. *Science, 331,* 1002–1004.

Schwedt, T. J., Guo, Y., & Rothner, A. D. (2006). "Benign" imaging abnormalities in children and adolescents with headache. *Headache, 46*(3), 387–398.

Semelka, R. C., Armao, D. M., Elias, J., Jr., & Huda, W. (2007). Imaging strategies to reduce the risk of radiation in CT studies, including selective substitution with MRI. *Journal of Magnetic Resonance Imaging, 25,* 900–909.

Sempere, A. P., Porta-Etessam, J., Medrano, V., Garcia-Morales, I., Concepción, L., Ramos, A., et al. (2005). Neuroimaging in the evaluation of patients with non-acute headache. *Cephalalgia, 25,* 30–35.

Silberstein, S. D. (2000). Practice parameter: Evidence-based guidelines for migraine headache (an evidence-based review): Report of the Quality Standards Subcommittee of the American Academy of Neurology. *Neurology, 55,* 754–762.

Silberstein, S. D. (2004). Headaches due to nasal and paranasal sinus disease. *Neurologic Clinics, 22,* 1–19.

Silverman, I. E., & Wityk, R. J. (1998). Transient migraine-like symptoms with internal carotid artery dissection. *Clinical Neurology and Neurosurgery, 100,* 116–120.

Soges, L. J., Cacayorin, E. D., Petro, G. R., & Ramachandran, T. S. (1988). Migraine: Evaluation by MR. *AJNR American Journal of Neuroradiology, 9,* 425–429.

Stagg, E. V. (2010, August 2). Medical societies demand insurers rethink doctor cost ratings. *American Medical News.* Retrieved from http://www.ama-assn.org/amednews/2010/08/02/bil20802.htm

Stosic, M., Ambrus, J., Garg, N., Weinstock-Guttman, B., Ramanathan, M., Kalman, B., et al. (2010). MRI characteristics of patients with antiphospholipid syndrome and multiple sclerosis. *Journal of Neurology, 257*(1), 63–71.

Swanson, J. W., & Sakai, F. (2006). Diagnosis and differential diagnosis of migraines. In J. Olesen, P. Tfelt-Hansen, K. M. A. Welch, P. J. Goadsby, N. M. Ramadan (Eds.), *The headaches* (3rd ed., pp. 423–428). Philadelphia: Lippincott Williams & Wilkins.

Tietjen, G. E. (1992). Migraine and antiphospholipid antibodies. *Cephalalgia, 12,* 69–74.

Tietjen, G. E., Day, M., Norris, L., Aurora, S., Halvorsen, A., Schultz, L. R. et al. (1998). Role of anticardiolipin antibodies in young persons with migraine and transient focal neurologic events. A prospective study. *Neurology, 50,* 1433–1440.

Tsushima, Y., & Endo, K. (2005). MR imaging in the evaluation of chronic or recurrent headache. *Radiology, 235,* 575–579.

Valentinis, L., Tuniz, F., Valent, F., Mucchiut, M., Little, D., Skrap, M., et al. (2010). Headache attributed to intracranial tumours. *Cephalalgia, 30*(4), 389–398.

Wang, H. Z., Simonson, T. M., Greco, W. R., & Yuh, W. T. (2001). Brain MR imaging in the evaluation of chronic headache in patients without other neurologic symptoms. *Academy of Radiology, 8,* 405–408.

Wöber-Bingöl, C., Wöber, C., Prayer, D., Wagner-Ennsgraber, C., Karwautz, A., Vesely, C., et al. (1996) Magnetic resonance imaging for recurrent headache in childhood and adolescence. *Headache, 36,* 83–90.

Wong, D. A., & Forese, L. L. (2010). Economic credentialing and physician performance measures: They know who you are. *Journal of Bone and Joint Surgery of America, 92*(5), 1305–1311.

Woolf, S. H., & Kamerow, D. B. (1990). Testing for uncommon conditions. The heroic search for positive test results. *Archives of Internal Medicine, 15,* 2451–2458.

Young, W. B., & Silberstein, S. D. (1997). Paroxysmal headache caused by colloid cyst of the third ventricle: Case report and review of the literature. *Headache, 37*(1), 15–20.

Ziegler, D. K., Batnitzky, S., Barter, R., & McMillan, J. H. (1991). Magnetic resonance image abnormality in migraine with aura. *Cephalalgia, 11,* 147–150.

9 Prophylaxis: What Measures?

STEPHEN D. SILBERSTEIN

INTRODUCTION

The treatment of migraine with pharmacologic agents may be acute (abortive) or preventive (prophylactic), and patients with frequent severe headaches often require both approaches. Preventive therapy is used to try to reduce the frequency, duration, or severity of attacks. Additional benefits include enhancement of response to acute treatments, improvement of a patient's ability to function, and reduction of disability (Lipton & Silberstein, 1994). Preventive treatment may also result in the reduction of health care costs (Silberstein et al., 2003). Recent US and European guidelines (Lipton et al., 2005; Silberstein, 2004) have established the circumstances that might warrant preventive treatment. These include (a) recurring migraine that significantly interferes with a patient's quality of life and daily routine despite acute treatment; (b) four or more attacks per month; (c) failure of, contraindication to, or troublesome side effects from acute medications; and (d) frequent, very long, or uncomfortable auras (Lipton et al., 2005; Silberstein, 2004). A migraine preventive drug is considered successful if it reduces migraine attack frequency by at least 50% within 3 months. A migraine diary is useful in evaluating response to treatment (Lipton et al., 2005; Silberstein, 2004) (see Fig. 9–1).

Prevention is not being utilized to the extent it should be; only 13% of all migraineurs currently use preventive therapy to control their attacks (Lipton et al., 2005). According to the American Migraine Prevalence and Prevention (AMPP) study, 38.8% of patients with migraine should be considered for (13.1%) or offered (25.7%) migraine preventive therapy (Silberstein, Diamond, et al., 2005).

The following classes of medications are used for migraine prevention: anticonvulsants, antidepressants, β-adrenergic blockers, calcium channel antagonists, serotonin antagonists, botulinum neurotoxins, nonsteroidal anti-inflammatory drugs, and others (including riboflavin, magnesium, and petasides). If preventive medication is indicated, the agent should be chosen from one of the first-line categories based on the drug's relative efficacy in double-blind, placebo-controlled trials; its side-effect profile; the patient's preference; and coexistent and comorbid conditions

(Tfelt-Hansen, 2000). The following are general principles of preventive therapy, based on the author's experience.

GENERAL GUIDELINES FOR INSTITUTING PREVENTIVE THERAPY

Start the chosen drug at a low dose and increase it slowly until therapeutic effects develop, the ceiling dose for the chosen drug is reached, or adverse events (AEs) become intolerable.

- Give each treatment an adequate trial. The full benefit of the drug may not be realized until 6 months have elapsed.
- Set realistic goals. Success is defined as a 50% reduction in attack frequency, a significant decrease in attack duration, or an improved response to acute medication.
- Set realistic expectations regarding AEs. The risk and extent of AEs vary greatly from patient to patient and we presently have no way of predicting the presence or severity of AEs for an individual patient. Most AEs are self-limited and dose dependent, and patients should be encouraged to tolerate the early AEs that may develop when a new medication is started.
- Avoid acute headache medication overuse and drugs that are contraindicated because of coexistent or comorbid illnesses.
- Re-evaluate therapy and, if possible, taper or discontinue the drug after a sustained period of remission (6 to 9 months).
- Be sure that a woman of childbearing potential is aware of any potential risks and choose the medication that will have the least potential for adverse effects on a fetus (Silberstein, 1997).
- To maximize compliance, involve patients in their own care. Take patient preferences into account when deciding between drugs of relatively equivalent efficacy and tolerability.
- Consider comorbidity, which is the presence of two or more disorders whose association is more likely than

1) Recurring migraine that significantly interferes with the patient's daily routine despite acute treatment (e.g., two or more attacks a month that produce disability that lasts three or more days, or headache attacks that are infrequent but produce profound disability)
2) Failure of, contraindication to, or troublesome side effects from acute medications
3) Overuse of acute medications
4) Special circumstances, such as hemiplegic migraine or attacks with a risk of permanent neurologic injury
5) Very frequent headaches (more than two a week) or a pattern of increasing attacks over time, with the risk of developing medication overuse headache
6) Patient preference, that is, the desire to have as few acute attacks as possible

FIGURE 9–1 *US evidence-based guidelines for migraine preventive treatment.*

TABLE 9–1 *Migraine Comorbid Disease*

CARDIOVASCULAR

Hyper-/hypotension

Raynaud

Patent foramen ovale (migraine with aura)

Atrial septal defects, pulmonary arteriovenous malformations

Mitral valve prolapse

Angina/myocardial infarction

Stroke

PSYCHIATRIC

Depression

Mania

Panic disorder

Anxiety disorder

NEUROLOGIC

Epilepsy

Essential tremor

Fibromyalgia

Positional vertigo

Restless legs syndrome

GASTROINTESTINAL

Irritable bowel syndrome

OTHER

Asthma

Allergies

chance. Conditions that are comorbid with migraine are shown in Table 9–1 (Diener, Kurth, et al., 2007; Ifergane, 2006; Olerud et al., 1986; Ryan, 1984; Ryan & Sudilovsky, 1983; Saunders et al., 2008; Schwedt, 2009; Silberstein, 2010; Sudilovsky et al., 1986).

Preventive treatment is often recommended for only 6 to 9 months, but until now no randomized, placebo-controlled trials have been performed to investigate migraine frequency after the preventive treatment has been discontinued. Diener et al. (Diener, Agosti, et al., 2007) assessed 818 migraine patients who were treated with topiramate for 6 months to see the effects of topiramate discontinuation. Patients received topiramate in a 26-week open-label phase. They were then randomly assigned to continue this dose or switch to placebo for a 26-week, double-blind phase. Of the 559 patients who completed the open-label phase, 514 entered the double-blind phase and were assigned to topiramate ($n = 255$) or placebo ($n = 259$). The mean increase in number of migraine days was greater in the placebo group (1.19 days in 4 weeks, 95% confidence interval [CI], 0.71–1.66; $p < .0001$) than in the topiramate group (0.10, −0.36 to 0.56; $p = .5756$). Patients in the placebo group had a greater number of days on acute medication than did those in the topiramate group (mean difference between groups −0.95, −1.49 to −0.41; $p = .0007$). Sustained benefit was reported after topiramate was discontinued, although the number of migraine days did increase. These findings suggest that patients should be treated for 6 months, with the option to continue to 12 months.

SPECIFIC MIGRAINE PREVENTIVE AGENTS

β-Adrenergic Blockers for the Prevention of Migraine

β-Blockers are the most widely used class of drugs in prophylactic migraine treatment, and are about 50%

effective in producing a greater than 50% reduction in attack frequency (Table 9–2). Evidence has consistently demonstrated the efficacy (Gray et al., 1999; Silberstein, 2000) of the nonselective β-blocker propranolol (Andersson & Vinge, 1990; Cortelli et al., 1985; Gray et al., 1999; Koella, 1985; Ramadan, 2004; Ryan, 1984; Ryan & Sudilovsky, 1983; Silberstein, 2000; Sudilovsky et al., 1986) and of the selective $β_1$-blocker metoprolol (Andersson & Vinge, 1990; Panerai et al., 1990; Ryan, 1984; Ryan & Sudilovsky, 1983; Sudilovsky et al., 1987; Tfelt-Hansen et al., 1984). Atenolol (Kishore-Kumar et al., 1990), bisoprolol (Feinmann, 1985; Panerai et al., 1990), nadolol (Baldessarini, 1990; Richelson, 1990), and timolol (Abramowicz, 1990; Gray et al., 1999) are also likely to be effective. β-Blockers with intrinsic sympathomimetic activity (acebutolol, alprenolol, oxprenolol, pindolol) are not effective for migraine prevention. Propranolol is effective for migraine prevention in a daily dose of 120 to 240

TABLE 9–2 *β-Blockers and Antidepressants in the Preventive Treatment of Migraine*

Agent	Daily Dose	Comment
β-BLOCKERS		
Atenolol	50–200 mg	• Use qid • Fewer side effects than propranolol
Metoprolol	100–200 mg	• Use the short-acting form bid • Use the long-acting form qid
Nadolol	20–160 mg	• Use qid • Fewer side effects than propranolol
Propranolol	40–400 mg	• Use the short-acting form bid or tid • Use the long-acting form qid or bid • 1–2 mg/kg in children
Timolol	20–60 mg	• Divide the dose • Short half-life
ANTIDEPRESSANTS		
Tertiary Amines		
Amitriptyline	10–400 mg	Start at 10 mg at bedtime
Doxepin	10–300 mg	Start at 10 mg at bedtime
Secondary Amines		
Nortriptyline	10–150 mg	• Start at 10–25 mg at bedtime • If insomnia, give early in the morning
Protriptyline	5–60 mg	Start at 10–25 mg at bedtime
SELECTIVE SEROTONIN AND NOREPINEPHRINE REUPTAKE INHIBITORS		
Venlafaxine	75–225 mg	Start 37.5 mg in the morning

mg, but no correlation has been found between its dose and its clinical efficacy.

The combination of propranolol and topiramate versus topiramate alone was recently examined as a preventive treatment for chronic migraineurs in the National Institute of Neurological Diseases and Stroke (NINDS) Clinical Research Collaboration Chronic Migraine Treatment Trial (CMTT). This was a randomized, double-blind, placebo-controlled, parallel study to examine the safety and efficacy of topiramate (up to 100 mg/day) and propranolol (up to 240 mg/day LA formulation) taken in combination, compared with treatment with topiramate (up to 100 mg/day) and placebo. The trial was terminated in September 2010, when an interim analysis determined that the combination of topiramate and propranolol offered no additional advantage over topiramate alone (Dodick et al., 2011).

The action of β-blockers is probably central and could be mediated by (a) inhibiting central β receptors that interfere with the vigilance-enhancing adrenergic pathways, (b) interaction with 5-HT receptors (but not all effective β-blockers bind to the 5-HT receptors), and (c) cross-modulation of the serotonin system (Koella, 1985). Propranolol inhibits nitrous oxide production by blocking inducible nitric oxide synthase. Propranolol also inhibits kainate-induced currents and is synergistic with *N*-methyl-d-aspartate blockers, which reduce neuronal activity and have membrane-stabilizing properties (Ramadan, 2004).

Contraindications to the use of β-blockers include asthma and chronic obstructive lung disease, congestive heart failure, atrioventricular conduction defects, Raynaud disease, peripheral vascular disease, and brittle diabetes. All β-blockers can produce behavioral AEs, such as drowsiness, fatigue, lethargy, sleep disorders, nightmares, depression, memory disturbance, and hallucinations (Gray et al., 1999). Other potential AEs include gastrointestinal complaints, decreased exercise tolerance, orthostatic hypotension, bradycardia, and impotence. Although stroke has been reported to occur after patients with migraine with aura were started on β-blockers, there is neither an absolute nor a relative contraindication to their use by patients with migraine, either with or without aura.

Summary: Evidence for β-blockers in the prevention of migraine (Pearlman et al., 2010)

There is strong evidence establishing the effectiveness of metoprolol, propranolol, and timolol (Level A: see Table 9–3 for definitions of levels of evidence).

Evidence exists (Level B) to suggest that the following are probably effective and should be considered: atenolol and nadolol.

The following are possibly effective (Level C) and may be considered: nebivolol and pindolol.

There is inadequate evidence to support or refute the use of the following: bisoprolol.

Antidepressant Medication for the Prevention of Migraine

Antidepressants consist of a number of different drug classes with different mechanisms of action (Table 9–2). Although the mechanism by which antidepressants work to prevent migraine headache is uncertain, it does not result from treating masked depression. Antidepressants are useful in treating many chronic pain states, including headache, independent of the presence of depression, and the response occurs sooner than the expected antidepressant effect (Kishore-Kumar et al., 1990; Panerai et al., 1990). In animal pain models, antidepressants potentiate the

TABLE 9–3 *Selected Calcium Channel Blockers and Selected Anticonvulsants in the Preventive Treatment of Migraine*

Level A = Established as effective, ineffective, or harmful (or established as useful/predictive or not useful/predictive) for the given condition in the specified population. (Level A rating requires at least two consistent Class I studies.[a])

Level B = Probably effective, ineffective, or harmful (or probably useful/predictive or not useful/predictive) for the given condition in the specified population. (Level B rating requires at least one Class I study or two consistent Class II studies.)

Level C = Possibly effective, ineffective, or harmful (or possibly useful/predictive or not useful/predictive) for the given condition in the specified population. (Level C rating requires at least one Class II study or two consistent Class III studies.)

Level U = Data inadequate or conflicting; given current knowledge, treatment (test, predictor) is unproven.

[a] In exceptional cases, one convincing Class I study may suffice for an "A" recommendation if (a) all criteria are met and (b) the magnitude of effect is large (relative rate improved outcome >5 and the lower limit of the confidence interval is >2).

effects of coadministered opioids (Feinmann, 1985). The antidepressants that are clinically effective in headache prevention either inhibit noradrenaline and 5-HT reuptake or are antagonists at the 5-HT_2 receptors (Richelson, 1990).

TRICYCLIC ANTIDEPRESSANTS

Tricyclic antidepressants (TCAs) are used for the prevention of migraine. Only one TCA (amitriptyline) has proven efficacy in migraine (Silberstein, 2000). Amitriptyline has been used for migraine prophylaxis for over 35 years (Couch, 2010). Jackson et al. (2010) performed a meta-analysis in which adults with migraine or tension-type headache were treated with a TCA as a single intervention for at least 4 weeks. Control groups included placebo or another preventive, such as β-blockers, serotonin reuptake inhibitors (SSRIs), or alternative/complementary strategies, such as spinal manipulation or behavioral therapy. Although the analyses were performed on studies that were heterogeneous with respect to study population, study design, and study quality, the study did demonstrate the effectiveness of amitriptyline over placebo for both migraine and tension-type headache. When pooling data from studies that compared TCAs and SSRIs, the authors found that TCAs were superior to SSRIs in subjects with both migraine and tension-type headache. The subjects in the tricyclic arms had higher rates of adverse effects than those on SSRIs, although the rates of study withdrawal did not differ in the two treatment arms. An analysis of studies that compared TCAs with β-blockers found no difference in the reduction of the number of headache days or attacks.

Couch (2010) published the results of a randomized, double-blind, placebo-controlled study (N = 391) on the efficacy of amitriptyline in the prevention of intermittent migraine and chronic daily headache. Although the study took place between 1976 and 1979, the results had not been reported previously. Results for the entire study group (i.e., both intermittent migraine and chronic daily headache) revealed that there was a statistically significant improvement in the frequency of headache from the end of the titration period (week 4) to the end of the first 4 weeks on maintenance dose (week 8) between the amitriptyline arm and placebo arm (p = .018 in favor of amitriptyline). However, when week 4 was compared with subsequent weeks of treatment (i.e., weeks 12, 16, and 20), the differences in the decrease in headache frequency between the amitriptyline and placebo groups did not persist, probably because of the large placebo effect that continued to increase with the duration of study participation. Additionally, there was a large attrition rate, whereby Couch suggests that subjects in the placebo group who did not improve may have preferentially withdrawn, thus diminishing the difference between the treatment and placebo groups. When subgroups were examined, there was no difference between the amitriptyline and placebo group in reduction of headache frequency for subjects with episodic migraine. Amitriptyline was effective in reducing headache frequency in subjects with chronic daily headache. When headaches did occur in subjects with either episodic migraine or chronic daily headache, there was no significant difference in pain intensity or duration between placebo and amitriptyline groups. This may have resulted because the duration of headache was assessed independently of severity (i.e., duration of a mild headache contributed the same as a disabling headache). The importance of this recently published older study is that it is the largest placebo-controlled study of amitriptyline for the prevention of migraine.

The dose range for TCAs is wide and must be individualized. Amitriptyline and doxepin are sedating TCAs. Patients with coexistent depression may require higher doses of these drugs to treat underlying depression. Start at a dose of 10 to 25 mg at bedtime. The usual effective dosage for migraine ranges from 25 to 200 mg. Nortriptyline, a major metabolite of amitriptyline, is a secondary amine that is less sedating than amitriptyline. Start at a dose of 10 to 25 mg at bedtime. The dose ranges from 10 to 150 mg/day. Protriptyline is a secondary amine that is similar to nortriptyline. Start at a dose of 5 mg in the morning. The dose ranges from 5 to 60 mg/day, as a single or split dose. Start with a low dose of the chosen TCA at bedtime, except when using protriptyline, which should be administered in the morning. If the TCA is too sedating, switch from a tertiary TCA (amitriptyline, doxepin) to a secondary TCA (nortriptyline, protriptyline). AEs are common with TCA use. Antimuscarinic AEs include dry mouth, a metallic taste, epigastric distress, constipation, dizziness, mental confusion, tachycardia, palpitations, blurred vision, and urinary retention. Other AEs include weight gain (rarely seen with protriptyline), orthostatic hypotension, reflex tachycardia, and palpitations. Antidepressant treatment may change depression to hypomania or frank mania (particularly in bipolar patients). Older patients may develop confusion or delirium (Baldessarini, 1990). The muscarinic and adrenergic effects of these agents may pose increased risks for cardiac conduction abnormalities, especially in the elderly, and these patients should be carefully monitored or other agents considered.

SELECTIVE SEROTONIN AND NOREPINEPHRINE REUPTAKE INHIBITORS

Evidence for the use of SSRIs or other antidepressants for migraine prevention is poor. Fluoxetine in doses between 10 and 40 mg was effective in three and not effective in one placebo-controlled trial (Mathew, Saper, Silberstein, Tolander, et al., 1995; Silberstein et al., 1995, 2001). Other antidepressants not effective in placebo-controlled trials were clomipramine and sertraline; for other antidepressants, only open or non-placebo-controlled trials are available. Because their tolerability profile is superior to that of tricyclics, SSRIs may be helpful for patients with comorbid depression (Lipton et al., 2002). The most common AEs include sexual dysfunction, anxiety, nervousness, insomnia, drowsiness, fatigue, tremor, sweating, anorexia, nausea, vomiting, and dizziness or lightheadedness. The combination of an SSRI and a TCA can be beneficial in treating refractory depression (Bowden et al., 1994) and, in our experience, resistant cases of migraine. The combination may require the TCA dose to be adjusted, because TCA plasma levels may significantly increase.

Recently, venlafaxine, a selective serotonin and norepinephrine reuptake inhibitor, has been shown to be effective in a double-blind, placebo-controlled trial (Ozyalcin et al., 2005) and a separate placebo- and amitriptyline-controlled trial (Bulut et al., 2004). The usual effective dose is 150 mg/day. Start with the extended-release tablet of 37.5 mg for 1 week, then 75 mg for 1 week, and then 150 mg extended release in the morning. AEs include insomnia, nervousness, mydriasis, and seizures.

Summary: Evidence for antidepressants in the prevention of migraine (Pearlman et al., 2010)

There is no strong evidence (Level A) for any.

The following are probably effective (Level B) and should be considered: amitriptyline, fluoxetine, and venlafaxine.

There is inadequate evidence to support or refute (Level U) the use of the following: fluvoxamine and protriptyline.

Calcium Channel Antagonists for the prevention of migraine

Two types of calcium channels exist: calcium entry channels, which allow extracellular calcium to enter the cell, and calcium release channels, which allow intracellular calcium (in storage sites in organelles) to enter the cytoplasm (Greenberg, 1997). Calcium entry channel subtypes include voltage gated, opened by depolarization; ligand gated, opened by chemical messengers, such as glutamate; and capacitative, activated by depletion of intracellular calcium stores. The mechanism of action of the calcium channel antagonists in migraine prevention is uncertain, but possibilities include inhibition of 5-HT release, neurovascular inflammation, or the initiation and propagation of cortical spreading depression (Table 9–4) (Altier & Zamponi, 2004; Cohen, 2005; Wauquier et al., 1985).

Flunarizine, a nonselective calcium channel antagonist with antidopaminergic properties, was superior to placebo in six of seven randomized clinical trials (Bulut et al., 2004; Cortelli et al., 1985; Greenberg, 1997; Markley et al., 1984; Ozyalcin et al., 2005; Reveiz-Herault et al., 2003; Riopelle & McCans, 1982; Smith & Schwartz, 1984; Solomon, 1986; Tfelt-Hansen et al., 1984; Wauquier et al., 1985). The dose is 5 to 10 mg at night (women seem to need lower doses than men). The most prominent AEs include weight gain, somnolence, dry mouth, dizziness, hypotension, occasional extrapyramidal reactions, and exacerbation of depression. Because of its side-effect profile, flunarizine should be considered as a second-line drug for migraine prevention, after β-blockers. Flunarizine is widely used in Europe but is not available in the United States, where verapamil is the recommended calcium channel antagonist.

Verapamil was more effective than placebo in two of three trials, but both positive trials were very small and dropout rates were high, rendering the findings uncertain (Hanston & Horn, 1985; Mathew et al., 2001; Rompel & Bauermeister, 1970). Nimodipine, nicardipine, diltiazem, and cyclandelate, other nonselective calcium channel antagonists, have not shown superiority over placebo in well-designed clinical trials and cannot be recommended for migraine prophylaxis.

> Summary: Evidence for calcium channel blockers in the prevention of migraine (Pearlman et al., 2010)
> One has strong evidence (Level A): flunarizine (European guidelines).
> The following are probably effective (Level B) and should be considered: cyclandelate, nimodipine, and verapamil.
> There is inadequate evidence (Level U) to support or refute the use of the following: nicardipine and nifedipine.

Anticonvulsants for the Prevention of Migraine

Anticonvulsants are increasingly recommended for migraine prevention because of well-conducted placebo-controlled trials. With the exception of valproic acid, topiramate (doses <200 mg/day), and zonisamide, anticonvulsants

TABLE 9–4 *Miscellaneous Medication in the Preventive Treatment of Migraine*

Agent	Daily Dose	Comment
SELECTED CALCIUM CHANNEL BLOCKERS		
Verapamil	120–640 mg	• Start 80 mg bid or tid • Sustained release can be given qid or bid
Flunarizine	5–10 mg	• qid at bedtime • Weight gain is the most common side effect.
SELECTED ANTICONVULSANTS		
Carbamazepine	600–1,200 mg	Give tid
Gabapentin	600–1,200 mg	• Dose can be increased to 3,000 mg
Topiramate	100 mg	• Start 15–25 mg at bedtime • Increase 15–25 mg per week • Attempt to reach 50–100 mg • Increase further if necessary • Associated with weight loss, not weight gain
Valproate/divalproex	500–1,500 mg/day	• Start 250–500 mg day • Monitor levels if compliance is an issue • Maximum dose is 60 mg/kg per day

may substantially interfere with the efficacy of oral contraceptives (Coulam & Annagers, 1979; Hanston & Horn, 1985).

CARBAMAZEPINE

The only placebo-controlled trial of carbamazepine that suggested a significant benefit suffered from methodologic issues in several respects, including the absence of a washout phase between the two treatment arms in the cross-over design (Table 9–4) (Rompel & Bauermeister, 1970). Carbamazepine, 600 to 1,200 mg/day, may be effective preventive migraine treatment, but it is rarely used in clinical practice for this purpose, because of the absence of rigorous data concerning efficacy and because of adverse hematologic, hepatic, and cardiovascular effects.

GABAPENTIN

Gabapentin (1,800 to 2,400 mg) showed efficacy in a placebo-controlled, double-blind trial only when a modified intent-to-treat analysis was used (Table 9–4). Migraine attack frequency was reduced by 50% in about one third of patients (Mathew et al., 2001). The most common AEs were dizziness or giddiness and drowsiness.

VALPROIC ACID

Valproic acid is a simple eight-carbon, two-chain fatty acid. Divalproex sodium (approved by the US Food and Drug Administration [FDA]) is a combination of valproic acid and sodium valproate. Both are effective (Klapper, 1995, 1997), as is an extended-release form of divalproex sodium (Freitag et al., 2003). In 1992, Hering and Kuritzky (1992) evaluated sodium valproate's efficacy in migraine treatment in a double-blind, randomized, cross-over study. Sodium valproate was effective in preventing migraine or reducing the frequency, severity, and duration of attacks in 86.2% of 29 patients, whose attacks were reduced from 15.6 to 8.8 a month. In 1994, Jensen et al. (1998) studied 43 patients with migraine without aura in a triple-blind, placebo- and dose-controlled, cross-over study of slow-release sodium valproate. In the valproate group, 50% of the patients had a reduction in migraine frequency to 50% or less, compared with 18% for placebo.

Several subsequent randomized, placebo-controlled studies have confirmed these results, with significant responder rates ranging between 43% and 48% (Jensen et al., 1994; Smith & Schwartz, 1984) with dosages ranging from 500 to 1,500 mg/day. Extended-release divalproex sodium has also been shown to be effective for migraine prevention, and compliance and side-effect profile may be more favorable with this formulation (Mathew, Saper, Silberstein, Rankin, et al., 1995).

Nausea, vomiting, and gastrointestinal distress are the AEs that occur most commonly; their incidence decreases, however, particularly after 6 months. Tremor and alopecia can, however, occur later. Valproate has little effect on cognitive functions and rarely causes sedation. Rare, severe AEs include hepatitis and pancreatitis. The frequency varies with the number of concomitant medications used, the patient's age, the presence of genetic and metabolic disorders, and the patient's general state of health. These idiosyncratic reactions are unpredictable (Pellock & Willmore, 1991). Valproate is teratogenic (Silberstein, 1996). Hyperandrogenism, ovarian cysts, and obesity are of concern in young women with epilepsy who use valproate (Vainionpaa et al., 1999). Absolute contraindications are pregnancy and a history of pancreatitis or a hepatic disorder. Other contraindications are thrombocytopenia, pancytopenia, and bleeding disorders.

Valproic acid is available as 250 mg capsules and as syrup (250 mg/5 mL) (Table 9–4). Divalproex sodium is available as 125-, 250-, and 500-mg capsules and a sprinkle formulation. Start with 250 to 500 mg/day in divided doses and slowly increase the dose. Monitor serum levels if there is a question of toxicity or compliance. The maximum recommended dose is 60 mg/kg per day.

TOPIRAMATE

Topiramate was originally synthesized as part of a research project to discover structural analogs of fructose-1, 6-diphosphate capable of inhibiting the enzyme fructose-1, 6-bisphosphatase, thereby blocking gluconeogenesis, but it has no hypoglycemic activity. Topiramate and divalproex sodium are the only two anticonvulsants that have FDA approval for migraine prevention. Topiramate is not associated with significant reductions in estrogen exposure at doses below 200 mg/day. At doses above 200 mg/day, there may be a dose-related reduction in exposure to the estrogen component of oral contraceptives.

Two large, pivotal, multicenter, randomized, double-blind, placebo-controlled clinical trials assessed the efficacy and safety of topiramate (50, 100, and 200 mg/day) in migraine prevention. In the first trial, the responder rate (patients with >50% reduction in monthly migraine frequency) was 52% with topiramate 200 mg/day ($p < .001$), 54% with topiramate 100 mg ($p < .001$), and 36% with topiramate 50 mg/day ($p = 0.039$), compared with 23% with placebo (Silberstein et al., 2004). The 200-mg dose was not significantly more effective than the 100-mg dose. The second pivotal trial (Brandes et al., 2004) had significantly more patients who exhibited at least a 50% reduction in mean monthly migraines in the groups treated with 50 mg/day of topiramate (39%, $p = .009$), 100 mg/day of topiramate (49%, $p = .001$), and 200 mg/day of topiramate (47%, $p = .001$).

A third randomized, double-blind, parallel-group, multicenter trial (Diener et al., 2004) compared two doses of topiramate (100 mg/day or 200 mg/day) to placebo or propranolol (160 mg/day). Topiramate 100 mg/day was superior to placebo as measured by average monthly migraine period rate, average monthly migraine days, rate of rescue medication use, and percentage of patients with a 50% or greater decrease in average monthly migraine period rate (responder rate 37%). The topiramate 100 mg/day and propranolol groups were similar in change from baseline to the core double-blind phase in average monthly migraine period rate and other secondary efficacy variables.

Topiramate's most common AE is paresthesia; other common AEs are fatigue, decreased appetite, nausea, diarrhea, weight decrease, taste perversion, hypoesthesia, and abdominal pain. In the migraine trials, body weight was reduced an average of 2.3% in the 50-mg group, 3.2% in the 100-mg group, and 3.8% in the 200-mg group. Patients on propranolol gained 2.3% of their baseline body weight. The most common central nervous system AEs were somnolence, insomnia, mood problems, anxiety, difficulty with memory, language problems, and difficulty with concentration. Renal calculi can occur with topiramate use. The reported incidence is about 1.5%, representing a two- to fourfold increase over the estimated occurrence in the general population (Sachedo et al., 1997).

A very rare AE is acute myopia associated with secondary angle closure glaucoma. No cases of this condition were reported in the clinical studies (Thomson Healthcare, 2003). Oligohidrosis has been reported in association with an elevation in body temperature. Most reports have involved children.

Start topiramate at a dose of 15 to 25 mg at bedtime (Table 9–4). Increase by a dose of 15 to 25 mg/week. Do not increase the dose if bothersome AEs develop; wait until they resolve (they usually do). If they do not resolve, decrease the drug to the last tolerable dose, and then increase by a lower dose more slowly. Attempt to reach a dose of 50 to 100 mg/day given twice a day. It is our experience that patients who tolerate the lower doses with only partial improvement often have increased benefit with higher doses. The dose can be increased to 600 mg/day or higher.

Dodick et al. (2009), in a multicenter, randomized, double-blind double-dummy, parallel-group, noninferiority trial comparing topiramate and amitriptyline for the prevention of episodic migraine, demonstrated that topiramate was as effective as amitriptyline in reducing the frequency of migraine headache. The primary efficacy variable, change from baseline in the mean monthly number of migraine episodes, was –2.6 in the topiramate arm and –2.7 in the amitriptyline arm (NS). There also was no significant difference between the two preventives, with respect to the prespecified secondary outcome measures. However, the topiramate group showed statistically greater improvement in mean functional disability during migraine attacks (least squares mean [LSM] change: –0.33 vs. –0.19; 95% CI, –0.3 to 0.0; $p = .040$) and experienced an improvement in weight satisfaction, while subjects on amitriptyline experienced weight satisfaction deterioration ($p < .001$).

Very recently, the National Institute of Neurological Diseases and Stroke (NINDS) Clinical Research Collaboration conducted the Chronic Migraine Treatment Trial to examine the safety and efficacy of topiramate (up to 100 mg/day) and propranolol (up to 240 mg/day LA formulation) taken in combination compared with treatment with topiramate (up to 100 mg/day) and placebo. This double-blind, placebo-controlled, randomized clinical trial was terminated in September 2010, when an interim analysis determined that the combination of topiramate and propranolol offered no additional advantage over topiramate alone (Silberstein et al., 2011).

LAMOTRIGINE

Lamotrigine blocks voltage-sensitive sodium channels, leading to inhibition of neuronal glutamate release. Chen et al. (2001) reported two patients with migraine with persistent auralike visual phenomena for months to years. After 2 weeks of lamotrigine treatment, both had resolution of the visual symptoms.

Although open-label studies have suggested that lamotrigine may have a select role in the treatment of patients with frequent or prolonged aura, results from a placebo-controlled study in migraine without aura was negative. Steiner et al. (1997) compared the safety and efficacy of lamotrigine (200 mg/day) and placebo in migraine prophylaxis in a double-blind, randomized, parallel-group trial. Although improvements were greater with placebo, these changes were not statistically significant and indicate that lamotrigine was ineffective for migraine prophylaxis. There were more AEs with lamotrigine than placebo, most commonly rash. With slow dose-escalation, their frequency was reduced and the rate of withdrawal due to AEs was similar in both treatment groups.

Open-label studies have suggested that lamotrigine may have a select role in the treatment of migraine with aura, but no placebo-controlled studies have yet been conducted in this patient population. Both lamotrigine and topiramate (Freitag, 2003) may have a special role in the treatment of migraine with aura. A more recent Class I (see Table 9–5) study comparing lamotrigine

50 mg/day to placebo or topiramate 50 mg/day reported that lamotrigine was not more effective than placebo (for both primary endpoints) and was less effective than topiramate in reducing frequency and intensity of migraine (Gupta et al., 2007). The primary outcome measure (responder rate of ≥50% reduction in monthly migraine frequency) was 46% for lamotrigine versus 34% for placebo ($p = .093$, CI 0.02–0.26), and 63% for topiramate versus 46% for lamotrigine ($p = .019$, CI 0.03–0.31).

Summary: Evidence for anticonvulsants in the prevention of migraine (Pearlman et al., 2010)

There is strong evidence (Level A) establishing the effectiveness of the following: divalproex sodium, sodium valproate, and topiramate.

Evidence exists (Level B) to suggest that the following is probably effective and should be considered: gabapentin.

The following anticonvulsant is possibly effective (Level C): carbamazepine.

Lamotrigine is ineffective (Level A negative) and should not be offered for migraine prevention, although there is anecdotal evidence that it may have some efficacy for patients with migraine with aura.

TABLE 9–5 *American Academy of Neurology Classification of Evidence for the Rating of a Therapeutic Study*

Class I: A randomized, controlled clinical trial of the intervention of interest with masked or objective outcome assessment, in a representative population. Relevant baseline characteristics are presented and substantially equivalent among treatment groups or there is appropriate statistical adjustment for differences.

The following are also required:

a. Concealed allocation

b. Primary outcome(s) clearly defined

c. Exclusion/inclusion criteria clearly defined

d. Adequate accounting for dropouts (with at least 80% of enrolled subjects completing the study) and cross-overs with numbers sufficiently low to have minimal potential for bias

e. For noninferiority or equivalence trials claiming to prove efficacy for one or both drugs, the following are also required[a]:

   1. The authors explicitly state the clinically meaningful difference to be excluded by defining the threshold for equivalence or noninferiority.

   2. The standard treatment used in the study is substantially similar to that used in previous studies establishing efficacy of the standard treatment (e.g., for a drug, the mode of administration, dose, and dosage adjustments are similar to those previously shown to be effective).

   3. The inclusion and exclusion criteria for patient selection and the outcomes of patients on the standard treatment are comparable to those of previous studies establishing efficacy of the standard treatment.

   4. The interpretation of the results of the study is based on a per protocol analysis that takes into account dropouts or cross-overs.

Class II: A randomized, controlled clinical trial of the intervention of interest in a representative population with masked or objective outcome assessment that lacks one criteria a–e above or a prospective matched cohort study with masked or objective outcome assessment in a representative population that meets b–e above. Relevant baseline characteristics are presented and substantially equivalent among treatment groups or there is appropriate statistical adjustment for differences.

Class III: All other controlled trials (including well-defined natural history controls or patients serving as own controls) in a representative population, where outcome is independently assessed, or independently derived by objective outcome measurement.[b]

Class IV: Studies not meeting Class I, II, or III criteria including consensus or expert opinion

[a] Note that numbers 1–3 in Class Ie are required for Class II in equivalence trials. If any one of the three is missing, the class is automatically downgraded to Class III.

[b] Objective outcome measurement: an outcome measure that is unlikely to be affected by an observer's (patient, treating physician, investigator) expectation or bias (e.g., blood tests, administrative outcome data).

Angiotensin-Converting Enzyme Inhibitors and Angiotensin II Receptor Antagonists

Schrader et al. (2001) conducted a double-blind, placebo-controlled, cross-over study of lisinopril, an angiotensin-converting enzyme inhibitor in migraine prophylaxis (Table 9–6). Days with migraine were reduced by at least 50% in 14 participants for active treatment versus placebo and 17 patients for active treatment versus runin period. Days with migraine were fewer by at least 50% in 14 participants for active treatment versus placebo. Tronvik et al. (2003) performed a randomized, double-blind, placebo-controlled, cross-over study of candesartan (16 mg), an angiotensin II receptor blocker, in migraine prevention. In a period of 12 weeks, the mean number of days with headache was 18.5 with placebo versus 13.6 with candesartan ($p = .001$) in the intention-to-treat analysis ($n = 57$). The number of candesartan responders (reduction of ≥50% compared with placebo) was 18 of 57 (31.6%) for days with headache and 23 of 57 (40.4%) for days with migraine. AEs were similar in the two periods. In this study, the angiotensin II receptor blocker candesartan was effective, with a tolerability profile comparable with that of placebo (Table 9–6).

> Summary: Evidence for ACE inhibitors/antagonists in the prevention of migraine (Pearlman et al., 2010)
> The following are possibly effective (Level C) and may be considered: candesartan, lisinopril, telmisartan.

While daily oral prophylactic treatments have proven effective for many patients, issues such as lack of compliance with daily dosing regimens and adverse effects have limited their usefulness (Blumenfeld et al., 2003; Silberstein, 2004) and resulted in looking for other modalities and agents, including botulinum toxins (botulinum neurotoxins; BoNTs), as potential preventive treatments.

Formulations of Botulinum Toxin

The seven BoNT serotypes (A, B, C1, D, E, F, and G) produced by *Clostridium botulinum* are synthesized as single-chain polypeptides. All serotypes inhibit acetylcholine release, although their intracellular target proteins, physiochemical characteristics, and potencies are different (Aoki & Guyer, 2001; Mauskop, 2004). Botulinum toxin type A (BoNTA) has been the most widely studied serotype for therapeutic purposes (Aoki & Guyer, 2001).

Currently, BoNT is available for clinical use in the United States as onabotulinumtoxinA (Botulinum toxin type A) branded as BOTOX (Allergan, Inc., Irvine, CA, USA) and abobotulinumtoxinA (another Botulinum toxin type A) branded as Dysport (Ipsen Ltd., Slough, UK), and the BoNTB product rimabotulinumtoxinB, branded as Myobloc/Neurobloc (Solstice Neurosciences, Inc., South San Francisco, CA, USA/Solstice Neurosciences Ltd., Dublin, Ireland). Lyophilized BOTOX is available in vials containing 100 U of BoNTA and is diluted with 2 or 4 mL of preservative-free 0.9% saline to yield a concentration of 5.0 or 2.5 U per 0.1 mL, respectively (BOTOX package insert, 2004). Reconstituted solutions of BOTOX can be refrigerated but must be used within 4 hours (BOTOX

TABLE 9–6 *Miscellaneous Medication in the Preventive Treatment of Migraine*

Agent	Daily Dose	Comment
ANGIOTENSIN-CONVERTING ENZYME AND ANGIOTENSIN RECEPTOR ANTAGONISTS		
Lisinopril	10–40 mg	Positive small controlled trial
Candesartan	16 mg	Positive small controlled trial
OTHERS		
Feverfew	50–82 mg	Controversial evidence
Petasites	50–100 mg	75 and 100 mg better than placebo in independent trials
Riboflavin	400 mg	Positive small controlled trial
Coenzyme Q	100–150 mg	Two positive controlled trials
Magnesium	400–600 mg	Controversial evidence

package insert, 2004). Myobloc is available in 0.5-, 1-, and 2-mL vials containing 5,000 U/mL (Mauskop, 2004).

Mechanism of Action of Botulinum Toxin in Headache

BoNT acts by inhibiting the release of acetylcholine at the neuromuscular junction by binding to motor or sympathetic nerve terminals, then entering the nerve terminals and inhibiting the release of acetylcholine, thereby blocking neuromuscular transmission. This inhibition occurs as the BoNT cleaves one of several proteins integral to the successful docking and release of acetylcholine from vesicles situated within nerve endings. Following intramuscular injection, BoNT produces partial chemical denervation of the muscle, resulting in a localized reduction in muscle activity (Aoki & Guyer, 2001; Mauskop, 2004).

The association between BoNTA use and the alleviation of migraine headache symptoms was discovered during initial clinical trials of BoNTA treatment for hyperfunctional lines of the face (Binder et al., 2000). BoNTA therapy has been used for a variety of disorders associated with painful muscle spasms. Because migraine attacks are frequently associated with muscle tenderness (Jensen et al., 1998), it was generally believed that intramuscular BoNTA might prevent abnormal sensory signals in the affected muscle from arriving to the central nervous system. If abnormal muscle physiology can trigger migraine, one would predict that BoNTA treatment would work prophylactically only in patients whose migraine attacks develop on the heels of episodic or chronic muscle tenderness.

Jakubowski et al. (2005) explored neurological markers that might distinguish migraine patients who benefited from BoNTA treatment from those who did not. The prevalence of neck tenderness, aura, photophobia, phonophobia, osmophobia, nausea, and throbbing was similar between responders and nonresponders. However, the two groups offered different accounts of their pain. Among nonresponders, 92% described a buildup of pressure inside their head (exploding headache). Among responders, 74% perceived their head to be crushed, or clamped, or stubbed by external forces (imploding headache), and 13% attested to an eye-popping pain (ocular headache). The finding that exploding headache is not as responsive to extracranial BoNTA injections is consistent with the view that migraine pain is mediated by intracranial innervation. The amenability of imploding and ocular headaches to BoNTA treatment suggests that these types of migraine pain involve extracranial innervation as well (Jakubowski et al., 2006). The precise mechanisms by which BoNTA alleviates headache pain are unclear. It inhibits the release of glutamate and the neuropeptides substance P and calcitonin gene–related peptide (CGRP) from nociceptive neurons, suggesting that its antinociceptive properties are distinct from its neuromuscular activity (Dodick et al., 2005).

Evidence from preclinical studies suggests that BoNTA may inhibit central sensitization of trigeminovascular neurons, which is believed to be key to migraine's development and maintenance (Aoki, 2003; Cui et al., 2004; Dodick et al., 2005; Oshinsky, 2004). Afferent–afferent communication happens in the nerve through axon–axon glutamate secretion, and at the level of the ganglion through nonsynaptic release of glutamate and peptides (CGRP and substance P). Oshinsky et al. (2004) used a preclinical model of sensitizing dorsal horn neurons in the trigeminal nucleus caudalis (TNC) following a 5-minute chemical stimulation of the dura as a model for testing the effects of BoNTA on central sensitization. It was hypothesized that botulinum toxin may block the axon-to-axon and interganglionic communication of the afferents and thus prevent central and peripheral sensitization outside of rat dura. Single-neuron electrophysiological recordings of second-order sensory neurons in the TNC with cutaneous receptive fields and microdialysis of the TNC were used to evaluate the effects of pretreatment of the periorbital region of the rat with BoNTA. In saline-treated animals, extracellular glutamate increased steadily after 100 minutes following the application of inflammatory soup to the dura. The increase of glutamate reached approximately three times the basal level at 3 hours after the inflammatory soup. Electrophysiological recordings of neurons in the TNC, before and after sensitization by the inflammatory soup, showed an increase in the magnitude of the response to sensory stimuli and an increase in the cutaneous receptive field of the second sensory neurons in the TNC.

Increases in glutamate were blocked by pretreating the face of the rat with BoNTA. Electrophysiological studies then confirmed that, unlike saline-treated animals, there was no change in the magnitude of the sensory response in the TNC neurons or their receptive field in the BoNTA rats following the inflammatory soup. These data show that peripheral application of BoNTA prevents central sensitization elicited by stimulation of the dura with inflammatory mediators (Oshinsky et al., 2004).

BoNT Treatment Techniques

Sterile technique should be observed for the entire BoNT injection procedure. Injections do not have to be intramuscular, but the muscles can be used as reference sites for injections, which are usually administered in the glabellar and frontal regions, the temporalis muscle, the occipitalis muscle, and the cervical paraspinal region.

The following injection protocols are commonly used: (a) the fixed-site approach, which uses fixed, symmetrical injection sites and a range of predetermined doses; (b) the follow-the-pain approach, which adjusts the sites and doses depending on where the patient feels pain and where the examiner can elicit pain and tenderness on palpation of the muscle and often employs asymmetrical injections; and (c) a combination approach, using injections at fixed frontal sites, supplemented with follow-the-pain injections (this approach typically uses higher doses of BoNTA) (Blumenfeld et al., 2003). Table 9–7 lists recommended anatomical sites of injection for headache and the BoNTA (BOTOX) dose per site used in the PREEMPT trials.

Clinical Studies of BoNT's Efficacy in Headache Disorders

Most studies of BoNT's efficacy and safety in headache treatment have used BOTOX (Schulte-Mattler & Leinisch, 2007). No large, well-controlled studies using other preparations of botulinum toxin have been published. Clinical trial results discussed below are summarized in Table 9–8 (Schulte-Mattler & Leinisch, 2007).

Some studies support the efficacy of BoNTA in migraine treatment. A double-blind, vehicle-controlled trial of 123 patients with moderate to severe migraine found that subjects treated with a single injection of 25 U BoNTA (but not those treated with 75 U) had significantly fewer migraine attacks per month, as well as reductions in migraine severity, number of days requiring acute medication, and incidence of migraine-induced vomiting (Silberstein et al., 2000). The lack of significant effect in the higher-dose group may be related to group differences at baseline (e.g., fewer migraines or a longer time since migraine onset in the higher dose group) (Silberstein et al., 2000). Another double-blind, placebo-controlled, region-specific study found a significant reduction in migraine pain among patients who received simultaneous injections of BoNTA in the frontal and temporal regions, as well as an overall trend toward BoNTA superiority to placebo in reducing migraine frequency and duration (Silberstein et al., 2000). A randomized, double-blind, placebo-controlled study compared the efficacy of placebo, 16 U BoNTA, and 100 U BoNTA as migraine prophylaxis when injected into the frontal and neck muscles (Evers et al., 2004). There were no statistically significant differences in reduction of migraine frequency among the groups, but the accompanying migraine symptoms were reduced in the 16-U BoNTA group (Evers et al., 2004).

New studies, however, have not demonstrated significant improvements over placebo. A recent study (Saper et al., 2007) of patients ($N = 232$) with moderate to severe episodic migraine (four to eight episodes per month) compared placebo with regional (frontal, temporal, or glabellar) or combined (frontal/temporal/glabellar) treatment with BoNTA. Reductions from baseline in migraine frequency, maximum severity, and duration occurred with BoNTA and placebo, but there were no significant between-group differences (Saper et al., 2007). Elkind et al. (2006) conducted a series of three sequential studies of 418 patients with a history of four to eight moderate to severe migraines per month with rerandomization at each stage, and BoNTA doses ranging from 7.5 to 50 U and placebo produced comparable decreases from baseline in migraine frequency at each time point examined, with no consistent, statistically significant, between-group differences observed (Elkind et al., 2006).

TABLE 9–7 *BOTOX Dosing for Chronic Migraine, by Muscle*

Head/Neck Area	Total Number of Units (U)	(Number of IM Injection Sites)
	Minimum Dose	Maximum Dose
Frontalis	20 U (4 sites)	20 U (4 sites)
Corrugator	10 U (2 sites)	10 U (2 sites)
Procerus	5 U (1 site)	5 U (1 site)
Occipitalis	30 U (6 sites)	≤40 U (5 U per site; ≤8 sites)
Temporalis	40 U (8 sites)	≤50 U (5 U per site; ≤10 sites)
Trapezius	30 U (6 sites)	≤50 U (5 U per site; ≤10 sites)
Cervical paraspinal muscle group	20 U (4 sites)	20 U (4 sites)
Total Dose Range:	**155 U**	**195 U**
	31 sites	**≤39 sites**

Note. Each IM injection site = 0.1 mL = 5 U onabotulinumtoxinA.

TABLE 9–8 *Summary of Randomized, Double-Blind, Controlled Studies of the Efficacy of Botulinum Toxin Type A (BoNTA) in the Treatment of Headache*

Headache Type	Study Outcome
MIGRAINE	
Silberstein et al. (2000)	Decreased migraine frequency and severity and acute medication use with BoNTA 25 U but not with BoNTA 75 U
Brin et al. (2000)	Decreased migraine pain compared with PBO with simultaneous frontal and temporal BoNTA injections
Evers et al. (2004)	• No difference from PBO in decreased frequency of migraine • Greater decrease in migraine-associated symptoms with BoNTA 16 U
Saper et al. (2007)	Decreased frequency and severity of migraine in BoNTA and PBO groups with no between-group differences
Elkind et al. (2006)	Comparable decreases in migraine frequency in both BoNTA and PBO groups with no between-group differences
CHRONIC MIGRAINE	
Mathew et al. (2005)	• No difference from PBO on primary efficacy endpoint. Change in headache-free days from baseline at day 180 • A significantly higher percentage of BoNTA patients had a ≥50% decrease in headache days per month at day 180 compared with PBO.
Dodick et al. (2005)	Greater decrease in headache frequency after 2 and 3 injections compared with PBO
Silberstein et al. (2005)	• No difference from PBO on primary efficacy endpoint. Change in headache frequency from baseline at day 180 • Greater decrease in headache frequency for BoNTA 225 U and 150 U than PBO
Aurora et al. (2010); Diener et al. (2010); Dodick et al. (2010)	• Two large P-C, D-B trials • Follow the pain • BoNTA both safe and effective
CHRONIC TENSION-TYPE HEADACHE	
Silberstein et al. (2006)	• No difference from PBO on primary efficacy endpoint. Mean change from baseline in CTTH headache days • Greater percentage of BoNTA patients than PBO with ≥50% reduction in headache frequency at 90 and 120 days for several doses of BoNTA

Note. PBO = placebo.

In contrast, several randomized, double-blind, placebo-controlled studies support the efficacy of BoNT for the treatment of chronic daily headache. In a large, placebo-controlled study ($N = 355$), Mathew et al.(2005) found that while BoNTA did not differ from placebo in the primary efficacy measure (change from baseline in headache-free days at day 180), there were significant differences in several secondary endpoints, including a greater percentage of patients with ≥50% decrease in headache frequency and a greater mean change from baseline in headache frequency at day 180. A subgroup analysis of patients not taking concomitant preventive agents ($n = 228$) found that BoNTA patients had a greater decrease in headache frequency compared with placebo after two and three injections, and at most time points from day 180 to 270 (Dodick et al., 2005). In a similar study ($N = 702$) by Silberstein, Stark, et al. (2005), which utilized several doses of BoNTA (75, 150, and 225 U), the primary efficacy endpoint (mean improvement from baseline in headache frequency at day 180) was also not met. However, all groups responded to treatment, and patients taking 150 and 225 U of BoNTA had a greater decrease in headache frequency at day 240 than those taking placebo (Silberstein, Stark, et al., 2005).

THE PREEMPT TRIALS

More recently, the PREEMPT clinical program confirmed onabotulinumtoxinA as an effective, safe, and well-tolerated headache prophylaxis treatment for adults with chronic migraine. Two phase 3, multicenter studies (PREEMPT 1 and 2), which each had a 24-week, double-blind, parallel-group, placebo-controlled phase followed by a 32-week open-label phase, enrolled 1,384 patients with chronic migraine. All patients received the minimum intramuscular (IM) dose of 155 U of onabotulinumtoxinA administered to 31 injection sites across seven head and neck muscles using a fixed-site, fixed-dose injection paradigm. In addition, up to 40 U of onabotulinumtoxinA, administered IM to eight injection sites across three head and neck muscles, was allowed using a modified follow-the-pain approach. Thus, the minimum dose was 155 U and the maximum dose was 195 U (Table 9–8). Statistically significant reductions from baseline for frequency of headache days after BoNTA treatment compared with placebo treatment in both PREEMPT 1 and 2 ($p = .006$; $p < .001$) were observed. Statistically significant improvement from baseline after onabotulinumtoxinA treatment compared with placebo treatment was seen for headache episodes in PREEMPT 2 ($p = .003$). Pooled analysis demonstrated that onabotulinumtoxinA treatment significantly reduced mean frequency of headache days (-8.4 onabotulinumtoxinA, -6.6 placebo; $p < .001$) and headache episodes (5.2 onabotulinumtoxinA, -4.9 placebo; $p = .009$). Additionally, for several other efficacy variables (migraine episodes, migraine days, moderate or severe headache days, cumulative hours of headache on headache days, and proportion of patients with severe disability), there were significant between-group differences favoring onabotulinumtoxinA. The PREEMPT results showed highly significant improvements in multiple headache symptom measures and demonstrated improvement in patients' functioning, vitality, psychological distress, and overall quality of life. Multiple treatments of 155 U up to 195 U per treatment cycle administered every 12 weeks were shown to be safe and well tolerated (Aurora et al., 2010; Diener et al., 2010; Dodick et al., 2010).

Studies evaluating the efficacy of BoNTA in chronic tension-type headache (CTTH) have been inconsistent. A double-blind, randomized, placebo-controlled study (Silberstein et al., 2006) of 300 patients found that while all treatment groups, including placebo, improved in mean change from baseline in CTTH-free days per month (primary endpoint: within-group comparison) at day 60, BoNTA did not demonstrate improvement compared with placebo at any dose or regimen (50 to 150 U—between-group comparison). However, a significantly greater percentage of patients in three BoNTA groups at day 90 and two BoNTA groups at day 120 had a ≥50% decrease in CTTH days than the placebo group (Silberstein et al., 2006). Furthermore, a review evaluating clinical studies of tension-type headache supports the benefit of BoNTA in reducing frequency and severity of headaches, improving quality of life and disability scales, and reducing the need for acute medication (Mathew & Kaup, 2002). In contrast, a later review, which also included studies with both BOTOX and Dysport, concluded that randomized, double-blind, placebo-controlled trials present contradictory results attributable to variable doses, injection sites, and frequency of treatment (Rozen & Sharma, 2006).

Adverse Events Associated With the Use of BoNT

More than two decades of clinical use have established BoNTA as a safe drug (Mauskop, 2004) with no systemic reactions in clinical trials for headache. Side effects have been extensively summarized by Mauskop (2004) and are highlighted below. Rash and flulike symptoms can rarely occur as a result of an allergic reaction. However, serious allergic reactions have never been reported. Injection of anterior neck muscles can cause dysphagia (swallowing difficulties) in some patients. Dysphagia and dry mouth appear to be more common with injections of BoNTB (Myobloc) because of its wider migration pattern. The most common side effects when treating facial muscles are cosmetic and include ptosis or asymmetry of the position of the eyebrows. Another possible, but rare, side effect is difficulty holding the head erect because of neck muscle weakness. Headache patients occasionally develop a headache following the injection procedure; however, some patients have immediate relief of an acute attack. The latter is most likely due to trigger-point injection effect. Worsening of headaches and neck pain can occur and last for several days or, rarely, weeks after the injections, because of the irritating effect of the needling and delay in the muscle relaxing effect of BoNT.

In summary, clinical studies suggest that BoNT is a safe treatment and is efficacious for the prevention of some forms of migraine: that is, chronic migraine and perhaps high-frequency episodic migraine. Further research is needed to understand the mechanism of action of BoNT in headache, establish its safety and efficacy for these indications, and fully develop its therapeutic potential.

PETASITES HYBRIDUS (BUTTERBUR)

Petasites hybridus root (butterbur) is a perennial shrub (Lipton et al., 2001). In a double-blind, placebo-controlled trial conducted by Grossmann and Schmidramsl (2000), 50 mg of a standardized extract of petasites was given twice a day, resulting in a statistically significant decrease in both frequency of migraine (primary endpoint) and pain intensity. A three-arm, parallel-group, double-blind, placebo-controlled trial by Lipton et al. (2004) compared petasites extract at doses of 75 mg bid, 50 mg bid, and placebo, concluding that the 75-mg bid dose was superior to placebo in reducing migraine frequency; however, the 50-mg bid dose was not statistically different from placebo (Table 9–6). The most common AE was belching.

Feverfew (*Tanacetum parthenium*) is a medicinal herb whose effectiveness has not been totally established (Vogler et al., 1998). Riboflavin (400 mg) was effective in one placebo-controlled, double-blind trial. Over half the patients responded (Schoenen et al., 1998). Coenzyme Q10 may be effective for the prevention of migraine. One small Class II study (see Table 9–5) showed that coenzyme Q10 100 mg tid was significantly more effective than placebo in reducing attack frequency from baseline to 4 months following treatment (Sandor et al., 2005). A phytoestrogen preparation of 60 mg soy isoflavones, 100 mg dong quai, and 50 mg black cohosh (each component standardized to its primary alkaloid) reduced migraine attack frequency versus placebo in a small Class II study (Burke et al., 2002).

> Summary: Evidence for medicinal herbs and vitamins in the prevention of migraine (Pearlman et al., 2010)
> Petasites (butterbur) is established as effective (Level A) and should be offered.
> Magnesium, MIG-99 (feverfew), and riboflavin are probably effective (Level B) and should be considered.
> Coenzyme Q10 and phytoestrogens are possibly effective (Level C) and may be considered.
> Omega-3 is possibly ineffective (Level C negative) and may not be considered.

Aspirin and Other Nonsteroidal Anti-Inflammatory Drugs

The following nonsteroidal anti-inflammatory drugs (NSAIDS) are probably effective (Level B) for the prevention of migraine: aspirin, fenoprofen, ibuprofen, ketoprofen, naproxen, or naproxen sodium (Bensenor et al., 2001; Diener et al., 2001; Pradalier et al., 1988). Regular or daily use of selected NSAIDs for the treatment of frequent migraine attacks may exacerbate headache due to development of a condition called medication overuse headache (Silberstein, Olesen, et al., 2005). Therefore, using aspirin, selected analgesics, and NSAIDs may exacerbate headache, which may confound the clinical interpretation of study results in migraine prevention.

> Summary: Evidence for aspirin and other NSAIDS in the prevention of migraine (Pearlman et al., 2010)
> Aspirin is probably effective for migraine prevention (multiple Class II studies—see Table 9–5). Caution against overuse and exacerbation of headache is warranted.

Setting Treatment Priorities

The goals of preventive treatment are to reduce the frequency, duration, or severity of attacks; improve responsiveness to acute attack treatment; improve function; and reduce disability (Table 9–9). The preventive medications with the best-documented efficacy are the β-blockers and amitriptyline, divalproex, and topiramate. Choice is made based on a drug's proven efficacy, the physician's informed belief about medications not yet evaluated in controlled trials, the drug's AEs, the patient's preferences and headache profile, and the presence or absence of coexisting

TABLE 9–9 *Preventive Drugs*

HIGH EFFICACY: LOW TO MODERATE AES
Propranolol, timolol, amitriptyline, valproate, topiramate, flunarizine
LOW EFFICACY: LOW TO MODERATE AES
NSAIDs—Aspirin, flurbiprofen, ketoprofen, naproxen sodium
β-Blockers—Atenolol, metoprolol, nadolol
Calcium channel blockers—Verapamil
Anticonvulsants—Gabapentin
Other—Fenoprofen, feverfew, vitamin B_2
Pizotifen
UNPROVEN EFFICACY: LOW TO MODERATE AES
Antidepressants—Doxepin, nortriptyline, imipramine, protriptyline, venlafaxine, fluvoxamine, mirtazapine, paroxetine, protriptyline, sertraline, trazodone
PROVEN NOT EFFECTIVE OR LOW EFFICACY
Acebutolol, carbamazepine, clomipramine, clonazepam, indomethacin, lamotrigine, nabumetone, nicardipine, nifedipine, pindolol

Note. AEs = adverse effects; NSAIDs = nonsteroidal anti-inflammatory drugs.

disorders (Table 9–1) (Silberstein et al., 2001). Coexistent diseases have important implications for treatment. The presence of a second illness provides therapeutic opportunities but also imposes certain therapeutic limitations. In some instances, two or more conditions may be treated with a single drug. If individuals have more than one disease, certain categories of treatment may be relatively contraindicated.

There are limitations to using a single medication to treat two illnesses. Giving a single medication may not treat two different conditions optimally: Although one of the conditions may be adequately treated, the second illness may require a higher or lower dose, and therefore the patient is at risk of the second illness not being adequately treated. Therapeutic independence may be needed should monotherapy fail. Avoiding drug interactions or increased AEs is a primary concern when using polypharmacy.

For some patients, a single medication may adequately manage comorbid conditions. However, this is likely to be the exception rather than the rule. Polytherapy may enable therapeutic adjustments based on the status of each illness. TCAs are often recommended for patients with migraine and depression (Silberstein et al., 1995). However, appropriate management of depression often requires higher doses of TCAs, which may be associated with more AEs. A better approach might be to treat the depression with an SSRI or serotonin-norepinephrine reuptake inhibitr and treat the migraine with an anticonvulsant. Migraine and epilepsy (Mathew, Saper, Silberstein, Tolander, et al., 1995) may both be controlled with an antiepileptic drug, such as topiramate or divalproex sodium. Divalproex and topiramate are the drugs of choice for the patient with migraine and bipolar illness (Bowden et al., 1994; Silberstein, 1996). When individuals have more than one disease, certain categories of treatment may be relatively contraindicated. For example, β-blockers should be used with caution for the depressed migraineur, while TCAs or neuroleptics may lower the seizure threshold and should be used with caution for the epileptic migraineur.

Although monotherapy is preferred, it often does not yield the desired therapeutic effect, and it may be necessary to combine preventive medications. Antidepressants are often used with β-blockers or calcium channel blockers, and topiramate or divalproex sodium may be used in combination with any of these medications.

CONCLUSION

Preventive therapy plays an important role in migraine management. With the addition of a preventive medication, patients may experience reduced attack frequency and improved response to acute treatment, which can result in reduced health care resource utilization and improved quality of life. Despite research suggesting that a large percentage of migraine patients are candidates for prevention, only a fraction of these patients are receiving or have ever received preventive migraine medication.

Many preventive medications are available, and guidelines for their selection and use have been established. Since comorbid medical and psychological illnesses are prevalent in patients with migraine, one must consider comorbidity when choosing preventive drugs. Drug therapy may be beneficial for both disorders; however, it is also a potential confounder of optimal treatment of either.

There are no biological markers or clinical characteristics that are predictive of response to a particular migraine preventive medication. The impact of prevention on the natural history of migraine remains to be fully investigated.

REFERENCES

Abramowicz, M. (1990). Fluoxetine (Prozac) revisited. *Drugs and Therapy Medical Letter*, 83–85.

Altier, C., & Zamponi, G. W. (2004). Targeting Ca2 + channels to treat pain: T-type versus N-type. *Trends in Pharmacological Sciences, 25*(9), 465–470.

Andersson, K., & Vinge, E. (1990). Beta-adrenoceptor blockers and calcium antagonists in the prophylaxis and treatment of migraine. *Drugs, 39,* 355–373.

Aoki, K. R. (2003). Evidence for antinociceptive activity of botulinum toxin Type A in pain management. *Headache, 43,* S109–S115.

Aoki, K. R., & Guyer, B. (2001). Botulinum toxin type A and other botulinum toxin serotypes; a comparative review of biochemical and pharmacological actions. *European Journal of Neurology, 8*(Suppl 5), 21–29.

Aurora, S. K., Dodick, D. W., Turkel, C. C., DeGryse, R. E., Silberstein, S. D., Lipton, R. B., et al. (2010). OnabotulinumtoxinA for treatment of chronic migraine: Results from the double-blind, randomized, placebo-controlled phase of the PREEMPT 1 trial. *Cephalalgia, 30,* 793–803.

Baldessarini, R. J. (1990). Drugs and the treatment of psychiatric disorders. In A. G. Gilman, T. W. Rall, A. S. Nies, & P. Taylor (Eds.), *The pharmacological basis of therapeutics* (pp. 383–435). New York: Pergamon.

Bensenor, I. M., Cook, N. R., Lee, I. M., Chown, M. J., Hennekens, C. H., & Buring, J. E. (2001). Low-dose aspirin for migraine prophylaxis in women. *Cephalalgia, 21,* 175–183.

Binder, W. J., Brin, M. F., Blitzer, A., Shoenrock, L. D., & Pogoda, J. M. (2000). Botulinum toxin type A (Botox) for treatment of migraine headaches: an open-label study. *Otolaryngology—Head and Neck Surgery, 123,* 669–676.

Blumenfeld, A. M., Binder, W., Silbrestein, S. D., & Blizter, A. (2003). Procedures for administering botulinum toxin type A for migraine and tension-type headache. *Headache, 43,* 884–891.

BOTOX *package insert.* (2004). Irvine, CA: Allergan, Inc.

Bowden, C. L., Brugger, A. M., & Swann, A. C. (1994). Efficacy of divalproex vs lithium and placebo in the treatment of mania. *Journal of the American Medical Association, 271*, 918–924.

Brandes, J. L., Saper, J. R., Diamond, M., Couch, J. R., Lewis, D. W., Schmitt, J., et al., MIGR-002 Study Group. (2004). Topiramate for migraine prevention: A randomized controlled trial. *Journal of the American Medical Association, 291*, 965–973.

Brin, M. F., Swope, D. M., O'Brien, C., Abbasi, S., & Pogoda, J. M. (2000). Botox for migraine: Double-blind, placebo-controlled, region-specific evaluation [Abstract]. *Cephalalgia, 20*, 421–422.

Bulut, S., Berilgen, M. S., Baran, A., Tekatas, A., Atmaca, M., & Mungen, B. (2004). Venlafaxine versus amitriptyline in the prophylactic treatment of migraine: Randomized, double-blind, crossover study. *Clinical Neurology and Neurosurgery, 107*, 44–48.

Burke, B. E., Olson, R. D., & Cusack, B. J. (2002). Randomized, controlled trial of phytoestrogen in the prophylactic treatment of menstrual migraine. *Biomedical Pharmacotherapy, 56*, 283–288.

Chen, W. T., Fuh, J. L., Lu, S. R., & Wang, S. J. (2001). Persistent migrainous visual phenomena might be responsive to lamotrigine. *Headache, 41*, 823–825.

Cohen, G. L. (2005). Migraine prophylactic drugs work via ion channels. *Medical Hypotheses, 65*(1), 114–122. doi:10.1016/j.mehy.2005.01.027

Cortelli, P., Sacquegna, T., Albani, F., Baldrati, A., D'Alessandro, R., Baruzi, A., et al. (1985). Propranolol plasma levels and relief of migraine. *Archives of Neurology, 42*, 46–48.

Couch, J. R., for the Amitriptyline Versus Placebo Study Group. (2010). Amitriptyline in the prophylactic treatment of migraine and chronic daily headache. *Headache, 51*(1), 33–51.

Coulam, C. B., & Annagers, J. R. (1979). New anticonvulsants reduce the efficacy of oral contraception. *Epilepsia, 20*, 519–525.

Cui, M., Khanijou, S., Rubino, J., & Aoki, K. R. (2004). Subcutaneous administration of botulinum toxin A reduces formalin-induced pain. *Pain, 107*, 125–133.

Diener, H. C., Agosti, R., Allais, G., Bergmans, P., Bussone, G., Davies, B., et al. (2007). Cessation versus continuation of 6-month migraine preventive therapy with topiramate (PROMPT): A randomised, double-blind, placebo-controlled trial. *Lancet Neurology, 6*, 1054–1062.

Diener, H. C., Dodick, D. W., Aurora, S. K., Turkel, C. C., DeGryse, R. E., Lipton, R. B., et al. (2010). OnabotulinumtoxinA for treatment of chronic migraine: Results from the double-blind, randomized, placebo-controlled phase of the PREEMPT 2 trial. *Cephalalgia, 30*, 804–814.

Diener, H. C., Hartung, E., Chrubasik, J., Evers, S., Schoenen, J., Eikermann, A., et al. (2001). A comparative study of oral acetylsalicylic acid and metoprolol for the prophylactic treatment of migraine. A randomized, controlled, double-blind, parallel group phase III study. *Cephalalgia, 21*, 120–128.

Diener, H. C., Kurth, T., & Dodick, D. (2007). Patent foramen ovale and migraine. *Current Pain and Headache Reports, 11*(3), 236–240.

Diener, H. C., Tfelt-Hansen, P., Dahlof, C., Lainez, M. J., Sandrini, G., Wang, S. J., et al. (2004). Topiramate in migraine prophylaxis—results from a placebo-controlled trial with propranolol as an active control. *Journal of Neurology, 251*, 943–950.

Dodick, D., Silberstein, S. D., Lindblad, A., Holroyd, K., Mathew, N., Cordell, J., et al. (2011). *Clinical trial design in chronic migraine: Lessons learned from the NINDS CRC Chronic Migraine Treatment Trial (CMTT)*. Abstract presented at the American Academy of Neurology, Honolulu, Hawaii, April 13, 2011.

Dodick, D. W. (2010). Prevention of migraine. *BMJ, 341*(7776), 740.

Dodick, D. W., Freitag, F., Banks, J., Saper, J., Xiang, J., Rupnow, M., et al. (2009). Topiramate versus amitriptyline in migraine prevention: A 26-week, multicenter, randomized, double-blind, double-dummy, parallel-group noninferiority trial in adult migraineurs. *Clinical Therapy, 31*(3), 542–559

Dodick, D. W., Mauskop, A., Elkind, A. H., deGryse, R., Brin, M. F., & Silberstein, S. D. (2005). Botulinum toxin type A for the prophylaxis of chronic daily headache: subgroup analysis of patients not receiving other prophylactic medications: A randomized double-blind, placebo-controlled study. *Headache, 45*, 315–324.

Dodick, D. W., Turkel, C. C., DeGryse, R. E., Aurora, S. K., Silberstein, S. D., Lipton, R. B., et al. (2010). OnabotulinumtoxinA for treatment of chronic migraine: Pooled results from the double-blind, randomized, placebo-controlled phases of the PREEMPT clinical program. *Headache, 50*, 921–936.

Elkind, A. H., O'Carroll, P., Blumenfeld, A., deGryse, R., & Dimitrova, R. (2006). A series of three sequential, randomized, controlled studies of repeated treatments with botulinum toxin type A for migraine prophylaxis. *Journal of Pain, 7*, 688–696.

Evers, S., Vollmer-Haase, J., Schwaag, S., Rahmann, A., Husstedt, I. W., & Frese, A. (2004). Botulinum toxin A in the prophylactic treatment of migraine—a randomized, double-blind, placebo-controlled study. *Cephalalgia, 24*, 838–843.

Feinmann, C. (1985). Pain relief by antidepressants: Possible modes of action. *Pain, 23*, 1–8.

Freitag, F. G. (2003). Topiramate prophylaxis in patients suffering from migraine with aura: Results from a randomized, double-blind, placebo-controlled trial. *Advanced Studies in Medicine, 3*, S562–S564.

Freitag, F. G., Collins, S. D., Carlson, H. A., Goldstein, J., Saper, J., Silberstein, S. D., et al. (2003). A randomized trial of divalproex sodium extended-release tablets in migraine prophylaxis. For the Depakote ER Migraine Study Group. *Neurology, 58*, 1652–1659.

Gray, R. N., Goslin, R. E., McCrory, D. C., Eberlein, K., Tulsky, J., & Hasselblad, V. (1999). *Drug treatments for the prevention of migraine headache*. Prepared for the Agency for Health Care Policy and Research, Contract No. 290-94-2025. Available from the National Technical Information Service Accession No. 127, 953.

Greenberg, D. A. (1997). Calcium channels in neurological disease. *Annals of Neurology, 42*, 275–282.

Grossmann, M., & Schmidramsl, H. (2000). An extract of Petasites hybridus is effective in the prophylaxis of migraine. *International Journal of Clinical Pharmacology and Therapeutics, 38*, 430–435.

Gupta, P., Singh, S., Goyal, V., Shukla, G., & Behari, M. (2007). Low-dose topiramate versus lamotrigine in migraine prophylaxis (the Lotolamp study). *Headache, 47*, 402–412

Hanston, P. P., & Horn, J. R. (1985). Drug interaction. *Newsletter, 5*, 7–10.

Hering, R., & Kuritzky, A. (1992). Sodium valproate in the prophylactic treatment of migraine: A double-blind study versus placebo. *Cephalalgia, 12*, 81–84.

Ifergane, G., Buskila, D., Simiseshvely, N., Zeev, K., & Cohen, H. (2006). Prevalence of fibromyalgia syndrome in migraine patients. *Cephalalgia, 26*(4), 451–456.

Jackson, J. L., Shimeall, W., Sessums, L., Dezee, K., Becker, D., Diemer, M., et al. (2010). Tricyclic antidepressants and headaches: Systematic review and meta-analysis. *BMJ, 341*, c5222.

Jakubowski, M., McAllister, P. J., Bajwa, Z. H., Ward, T. N., Smith, P., & Burstein, R. (2006). Exploding vs. imploding headache in migraine prophylaxis with Botulinum toxin A. *Pain, 24*, 1872–6623.

Jakubowski, M., Silberstein, S., Ashkenazi, A., & Burstein, R. (2005). Can allodynic migraine patients be identified interictally using a questionnaire? *Neurology, 65,* 1419–1422.

Jensen, R., Bendtsen, L., & Olesen, J. (1998). Muscular factors are of importance in tension-type headache. *Headache, 38,* 10–17.

Jensen, R., Brinck, T., & Olesen, J. (1994). Sodium valproate has prophylactic effect in migraine without aura: A triple-blind, placebo-controlled crossover study. *Neurology, 44,* 241–244.

Kishore-Kumar, R., Max, M. B., Schafer, S. C., Gaughan, A. M., Smoller, B., Gracely, R. H., et al. (1990). Desipramine relieves post-herpetic neuralgia. *Clinical Pharmacology and Therapeutics, 47,* 305–312.

Klapper, J. A. (1995). An open label crossover comparison of divalproex sodium and propranolol HCl in the prevention of migraine headaches. *Headache Quarterly, 5,* 50–53.

Klapper, J. A. (1997). Divalproex sodium in migraine prophylaxis: A dose-controlled study. *Cephalalgia, 17,* 103–108.

Koella, W. P. (1985). CNS-related (side-)effects of b-blockers with special reference to mechanisms of action. *European Journal of Clinical Pharmacology, 28,* 55–63.

Lipton, R. B., Diamond, M., Freitag, F., Bigal, M., Stewart, W. F., & Reed, M. L. (2005). Migraine prevention patterns in a community sample: Results from the American migraine prevalence and prevention (AMPP) study [Abstract]. *Headache, 45,* 792–793.

Lipton, R. B., Gobel, H., Einhaupl, K. M., Wilks, K., & Mauskop, A. (2004). Petasites hybridus root (butterbur) is an effective preventive treatment for migraine. *Neurology, 63,* 2240–2244.

Lipton, R. B., Gobel, H., Wilks, K., & Mauskop, A. (2002). Efficacy of petasites (an extract from petasites rhizone) 50 and 75mg for prophylaxis of migraine: results of a randomized, double-blind, placebo-controlled study [Abstract]. *Neurology, 58,* A472.

Lipton, R. B., Hamelsky, S. W., & Stewart, W. F. (2001). Epidemiology and impact of headache. In: S. D. Silberstein, R. B. Lipton, & D. J. Dalessio (Eds.), *Wolff's headache and other head pain* (pp. 85–107). New York: Oxford University Press.

Lipton, R. B., & Silberstein, S. D. (1994). Why study the comorbidity of migraine? *Neurology, 44,* 4–5.

Markley, H. G., Cleronis, J. C. D., & Piepko, R. W. (1984). Verapamil prophylactic therapy of migraine. *Neurology, 34,* 973–976.

Mathew, N. T., Frishberg, B. M., Gawel, M., Dimitrova, R., Gibson, J., & Turkel, C. (2005). Botulinum toxin type A (BOTOX) for the prophylactic treatment of chronic daily headache: A randomized, double-blind, placebo-controlled trial. *Headache, 45,* 293–307.

Mathew, N. T., & Kaup, A. O. (2002). The use of botulinum toxin type A in headache treatment. *Current Treatment Options in Neurology, 4,* 365–373.

Mathew, N. T., Rapoport, A., Saper, J., Magnus, L., Klapper, J., Ramadan, N., et al. (2001). Efficacy of gabapentin in migraine prophylaxis. *Headache, 41,* 119–128.

Mathew, N. T., Saper, J. R., Silberstein, S. D., Rankin, L., Markley, H. G., Solomon, S., et al. (1995). Migraine prophylaxis with divalproex. *Archives of Neurology, 52,* 281–286.

Mauskop, A. (2004). The use of botulinum toxin in the treatment of headaches. *Pain Physician, 7,* 377–387.

Olerud, B., Gustavsson, C. L., & Furberg, B. (1986). Nadolol and propranolol in migraine management. *Headache, 26,* 490–493.

Oshinsky, M., Poso-Rosich, P., Luo, J., Hyman, S., & Silberstein, S. D. (2004). Botulinum toxin A blocks sensitization of neurons in the trigeminal nucleus caudalis [Abstract]. *Cephalalgia, 24,* 781.

Oshinsky, M. L. (2004). Botulinum toxins and migraine: How does it work? *Practical Neurology,* (Suppl), 10–13.

Ozyalcin, S. N., Talu, G. K., Kiziltan, E., Yucel, B., Ertas, M., & Disci, R. (2005). The efficacy and safety of venlafaxine in the prophylaxis of migraine. *Headache, 45,* 144–152.

Panerai, A. E., Monza, G., Movilia, P., Bianchi, M., Francussi, B. M., & Tiengo, M. (1990). A randomized, within-patient, cross-over, placebo-controlled trial on the efficacy and tolerability of the tricyclic antidepressants chlorimipramine and nortriptyline in central pain. *Acta Neurologica Scandinavica, 82,* 34–38.

Pellock, J. M., & Willmore, L. J. (1991). A rational guide to routine blood monitoring in patients receiving antiepileptic drugs. *Neurology, 41,* 961–964.

Pearlman, S., Silberstein, S., Freitag, F., Dodick, D., & Ashman, E. (2010). Evidence-based guideline update: OTC treatments for migraine prevention in adults. Report of the Quality Standards Subcommittee of the American Academy of Neurology and the American Headache Society. *Neurology.*

Pradalier, A., Clapin, A., & Dry, J. (1988). Treatment review: Nonsteroid antiinflammatory drugs in the treatment and long-term prevention of migraine attacks. *Headache, 28,* 550–557.

Ramadan, N. M. (2004). Prophylactic migraine therapy: Mechanisms and evidence. *Current Pain and Headache Reports, 8,* 91–95.

Reveiz-Herault, L., Cardona, A. F., Ospina, E. G., & Carrillo, P. (2003). [Effectiveness of flunarizine in the prophylaxis of migraine: a meta-analytical review of the literature]. *Review Neurologique, 36,* 907–912.

Richelson, E. (1990). Antidepressants and brain neurochemistry. *Mayo Clinic Proceedings, 65,* 1227–1236.

Riopelle, R., & McCans, J. L. (1982). A pilot study of the calcium channel antagonist diltiazem in migraine syndrome prophylaxis. *Canadian Journal of Neurological Sciences, 9,* 269.

Rompel, H., & Bauermeister, P. W. (1970). Aetiology of migraine and prevention with carbamazepine (Tegretol). *South Africa Medical Journal, 44,* 75–80.

Rozen, D., & Sharma, J. (2006). Treatment of tension-type headache with Botox: A review of the literature. *Mount Sinai Journal of Medicine, 73,* 493–498.

Ryan, R. E. (1984). Comparative study of nadolol and propranolol in prophylactic treatment of migraine. *American Heart Journal, 108,* 1156–1159.

Ryan, R. E., & Sudilovsky, A. (1983). Nadolol: Its use in the prophylactic treatment of migraine. *Headache, 23,* 26–31.

Sachedo, R. C., Reife, R. A., Lim, P., & Pledger, G. (1997). Topiramate monotherapy for partial onset seizures. *Epilepsia, 38,* 294–300.

Sandor, P. S., Di, C. L., Coppola, G., Saenger, U., Fumal, A., Magis, D., et al. (2005). Efficacy of coenzyme Q10 in migraine prophylaxis: A randomized controlled trial. *Neurology, 64,* 713–715.

Saper, J. R., Mathew, N. T., Loder, E. W., deGryse, R., & VanDenburgh, A. M. (2007). A double-blind, randomized, placebo-controlled comparison of botulinum toxin type A injection sites and doses in the prevention of episodic migraine. *Pain Medicine, 8,* 478–485.

Saunders, K., Merikangas, K., Low, N. C. P., Von Korff, M., & Kessler, R. C. (2008). Impact of comorbidity on headache-related disability. *Neurology, 70*(7), 538–547. Retrieved from SCOPUS database.

Schoenen, J., Jacquy, J., & Lenaerts, M. (1998). Effectiveness of high-dose riboflavin in migraine prophylaxis. A randomized controlled trial. *Neurology, 50,* 466–470.

Schrader, H., Stovner, L. J., Helde, G., Sand, T., & Bovim, G. (2001). Prophylactic treatment of migraine with angiotensin converting enzyme inhibitor (lisinopril): Randomized, placebo-controlled, crossover study. *BMJ, 322,* 19–22.

Schulte-Mattler, W. J., & Leinisch, E. (2007). Evidence based medicine on the use of botulinum toxin for headache disorders. *Journal of Neural Transmission, 47,* 402–412.

Schwedt, T. J. (2009). The migraine association with cardiac anomalies, cardiovascular disease, and stroke. *Neurologic Clinics, 27*(2), 513–523. doi:10.1016/j.ncl.2008.11.006

Silberstein, S., Dodick, D., Lindblad, A., Holroyd, K., Mathew, N., Cordell, J., & Hirtz, D. (2011). A randomized, double-blind, placebo-controlled clinical trial of adding propranolol to topiramate in subjects with suboptimal response to topiramate alone: Results from the NINDS CRC Chronic Migraine Treatment Trial (CMTT). Abstract presented at the American Academy of Neurology Annual Meeting, Honolulu, Hawaii, April 14, 2011.

Silberstein, S., Diamond, S., Loder, E., Reed, M. L., & Lipton, R. B. (2005). Prevalence of migraine sufferers who are candidates for preventive therapy: Results from the American migraine study (AMPP) study [Abstract]. *Headache, 45,* 770–771.

Silberstein, S. D. (1996). Divalproex sodium in headache—literature review and clinical guidelines. *Headache, 36,* 547–555.

Silberstein, S. D. (1997). Migraine and pregnancy. *Neurologic Clinics, 15,* 209–231.

Silberstein, S. D. (2000). Practice parameter—Evidence-based guidelines for migraine headache (an evidence-based review): Report of the Quality Standards Subcommittee of the American Academy of Neurology for the United States Headache Consortium. *Neurology, 55,* 754–762.

Silberstein, S. D. (2004). Headaches in pregnancy. *Neurologic Clinics, 22,* 727–756.

Silberstein, S. D. (2010). Association between restless legs syndrome and migraine. *Journal of Neurology, Neurosurgery, and Psychiatry, 81*(5), 473–475.

Silberstein, S. D., Gobel, H., Jensen, R., Elkind, A. H., deGryse, R., Walcott, J. M., et al. (2006). Botulinum toxin type A in the prophylactic treatment of chronic tension-type headache: A multicentre, double-blind, randomized, placebo-controlled, parallel-group study. *Cephalalgia, 26,* 790–800.

Silberstein, S. D., Lipton, R. B., & Breslau, N. (1995). Migraine: Association with personality characteristics and psychopathology. *Cephalalgia, 15,* 337–369.

Silberstein, S. D., Mathew, N., Saper, J., & Jenkin, S. (2000). Botulinum toxin type A as a migraine preventive treatment: For the Botox® Migraine Clinical Research Group. *Headache, 40,* 445–450.

Silberstein, S. D., Neto, W., Schmitt, J., & Jacobs, D. (2004). Topiramate in the prevention of migraine headache: A randomized, double-blind, placebo-controlled, multiple-dose study. For the MIGR-001 Study Group. *Archives of Neurology, 61,* 490–495.

Silberstein, S. D., Olesen, J., Bousser, M. G., Diener, H. C., Dodick, D., First, M., et al. (2005). The international classification of headache disorders, 2nd edition (ICHD-II)—revision of criteria for 8.2 medication-overuse headache. *Cephalalgia, 25,* 460–465.

Silberstein, S. D., Saper, J. R., & Freitag, F. (2001). Migraine: Diagnosis and treatment. In: S. D. Silberstein, R. B. Lipton, & D. J. Dalessio (Eds.), *Wolff's headache and other head pain* (pp. 121–237). New York: Oxford University Press.

Silberstein, S. D., Stark, S. R., Lucas, S. M., Christie, S. N., DeGryse, R. E., & Turkel, C. C. (2005). Botulinum toxin type A for the prophylactic treatment of chronic daily headache: A randomized, double-blind, placebo-controlled trial. *Mayo Clinic Proceedings, 80,* 1126–1137.

Silberstein, S. D., Winner, P. K., & Chmiel, J. J. (2003). Migraine preventive medication reduces resource utilization. *Headache: The Journal of Head and Face Pain, 43,* 171–178.

Smith, R., & Schwartz, A. (1984). Diltiazem prophylaxis in refractory migraine. *New England Journal of Medicine, 310,* 1327–1328.

Solomon, G. D. (1986). Verapamil and propranolol in migraine prophylaxis: A double-blind crossover study. *Headache, 26,* 325.

Steiner, T. J., Findley, L. J., & Yuen, A. W. (1997). Lamotrigine versus placebo in the prophylaxis of migraine with and without aura. *Cephalalgia, 17,* 109–112.

Sudilovsky, A., Elkind, A. H., Ryan, R. E., Saper, J. R., Stern, M. A., & Meyer, J. H. (1987). Comparative efficacy of nadolol and propranolol in the management of migraine. *Headache, 27,* 421–426.

Sudilovsky, A., Stern, M. A., & Meyer, J. H. (1986). Nadolol: The benefits of an adequate trial duration in the prophylaxis of migraine. *Headache, 26,* 325.

Tfelt-Hansen, P. (2000). Prioritizing acute pharmacotherapy of migraine. In: J. Olesen, P. Tfelt-Hansen, & K. M. A. Welch (Eds.), *The headaches* (pp. 453–456). New York: Lippincott Williams & Wilkins.

Tfelt-Hansen, P., Standnes, B., Kangasniemi, P., Hakkarainen, H., & Olesen, J. (1984). Timolol vs propranolol vs placebo in common migraine prophylaxis: A double-blind multicenter trial. *Acta Neurologica Scandinavica, 69,* 1–8.

Thomson Healthcare. (2003). *Physicians' desk reference.* Montvale: Author.

Tronvik, E., Stovner, L. J., Helde, G., Sand, T., & Bovim, G. (2003). Prophylactic treatment of migraine with an angiotensin II receptor blocker: A randomized controlled trial. *Journal of the American Medical Association, 289,* 65–69.

Vainionpaa, L. K., Rattya, J., Knip, M., Tapanainen, J. S., Pakarinen, A. J., Lanning, P., et al. (1999). Valproate-induced hyperandrogenism during pubertal maturation in girls with epilepsy. *Annals of Neurology, 45,* 444–450.

Vogler, B. K., Pittler, M. H., & Ernst, E. (1998). Feverfew as a preventive treatment for migraine: A systematic review. *Cephalalgia, 18,* 704–708.

Wauquier, A., Ashton, D., & Marranes, R. (1985). The effects of flunarizine in experimental models related to the pathogenesis of migraine. *Cephalalgia, 5,* 119–120.

10 Iron Accumulation in Migraine

INGE H. PALM-MEINDERS, MICHEL D. FERRARI, AND

MARK C. KRUIT

IRON HOMEOSTASIS

Iron plays an important role in many biochemical processes. In general, iron is essential for proper functioning of the body due to its involvement in oxygen transport, oxygen storage, transportation of electrons, glucose metabolism, synthesis of neurotransmitters and myelin, and DNA replication (Connor & Benkovic, 1992; Kell, 2009; Rouault & Cooperman, 2006). The body needs to maintain stable iron concentrations, because both iron shortage and iron excess lead to dysfunction. Excess of iron is harmful because of its role in the formation of highly reactive hydroxyl radicals, which cause damage to all components of a cell, including proteins, lipids, and DNA. The imbalance between reactive oxygen species and the ability of the body to detoxify the reactive intermediates, or to repair the resulting damage, is called oxidative stress. Oxidative stress is involved in many diseases, including neurological diseases. To prevent an excess of iron, the body regulates the amount of it by changes in uptake, storage, and release in relation to its need. Recently, the protein hepcidin was found to play an important role in this process of iron homeostasis by regulating intestinal iron absorption (Ganz & Nemeth, 2011). Ferritin is the protein that serves to store iron in a soluble and nontoxic form, to deposit it in a safe form, and to transport it to areas where it is required (Maguire et al., 1982). Ferritin is also involved as a delivery protein in the brain (Hulet et al., 1999) and is especially present in larger concentrations in the basal ganglia (Aquino et al., 2009). Iron is important for the brain, as the brain requires relatively much energy, and iron is an essential component of ATP synthesis (Gordon, 2003). In addition, iron is essential for the production of lipids and cholesterol and is therefore important in the synthesis and metabolism of myelin and neurotransmitters (Levenson & Tassabehji, 2004; Thomas & Jankovic, 2004). Brain iron homeostasis is different from other organs because of several brain-specific characteristics. First, brain tissue is protected from free influx of iron from the plasma by the blood-brain barrier (Burdo & Connor, 2003; Burdo et al., 2003). This barrier, together with the ventricular system, actively regulates iron transportation by transferring receptors on capillary endothelial cells (Connor, 1994) as well as on endothelial cells of the choroid plexus (Moos, 1996). Second, the concentration of iron varies between different parts of the brain. Brain regions with motor function (extrapyramidal regions) contain more iron than nonmotor parts (Koeppen et al., 1995).

IRON AND THE BRAIN

In 1922, Spatz recorded the distribution of iron in the different areas of the brain by immersion of brain slices in a staining solution (Perl stain or the Prussian blue stain). Today, iron in the brain can be detected by using magnetic resonance imaging (MRI) and is visible on T2-weighted and T2*-weighted images as hypointensity caused by field heterogeneity and magnetic susceptibility effects (Drayer, Burger, et al., 1986; Haacke et al., 2005). A higher iron load is associated with more hypointensity on the MRI (Haacke et al., 2005; Schenck, 1995). Recent evidence shows a good correlation between conclusions on iron distribution in brain areas from postmortem data and MRI (Peran et al., 2009). In adults, the largest concentration of iron is found in the globus pallidus, red nucleus, and substantia nigra (including pars reticularis), followed by the caudate nucleus and putamen. Through staining of brain slices as well as by MRI, infants have been shown to have only minimal concentrations of iron in the brain (Diezel, 1955; Drayer, Olanow, et al., 1986). The increase in iron concentration in the brain is speculated to be associated with a change in vascularization (Faucheux et al., 1999).

Age-specific iron accumulation in the human brain was described as early as 1958 by Hallgren (Hallgren & Sourander, 1958). He demonstrated, by staining of brain slices, an increase of especially ferritin in specific brain structures, including the globus pallidus and putamen, as preferred sites during the first three decades of human life (Hallgren & Sourander, 1958). More recent postmortem studies have shown higher ferritin levels at older age in several basal ganglia, including the caudate nucleus, putamen, substantia nigra, and globus pallidus (Connor et al., 1995; Zecca et al., 2001). These findings have been confirmed by MRI results demonstrating age-related iron increases among these basal ganglia (Bartzokis et al., 1997). Two recent MRI studies on changes in brain iron concentration related to aging showed an increase of iron in all basal ganglia with increasing age, with specific age-related iron deposition patterns for the different structures (Cherubini et al., 2009; Peran et al., 2009). For instance, the globus pallidus shows a clear increase of iron concentration from childhood into adulthood. The substantia nigra already contains more iron than the globus pallidus at a younger age and the increase follows a steeper curve, whereas both the putamen and caudate nucleus show a much slower rate of iron increase with aging (Aquino et al., 2009). Furthermore, iron increase follows a precise accumulation direction from posterior to anterior and from medial to lateral parts of the basal ganglia (Aquino et al., 2009). Below the age of 15 years, iron accumulation is largest in the medial part of the internal globus pallidus, whereas it is largest in the lateral part between the ages of 15 and 30 years (Aquino et al., 2009). Mechanisms responsible for early accumulation in the substantia nigra and globus pallidus are not clear, but it could be the result of preferential or abnormal local neuronal uptake of iron (Bartzokis et al., 1997) or abnormal transportation of iron along white matter pathways connecting these nuclei (Aoki et al., 1989; Drayer et al., 1986a), or it could be based on a decreased efficiency of the usual iron transport from the basal ganglia to areas elsewhere due to age-related loss of neurons (Cross et al., 1990; Dietrich & Bradley, 1988).

After the age of 50 years, all basal ganglia show a large variability between subjects for hypointensity on MRI, because the T2 values of deep nuclei are significantly influenced by non-iron-related tissue changes, such as myelin loss or an increase in water content associated with microvascular changes (Aquino et al., 2009; Bartzokis et al., 1997; Schenker et al., 1993). Despite the large variability of brain iron accumulation among elderly subjects, it has been suggested that if hypointensity is found in the caudate nucleus, this could be a sign of central nervous system disease instead of being part of the normal aging process (Milton et al., 1991). This was confirmed by a recent MRI study among elderly subjects, which described hypointensity of the caudate nucleus as associated with the presence of a higher load of age-related cerebral changes, such as more atrophy and a higher load of white matter hyperintensities (van Es et al., 2008). Iron excess in the basal ganglia is damaging, because it increases the tissue's susceptibility for apoptosis and inflammation, it could lead to basal ganglia dysfunction due to decreased

protein synthesis, and the tissue becomes more vulnerable to the damaging effect of reactive oxygen species. This destructive process was summarized by Zecca et al. (2004) as iron accumulation, invasion, and increased reactivity.

IRON AND NEUROLOGICAL DISORDERS

Increased iron levels in pathological relevant brain structures and iron-mediated oxidative stress are associated with several neurological disorders, including Parkinson disease, Alzheimer disease, Huntington disease, Friedreich ataxia, amyotrophic lateral sclerosis (ALS), neurodegeneration with brain iron accumulation (formerly Hallervorden-Spatz syndrome), and migraine. Every disorder has its specific mechanisms and locations of brain iron accumulation.

In Parkinson disease, iron excess has been demonstrated in the substantia nigra (Bartzokis et al., 1997; Gorell et al., 1995; Gotz et al., 1990; Kell, 2010; Ryvlin et al., 1995; Sian-Hulsmann et al., 2010) and was found to be associated with local oxidative stress, as indicated by protein disruption (Goodwin et al., 2000) and oxidative DNA damage (Alam et al., 1997; Poon et al., 2004a, 2004b; Sanchez-Ramos et al., 1987).

In the brains of patients suffering from Alzheimer disease, iron accumulation occurs without the normal age-related increase in ferritin, thereby increasing the risk of oxidative stress (Zecca et al., 2004). Iron excess is found early in the disease process in several brain structures, including the basal ganglia (Bartzokis & Tishler, 2000; Bartzokis et al., 1997, 2000; Connor & Benkovic, 1992). Although the origin of elevated brain iron levels is unclear, the role of iron is apparent: Both senile plaques and neurofibrillary tangles, characteristic for the disease, have been shown to accumulate iron (Good et al., 1992; Levine, 1997; Rottkamp et al., 2000; Sayre et al., 2000).

In Huntington disease, iron accumulation has been demonstrated in the putamen, caudate nucleus, and globus pallidus by postmortem studies and MRI studies (Bartzokis & Tishler, 2000; Chen et al., 1993; Dexter et al., 1992; Rutledge et al., 1987). The iron excess contributes to oxidative stress, as indicated by protein disruption (Marnett, 2000; Stadtman, 2001) and oxidative DNA damage (Alam et al., 1997; Marnett, 2000; Poon et al., 2004a; Sanchez-Ramos et al., 1987).

Friedreich ataxia was first described by the German physician Nikolaus Friedreich in 1860 (Friedreich, 1863) and is marked by a genetic mutation causing the mitochondrial protein frataxin to be lacking, leading to impaired iron export from the mitochondria, cytoplasmic depletion, induction of plasma membrane proteins involved in iron uptake, and consequent iron overload (Berg & Youdim, 2006), including iron excess in the dentate nucleus (Koeppen et al., 2007; Waldvogel et al., 1999).

In ALS, increased serum levels of ferritin have been reported (Goodall et al., 2008) and MRIs of the brains of ALS patients show iron accumulation in the dentate nucleus (Langkammer et al., 2010). Although the origin of iron excess in ALS is not yet clear, increased oxidative damage to DNA, lipids, and proteins can be seen early in the disease process, which makes it plausible that iron is at least partly involved (Berg & Youdim, 2006).

Brain MRI evaluation of patients suffering from neuro-degeneration with brain iron accumulation usually shows iron accumulation in the globus pallidus (typical but non-specific eye-of-the-tiger sign), the substantia nigra, and the dentate nucleus (Halliday, 1995; Hayflick et al., 2003; Savoiardo et al., 1993; Swaiman, 1991), and histopathology demonstrates iron excess accompanied by neuronal loss and gliosis (Galvin et al., 2000; Savoiardo et al., 1993). It has been proposed that accumulation of cysteine, which chelates iron, causes oxidative stress and leads to the increase of iron in the basal ganglia (Berg & Youdim, 2006; Perry et al., 1985).

IRON AND MIGRAINE

Few studies have been published describing the association between migraine and iron levels in the brain. After earlier reports describing functional blood oxygenation level–dependent MRI demonstrating the involvement of pain in several specific brain structures, Welch and colleagues (2001) focused their attention on the peri-aqueductal gray matter, red nucleus, and substantia nigra in relation to migraine. It was speculated that, since these brain structures in particular show high iron levels and are densely populated with neurotransmitters that can generate free radicals, repeated migraine attacks and associated repeated hypoxia could result in release of free radicals and cell damage. This mechanism could be seen in those brain areas as accumulation of iron, similar to the processes already known in other neurodegenerative diseases as mentioned above.

To test this hypothesis, a clinic-based cross-sectional brain MRI study was carried out to assess iron levels by measuring transverse relaxation rates (Welch et al., 2001). This study included 17 migraine patients (diagnosed using International Headache Society [IHS] criteria), 17 patients with chronic daily headache, and 17 control participants, aged 20 to 64 years. Compared with controls, significant higher iron levels were found in the periaqueductal gray

matter of the patients with migraine and chronic daily headache. No differences were found between men and women, nor between migraine with and without aura. In addition, an association between iron accumulation and illness duration was found.

Because no relation was found between increased iron levels and age in this study, the authors speculated that iron accumulation must be related to repeated headache attacks. Several explanations for the high iron content of the periaqueductal gray matter among migraineurs were given by the authors. First, as a result of the migraine-related pain combined with oxidative stress, this structure could be abnormally highly metabolic active in migraineurs, since transferring-receptor binding is proportional to the metabolic activity of the neuron, and in turn may be influenced by nociceptive function. Overexpression of transferrin receptors might result in iron accumulation and free radical cell damage, a process that may be aggravated by eventual hypoperfusion during migraine attacks. As a consequence, metabolism and iron uptake in the remaining neurons would be increased, leading to even more iron accumulation. The second explanation for high iron concentration is the presence of gliosis, since glial cells have high iron content, but the authors found no evidence of gliosis on MRIs of these participants. From this study, it was concluded that iron accumulation in the periaqueductal gray matter among migraineurs was the result of an impaired iron homeostasis, possibly associated with neuronal dysfunction or damage (Welch et al., 2001).

To evaluate these interesting findings in a larger, population-based group of migraineurs, brain MRIs of 138 migraineurs (IHS criteria) and 75 matched controls were analyzed for iron concentration in deep brain nuclei as part of the CAMERA study (Cerebral Abnormalities in Migraine, an Epidemiological Risk Analysis) (Kruit et al., 2009). Because measurements in older subjects are increasingly influenced by non-iron-related factors, analyses were separated into subjects younger than 50 years and older than 50 years. In the younger group, compared to controls, migraineurs demonstrated higher iron concentrations in several nuclei, including the putamen, globus pallidus, and red nucleus. No differences were found between men and women, nor between migraine with and without aura. Among the participants younger than 50 years of age, an association was found between longer migraine duration and higher iron concentration in the putamen, caudate nucleus, and red nucleus (Kruit et al., 2009). These structures are all known to be involved in the normal central nociceptive network (Iadarola et al., 1998).

Data from both studies suggest that repeated migraine attacks, or the accompanying pain, are associated with higher iron concentration in several brain structures involved in central pain processing and migraine pathology. It is not known whether the increase in iron is caused by repetitive activation of the pain nuclei or whether the increased iron itself inflicts damage to these structures via free radicals in oxidative stress. Furthermore, it could be hypothesized that damage of these pain-processing nuclei could lead to chronification of migraine in specific patients. To date, studies on this subject have a cross-sectional design; the assumption that recurring attacks lead to accumulation of iron cannot be verified. A longitudinal study is needed to follow up on migraineurs and controls to carefully evaluate their general health status, headache history, course of migraine over the years, and measurements of brain iron concentration.

CONCLUSIONS

During aging, iron accumulates in the brain, specifically in the basal ganglia, following a certain distribution pattern. Iron accumulation could be the result of neuronal loss, followed by substitution by cells with higher iron loads, or of leakage of the blood-brain barrier, allowing iron to access the brain in higher concentrations. Several neurological disorders, as well as migraine, are associated with iron excess in the brain. Higher brain iron concentration generates a reactive iron overload, which invades and damages neurons and other cells. It is not clear yet whether iron accumulation in the basal ganglia plays a primary or secondary role in the pathogenesis.

REFERENCES

Alam, Z. I., Jenner, A., Daniel, S. E., Lees, A. J., Cairns, N., Marsden, C. D., et al. (1997). Oxidative DNA damage in the parkinsonian brain: An apparent selective increase in 8-hydroxyguanine levels in substantia nigra. *Journal of Neurochemistry, 69*, 1196–1203.

Aoki, S., Okada, Y., Nishimura, K., Barkovich, A. J., Kjos, B. O., Brasch, R. C., et al. (1989). Normal deposition of brain iron in childhood and adolescence: MR imaging at 1.5 T. *Radiology, 172*, 381–385.

Aquino, D., Bizzi, A., Grisoli, M., Garavaglia, B., Bruzzone, M. G., Nardocci, N., et al. (2009). Age-related iron deposition in the basal ganglia: Quantitative analysis in healthy subjects. *Radiology, 252*, 165–172.

Bartzokis, G., Beckson, M., Hance, D. B., Marx, P., Foster, J. A., & Marder, S. R. (1997). MR evaluation of age-related increase of brain iron in young adult and older normal males. *Magnetic Resonance Imaging, 15*, 29–35.

Bartzokis, G., Sultzer, D., Cummings, J., Holt, L. E., Hance, D. B., Henderson, V. W., et al. (2000). In vivo evaluation of brain iron in Alzheimer disease using magnetic resonance imaging. *Archives of General Psychiatry, 57*, 47–53.

Bartzokis, G., & Tishler, T. A. (2000). MRI evaluation of basal ganglia ferritin iron and neurotoxicity in Alzheimer's and Huntingon's disease. *Cellular and Molecular Biology (Noisy-le-Grand, France), 46*, 821–833.

Berg, D., & Youdim, M. B. (2006). Role of iron in neurodegenerative disorders. *Topics in Magnetic Resonance Imaging, 17*, 5–17.

Burdo, J. R., Antonetti, D. A., Wolpert, E. B., & Connor, J. R. (2003). Mechanisms and regulation of transferrin and iron transport in a model blood-brain barrier system. *Neuroscience, 121*, 883–890.

Burdo, J. R., & Connor, J. R. (2003). Brain iron uptake and homeostatic mechanisms: An overview. *Biometals, 16*, 63–75.

Chen, J. C., Hardy, P. A., Kucharczyk, W., Clauberg, M., Joshi, J. G., Vourlas, A., et al. (1993). MR of human postmortem brain tissue: Correlative study between T2 and assays of iron and ferritin in Parkinson and Huntington disease. *AJNR American Journal of Neuroradiology, 14*, 275–281.

Cherubini, A., Peran, P., Caltagirone, C., Sabatini, U., & Spalletta, G. (2009). Aging of subcortical nuclei: Microstructural, mineralization and atrophy modifications measured in vivo using MRI. *Neuroimage, 48*, 29–36.

Connor, J. R. (1994). Iron regulation in the brain at the cell and molecular level. *Advances in Experimental Medicine and Biology, 356*, 229–238.

Connor, J. R., Snyder, B. S., Arosio, P., Loeffler, D. A., & LeWitt, P. (1995). A quantitative analysis of isoferritins in select regions of aged, parkinsonian, and Alzheimer's diseased brains. *Journal of Neurochemistry, 65*, 717–724.

Connor, J. R., & Benkovic, S. A. (1992). Iron regulation in the brain: Histochemical, biochemical, and molecular considerations. *Annals of Neurology, 32*(Suppl):S51–S61.

Cross, P. A., Atlas, S. W., & Grossman, R. I. (1990). MR evaluation of brain iron in children with cerebral infarction. *AJNR American Journal of Neuroradiology, 11*, 341–348.

Dexter, D. T., Jenner, P., Schapira, A. H., & Marsden, C. D. (1992). Alterations in levels of iron, ferritin, and other trace metals in neurodegenerative diseases affecting the basal ganglia. The Royal Kings and Queens Parkinson's Disease Research Group. *Annals of Neurology, 32*(Suppl), S94–S100.

Dietrich, R. B., & Bradley, W. G., Jr. (1988). Iron accumulation in the basal ganglia following severe ischemic-anoxic insults in children. *Radiology, 168*, 203–206.

Diezel, P. D. (1955). Iron in the brain: A chemical and histochemical examination. In: H. Waelsch (Ed.), *Biochemistry of the developing nervous system* (pp. 145–152). New York: Academic Press.

Drayer, B., Burger, P., Darwin, R., Riederer, S., Herfkens, R., & Johnson, G. A. (1986). MRI of brain iron. *AJR American Journal of Roentgenology, 147*, 103–110.

Drayer, B. P., Olanow, W., Burger, P., Johnson, G. A., Herfkens, R., & Riederer, S. (1986). Parkinson plus syndrome: Diagnosis using high field MR imaging of brain iron. *Radiology, 159*, 493–498.

Faucheux, B. A., Bonnet, A. M., Agid, Y., & Hirsch, E. C. (1999). Blood vessels change in the mesencephalon of patients with Parkinson's disease. *Lancet, 353*, 981–982.

Friedreich, N. (1863). Über degenerative Atrophie der spinalen Hinterstränge. *Virchows Archiv für pathologische Anatomie und Physiologie und für klinische Medizin, 26*, 391–419.

Galvin, J. E., Giasson, B., Hurtig, H. I., Lee, V. M., & Trojanowski, J. Q. (2000). Neurodegeneration with brain iron accumulation, type 1 is characterized by alpha-, beta-, and gamma-synuclein neuropathology. *American Journal of Pathology, 157*, 361–368.

Ganz, T., & Nemeth, E. (2011). Hepcidin and disorders of iron metabolism. *Annual Review of Medicine, 62*, 347–360.

Good, P. F., Perl, D. P., Bierer, L. M., & Schmeidler, J. (1992). Selective accumulation of aluminum and iron in the neurofibrillary tangles of Alzheimer's disease: A laser microprobe (LAMMA) study. *Annals of Neurology, 31*, 286–292.

Goodall, E. F., Haque, M. S., & Morrison, K. E. (2008). Increased serum ferritin levels in amyotrophic lateral sclerosis (ALS) patients. *Journal of Neurology, 255*, 1652–1656.

Goodwin, D. C., Rowlinson, S. W., & Marnett, L. J. (2000). Substitution of tyrosine for the proximal histidine ligand to the heme of prostaglandin endoperoxide synthase 2: Implications for the mechanism of cyclooxygenase activation and catalysis. *Biochemistry, 39*, 5422–5432.

Gordon, N. (2003). Iron deficiency and the intellect. *Brain Development, 25*, 3–8.

Gorell, J. M., Ordidge, R. J., Brown, G. G., Deniau, J. C., Buderer, N. M., & Helpern, J. A. (1995). Increased iron-related MRI contrast in the substantia nigra in Parkinson's disease. *Neurology, 45*, 1138–1143.

Gotz, M. E., Freyberger, A., & Riederer, P. (1990). Oxidative stress: A role in the pathogenesis of Parkinson's disease. *Journal of Neural Transmission Supplementum, 29*, 241–249.

Haacke, E. M., Cheng, N. Y., House, M. J., Liu, Q., Neelavalli, J., Ogg, R. J., et al. (2005). Imaging iron stores in the brain using magnetic resonance imaging. *Magnetic Resonance Imaging, 23*, 1–25.

Hallgren, B., & Sourander, P. (1958). The effect of age on the non-haemin iron in the human brain. *Journal of Neurochemistry, 3*, 41–51.

Halliday, W. (1995). The nosology of Hallervorden-Spatz disease. *Journal of the Neurological Sciences, 134*(Suppl), 84–91.

Hayflick, S. J., Westaway, S. K., Levinson, B., Zhou, B., Johnson, M. A., Ching, K. H., et al. (2003). Genetic, clinical, and radiographic delineation of Hallervorden-Spatz syndrome. *New England Journal of Medicine, 348*, 33–40.

Hulet, S. W., Powers, S., & Connor, J. R. (1999). Distribution of transferrin and ferritin binding in normal and multiple sclerotic human brains. *Journal of the Neurological Sciences, 165*, 48–55.

Iadarola, M. J., Berman, K. F., Zeffiro, T. A., Byas-Smith, M. G., Gracely, R. H., Max, M. B., et al. (1998). Neural activation during acute capsaicin-evoked pain and allodynia assessed with PET. *Brain, 121*(Pt 5), 931–947.

Kell, D. B. (2009). Iron behaving badly: Inappropriate iron chelation as a major contributor to the aetiology of vascular and other progressive inflammatory and degenerative diseases. *BMC Medical Genomics, 2*, 2.

Kell, D. B. (2010). Towards a unifying, systems biology understanding of large-scale cellular death and destruction caused by poorly liganded iron: Parkinson's, Huntington's, Alzheimer's, prions, bactericides, chemical toxicology and others as examples. *Archives of Toxicology, 84*, 825–889.

Koeppen, A. H., Dickson, A. C., & McEvoy, J. A. (1995). The heterogeneous distribution of brain transferrin. *Journal of Neuropathology and Experimental Neurology, 54*, 395–403.

Koeppen, A. H., Michael, S. C., Knutson, M. D., Haile, D. J., Qian, J., Levi, S., et al. (2007). The dentate nucleus in Friedreich's ataxia: The role of iron-responsive proteins. *Acta Neuropathologique, 114*, 163–173.

Kruit, M. C., Launer, L. J., Overbosch, J., van Buchem, M. A., & Ferrari, M. D. (2009). Iron accumulation in deep brain nuclei in migraine: A population-based magnetic resonance imaging study. *Cephalalgia, 29*, 351–359.

Langkammer, C., Enzinger, C., Quasthoff, S., Grafenauer, P., Soellinger, M., Fazekas, F., et al. (2010). Mapping of iron deposition in conjunction with assessment of nerve fiber tract integrity in amyotrophic lateral sclerosis. *Journal of Magnetic Resonance Imaging, 31*, 1339–1345.

Levenson, C. W., & Tassabehji, N. M. (2004). Iron and ageing: An introduction to iron regulatory mechanisms. *Ageing Research Reviews, 3*, 251–263.

Levine, S. M. (1997). Iron deposits in multiple sclerosis and Alzheimer's disease brains. *Brain Research, 760*, 298–303.

Maguire, J. J., Kellogg, E. W., III, & Packer, L. (1982). Protection against free radical formation by protein bound iron. *Toxicology Letters, 14*, 27–34.

Marnett, L. J. (2000). Oxyradicals and DNA damage. *Carcinogenesis, 21*, 361–370.

Milton, W. J., Atlas, S. W., Lexa, F. J., Mozley, P. D., & Gur, R. E. (1991). Deep gray matter hypointensity patterns with aging in healthy adults: MR imaging at 1.5 T. *Radiology, 181*, 715–719.

Moos, T. (1996). Immunohistochemical localization of intraneuronal transferrin receptor immunoreactivity in the adult mouse central nervous system. *Journal of Comparative Neurology, 375*, 675–692.

Peran, P., Cherubini, A., Luccichenti, G., Hagberg, G., Demonet, J. F., Rascol, O., et al. (2009). Volume and iron content in basal ganglia and thalamus. *Human Brain Mapping, 30*, 2667–2675.

Perry, T. L., Norman, M. G., Yong, V. W., Whiting, S., Crichton, J. U., Hansen, S., et al. (1985). Hallervorden-Spatz disease: Cysteine accumulation and cysteine dioxygenase deficiency in the globus pallidus. *Annals of Neurology, 18*, 482–489.

Poon, H. F., Calabrese, V., Scapagnini, G., & Butterfield, D. A. (2004a). Free radicals and brain aging. *Clinics in Geriatric Medicine, 20*, 329–359.

Poon, H. F., Calabrese, V., Scapagnini, G., & Butterfield, D. A. (2004b). Free radicals: Key to brain aging and heme oxygenase as a cellular response to oxidative stress. *Journal of Gerontology Series A, Biological Sciences and Medical Sciences, 59*, 478–493.

Rottkamp, C. A., Nunomura, A., Raina, A. K., Sayre, L. M., Perry, G., & Smith, M. A. (2000). Oxidative stress, antioxidants, and Alzheimer disease. *Alzheimer Disease and Associated Disorders, 14*(Suppl 1), S62–S66.

Rouault, T. A., & Cooperman, S. (2006). Brain iron metabolism. *Seminars in Pediatric Neurology, 13*, 142–148.

Rutledge, J. N., Hilal, S. K., Silver, A. J., Defendini, R., & Fahn, S. (1987). Study of movement disorders and brain iron by MR. *AJR American Journal of Roentgenology, 149*, 365–379.

Ryvlin, P., Broussolle, E., Piollet, H., Viallet, F., Khalfallah, Y., & Chazot, G. (1995). Magnetic resonance imaging evidence of decreased putamenal iron content in idiopathic Parkinson's disease. *Archives of Neurology, 52*, 583–588.

Sanchez-Ramos, J. R., Hefti, F., & Weiner, W. J. (1987). Paraquat and Parkinson's disease. *Neurology, 37*, 728.

Savoiardo, M., Halliday, W. C., Nardocci, N., Strada, L., D'Incerti, L., Angelini, L., et al. (1993). Hallervorden-Spatz disease: MR and pathologic findings. *AJNR American Journal of Neuroradiology, 14*, 155–162.

Sayre, L. M., Perry, G., Atwood, C. S., & Smith, M. A. (2000). The role of metals in neurodegenerative diseases. *Cellular and Molecular Biology (Noisy-le-Grand, France), 46*, 731–741.

Schenck, J. F. (1995). Imaging of brain iron by magnetic resonance: T2 relaxation at different field strengths. *Journal of the Neurological Sciences, 134*(Suppl), 10–18.

Schenker, C., Meier, D., Wichmann, W., Boesiger, P., & Valavanis, A. (1993). Age distribution and iron dependency of the T2 relaxation time in the globus pallidus and putamen. *Neuroradiology, 35*, 119–124.

Sian-Hulsmann, J., Mandel, S., Youdim, M. B., & Riederer, P. (2010). The relevance of iron in the pathogenesis of Parkinson's disease. *Journal of Neurochemistry, 118*(6), 939–957.

Stadtman, E. R. (2001). Protein oxidation in aging and age-related diseases. *Annals of the New York Academy of Sciences, 928*, 22–38.

Swaiman, K. F. (1991). Hallervorden-Spatz syndrome and brain iron metabolism. *Archives of Neurology, 48*, 1285–1293.

Thomas, M., & Jankovic, J. (2004). Neurodegenerative disease and iron storage in the brain. *Current Opinions in Neurology, 17*, 437–442.

Waldvogel, D., van, G. P., & Hallett, M. (1999). Increased iron in the dentate nucleus of patients with Friedrich's ataxia. *Annals of Neurology, 46*, 123–125.

Welch, K. M., Nagesh, V., Aurora, S. K., & Gelman, N. (2001). Periaqueductal gray matter dysfunction in migraine: Cause or the burden of illness? *Headache, 41*, 629–637.

Zecca, L., Gallorini, M., Schunemann, V., Trautwein, A. X., Gerlach, M., Riederer, P., et al. (2001). Iron, neuromelanin and ferritin content in the substantia nigra of normal subjects at different ages: Consequences for iron storage and neurodegenerative processes. *Journal of Neurochemistry, 76*, 1766–1773.

Zecca, L., Youdim, M. B., Riederer, P., Connor, J. R., & Crichton, R. R. (2004). Iron, brain ageing and neurodegenerative disorders. *Nature Reviews Neuroscience, 5*, 863–873.

van Es, A. C., van der, G. J., de Craen, A. J., Admiraal-Behloul, F., Blauw, G. J., & van Buchem, M. A. (2008). Caudate nucleus hypointensity in the elderly is associated with markers of neurodegeneration on MRI. *Neurobiology of Aging, 29*, 1839–1846.

11 Migraine and Brain Lesions

INGE H. PALM-MEINDERS, MICHEL D. FERRARI, AND

MARK C. KRUIT

INTRODUCTION

Migraine is a common, chronic, multifactorial neurovascular brain disorder, affecting over 10% of the general population, and is characterized by recurrent attacks of disabling headache and autonomic nervous system dysfunction (migraine without aura, MO); up to one third of patients also have neurological aura symptoms (migraine with aura, MA) (Ferrari, 1998; Headache Classification Committee of the International Headache Society, 1988). Migraine was known to be highly disabling (Leonardi et al., 2005; Lipton et al., 1997; Nash & Thebarge, 2006; Nash et al., 2006) but was for a long time believed to be an episodic disorder without permanent effects on the brain. However, in several studies during the last two to three decades, associations have been reported between migraine and ischemic cerebrovascular disease.

Below, we first describe different lines of evidence from earlier clinic-based studies linking migraine to ischemic cerebrovascular disease. Second, we summarize the various methodological issues in these earlier studies that prohibited the scientific field to draw definite answers to the question of whether migraine is an independent risk factor for permanent brain lesions, which was the reason for us to organize and perform an unbiased, population-based magnetic resonance imaging (MRI) study in migraineurs and controls. Thereafter, we focus on the results of our CAMERA MRI study.

CLINIC-BASED EVIDENCE FOR A LINK BETWEEN MIGRAINE AND ISCHEMIC BRAIN LESIONS

Migrainous Infarction

Several case reports described that migraine can act as a direct cause of ischemic stroke (migrainous infarction). In such cases stroke is assumed to be directly and causally related to an acute migraine attack. According to International Headache Society (IHS) criteria, the diagnosis "migrainous cerebral infarction" can be applied in known MA patients when in a typical attack, one or more aura symptoms are not fully reversible within 7 days, or when there are neuroimaging findings consistent with ischemic stroke and other causes of infarction are ruled out (Headache Classification Committee of the International Headache Society, 1988). It was suggested that a prolongation of the migrainous process beyond usual limits may explain most migrainous infarctions (Bogousslavsky et al., 1988). The annual incidence of migrainous infarction was estimated in a few studies, and ranged between 1.4 and 3.4 per 100.000 (Broderick & Swanson, 1987; Henrich et al., 1986; Welch, 1994). Migrainous infarction is estimated to account for up to 40% of ischemic strokes in women with migraine (Chang et al., 1999). But, because the strict definition for migrainous infarction has been inconsistently applied in several studies, this rare condition is likely to be overdiagnosed (Bousser, 2004).

Risk of Clinical Ischemic Stroke

Extensive observational studies (Bono et al., 2006; Kern, 2004; Welch, 1994; Welch & Levine, 1990) as well as hospital-based stroke case-control studies suggested that migraine is—at least—an independent risk factor for ischemic stroke (Buring et al., 1995; Carolei et al., 1996; Chang et al., 1999; Collaborative Group for the Study of Stroke in Young Women, 1975; Donaghy et al., 2002; Etminan et al., 2005; Haapaniemi et al., 1997; Henrich & Horwitz, 1989; Lidegaard, 1995; Marini et al., 1993; Merikangas et al., 1997; Nightingale & Farmer, 2004; Schwaag et al., 2003; Tzourio et al., 1993, 1995; 2000; Katsarava & Weimar, 2010). A meta-analysis based on 14 studies summarized the evidence for migraine as a risk factor for clinical ischemic stroke and calculated a pooled relative risk of 2.2 (95% confidence interval [CI]: 1.9–2.6) for migraineurs compared to controls (Etminan et al., 2005). Six studies provided data specified by migraine subtype, resulting in a pooled relative risk of 2.3 (95% CI: 1.6–3.2) for those with MA and 1.8 (95% CI: 1.1–3.2) for those with MO, compared to controls. These data did not change in stratified analyses by age, but it needs to be considered that a number of the pooled studies only included younger (younger than 45 years of age) women (Chang et al., 1999; Lidegaard,

1995; Marini et al., 1993; Merikangas et al., 1997; Schurks et al., 2009; Schwaag et al., 2003; Tzourio et al., 2000).

For this younger subgroup of female migraine patients, the recent case-control studies of migraine and stroke show a consistent, significant, and homogeneous increase in the risk of about three times compared to controls of the same age (Carolei et al., 1996; Chang et al., 1999; Donaghy et al., 2002; Lidegaard, 1995; Schwaag et al., 2003; Tzourio et al., 1995). In women younger than age 45 with migraine who smoked, the risk of ischemic stroke was found to be higher than the product of migraine-associated risk times smoking-associated risk (odds ratio [OR] for those migraine patients who smoked ranging from 7.4 to 10.2). Among current heavy smokers, migraine increased the risk by a factor of 3.4 (Chang et al., 1999; Tzourio et al., 2000). Similarly, the coexistence of migraine and high blood pressure had a greater than multiplicative effect in one study (Chang et al., 1999). In three studies the effect of oral contraceptive use was evaluated (Chang et al., 1999; Collaborative Group for the Study of Stroke in Young Women, 1975; Tzourio et al., 1995), summarized in a pooled relative risk of 8.7 (95% CI: 5.1–15.1) among female migraineurs using oral contraceptives (Etminan et al., 2005). ORs were lower in those using low-dose (<50 μg estrogen) oral contraceptives than in those using higher doses. These relationships and probable interactions are complex, and the available data are relatively limited. Further study in large samples is needed to explore the effects in detail. Significantly increased ORs have further been found among female migraine patients with a family history of migraine (Chang et al., 1999). One study investigated the effect of duration, frequency, and recency of migraine on the risk of ischemic stroke (Donaghy et al., 2002). They found higher risks in those with migraine with more than 12 years' duration, those with initial MA, and those with more than 12 attacks per year (OR: 10.4; 95% CI: 2.2–49). Further, a relation between increased frequency of MA during the months preceding ischemic stroke was observed. A subsequent meta-analysis confirmed the finding of relative ischemic stroke risk being doubled among migraineurs, although this publication suggested that this increased risk may only be apparent in those migraine patients with aura (Schurks et al., 2009). Few structured data exist on the topography of infarcts in stroke patients with migraine. In a large series of 3,500 patients with acute stroke, 130 (3.7%) had active migraine, and 66 of these were younger than 45 years. In the younger patients, posterior circulation involvement (55%) was characteristic (Milhaud et al., 2001). Also, other case reports and small series suggested an overrepresentation of clinical stroke in the occipital lobe and/or the posterior cerebral artery territory in migraine patients (Hoekstra-van Dalen et al., 1996).

In summary, data from observational clinical studies suggested that migraine is an independent risk factor for clinical ischemic stroke, notably in younger women. Those with higher attack frequency and those with MA seem to be at higher risk. The coexistence of migraine and oral contraceptive use, high blood pressure, or smoking seems to increase the risk. The combined effect of risk factors must be investigated further. Given the very low absolute risk of stroke in young women (estimated at 5.5 per 100.000 annually) (WHO Collaborative Study of Cardiovascular Disease and Steroid Hormone Contraception, 1996), there is no strict contraindication to oral contraceptive use for young female migraine patients; however, patients (as everyone) should be recommended to quit smoking and to use low-estrogen-content pills or progestogens only, particularly those with MA (Bousser, 2004). The consistency of case-control findings from several countries suggests that the association is not an artifact of study design or execution. However, due to methodological limitations (see below), none of the studies mentioned above can be considered definite proof of the association between migraine and (clinical) ischemic stroke (Tzourio et al., 2000).

Risk of Silent Infarction

Silent infarcts are defined by the presence of a brain parenchymal defect of vascular origin (confirmed by computed tomography [CT] or MRI), in the absence of a history of clinical stroke or transient ischemic attack (TIA), and in the absence of neurological symptoms and signs. Old infarcts seen on CT are common in acute stroke patients who have no history of clinical stroke (Kase et al., 1989). Silent brain infarcts are frequently seen on MRI in healthy elderly people and are associated with an increased risk of dementia and a steeper decline in cognitive function (Vermeer, Prins, et al., 2003). Furthermore, those with silent brain infarcts and white matter lesions are at considerable increased risk of having a stroke, which could not be explained by the common stroke risk factors (Bernick et al., 2001; Vermeer, Hollander, et al., 2003). Little is known about the prevalence of silent infarcts in the general population. In those aged 55 to 70 years, the prevalence ranges from 11% to 15% (Bryan et al., 1999; Howard et al., 1998), and it increases with age, from 8% in those aged 55 to 59 years to 23% in those aged 65 to 72 years (Bryan et al., 1999). To our knowledge, there are no population-based prevalence data available on silent cerebral infarcts in a population aged younger than 50 years. Consequently, we do not know whether the presence of silent infarcts in the younger population also implies increased risk of future stroke and/or cognitive decline. With respect to migraine, until we reported the results of the CAMERA study (see below), there were no previous studies specifically assessing the prevalence of silent infarcts.

EARLIER MAGNETIC RESONANCE IMAGING STUDIES ON WHITE MATTER HYPERINTENSE LESIONS

From the moment MRI became available for the evaluation of the brains of migraine patients, reports exist on the presence of white matter hyperintense signal abnormalities on T2-weighted MRI sequences in these cases (Kaplan et al., 1987; Soges et al., 1988). Numerous clinic-based studies have reported on white matter lesions (WMLs) in migraine patients, but results are inconsistent or conflicting (Cooney et al., 1996; De Benedittis et al., 1995; Fazekas et al., 1992; Ferbert et al., 1991; Gozke et al., 2006; Igarashi et al., 1991; Osborn et al., 1991; Pavese et al., 1994; Robbins & Friedman, 1992; Rovaris et al., 2001; Ziegler et al., 1991). Some only reported prevalence of WMLs in migraine patients, without the use of a control group (Cooney et al., 1996; Gozke et al., 1994; Osborn et al., 1991); most reported an increased prevalence among migraine patients compared to controls (De Benedittis et al., 1995; Igarashi et al. 1991; Pavese et al., 1994; Robbins & Friedman, 1992; Rovaris et al., 2001); and few did not find a statistically significant difference (Fazekas et al., 1992; Ferbert et al., 1991; Ziegler et al., 1991). Some found no difference in prevalence between MO and MA (Cooney et al., 1996; Fazekas et al., 1992; Igarashi et al., 1991; Pavese et al., 1994), but two studies found a higher WML prevalence in MA (Ferbert et al., 1991; Gozke et al., 2004). Only one study found an increased prevalence with increasing migraine attack frequency, but it has to be noted that none of the other studies assessed the influence of attack frequency as an indicator of migraine severity (Gozke et al., 2004).

Despite the various limitations and discrepancies in the previous MRI studies, a meta-analysis based on the results of seven case-control studies (De Benedittis et al., 1995; Fazekas et al., 1992; Igarashi et al., 1991; Pavese et al., 1994; Robbins & Friedman, 1992; Rovaris et al., 2001; Ziegler et al., 1991) was published (Swartz & Kern, 2004). The authors concluded that subjects with migraine (compared to controls) are at higher risk (OR: 3.9; 95% CI: 2.3–6.7) for having WMLs, regardless of comorbidities (such as cardiovascular risk factors, demyelinating disease, inflammatory conditions, and valvular heart disease). The increased risk was also found among younger subjects without co-occurring cerebrovascular disease risk factors. None of these studies was population based,

so much of the reported data is probably based on a more than average severe subgroup of migraine patients.

Methodological Issues in Earlier Clinic-Based Studies

In both clinical stroke case-control studies and clinic-based MRI studies, conflicting results made the interpretation difficult. Concomitant (cardiovascular) risk factors were not taken into account properly in a majority of the previous work, leaving potential associations uncorrected for important confounders. The observed associations are likely to be restricted to certain subpopulations or age groups of patients and cannot be generalized to the general population. Further, not all studies used IHS criteria for migraine diagnosis, and often there was no standard diagnosis of migraine subtype, thus allowing for the potential of misclassification.

In a number of studies, migraine prevalence was compared between patients with (clinical) stroke and those without stroke. In these hospital-based stroke case-control studies, migraine was almost always diagnosed retrospectively, which makes this procedure vulnerable to misclassification and recall bias. In these clinical case-control studies, referral bias might have played a role when migraine patients with symptoms of ischemic stroke have been preferentially referred to centers specialized in migraine or stroke and cases of stroke with migraine are then more likely to be detected. In such studies, a different type of classification bias might occur with respect to the diagnosis of a qualifying ischemic event. For instance, TIAs might be difficult to discriminate from migraine aura, particularly in cases with prolonged aura (Dennis & Warlow, 1992). Migraine might then be both overestimated (aura misclassified as ischemia) and underestimated (real ischemia misclassified as aura) as a risk factor for TIAs or stroke. To overcome this classification problem, neuroimaging proof consistent with cerebral ischemia is mandatory in such studies. In our opinion, a standard brain CT scan used in previous hospital-based case-control studies is not suitable for detecting acute cerebral ischemia and only has a place in excluding hemorrhagic strokes.

Whereas even in cases with clinical symptoms of stroke or TIA there is a need for objective neuroimaging proof of brain ischemia, accurate MRI of the brain is obviously the only way to be informed about the presence and extent of subclinical brain lesions in migraine patients. In addition to the inherent potential types of bias and other shortcomings described above, the most important problem with these MRI studies is the presence of selection bias: All studies included migraine patients visiting migraine-specialized neurologists. In this way, only the more severe migraine cases were included. Results of those studies can therefore not be generalized to a common (population-based) migraine population.

Variability in the detection rate of WMLs may be due to differences in populations with respect to clinical factors, which needs to be controlled for. In addition, diagnostic criteria for white matter disease can vary markedly, and without a clear definition of diagnostic criteria, for instance, dilated perivascular cerebrospinal fluid spaces could have been misclassified as lesions. None of the previous studies used fluid-attenuated inversion recovery (FLAIR) sequences to eliminate the latter problem. Only one study differentiated between deep and periventricular WMLs (Pavese et al., 1994) and found only the deep white matter affected; most other series just described "multiple small focal areas of increased T2 signal in the white matter," without indication of site or total lesion volume.

THE POPULATION-BASED CAMERA MAGNETIC RESONANCE IMAGING STUDY

As becomes clear from the text above, various reasons prohibited the scientific field to draw definite conclusions from the described clinic-based studies. It remained uncertain whether migraineurs are at independent risk for permanent brain changes, and, if so, there remained still controversies whether specific subgroups of patients would be most at risk and what etiologic mechanisms are involved. Since studies in nonmigraine cases have shown that both clinical and subclinical brain lesions increase the risk of (new) clinical stroke events, physical limitations, and cognitive impairment, it was important to establish whether migraine—as a highly prevalent condition—is a true and independent risk factor for clinical and subclinical brain lesions.

To find answers to these questions, we planned and performed a cross-sectional MRI study in an already existing population-based sample of adults with migraine and controls without a headache history: the Cerebral Abnormalities in Migraine, an Epidemiological Risk Analysis (CAMERA) study (Kruit et al., 2004). In this study we assessed (a) whether unselected migraine cases from the general population are at increased risk of several types of brain changes (see below), (b) whether this risk varies by migraine subtype and attack frequency, (c) whether certain areas of the brain are particularly vulnerable, and (d) whether traditional cardiovascular risk factors modify the risk of brain changes. In addition, we collected data from neurological physical examination and cognitive tests, to correlate these data with lesion load. The overall design of the study aimed as far as possible to exclude potential sources of bias, to minimize the risk of finding false associations, and to remain with unequivocal answers about migraine as a risk factor for brain lesions.

Study Population

Participants in the CAMERA study were 295 migraineurs ($n = 161$ MA; $n = 134$ MO) and 140 age- and scx-matched nonmigraine controls, who were randomly selected from a previously diagnosed sample ($n = 6,039$) from the Dutch general population. This epidemiological approach minimized the role of potential selection bias, and a proper, multistep method to establish the migraine diagnosis minimized the possibility of diagnostic misclassification and recall bias. The complete description of the cohort, with several baseline measurements available from the MORGEN study, allowed us to statistically control for relevant confounders. These rigid measures resulted in a study population that is representative for the general population and consists of a group of migraine sufferers with general migraine symptomatology and average migraine severity. Through these guarantees, the acquired results are robust and can be generalized to the general population. Nearly 50% of the migraine cases had not been previously diagnosed by a physician (Kruit et al., 2004).

Sensitive imaging and lesion rating methods, including full brain covering with thin (3-mm) T2 and FLAIR slices, blinded expert reading, and semiquantitative lesion volume quantification, minimized the possibility of lesion misclassification. Brain MRIs were evaluated for infarcts, by location and vascular supply territory, for periventricular WMLs (PVWMLs) and deep WMLs (DWMLs), and for infratentorial hyperintense lesions (IHLs). The risks (ORs) and 95% CIs of having these brain lesions compared to controls were examined by migraine subtype (with or without aura) and average monthly attack frequency (less than one attack, one or more attacks), controlling for cardiovascular risk factors and use of vasoconstrictor migraine agents. All participants underwent a standard neurological examination and a structured interview to be able to evaluate and control for confounding factors.

Magnetic Resonance Imaging Findings: Infarcts

None of the participants reported a history of stroke or transient ischemic attack or showed relevant abnormalities at standard neurological examination. In total, 60 brain infarcts were detected in 31 individuals. Infarct size ranged from 2 to 21 mm. We found no significant difference between migraineurs and controls in overall infarct prevalence (8% vs. 5%; $p = .2$). However, 65% of all infarcts were located in the posterior circulation territory (44% of all infarcts in controls; 47% in MO; 81% in MA), and

85% of the posterior circulation infarcts were located in the cerebellum. Of these cerebellar infarcts, 88% were located in a borderzone location. The average number of lesions per subject was 1.8. Lesion sizes and number of lesions per subject did not differ between the diagnostic groups. Prevalence of these posterior circulation infarcts differed significantly between controls (0.7%), MO (2%), and MA (8%; p <.005). The adjusted OR for posterior territory infarct varied by migraine subtype and attack frequency: Adjusted OR was 13.7 (95% CI: 1.7–112) for MA compared to controls. In patients with migraine with one or more attacks per month, the adjusted OR was 9.3 (95% CI: 1.1–76). The highest risk was found in MA with one or more attacks per month (OR, 15.8; 95% CI: 1.8–140).

Migraine patients with posterior circulation infarcts were significantly older, but cardiovascular risk factors were not more prevalent, and the presence of these lesions was not significantly associated with supratentorial brain changes, such as white matter lesions. These two observations suggest that the lesions are not atherosclerotic in origin. The combination of vascular distribution, deep borderzone location, shape, size, and imaging characteristics on MRI makes it likely that the lesions have an infarctious origin. The most likely etiological mechanism seems to be hypoperfusion and/or embolism, rather than atherosclerosis or small vessel disease. During and after migraine attacks, sluggish low cerebral flow below an ischemic threshold has been described (Bednarczyk et al., 1998; Cutrer et al., 1998; Olesen et al., 1990; Sanchez del Rio et al., 1999; Woods et al., 1994). A decrease in brain perfusion pressure (e.g., during migraine) theoretically affects the clearance and destination of embolic particles; narrowing of the arterial lumen and endothelial abnormalities stimulate formation of thrombi; and occlusive thrombi further reduce blood flow and brain perfusion (Caplan & Hennerici, 1998). Because the deep cerebellar territories have a pattern of progressively tapering arteries with only few anastomoses present, they are likely to be particularly vulnerable to hypoperfusion-related borderzone infarct mechanisms (Duvernoy et al., 1983; Fessatidis et al., 1993). This hypoperfusion-related concept matches the findings of previous studies in which the small cerebellar borderzone infarcts, in particular when multiple, were strongly associated with severe occlusive and/or (artery-to-artery) embolic disease based on vertebrobasilar atherosclerosis, likely to result in hypoperfusion and infarction (Amarenco et al., 1993; 1994; Barth et al., 1993; Canaple & Bogousslavsky, 1991).

Recently, the population-based AGES-Reykjavik Study confirmed a significantly higher prevalence of cerebellar infarcts among migraineurs (Scher et al., 2009), and the Epidemiology of Vascular Ageing study reported a higher risk of (multiple) infarcts among migraineurs with aura (Kurth et al., 2011). Although migraine-related clinical strokes are reported to occur most often supratentorially, in the occipital lobes (Bogousslavsky et al., 1988; Broderick & Swanson, 1987; Caplan, 1991; Featherstone, 1986; Hoekstra-van Dalen et al., 1996; Milhaud et al., 2001; Rothrock et al., 1993, 1988; Sacquegna et al., 1989; Shuaib & Lee, 1988), we did not find any infarcts in these areas of the posterior circulation territory. An association between migraine and (subclinical) infarcts is well established by now, but the exact mechanisms and potential consequences need evaluation and further research (Figs. 11–1 and 11–2).

Magnetic Resonance Imaging Findings: Supratentorial White Matter Hyperintense Lesions

Among women of the CAMERA cohort, the risk of having a high DWML load (top 20th percentile of the distribution of DWML load) was increased in patients with migraine compared to controls (OR, 2.1; 95% CI: 1.0–4.1). This risk was higher in those with higher attack frequency (in those with one or more attacks per month: OR, 2.6; 95% CI: 1.2–5.7) but was similar among MA and MO. Among men on the other hand, prevalence of DWMLs did not differ between controls and migraineurs. No association was found between severity of PVWMLs and migraine, irrespective of gender or migraine frequency or subtype.

Although the pathologic substrate of WMLs in migraine remains unknown, the most likely histological substrate of these abnormalities is incomplete infarction with changes such as gliosis and demyelination (Rocca et al., 2000). These changes probably result from reduced blood flow in large and/or small arteries (Bednarczyk et al., 1998; Sanchez del Rio et al., 1999) during migraine attacks (possibly accompanying cortical spreading depression, the underlying mechanism for migraine aura). Vasoconstriction or activation of the clotting system/platelets (Crassard et al., 2001; Tietjen et al., 2001) might also contribute, possibly leading to formation of local thrombi. An alternative explanation is that local tissue changes during migraine attacks, such as excessive neuronal activation, neurogenic inflammation, neuropeptide and cytokine release (Goadsby, 1997), or excitotoxity (Eggers, 2001), occur and that these changes directly lead to tissue damage. Reversible MRI abnormalities during migraine aura, including regions of cerebral vasogenic edema (Resnick et al., 2006) and evidence of vasogenic blood-brain barrier leakage in prolonged aura (Iizuka et al., 2004; Smith et al., 2002), have been reported. These abnormalities were linked to (temporal) impairment of the blood-brain barrier integrity and enhanced permeability

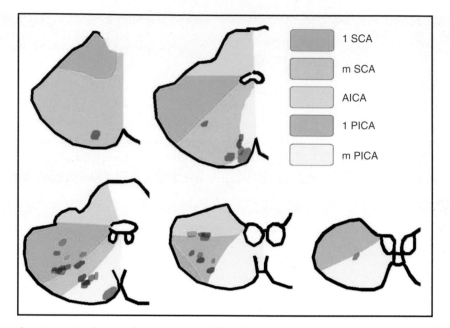

FIGURE 11–1 *Infratentorial posterior circulation infarcts in the cerebellum* (n = 33) *superimposed over a diagram with arterial territories indicated. Size and position of all cerebellar infarcts in a vascular territories template of the cerebellum. Most lesions were located at deep borderzone location. Territories are supplied by the posterior inferior cerebellar artery (PICA), the medial branch of the PICA (m PICA), the lateral branch of the PICA (l PICA), the territory of the superior cerebellar artery (SCA), the medial branch of the SCA (m SCA), the lateral branch of the SCA (l SCA), or the territory of the anterior inferior cerebellar artery (AICA). Left-sided lesions (red colored) are mirrored to the right hemisphere for presentation purposes. Source: Kruit, Launer, Ferrari, and van Buchem, 2005.*

of dura mater microvessels (Ghabriel et al., 1999; Smith et al., 2002). Cortical spreading depression may cause disruption of the blood-brain barrier through a matrix metalloproteinase-9-dependent cascade mechanism, possibly resulting in local tissue damage (Gursoy-Ozdemir et al., 2004). In addition, population-based evidence that migraine (with aura) is associated with a higher cardiovascular risk profile and the MTHFR C677T genotype, which is a risk factor for stroke, might contribute to the risk of (ischemic) brain lesions (Scher et al., 2005; Scher, Stewart, et al., 2006; Scher, Terwindt, et al., 2006). The exact cause and possible consequences of these brain lesions are unknown (Fig. 11–3).

Magnetic Resonance Imaging Findings: Infratentorial Hyperintense Lesions

IHLs are high-signal areas found on brain MRI in infratentorial regions. IHLs were identified in 13 of 295 (4.4%) patients with migraine and in 1 of 140 (0.7%) controls (p = .04) (Kruit et al., 2006). All subjects had a normal standard neurological examination and no history of transient ischemic attack or stroke. The majority of the cases (n = 12) showed hyperintensities in the brainstem. All IHLs were located in the dorsal basis pontis, adjacent to the tegmentum,

at the level of, and slightly cranial to, the entry zone of the trigeminal nerve. In nearly all cases lesions were located bilaterally, sometimes extending to the midline; none reached the surface of the pons. Hyperintensities seem to involve the pontocerebellar fibers, the pontine nuclei, or the nucleus reticularis tegmenti pontis and, in some cases, parts of the corticopontine (pyramidal tract) or medial lemniscus fibers. These anatomical locations are supplied by the anteromedial and anterolateral groups arising from the basilar artery.

Cases with IHLs also had more often supratentorial white matter lesions (p < .05). Migraine cases with and without IHLs were similar with respect to migraine type, attack frequency, age at onset, or treatment status. These findings extended the knowledge about vulnerable brain regions and type of lesions in migraine brains.

Not many studies have reported on IHLs; therefore, etiology and consequences of these lesions in general are uncertain. Both ischemia (Bastos Leite et al., 2006; Goadsby, 2002; Kwa et al., 1997; Salomon et al., 1987) and edema (de Seze et al., 2000; Tortorella et al., 2006) have been suggested as a cause for the presence of IHLs. The increased prevalence of IHLs among patients with atherosclerosis (Kwa et al., 1997), hypertension (de Seze et al., 2000), diabetes mellitus (Ichikawa et al., 2008), chronic

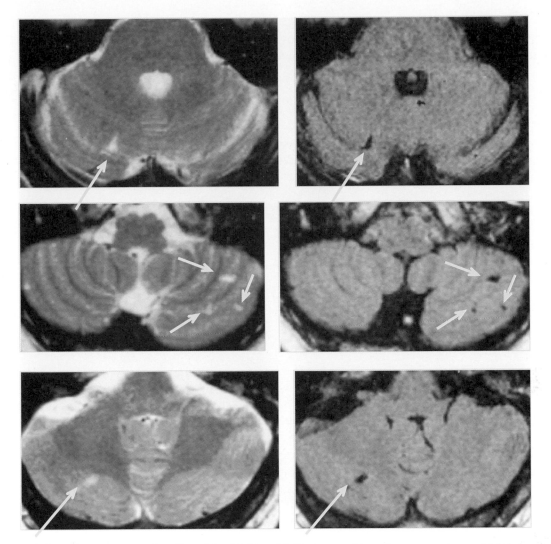

FIGURE 11–2 *Cerebellar infarcts. Corresponding T2-weighted* (left) *and fluid-attenuated inversion recovery images* (right) *showing (multiple) cerebellar infarcts* (arrows) *in three representative cases.*

kidney disease (Ichikawa et al., 2008), and cerebral autosomal dominant arteriopathy with subcortical infarcts and leukoencephalopathy (CADASIL) (Chabriat et al., 1999) suggests that small vessel disease lies at the origin of IHLs. In CADASIL, migraine with aura is often the presenting symptom, and similar brainstem hyperintensities are frequent (Chabriat et al., 1999), likely due to decreased tissue perfusion secondary to changes in the wall of cerebral arteries. In CADASIL, this leads to early ischemic damage, notably in regions that are irrigated by

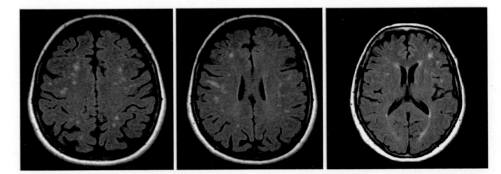

FIGURE 11–3 *Examples of small to medium focal deep WMLs in representative migraine patients (fluid-attenuated inversion recovery images).*

the longest perforating arteries, which are most vulnerable to hypoperfusion. This is particularly the case for the central part of the pons. Repeated or prolonged reduced perfusion has been described during migraine attacks, although not specifically in the pons (Bednarczyk et al., 1998). Besides possible effects of repetitive perfusion deficits (Kwa et al., 1997; Pullicino et al., 1995; Tortorella et al., 2006;), endothelial dysfunction (Ichikawa et al., 2008), which is known to be related to both small vessel disease and migraine, could explain the increased small vessel vulnerability. The clinical relevance of having IHLs is largely unknown. Although the brainstem is involved in migraine pathophysiology, and specific activation of the dorsal rostral pons and periaqueductal gray matter have been reported during migraine (Kaplan et al., 1987), IHLs did not involve the specific "migraine areas" in our cases (Fig. 11–4).

POSSIBLE CONSEQUENCES

Cognitive Dysfunction

The association between WMLs and cognitive deficits is known from nonmigraine elderly population studies (Longstreth et al., 1996; Prins et al., 2005; Vermeer, Hollander, et al., 2003). A recent meta-analysis describes the association between the presence of WMLs and an increased risk of cognitive dysfunction, especially in the executive function and processing speed domains, and dementia (hazard ratio 1.9, 95% CI: 1.3–2.8) (Debette & Markus, 2010). In addition, many papers have described cognitive dysfunction among migraine patients (Ardila & Sanchez, 1988; Farmer et al., 2000; Hooker & Raskin, 1986; Le Pira et al., 2000; Mulder et al., 1999), For example, O'Bryant et al. (2006) concluded in a recent review on the neuropsychology of recurrent headaches that there is a trend for subtle deficits in verbal and visual memory as well as executive processes across studies on cognitive dysfunction in migraine. The authors concluded that migraine patients with aura appeared to experience more neuropsychological deficits than migraine patients without aura (Ardila & Sanchez, 1988; Martins & Cunha e Sa, 1999; Mulder et al., 1999). Furthermore, when directly compared, migraineurs with aura performed more poorly on motor tests as well as on measures of sustained attention and information-processing speed than migraineurs without aura (Hooker & Raskin, 1986; Mulder et al., 1999). A satisfying explanation for the found differences between migraine with and without aura is lacking. Additional deficits have been found in verbal expression and reception, information-processing speed, and recognition memory among migraine patients in general (Hooker & Raskin, 1986; Waldie et al., 2002; Zeitlin & Oddy, 1984). On the other hand, several studies were not able to confirm these findings of cognitive dysfunction among migraineurs (Bell et al., 1999; Gaist et al., 2005; Jelicic et al., 2000; Pearson et al., 2006). It has to be noted that differences in study design, participant populations, and methods make it rather difficult to directly compare results across publications. Very little is known about the effect of having both WMLs and migraine in association with cognitive dysfunction. Recently, the Epidemiology of Vascular Aging study has evaluated this complex relation and demonstrated no evidence that migraine in itself, or in combination with structural brain lesions, results in cognitive impairment (Kurth et al., 2011). The question whether migraine and (the accumulation of) brain lesions lead to (progression of) cognitive dysfunction needs to be further clarified in the future. As of today, it is not clear whether having brain lesions and migraine is associated with impaired cognition and to what extent the amount of lesions and, for instance, migraine severity play a role.

Cerebellar Dysfunction

Cerebellar dysfunction is a known entity in familial hemiplegic migraine, a rare type of inherited migraine; however, even in common forms of migraine, evidence has been found for dysfunction of cerebellum-controlled actions. A study assessing stabilimetric parameters reported a significant increase in body sway among migraine

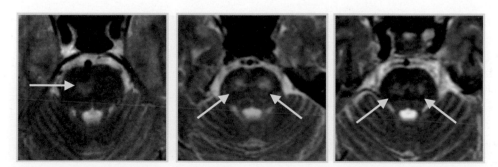

FIGURE 11–4 *Detailed T2-weighted images at the midpontine level showing pontine hyperintense lesions in three cases.*

patients (Ishizaki et al., 2002). The observed patients had no clinically apparent equilibrium dysfunction. One explanation for the findings is that repeated ischemic episodes during migraine attacks could cause irreversible changes in the central and/or peripheral vestibulospinal systems (Ishizaki et al., 2002). Another study reported evidence for subclinical cerebellar dysfunction in the common forms of migraine (Sandor et al., 2001). Using a pointing paradigm and infrared optoelectronic tracking system, subclinical hypermetria and other subtle cerebellar signs were identified, with more pronounced abnormalities among the migraineurs with aura subgroup. The results indicated abnormal functioning of the lateral cerebellum, leading to impaired braking (and thus to hypermetria) compensated for by particularly accurate targeting. The cause of subclinical dysfunction of the lateral cerebellum in migraine patients is unknown. The authors suggested these findings to be related to a possible calcium channelopathy, although there is no direct evidence for this statement. However, recent findings of specifically increased vulnerability of the posterior circulation territory for tissue damage in migraine, as reflected by the high prevalence of (subclinical) infarctlike cerebellar lesions and pontine and cerebellar hyperintense lesions in migraineurs (Kruit et al., 2005, 2006), might provide a possible explanation for the observed cerebellar dysfunction and needs further evaluation.

REMARKS

The data from the CAMERA study support and extend the results from earlier studies on the association between migraine and brain lesions, and the robustness of the methods and validity of the findings have been acknowledged (Lipton & Pan, 2004; Tietjen, 2004; Welch, 2008). Studies published in later years confirmed and expanded CAMERA study findings (Scher et al., 2009; Swartz & Kern, 2004). The higher risk of brain changes in those with a higher migraine attack frequency suggested (but did not prove) a causal relationship between migraine severity and lesion load. If true, this might imply that recurrent migraine attacks could be directly responsible for progressive brain damage. Because of the cross-sectional designs of studies on this subject, it is impossible to evaluate any kind of causality. To further evaluate the speculations about accumulation of brain lesions associated with repetitive migraine attacks, and to investigate whether progression of lesions has functional consequences, follow-up data are needed. These follow-up data will help us determine whether migraineurs show a higher rate of brain lesion progression over time compared to (age-related physiological) progression among controls. They will also further clarify the role of migraine activity or severity and brain lesion accumulation. Furthermore, numerous studies have demonstrated that brain lesions, similar to those found among the CAMERA study participants, are associated with adverse functional consequences. Therefore, careful follow-up study of this cohort, using repeated neuropsychological testing and cerebellar functioning evaluation, will assess possible consequences of being a migraine patient and having these brain lesions. In view of the high prevalence of migraine, confirmation that recurrence of migraine attacks is indeed associated with an increased risk of brain lesion accumulation, and possibly brain dysfunction, is a matter of public health importance. At this moment, extensive and careful follow-up study, including MRI, cognitive testing, cerebellar function evaluation, and neurological physical examination, on the CAMERA cohort is under way, and will likely give answers to these important questions. Results of this follow-up study will be published shortly.

If future studies confirm that recurrence of migraine attacks is indeed associated with an increasing risk of brain lesions or brain dysfunction, this will change the concept of migraine from an episodic disorder to a chronic-episodic or chronic progressive disorder (Ophoff et al., 1996). Such a shift in conceptualization of the disease also will change goals of treatments, and prevention of migraine may then potentially need to become an important target for secondary prevention in the general population. This should boost the interest of academic institutes and pharmaceutical companies to invest in the development of specific, effective prophylactic (rather than symptomatic) migraine agents, which are currently lacking. Such new therapeutic strategies have to be tested in randomized controlled trials.

Identification of specific factors that increase the risk of brain lesions in migraine patients, such as migraine type, migraine severity, sympathetic nervous system dysfunction, cardiovascular risk factors, and the presence of a patent foramen ovale (PFO), may allow identification of specific subgroups to be treated. For instance, demonstration of an association between MRI lesions and the presence of a PFO would promote the (renewed) initiation of prospective randomized clinical trials on the effect of closure of PFO on migraine severity and associated brain lesions.

NEURORADIOLOGICAL CONSIDERATIONS

The knowledge that migraine is an independent risk factor for high DWML load and posterior circulation infarcts cannot be translated directly to an individual patient or MRI scan. In routine neuroradiological practice, on FLAIR and/or T2 images hyperintense lesions in the white matter are frequently encountered in subjects older than age 50, but can also appear in younger individuals. The clinical context; the number, aspect, and distribution of lesions; and the age of the patient together enable the neuroradiologist only in a limited number of cases to identify a cause of the lesions, but mostly lesions remain "aspecific" and/or "probably based on vasculo-ischemic processes." The identified white matter hyperintense lesions in the migraineurs in the CAMERA study appeared not to present in a specific pattern, on a preferential location, or after a certain age. Therefore, in our opinion, WMLs in individual patients cannot be attributed to migraine directly. Because data are lacking so far on functional consequences of such lesions, the identification of a limited number of small to medium-sized lesions does not need further medical attention in general. In other cases, evaluation of potential causes of lesions should be considered.

Incidentally, WMLs are observed in MRIs from relatively young patients (e.g., younger than age 35 to 40 years). In such cases, number, location, aspect, and distribution of the lesions have to be carefully evaluated, and based on the images and clinical history together, the likelihood of diseases (e.g., multiple sclerosis, vasculitis, CADASIL, MELAS, coagulation disorders, cardiac abnormalities, etc.) associated with WMLs has to be considered. With the observations from the CAMERA study, "migraine" has to be added to this list, but this does not imply that other options can be disregarded, or that migraine is "the cause" of the lesions in a patient with migraine.

Similarly, the identification of one or more silent cerebellar infarcts on an MRI scan cannot directly be attributed to migraine, although this finding—with the data from the CAMERA study, showing 8% affected—is not so unusual in migraine patients with aura. In such cases, if the observation is incidental, no direct clinical consequence seems to be necessary, until data are available regarding potential progression or functional consequences of small cerebellar infarcts. If future research indicates that there is a risk of progression of number or size of lesions or if there are associated functional consequences, additional study of causes and evaluation of usefulness of preventive therapy has to be initiated. However, a patient who presents with an acute cerebellar infarct, irrespective of the size of the lesion or presence of migraine, has to be screened for (embolic) sources of the infarction and treated accordingly.

REFERENCES

Amarenco, P., Kase, C. S., Rosengart, A., Pessin, M. S., Bousser, M. G., & Caplan, L. R. (1993). Very small (border zone) cerebellar infarcts. Distribution, causes, mechanisms and clinical features. *Brain, 116*(Pt 1), 161–186.

Amarenco, P., Levy, C., Cohen, A., Touboul, P. J., Roullet, E., & Bousser, M. G. (1994). Causes and mechanisms of territorial and nonterritorial cerebellar infarcts in 115 consecutive patients. *Stroke, 25*(1), 105–112.

Ardila, A., & Sanchez, E. (1988). Neuropsychologic symptoms in the migraine syndrome. *Cephalalgia, 8*(2), 67–70.

Barth, A., Bogousslavsky, J., & Regli, F. (1993). The clinical and topographic spectrum of cerebellar infarcts: A clinical-magnetic resonance imaging correlation study. *Annals of Neurology, 33*(5), 451–456.

Bastos Leite, A. J., van der Flier, W. M., van Straaten, E. C., Scheltens, P., & Barkhof, F. (2006). Infratentorial abnormalities in vascular dementia. *Stroke, 37*(1), 105–110.

Bednarczyk, E. M., Remler, B., Weikart, C., Nelson, A. D., & Reed, R. C. (1998). Global cerebral blood flow, blood volume, and oxygen metabolism in patients with migraine headache. *Neurology, 50*(6), 1736–1740.

Bell, B. D., Primeau, M., Sweet, J. J., & Lofland, K. R. (1999). Neuropsychological functioning in migraine headache, non-headache chronic pain, and mild traumatic brain injury patients. *Archives of Clinical Neuropsychology, 14*(4), 389–399.

Bernick, C., Kuller, L., Dulberg, C., Longstreth Jr., W. T., Manolio, T., Beauchamp, N., & Price, T. (2001). Silent MRI infarcts and the risk of future stroke: The cardiovascular health study. *Neurology, 57*(7), 1222–1229.

Bogousslavsky, J., Regli, F., Van Melle, G., Payot, M., & Uske, A. (1988). Migraine stroke. *Neurology, 38*(2), 223–227.

Bono, G., Minonzio, G., Mauri, M., & Clerici, A. M. (2006). Complications of migraine: Migrainous infarction. *Clinical and Experimental Hypertension, 28*(3–4), 233–242.

Bousser, M. G. (2004). Estrogens, migraine, and stroke. *Stroke, 35*(11 Suppl 1), 2652–2656.

Broderick, J. P., & Swanson, J. W. (1987). Migraine-related strokes. Clinical profile and prognosis in 20 patients. *Archives of Neurology, 44*(8), 868–871.

Bryan, R. N., Cai, J., Burke, G., Hutchinson, R. G., Liao, D., Toole, J. F., Dagher, A. P., Cooper, L. (1999). Prevalence and anatomic characteristics of infarct-like lesions on MR images of middle-aged adults: The atherosclerosis risk in communities study. *AJNR American Journal of Neuroradiology, 20*(7), 1273–1280.

Buring, J. E., Hebert, P., Romero, J., Kittross, A., Cook, N., Manson, J., Peto, R., & Hennekens, C. (1995). Migraine and subsequent risk of stroke in the Physicians' Health Study. *Archives of Neurology, 52*(2), 129–134.

Canaple, S., & Bogousslavsky, J. (1999). Multiple large and small cerebellar infarcts. *Journal of Neurology, Neurosurgery, and Psychiatry, 66*(6), 739–745.

Caplan, L. R. (1991). Migraine and vertebrobasilar ischemia. *Neurology, 41*(1), 55–61.

Caplan, L. R., & Hennerici, M. (1998). Impaired clearance of emboli (washout) is an important link between hypoperfusion, embolism, and ischemic stroke. *Archives of Neurology, 55*(11), 1475–1482.

Carolei, A., Marini, C., & De Matteis, G. (1996). History of migraine and risk of cerebral ischaemia in young adults. The Italian

National Research Council Study Group on Stroke in the Young. *Lancet, 347*(9014), 1503–1506.

Chabriat, H., Mrissa, R., Levy, C., Vahedi, K., Taillia, H., Iba-Zizen, M. T., et al. (1999). Brain stem MRI signal abnormalities in CADASIL. *Stroke, 30*(2), 457–459.

Chang, C. L., Donaghy, M., & Poulter, N. (1999). Migraine and stroke in young women: Case-control study. The World Health Organisation Collaborative Study of Cardiovascular Disease and Steroid Hormone Contraception. *BMJ, 318*(7175), 13–18.

Collaborative Group for the Study of Stroke in Young Women. (1975). Oral contraceptives and stroke in young women. Associated risk factors. *Journal of the American Medical Association, 231*(7), 718–722.

Cooney, B. S., Grossman, R. I., Farber, R. E., Goin, J. E., & Galetta, S. L. (1996). Frequency of magnetic resonance imaging abnormalities in patients with migraine. *Headache, 36*(10), 616–621.

Crassard, I., Conard, J., & Bousser, M. G. (2001). Migraine and haemostasis. *Cephalalgia, 21*(6), 630–636.

Cutrer, F. M., Sorensen, A. G., Weisskoff, R. M., Ostergaard, L., Sanchez del Rio, M., Lee, E. J., Rosen, B. R., & Moskowitz, M. A. (1998). Perfusion-weighted imaging defects during spontaneous migrainous aura. *Annals of Neurology, 43*(1), 25–31.

De Benedittis, G., Lorenzetti, A., Sina, C., & Bernasconi, V. (1995). Magnetic resonance imaging in migraine and tension-type headache. *Headache, 35*(5), 264–268.

de Seze, J., Mastain, B., Stojkovic, T., et al. (2000). Unusual MR findings of the brain stem in arterial hypertension. *AJNR American Journal of Neuroradiology, 21*(2), 391–394.

Debette, S., & Markus, H. S. (2010). The clinical importance of white matter hyperintensities on brain magnetic resonance imaging: Systematic review and meta-analysis. *BMJ, 341*, c3666.

Dennis, M., & Warlow, C. (1992). Migraine aura without headache: Transient ischaemic attack or not? *Journal of Neurology, Neurosurgery, and Psychiatry, 55*(6), 437–440.

Donaghy, M., Chang, C. L., & Poulter, N. (2002). Duration, frequency, recency, and type of migraine and the risk of ischaemic stroke in women of childbearing age. *Journal of Neurology, Neurosurgery, and Psychiatry, 73*(6), 747–750.

Duvernoy, H., Delon, S., & Vannson, J. L. (1983). The vascularization of the human cerebellar cortex. *Brain Research Bulletin, 11*(4), 419–480.

Eggers, A. E. (2001). New neural theory of migraine. *Medical Hypotheses, 56*(3), 360–363.

Etminan, M., Takkouche, B., Isorna, F. C., & Samii, A. (2005). Risk of ischaemic stroke in people with migraine: Systematic review and meta-analysis of observational studies. *British Medical Journal, 330*(7482), 63.

Farmer, K., Cady, R., Bleiberg, J., & Reeves, D. (2000). A pilot study to measure cognitive efficiency during migraine. *Headache, 40*(8), 657–661.

Fazekas, F., Koch, M., Schmidt, R., Offenbacher, H., Payer, F., Freidl, W., Lechner, H., Schmidt, R., et al. (1992). The prevalence of cerebral damage varies with migraine type: A MRI study. *Headache, 32*(6), 287–291.

Featherstone, H. J. (1986). Clinical features of stroke in migraine: A review. *Headache, 26*(3), 128–133.

Ferbert, A., Busse, D., & Thron, A. (1991). Microinfarction in classic migraine? A study with magnetic resonance imaging findings. *Stroke, 22*(8), 1010–1014.

Ferrari, M. D. (1998). Migraine. *Lancet, 351*(9108), 1043–1051.

Fessatidis, I. T., Thomas, V. L., Shore, D. F., Hunt, R. H., Weller, R. O., Goodland, F., et al. (1993). Assessment of neurological injury due to circulatory arrest during profound hypothermia. An experimental study in vertebrates. *European Journal of Cardiothoracic Surgery, 7*(9), 465–472.

Gaist, D., Pedersen, L., Madsen, C., Tsiropoulos, I., Bak, S., Sindrup, S., et al. (2005). Long-term effects of migraine on cognitive function: A population-based study of Danish twins. *Neurology, 64*(4), 600–607.

Ghabriel, M. N., Lu, M. X., Leigh, C., Cheung, W. C., & Allt, G. (1999). Substance P-induced enhanced permeability of dura mater microvessels is accompanied by pronounced ultrastructural changes, but is not dependent on the density of endothelial cell anionic sites. *Acta Neuropathologica (Berlin), 97*(3), 297–305.

Goadsby, P. J. (2002). Neurovascular headache and a midbrain vascular malformation: Evidence for a role of the brainstem in chronic migraine. *Cephalalgia, 22*(2), 107–111.

Goadsby, P. J. (1997). Pathophysiology of migraine: A disease of the brain. In: P. J. Goadsby & S. D. Silberstein (Eds.), *Headache* (pp. 5–25). Boston: Butterworth-Heinemann.

Gozke, E., Ore, O., Dortcan, N., Unal, Z., & Cetinkaya, M. (2004). Cranial magnetic resonance imaging findings in patients with migraine. *Headache, 44*(2), 166–169.

Gursoy-Ozdemir, Y., Qiu, J., Matsuoka, N., Bolay, H., Bermpohl, D., Jin, H., et al. (2004). Cortical spreading depression activates and upregulates MMP-9. *Journal of Clinical Investigation, 113*(10), 1447–1455.

Haapaniemi, H., Hillbom, M., & Juvela, S. (1997). Lifestyle-associated risk factors for acute brain infarction among persons of working age. *Stroke, 28*(1), 26–30.

Headache Classification Committee of the International Headache Society. (1988). Classification and diagnostic criteria for headache disorders, cranial neuralgias and facial pain. *Cephalalgia, 8*(Suppl 7), 1–96.

Henrich, J. B., & Horwitz, R. I. (1989). A controlled study of ischemic stroke risk in migraine patients. *Journal of Clinical Epidemiology, 42*(8), 773–780.

Henrich, J. B., Sandercock, P. A., Warlow, C. P., & Jones, L. N. (1986). Stroke and migraine in the Oxfordshire Community Stroke Project. *Journal of Neurology, 233*(5), 257–262.

Hoekstra-van Dalen, R. A., Cillessen, J. P., Kappelle, L. J., & van Gijn, J. (1996). Cerebral infarcts associated with migraine: Clinical features, risk factors and follow-up. *Journal of Neurology, 243*(7), 511–515.

Hooker, W. D., & Raskin, N. H. (1986). Neuropsychologic alterations in classic and common migraine. *Archives of Neurology, 43*(7), 709–712.

Howard, G., Wagenknecht, L. E., Cai, J., Cooper, L., Kraut, M. A., & Toole, J. F. (1998). Cigarette smoking and other risk factors for silent cerebral infarction in the general population. *Stroke, 29*(5), 913–917.

Ichikawa, H., Takahashi, N., Mukai, M., Akizawa, T., & Kawamura, M. (2008). Asymptomatic large T2 high-signal pontine lesions that are different from ischemic rarefaction. *Journal of Stroke and Cerebrovascular Diseases, 17*(6), 394–400.

Igarashi, H., Sakai, F., Kan, S., Okada, J., & Tazaki, Y. (1991). Magnetic resonance imaging of the brain in patients with migraine. *Cephalalgia, 11*(2), 69–74.

Iizuka, T., Sakai, F., Yamakawa, K., Suzuki, K., & Suzuki, N. (2004). Vasogenic leakage and the mechanism of migraine with prolonged aura in Sturge-Weber syndrome. *Cephalalgia, 24*(9), 767–770.

Ishizaki, K., Mori, N., Takeshima, T., Fukuhara, Y., Ijiri, T., Kusumi, M., et al. (2002). Static stabilometry in patients with migraine and tension-type headache during a headache-free period. *Psychiatry and Clinical Neuroscience, 56*(1), 85–90.

Jelicic, M., van Boxtel, M. P., Houx, P. J., & Jolles, J. (2000). Does migraine headache affect cognitive function in the elderly? Report from the Maastricht Aging Study (MAAS). *Headache, 40*(9), 715–719.

Kaplan, R. D., Solomon, G. D., Diamond, S., & Freitag, F. G. (1987). The role of MRI in the evaluation of a migraine population: Preliminary data. *Headache, 27*(6), 315–318.

Kase, C. S., Wolf, P. A., Chodosh, E. H., Zacker, H. B., Kelly-Hayes, M., Kannel, W. B., et al. (1989). Prevalence of silent stroke in patients presenting with initial stroke: The Framingham Study. *Stroke, 20*(7), 850–852.

Katsarava, Z., & Weimar, C. (2010). Migraine and stroke. *Journal of the Neurological Sciences, 299*(1–2), 42–44.

Kern, R. Z. (2004). Progress in clinical neurosciences: Migraine-stroke: a causal relationship, but which direction? *Canadian Journal of Neurological Sciences, 31*(4), 451–459.

Kruit, M. C., Launer, L. J., Ferrari, M. D., & van Buchem, M. A. (2006). Brain stem and cerebellar hyperintense lesions in migraine. *Stroke, 37*(4), 1109–1112.

Kruit, M. C., Launer, L. J., Ferrari, M. D., & van Buchem, M. A. (2005). Infarcts in the posterior circulation territory in migraine. The population-based MRI CAMERA study. *Brain, 128*(Pt 9), 2068–2077.

Kruit, M. C., van Buchem, M. A., Hofman, P. A., Bakkers, J. T., Terwindt, G. M., Ferrari, M. D., & Launer, L. J. (2004). Migraine as a risk factor for subclinical brain lesions. *Journal of the American Medical Association, 291*(4), 427–434.

Kurth, T., Mohamed, S., Maillard, P., Zhu, Y. C., Chabriat, H., Mazoyer, B., Bousser, M. G., et al. (2011). Headache, migraine, and structural brain lesions and function: Population based Epidemiology of Vascular Ageing-MRI study. *British Medical Journal, 342*, c7357.

Kwa, V. I., Stam, J., Blok, L. M., & Verbeeten, B., Jr. (1997). T2-weighted hyperintense MRI lesions in the pons in patients with atherosclerosis. Amsterdam Vascular Medicine Group. *Stroke, 28*(7), 1357–1360.

Le Pira, F., Zappala, G., Giuffrida, S., Lo Bartolo, M. L., Reggio, E., Morana, R., & Lanaia, F. (2000). Memory disturbances in migraine with and without aura: A strategy problem? *Cephalalgia, 20*(5), 475–478.

Leonardi, M., Steiner, T. J., Scher, A. T., & Lipton, R. B. (2005). The global burden of migraine: Measuring disability in headache disorders with WHO's Classification of Functioning, Disability and Health (ICF). *Journal of Headache and Pain, 6*(6), 429–440.

Lidegaard, O. (1995). Oral contraceptives, pregnancy and the risk of cerebral thromboembolism: The influence of diabetes, hypertension, migraine and previous thrombotic disease. *British Journal of Obstetrics and Gynaecology, 102*(2), 153–159.

Lipton, R. B., & Pan, J. (2004). Is migraine a progressive brain disease? *Journal of the American Medical Association, 291*(4), 493–494.

Lipton, R. B., Stewart, W. F., & von Korff, M. (1997). Burden of migraine: Societal costs and therapeutic opportunities. *Neurology, 48*(3 Suppl 3), S4–S9.

Longstreth, W. T., Jr., Manolio, T. A., Arnold, A., Burke, G. L., Bryan, N., Jungreis, C. A., et al. (1996). Clinical correlates of white matter findings on cranial magnetic resonance imaging of 3301 elderly people. The Cardiovascular Health Study. *Stroke, 27*(8), 1274–1282.

Marini, C., Carolei, A., Roberts, R. S., Prencipe, M., Gandolfo, C., Inzitari, D., et al. (1993). Focal cerebral ischemia in young adults: A collaborative case-control study. The National Research Council Study Group. *Neuroepidemiology, 12*(2), 70–81.

Martins, I. P., & Cunha e Sa, M. (1999). Loss of topographic memory and prosopagnosia during migraine aura. *Cephalalgia, 19*(9), 841–843.

Merikangas, K. R., Fenton, B. T., Cheng, S. H., Stolar, M. J., & Risch, N. (1997). Association between migraine and stroke in a large-scale epidemiological study of the United States. *Archives of Neurology, 54*(4), 362–368.

Milhaud, D., Bogousslavsky, J., Van Melle, G., & Liot, P. (2001). Ischemic stroke and active migraine. *Neurology, 57*(10), 1805–1811.

Mulder, E. J., Linssen, W. H., Passchier, J., Orlebeke, J. F., & de Geus, E. J. (1999). Interictal and postictal cognitive changes in migraine. *Cephalalgia, 19*(6), 557–565.

Nash, J. M., & Thebarge, R. W. (2006). Understanding psychological stress, its biological processes, and impact on primary headache. *Headache, 46*(9), 1377–1386.

Nash, J. M., Williams, D. M., Nicholson, R., & Trask, P. C. (2006). The contribution of pain-related anxiety to disability from headache. *Journal of Behavioral Medicine, 29*(1), 61–67.

Nightingale, A. L., & Farmer, R. D. (2004). Ischemic stroke in young women: A nested case-control study using the UK General Practice Research Database. *Stroke, 35*(7), 1574–1578.

O'Bryant, S. E., Marcus, D. A., Rains, J. C., & Penzien, D. B. (2006). The neuropsychology of recurrent headache. *Headache, 46*(9), 1364–1376.

Olesen, J., Friberg, L., Olsen, T. S., Iversen, H. K., Lassen, N. A., Andersen, A. R., & Karle, A. (1990). Timing and topography of cerebral blood flow, aura, and headache during migraine attacks. *Annals of Neurology, 28*(6), 791–798.

Ophoff, R. A., Terwindt, G. M., Vergouwe, M. N., van Eijk, R., Oefner, P. J., Hoffman, S. M., et al. (1996). Familial hemiplegic migraine and episodic ataxia type-2 are caused by mutations in the Ca2 + channel gene CACNL1A4. *Cell, 87*(3), 543–552.

Osborn, R. E., Alder, D. C., & Mitchell, C. S. (1991). MR imaging of the brain in patients with migraine headaches. *AJNR American Journal of Neuroradiology, 12*(3), 521–524.

Pavese, N., Canapicchi, R., Nuti, A., Bibbiani, F., Lucetti, C., Collavoli, P., & Bonuccelli, U. (1994). White matter MRI hyperintensities in a hundred and twenty-nine consecutive migraine patients. *Cephalalgia, 14*(5), 342–345.

Pearson, A. J., Chronicle, E. P., Maylor, E. A., & Bruce, L. A. (2006). Cognitive function is not impaired in people with a long history of migraine: A blinded study. *Cephalalgia, 26*(1), 74–80.

Prins, N. D., van Dijk, E. J., den Heijer, T., Vermeer, S. E., Jolles, J., Koudstaal, P. J., et al. (2005). Cerebral small-vessel disease and decline in information processing speed, executive function and memory. *Brain, 128*(Pt 9), 2034–2041.

Pullicino, P., Ostrow, P., Miller, L., Snyder, W., & Munschauer, F. (1995). Pontine ischemic rarefaction. *Annals of Neurology, 37*(4), 460–466.

Resnick, S., Reyes-Iglesias, Y., Carreras, R., & Villalobos, E. (2006). Migraine with aura associated with reversible MRI abnormalities. *Neurology, 66*(6), 946–947.

Robbins, L., & Friedman, H. (1992). MRI in migraineurs. *Headache, 32*(10), 507–508.

Rocca, M. A., Colombo, B., Pratesi, A., Comi, G., & Filippi, M. (2000). A magnetization transfer imaging study of the brain in patients with migraine. *Neurology, 54*(2), 507–509.

Rothrock, J., North, J., Madden, K., Lyden, P., Fleck, P., & Dittrich, H. (1993). Migraine and migrainous stroke: Risk factors and prognosis. *Neurology, 43*(12), 2473–2476.

Rothrock, J. F., Walicke, P., Swenson, M. R., Lyden, P. D., & Logan, W. R. (1988). Migrainous stroke. *Archives of Neurology, 45*(1), 63–67.

Rovaris, M., Bozzali, M., Rocca, M. A., Colombo, B., & Filippi, M. (2001). An MR study of tissue damage in the cervical cord of patients with migraine. *Journal of the Neurological Sciences, 183*(1), 43–46.

Sacquegna, T., Andreoli, A., Baldrati, A., et al. (1989). Ischemic stroke in young adults: The relevance of migrainous infarction. *Cephalalgia, 9*(4), 255–258.

Salomon, A., Yeates, A. E., Burger, P. C., & Heinz, E. R. (1987). Subcortical arteriosclerotic encephalopathy: Brain stem findings with MR imaging. *Radiology, 165*(3), 625–629.

Sanchez del Rio, M., Bakker, D., Wu, O., Agosti, R., Mitsikostas, D. D., Ostergaard, L., et al. (1999). Perfusion weighted imaging during migraine: Spontaneous visual aura and headache. *Cephalalgia, 19*(8), 701–707.

Sandor, P. S., Mascia, A., Seidel, L., De P, V., & Schoenen, J. (2001). Subclinical cerebellar impairment in the common types of migraine: A three-dimensional analysis of reaching movements. *Annals of Neurology, 49*(5), 668–672.

Scher, A. I., Gudmundsson, L. S., Sigurdsson, S., Ghambaryan, A., Aspelund, T., Eiriksdottir, G., et al. (2009). Migraine headache in middle age and late-life brain infarcts. *Journal of the American Medical Association, 301*(24), 2563–2570.

Scher, A. I., Stewart, W. F., & Lipton, R. B. (2006). The comorbidity of headache with other pain syndromes. *Headache, 46*(9), 1416–1423.

Scher, A. I., Terwindt, G. M., Picavet, H. S., Verschuren, W. M., Ferrari, M. D., & Launer, L. J. (2005). Cardiovascular risk factors and migraine: The GEM population-based study. *Neurology, 64*(4), 614–620.

Scher, A. I., Terwindt, G. M., Verschuren, W. M., Kruit, M. C., Blom, H. J., Kowa, H., Frants, R. R., et al. (2006). Migraine and MTHFR C677T genotype in a population-based sample. *Annals of Neurology, 59*(2), 372–375.

Schurks, M., Rist, P. M., Bigal, M. E., Buring, J. E., Lipton, R. B., & Kurth, T. (2009). Migraine and cardiovascular disease: Systematic review and meta-analysis. *BMJ, 339*, b3914.

Schwaag, S., Nabavi, D. G., Frese, A., Husstedt, I. W., & Evers, S. (2003). The association between migraine and juvenile stroke: A case-control study. *Headache, 43*(2), 90–95.

Shuaib, A., & Lee, M. A. (1988). Cerebral infarction in patients with migraine accompaniments. *Headache, 28*(9), 599–601.

Smith, M., Cros, D., & Sheen, V. (2002). Hyperperfusion with vasogenic leakage by fMRI in migraine with prolonged aura. *Neurology, 58*(8), 1308–1310.

Soges, L. J., Cacayorin, E. D., Petro, G. R., & Ramachandran, T. S. (1988). Migraine: Evaluation by MR. *AJNR American Journal of Neuroradiology, 9*(3), 425–429.

Swartz, R. H., & Kern, R. Z. (2004). Migraine is associated with magnetic resonance imaging white matter abnormalities: A meta-analysis. *Archives of Neurology, 61*(9), 1366–1368.

Tietjen, G. E. (2004). Stroke and migraine linked by silent lesions. *Lancet Neurology, 3*(5), 267.

Tietjen, G. E., Al Qasmi, M. M., Athanas, K., Dafer, R. M., & Khuder, S. A. (2001). Increased von Willebrand factor in migraine. *Neurology, 57*(2), 334–336.

Tortorella, P., Rocca, M. A., Colombo, B., Annovazzi, P., Comi, G., & Filippi, M. (2006). Assessment of MRI abnormalities of the brainstem from patients with migraine and multiple sclerosis. *Journal of the Neurological Sciences, 244*(1–2), 137–141.

Tzourio, C., Iglesias, S., Hubert, J. B., Visy, J. M., Alpérovitch, A., Tehindrazanarivelo, A., et al. (1993). Migraine and risk of ischaemic stroke: A case-control study. *British Medical Journal, 307*(6899), 289–292.

Tzourio, C., Kittner, S. J., Bousser, M. G., & Alperovitch, A. (2000). Migraine and stroke in young women. *Cephalalgia, 20*(3), 190–199.

Tzourio, C., Tehindrazanarivelo, A., Iglesias, S., Alpérovitch, A., Chedru, F., d'Anglejan-Chatillon, J., & Bousser, M. G. (1995). Case-control study of migraine and risk of ischaemic stroke in young women. *BMJ, 310*(6983), 830–833.

Vermeer, S. E., Hollander, M., van Dijk, E. J., Hofman, A., Koudstaal, P. J., & Breteler, M. M. (2003). Silent brain infarcts and white matter lesions increase stroke risk in the general population: The Rotterdam Scan Study. *Stroke, 34*(5), 1126–1129.

Vermeer, S. E., Prins, N. D., den Heijer, T., Hofman, A., Koudstaal, P. J., & Breteler, M. M. (2003). Silent brain infarcts and the risk of dementia and cognitive decline. *New England Journal of Medicine, 348*(13), 1215–1222.

Waldie, K. E., Hausmann, M., Milne, B. J., & Poulton, R. (2002). Migraine and cognitive function: a life-course study. *Neurology, 59*(6), 904–908.

Welch, K. M. (2008). Iron in the migraine brain; a resilient hypothesis. *Cephalalgia.* 2009 Mar; *29*(3), 283–285.

Welch, K. M. (1994). Relationship of stroke and migraine. *Neurology, 44*(Suppl 7)(10):S33–S36.

Welch, K. M., & Levine, S. R. (1990). Migraine-related stroke in the context of the International Headache Society classification of head pain [Review] [20 refs]. *Archives of Neurology, 1990, 47*(4), 458–462.

WHO Collaborative Study of Cardiovascular Disease and Steroid Hormone Contraception. (1996). Ischaemic stroke and combined oral contraceptives: Results of an international, multicentre, case-control study. *Lancet, 348*(9026), 498–505.

Woods, R. P., Iacoboni, M., & Mazziotta, J. C. (1994). Brief report: Bilateral spreading cerebral hypoperfusion during spontaneous migraine headache. *New England Journal of Medicine, 331*(25), 1689–1692.

Zeitlin, C., & Oddy, M. (1984). Cognitive impairment in patients with severe migraine. *British Journal of Clinical Psychology, 23*(Pt 1), 27–35.

Ziegler, D. K., Batnitzky, S., Barter, R., & McMillan, J. H. (1991). Magnetic resonance image abnormality in migraine with aura. *Cephalalgia, 11*(3), 147–150.

12 Clinical Utility of Objective Measures

FRANZ RIEDERER, ANDREAS R. GANTENBEIN, AND

PETER S. SÁNDOR

INTRODUCTION

Migraine and other primary headache types such as tension-type headache or trigemino-autonomic headaches are clinical diagnoses that can be made based on diagnostic criteria (International Headache Society [IHS], 2004). Investigations may be necessary in cases of unusual clinical presentation, the first appearance of focal neurological signs, or a recent change in attack pattern to exclude secondary headaches. It may also be difficult to make the diagnosis of migraine if precise history taking is confounded by a comorbid affective disorder or language difficulties. Also, in the case of chronic daily headache, the diagnosis of migraine may be difficult to make unless the patient is able to provide sufficient—ideally, headache diary based—information. Thus, objective measures to support the diagnosis of migraine in these instances may be useful. Ideally, these measures should have sufficient sensitivity and specificity to be of diagnostic value and be cost efficient. In recent years, substantial advances in our understanding of migraine pathophysiology have been achieved. The following chapter will review whether these advances may be used to support the migraine diagnosis. Because of the clinical relevance, some examples where instrumental investigations help to exclude secondary headaches that mimic migraine will also be mentioned.

NEUROIMAGING

In the past decade several neuroimaging modalities have demonstrated structural, functional, and metabolic abnormalities in primary headaches (May, 2009; Reyngoudt et al., 2011). However, it remains to be elucidated whether there are migraine-specific abnormalities or these changes are associated with chronic pain states in general. Although most findings are based on group statistics, some of the abnormalities could support the diagnosis of migraine. In a recent proton magnetic resonance spectroscopy study, migraine patients and controls were separated by means of linear discriminant analysis based

on the metabolites N-acetylaspartylglutamate and glutamine in the anterior cingulate cortex and insula (Prescot et al., 2009).

Theoretically, structural gray matter as detected by voxel-based morphometry could be used for automated diagnostic classification, as has been demonstrated for different types of dementias (Kloppel et al., 2008) and obsessive-compulsive disorder (Soriano-Mas et al., 2007).

The clinical value of magnetic resonance imaging (MRI) is well established for the differential diagnosis of acute diseases that may mimic migraine attacks. If focal neurological signs associated with migrainelike headache are unusual or last unusually long, diffusion-weighted imaging (DWI) can differentiate ischemic lesions (migrainous infarction) from a migraine aura. Migrainous infarction is considered a rare complication of migraine that may present with similar symptoms as migraine with aura (Wolf et al., 2011). This may be the reason why patients with migrainous infarction seek help late and rarely get thrombolyzed, as evidenced in a recent study (Wolf et al., 2011). Another clinical indication for MRI is the suspicion of sinus venous thrombosis. Headache may be the only clinical manifestation of sinus venous thrombosis (Chen et al., 2007) and may be associated with migrainelike visual disturbances (Newman et al., 1989). It may develop subacutely and may be worse in the supine position. Symptoms and signs of intracranial hypertension such as nausea and vomiting or papilledema may be present. Risk factors include hypercoagulable states, oral contraception, the peripartal period, malignant diseases, and dehydration (Chen et al., 2007).

Recently an updated version of the guidelines of the European Federation of Neurological Societies (EFNS) on neurophysiological tests and neuroimaging procedures in nonacute headache was published (Sandrini et al., 2011). These guidelines summarize current evidence from the literature on the clinical value of instrumental investigations including neuroimaging in the clinical setting in nonacute headache. It is suggested that in patients with a recent change in attack pattern, atypical headache patterns, a history of seizures, or symptomatic illness such as tumors, acquired immunodeficiency syndrome (AIDS), and neurofibromatosis, MRI may be indicated.

Finally, there is consensus that neuroimaging with MRI should be performed in patients with trigemino-autonomic headaches (Sandrini et al., 2011).

Positron emission tomography (PET) studies have shown increased blood flow in the brainstem during spontaneous migraine attacks (Afridi et al., 2005; Weiller et al., 1995), suggesting a pivotal role in migraine patho-physiology. According to EFNS guidelines, studies of cerebral blood flow with single-photon emission computed tomography or PET might be of value in patients in whom the standard IHS classification cannot be fully applied, when patients experience unusually severe attacks, or when the quality or severity of attacks has changed (Sandrini et al., 2011). In these rare cases, according to the above guidelines, measurements of cerebral blood flow should be performed both during the attacks and interictally.

However, even though PET has contributed substantially to our understanding of migraine, we consider it unlikely that PET studies will become a widely used tool for migraine diagnosis, among others, because of its limited availability. Also, exposure to radiation may be a limiting factor in the clinical setting.

EVOKED POTENTIALS

Probably the most and best evidence for neurophysiological changes comes from studies with evoked potentials. Although the results show some variation, and comparisons may be difficult due to methodological differences (stimulus design, recording set-up, patient selection), they mostly show that information processing is abnormal in migraineurs (Ambrosini, Rossi et al., 2003; Giffin & Kaube, 2002). The earliest findings come from routine visual evoked potentials (VEPs) showing higher amplitudes in migraine patients than healthy controls (Diener et al., 1989). P1 and N2 latencies were prolonged in some (Mariani et al., 1990, Tsounis et al., 1993) but not in other studies (Afra, Proietti et al., 2000; Judit et al., 2000).

The lack of habituation was first described by Schoenen (for review see Schoenen, 1996) in visual evoked potentials. Habituation is a gradual decrease in the magnitude of a cortical response usually observed after repeated exposition to a stimulus. A lack of habituation means that this decrease in response is absent. As habituation is known as a physiological process and probably one of the most basic mechanisms of learning (Carew et al., 1979), it may well be

a protective mechanism preventing the brain from sensory overload and therefore economizing energy balance in a normally functioning brain (Schoenen, 1994).

This might be the most salient characteristic of the migrainous brain between attacks. Habituation deficits can be found not only in VEPs, but also in cortical auditory evoked potentials (AEPs) (Ambrosini, Rossi et al., 2003; Judit et al., 2000); intensity dependence of auditory evoked potentials (IDAP) (Afra, Proietti et al., 2000; Wang et al., 1996); CO_2 laser-evoked potentials (LEPs) (de Tommaso et al., 2005); event-related potentials, "oddball" paradigm (P300) (Evers et al., 1998, Wang & Schoenen, 1998); and contingent negative variation (CNV) (Siniatchkin et al., 2003). Furthermore, the nociception-specific blink reflex (nBR) shows deficient habituation (for details see below) (Katsarava et al., 2003).

Altogether the deficient habituation most probably reflects an interictal trait of migraine patients and is, as consistent in nearly all studies, well accepted in the community (Ambrosini, Rossi et al., 2003). Although sensitivity and specificity of these electrophysiological surrogate markers would not allow using them as diagnostic tests for the individual, the abnormal sensory information processing qualifies as probably the best objective measure.

Some recent studies of AEPs (Judit et al., 2000) and CNV (see also below) (Kropp & Gerber, 1995, 1998, Siniatchkin et al., 1999) showed a normalization of the interictal lack of habituation before, during, and shortly after the migraine attack. This may represent a changing state of cortical information processing, correlating with the timing of the migraine cycle.

Two other studies (Sandor et al., 1999, Siniatchkin, Kirsch et al., 2000) demonstrate a familial character to the habituation deficit, which may predict, as a trait marker, subjects at risk of developing migraine.

VEPs and IDAP have also been studied during prophylactic treatment. Diener et al. (1989) showed a significant reduction of the VEP amplitude after treatment with β-blockers. Sandor et al. (2000) showed the same for the IDAP. In the latter study, a group of patients treated with riboflavin (vitamin B_2) had a reduction of the migraine frequency but no significant reduction of IDAP, implying different modes of action of the two drugs.

Habituation deficits of AEPs have been suggested in other disorders such as tinnitus (Walpurger et al., 2003), challenging the assumption that habituation deficits are specific for migraine (Stankewitz & May, 2009). However, in the study mentioned above, (Walpurger et al., 2003) significant differences in habituation between tinnitus complainers and non-complainers were found only in post hoc comparisons, so these results need to be further substantiated.

Despite these interesting findings, the literature data do not support the usefulness of EPs as a diagnostic tool in migraine (Sandrini et al., 2011).

Event-Related Potentials: Contingent Negative Variation and P300

CNV is a slow negative cortical brain potential that occurs after presentation of warning stimuli followed by "imperative" stimuli to which the subject has to respond. Thus, it reflects expectancy and motor preparation and seems hierarchically higher compared to the above-described evoked potentials. A higher amplitude and reduced habituation have been described in migraine (Maertens de Noordhout et al., 1986). Migraineurs, but also about up to two thirds of healthy children and about one third of nonmigrainous adults, show a lack of CNV habituation (Kropp & Gerber, 1993, Schoenen & Timsit-Berthier, 1993). This change may be a developmental feature of information processing and to some extent represent a risk factor for the development of migraine (Siniatchkin, Kirsch et al., 2000). CNV amplitude has been shown to normalize on successful prophylaxis with β-blockers (Maertens de Noordhout et al., 1987). CNV habituation also has been shown to normalize after prophylaxis with topiramate or levetiracetam (de Tommaso et al., 2008) in patients with migraine without aura. Even though CNV currently cannot be recommended as a diagnostic tool for migraine, it may have potential as a surrogate marker for treatment response (de Tommaso et al., 2008).

The P300 is an event-related potential that can be obtained from background electroencephalographic activity in the so-called oddball paradigm. In this paradigm, the subject has to respond after auditory target stimuli, which are intermingled in a random fashion with standard stimuli that demand no response. P300 refers to a surface-positive deflection in cortical activity, occurring about 300 to 600 milliseconds after the target stimulus. Studies in migraine showed conflicting results (Drake et al., 1989; Evers et al., 1997, 1998, 1999; Wang & Schoenen, 1998).

Electroencephalogram and Photic Driving Response

A suppression of α-rhythm has been found in patients with migraine during the attack (de Tommaso et al., 1998; Schoenen et al., 1987). Some changes in electroencephalogram (EEG) power spectra during sleep, the night before the attack, suggest a decrease in cortical activation preceding migraine attacks (Goder et al., 2001). In the late 1950s Golla and Winter (1959) studied photic driving responses in the EEG of headache patients and healthy controls. The photic driving response in healthy controls was limited at stimulation frequencies of about 14 Hz, whereas the responses in patients with headache were still present above 18 Hz. They named this phenomenon the "headache" or "H" response. Later studies confirmed the results applying IHS diagnostic criteria for migraine (Chorlton & Kane, 2000; Gantenbein et al., 2005). However, de Tommaso et al. (1999) found no distinction between migraine and other headache types, and a recent longitudinal controlled study showed that earlier results may have overestimated the driving response in migraine, neglecting the relation to the migraine attack (Bjork, 2011). Interestingly, the photic driving response might also be reproduced using faster changing flash frequencies instead of conventional photic driving, and therefore be less prone to habituation deficits in migraine patients (Gantenbein et al., 2005).

Findings using EEG and magnetoencephalography during the migraine attack as well as interictally are controversial, and by far do not qualify as objective measures for migraine.

According to EFNS guidelines (Sandrini et al., 2011), interictal EEG is indicated if the history suggests a possible diagnosis of epilepsy by unusual brief headache episodes, unusual aura symptoms such as gastric/olfactory symptoms, circular visual symptoms, and headache associated with severe neurological deficits. Ictal EEG is indicated during episodes with complicated auras and auras with alterations in consciousness or confusion. Although "acute confusional migraine" may be a migraine variant (Gantenbein et al., 2010), this remains a diagnosis of exclusion after careful diagnostic workup.

The differential diagnosis of visual seizures should be carefully evaluated in patients with unusual visual auras. Of note, occipital lobe epilepsy is often accompanied by severe headache and vomiting (Panayiotopoulos, 2010). Elementary visual hallucinations in occipital lobe epilepsy typically develop within seconds, are brief (<1 minute), and may occur daily (Panayiotopoulos, 1999). In contrast to migraine visual auras, they present with predominantly colored and circular patterns. EEGs may be normal or unspecific and high-resolution MRI is recommended (Panayiotopoulos, 2010).

Blink Reflex

The blink reflex is a trigeminofacial brainstem reflex. In the surface electromyogram three successive responses may be distinguished after electrical stimulation of the supraorbital nerve: an ipsilateral oligosynaptic pontine component (R1), a bilateral polysynaptic medullary response (R2), and a less distinct R3 component (de Tommaso et al., 2000).

Involvement of trigeminal dysfunction in the migraine pathophysiology has already been suggested when prolonged latencies were found in a group of migraine patients compared to healthy controls. Studies with a small concentric electrode, which elicits mostly the nociception-specific R2 component (nBR), have shown increased amplitudes on the headache side only in migraine but not in frontal sinus pain (Katsarava et al., 2002). Furthermore, a lack of habituation has been demonstrated in the interictal phase, which supports abnormal trigeminal nociceptive processing in migraine patients (Katsarava et al., 2003).

In a recent study a significantly positive correlation between habituation parameters of VEP and nBR was found in migraine without aura but not in healthy controls (Di Clemente et al., 2005), suggesting deficient habituation at the cortical as well as the brainstem level. The authors suggested that this could be explained by dysfunction in serotonergic brainstem nuclei.

Currently there are not enough data to support the use of the nBR as a diagnostic tool in migraine (Sandrini et al., 2011).

ABNORMALITIES IN COORDINATION AND THE MOTOR SYSTEM

The abnormalities described above have been suggested to be associated with mechanisms of attack generation, such as an increased consumption of cellular energy (Schoenen, 1998), and considered as "pathogenetic abnormalities." In contrast, the dysfunctions described below in migraineurs could be conceptualized more as a consequence of the underlying neurobiological abnormality than being directly involved in the generation of migraine attacks and could be called "incidental."

Subclinical hypermetria and other subtle cerebellar signs in the common forms of migraine have been described using a pointing paradigm (similar to a finger–nose test) with an infrared optoelectronic tracking system (Sandor et al., 2001). The abnormalities were more pronounced in migraine with aura than in migraine without aura.

Also, abnormalities in neuromuscular transmission have been described in a subgroup of migraine with aura patients. Several studies described single-fiber electromyelography abnormalities (abnormal jitter or impulse blocking) in patients with migraine and prolonged aura, sensorimotor symptoms, aphasia, or dysbalance during the aura (Ambrosini, de Noordhout, et al., 2001; Ambrosini, Maertens de Noordhout, et al., 2001; Ambrosini, Pierelli et al., 2003). An association with genetically modified P/Q-type Ca^{2+} channels has been suggested.

TRANSCRANIAL MAGNETIC STIMULATION

VEPs were studied using repetitive transcranial magnetic stimulation (rTMS) in migraine as an intervention combined with VEP recording (Bohotin et al., 2002). After repetitive stimulation at 1 Hz, the habituation of the VEPs disappeared in healthy controls, whereas there was no difference in migraine patients. Conversely, migraine patients showed a habituation pattern after stimulation at 10 Hz, whereas there was no change in healthy volunteers.

TMS has been used to study motor cortex excitability and phosphene thresholds over the occipital cortex in migraine (Schoenen et al., 2003). Also, the modulatory effect of transcranial direct current stimulation (tDCS) on cortical excitability seems to differ between patients and controls (Chadaide et al., 2007). The increase of the phosphene threshold after cathodal stimulation observed in healthy controls was absent in migraine patients.

However, because of inconsistent results probably related to different methodologies for TMS or fluctuations in cortical excitability in the migraine cycle, magnetic stimulation currently has no application as a diagnostic test (Mirza et al., 1998). A summary of ictal and interictal neurophysiological findings in migraine is given in Table 12–1.

ULTRASOUND OF CRANIAL ARTERIES AND ECHOCARDIOGRAPHY

Ultrasound investigations are not routinely used to support the diagnosis of migraine. Transcranial Doppler examination is not helpful for establishing the migraine diagnosis but may be a valuable tool to study vasoreactivity in migraine (Nedeltchev et al., 2004). In addition, transcranial Doppler is useful to detect cardiac shunts and should be used when paradoxical embolism is suspected (see below).

Headache is a frequent symptom in cervical artery dissection and may be the sole presenting symptom (Arnold et al., 2006). It is usually of sudden onset and may be associated with neck pain and accompanied by pulsatile tinnitus. However, it has occasionally been described to mimic migraine (Mirza et al., 1998; Morelli et al., 2008; Sharif et al., 2010; Young & Humphrey, 1995). In these cases new-onset transient or permanent neurological signs such as Horner syndrome (Sharif et al., 2010), weakness of the extremities, or speech disturbance (Mirza et al., 1998) were also present. In two cases with vertebral artery dissection, presenting symptoms were a scintillating scotoma mimicking migraine aura followed by headache in patients without migraine history (Morelli et al., 2008; Young & Humphrey, 1995). One case developed no other neurological symptoms and had a mild diffuse headache

TABLE 12–1 *Ictal and Interictal Findings of Electrophysiological Tests in Migraine Patients*

METHOD	FINDINGS	
	Ictal (headache phase)	Interictal
EEG	Alpha suppression	H response in photic driving
VEP	Normal latencies	Latencies ↑
		Amplitudes ↑ (↓)
		Lack of habituation
AEP	Normalized habituation	Lack of habituation of IDAP
CNV, P300	Normal amplitudes	Amplitudes ↑
	Normalized habituation	Lack of habituation
BR	AUC ↑ (facilitation of nBR)	Lack of habituation
Single-fiber EMG	Abnormal jitter or impulse blocking	
TMS	Phosphene thresholds ↑↓	
	Paradoxical behavior in rTMS	

Notes: EEG = electroencephalogram; VEP = visual evoke potential; AEP = auditory evoked potential; IDAP = intensity dependence of auditory evoked potentials; CNV = contingent negative variation; BR = blink reflex; AUC = areas under the curve; nBR = nociception-specific blink reflex; EMG = electromyelogram; TMS = transcranial magnetic stimulation; rTMS = repetitive transcranial magnetic stimulation.

Modified from Gantenbein, A. R., & Sandor, P. S. (2006). Physiological parameters as biomarkers of migraine. *Headache, 46*(7), 1069–1074.

and a stiff neck (Young & Humphrey, 1995). Migraine aura–like visual disturbances have also been described in carotid artery dissection, but seemed less typical (Ramadan et al., 1991) (followed sudden-onset headache, were monocular, or lasted for 3 days). Sonography of cervical arteries is appropriate to diagnose cervical artery dissection, although MRI is probably more sensitive.

Given that there is an association between migraine and cervical artery dissection (Rist et al., 2011), it should not be overlooked in migraine patients presenting with new or unusual neurological symptoms or a new headache type.

Although an association between migraine and cardiac abnormalities or peculiarities such as persistent foramen ovale, atrial septum defect, and mitral valve prolapse has been described (Anzola et al., 1999; Riederer et al., 2011; Spence et al., 1984), there is currently no indication to perform echocardiography routinely in migraine patients. Emboli of cardiac origin or paradoxical embolism through a cardiac shunt can probably trigger migraine attacks under special circumstances, establishing a link between cardiac peculiarities and migraine (Dalkara et al., 2010). The same is probably true for other sources of embolism such as cervical artery dissection. This could be called "symptomatic migraine" related to embolism.

Cessation of migraine with aura after removal of an atrial myxoma, a rare cardiac tumor, has been described in several cases (for review see de Ceuster et al., 2010; Riederer et al., 2010). In some of the cases, a significant

increase in the frequency of attacks of migraine with aura and triggering of attacks by exercise has been described.

We conclude that embolus detection by transcranial Doppler, ultrasound of cranial arteries, or echocardiography may be used in patients with unusual migraine aura that is prolonged, starts late in life, is complex, increases dramatically in frequency, or is triggered by exercise. In those instances MRI of the brain should also be performed.

CONCLUSION

In conclusion, a large number of investigations have contributed substantially to our current understanding of migraine pathophysiology. Neuroimaging has shown changes in pain processing and pain modulatory regions, and neurophysiological methods have demonstrated a lack of habituation to a variety of sensory modalities in migraine. This could have an impact on pharmacotherapy as well as nonpharmacological management of migraine.

Most findings are based on group statistics, and none of the methods can currently be recommended as a diagnostic tool for migraine. Possibly dynamic changes within the migraine cycle can explain some of the heterogeneity between studies.

Some of these investigations have some potential to monitor treatment response. Their mainstay currently remains the exclusion of secondary headaches that may mimic migraine.

REFERENCES

Afra, J., Proietti Cecchini, A., Sandor, P. S., & Schoenen, J. (2000). Comparison of visual and auditory evoked cortical potentials in migraine patients between attacks. Clinical Neurophysiology, 2000, 111(6), 1124–1129.

Afra, J., Sandor, P. S., & Schoenen, J. (2000). Habituation of visual and intensity dependence of auditory evoked cortical potentials tends to normalize just before and during the migraine attack. Cephalalgia, 20(8), 714–719.

Afridi, S. K., Giffin, N. J., Kaube, H., Friston, K. J., Ward, N. S., Frackowiak, R. S., et al. (2005). A positron emission tomographic study in spontaneous migraine. Archives of Neurology, 62(8), 1270–1275.

Ambrosini, A., de Noordhout, A. M., Sandor, P. S., & Schoenen, J. (2003). Electrophysiological studies in migraine: A comprehensive review of their interest and limitations. Cephalalgia, 23(Suppl 1), 13–31.

Ambrosini, A., de Noordhout, A. M., & Schoenen, J. (2001). Neuromuscular transmission in migraine patients with prolonged aura. Acta Neurologica Belgium, 101(3), 166–170.

Ambrosini, A., Maertens de Noordhout, A., & Schoenen, J. (2001). Neuromuscular transmission in migraine: A single-fiber EMG study in clinical subgroups. Neurology, 56(8), 1038–1043.

Ambrosini, A., Pierelli, F., & Schoenen, J. (2003). Acetazolamide acts on neuromuscular transmission abnormalities found in some migraineurs. Cephalalgia, 23(2), 75–78.

Ambrosini, A., Rossi, P., De Pasqua, V., Pierelli, F., & Schoenen, J. (2003). Lack of habituation causes high intensity dependence of auditory evoked cortical potentials in migraine. Brain, 126(Pt 9), 2009–2015.

Anzola, G. P., Magoni, M., Guindani, M., Rozzini, L., & Dalla Volta, G. (1999). Potential source of cerebral embolism in migraine with aura: A transcranial Doppler study. Neurology, 52(8), 1622–1625.

Arnold, M., Cumurciuc, R., Stapf, C., Favrole, P., Berthet, K., & Bousser, M. G. (2006). Pain as the only symptom of cervical artery dissection. Journal of Neurology, Neurosurgery, and Psychiatry, 77(9), 1021–1024.

Bohotin, V., Fumal, A., Vandenheede, M., Gerard, P., Bohotin, C., Maertens de Noordhout, A., et al. (2002). Effects of repetitive transcranial magnetic stimulation on visual evoked potentials in migraine. Brain, 125(Pt 4), 912–922.

Bjork, M., Hagen, K., Stovner, L. J., & Sand, T. (2011). Photic EEG-driving responses related to ictal phases and trigger sensitivity in migraine: a longitudinal, controlled study. Cephalalgia, 31(4), 444–455.

Carew, T., Castellucci, V. F., & Kandel, E. R. (1979). Sensitization in Aplysia: Restoration of transmission in synapses inactivated by long-term habituation. Science, 205(4404), 417–419.

Chadaide, Z., Arlt, S., Antal, A., Nitsche, M. A., Lang, N., & Paulus, W. (2007). Transcranial direct current stimulation reveals inhibitory deficiency in migraine. Cephalalgia, 27(7), 833–839.

Chen, W. L., Chang, S. H., Chen, J. H., & Wu, Y. L. (2007). Isolated headache as the sole manifestation of dural sinus thrombosis: A case report with literature review. American Journal of Emergency Medicine, 25(2), 218–219.

Chorlton, P., & Kane, N. (2000). Investigation of the cerebral response to flicker stimulation in patients with headache. Clinical Electroencephalography, 31(2), 83–87.

Dalkara, T., Nozari, A., & Moskowitz, M. A. (2010). Migraine aura pathophysiology: The role of blood vessels and microembolisation Lancet Neurology, 9(3), 309–317.

de Ceuster, L., van Diepen, T., & Koehler, P. J (2010). Migraine with aura triggered by cardiac myxoma: Case report and literature review. Cephalalgia, 30(11), 1396–1399.

de Tommaso, M., Sciruicchio, V., Bellotti, R., Guido, M., Sasanelli, G., Specchio, L. M., et al. (1999). Photic driving response in primary headache: Diagnostic value tested by discriminant analysis and artificial neural network classifiers. Italian Journal of Neurological Sciences, 20(1), 23–28.

de Tommaso, M., Guido, M., Libro, G., Sciruicchio, V., & Puca, F. (2000). The three responses of the blink reflex in adult and juvenile migraine. Acta Neurologica Belgium, 100(2), 96–102.

de Tommaso, M., Guido, M., Sardaro, M., Serpino, C., Vecchio, E., De Stefano, G., et al. (2008). Effects of topiramate and levetiracetam vs placebo on habituation of contingent negative variation in migraine patients. Neuroscience Letters, 442(2), 81–85.

de Tommaso, M., Libro, G., Guido, M., Losito, L., Lamberti, P., & Livrea, P. (2005). Habituation of single CO_2 laser-evoked responses during interictal phase of migraine. Journal of Headache and Pain, 6(4), 195–198.

de Tommaso, M., Sciruicchio, V., Guido, M., Sasanelli, G., Specchio, L. M., & Puca, F. M. (1998). EEG spectral analysis in migraine without aura attacks. Cephalalgia, 18(6), 324–328.

Di Clemente, L., Coppola, G., Magis, D., Fumal, A., De Pasqua, V., & Schoenen, J. (2005). Nociceptive blink reflex and visual evoked potential habituations are correlated in migraine. Headache, 45(10), 1388–1393.

Diener, H. C., Scholz, E., Dichgans, J., Gerber, W. D., Jack, A., Bille, A., et al. (1989). Central effects of drugs used in migraine prophylaxis evaluated by visual evoked potentials. Annals of Neurology, 25(2), 125–130.

Drake, M. E., Jr., Pakalnis, A., & Padamadan, H. (1989). Long-latency auditory event related potentials in migraine. Headache, 29(4), 239–241.

Evers, S., Bauer, B., Grotemeyer, K. H., Kurlemann, G., & Husstedt, I. W. (1998). Event-related potentials (P300) in primary headache in childhood and adolescence. Journal of Child Neurology, 13(7), 322–326.

Evers, S., Bauer, B., Suhr, B., Husstedt, I. W., & Grotemeyer, K. H. (1997). Cognitive processing in primary headache: A study on event-related potentials. Neurology, 48(1), 108–113.

Evers, S., Quibeldey, F., Grotemeyer, K. H., Suhr, B., & Husstedt, I. W. (1999). Dynamic changes of cognitive habituation and serotonin metabolism during the migraine interval. Cephalalgia, 19(5), 485–491.

Gantenbein, A. R., Goadsby, P. J., & Kaube, H. (2005). Chirp stimulation—H-response short and dynamic. Cephalalgia, 25(12), 1196–1197.

Gantenbein, A. R., Riederer, F., Mathys, J., Biethahn, S., Gossrau, G., Waldvogel, D., et al. (2011). Confusional migraine is an adult as well as a childhood disease. Cephalalgia, 31(2), 206–212.

Gantenbein, A. R., & Sandor, P. S. (2006). Physiological parameters as biomarkers of migraine. Headache, 46(7), 1069–1074.

Giffin, N. J., & Kaube, H. (2002). The electrophysiology of migraine. Current Opinion in Neurology, 15(3), 303–309.

Goder, R., Fritzer, G., Kapsokalyvas, A., Kropp, P., Niederberger, U., Strenge, H., et al. (2001). Polysomnographic findings in nights preceding a migraine attack. Cephalalgia, 21(1), 31–37.

Golla, F. L., & Winter, A. L. (1959). Analysis of cerebral responses to flicker in patients complaining of episodic headache. *Electroencephalography and Clinical Neurophysiological Supplement, 11*(3), 539–549.

International Headache Society. (2004). The international classification of headache disorders: 2nd edition. *Cephalalgia, 24*(Suppl 1), 9–160.

Judit, A., Sandor, P. S., & Schoenen, J. (2000). Habituation of visual and intensity dependence of auditory evoked cortical potentials tends to normalize just before and during the migraine attack. *Cephalalgia, 20*(8), 714–719.

Katsarava, Z., Giffin, N., Diener, H. C., & Kaube, H. (2003). Abnormal habituation of "nociceptive" blink reflex in migraine—evidence for increased excitability of trigeminal nociception. *Cephalalgia, 23*(8), 814–819.

Katsarava, Z., Lehnerdt, G., Duda, B., Ellrich, J., Diener, H. C., & Kaube, H. (2002). Sensitization of trigeminal nociception specific for migraine but not pain of sinusitis. *Neurology, 59*(9), 1450–1453.

Kloppel, S., Stonnington, C. M., Barnes, J., Chen, F., Chu, C., Good, C. D., et al. (2008). Accuracy of dementia diagnosis: A direct comparison between radiologists and a computerized method. *Brain, 131*(Pt 11), 2969–2974.

Kropp, P., & Gerber, W. D. (1993). Is increased amplitude of contingent negative variation in migraine due to cortical hyperactivity or to reduced habituation? *Cephalalgia, 13*(1), 37–41.

Kropp, P., & Gerber, W. D. (1995). Contingent negative variation during migraine attack and interval: Evidence for normalization of slow cortical potentials during the attack. *Cephalalgia, 15*(2), 123–128; discussion 78–79.

Kropp, P., & Gerber, W. D. (1998). Prediction of migraine attacks using a slow cortical potential, the contingent negative variation. *Neuroscience Letters, 257*(2), 73–76.

Maertens de Noordhout, A., Timsit-Berthier, M., Timsit, M., & Schoenen, J. (1986). Contingent negative variation in headache. *Annals of Neurology, 19*(1), 78–80.

Maertens de Noordhout, A., Timsit-Berthier, M., Timsit, M., & Schoenen, J. (1987). Effects of beta blockade on contingent negative variation in migraine [Letter]. *Annals of Neurology, 21*(1), 111–112.

Mariani, E., Moschini, V., Pastorino, G. C., Rizzi, F., Severgnini, A., & Tiengo, M. (1990). Pattern reversal visual evoked potentials (VEP-PR) in migraine subjects with visual aura. *Headache, 30*(7), 435–438.

May, A. (2009). Morphing voxels: The hype around structural imaging of headache patients. *Brain, 132*(Pt 6), 1419–1425.

Mirza, Z., Hayward, P., & Hulbert, D. (1998). Spontaneous carotid artery dissection presenting as migraine—a diagnosis not to be missed. *Journal of Accidental and Emergency Medicine, 15*(3), 187–189.

Morelli, N., Mancuso, M., Gori, S., Maluccio, M. R., Cafforio, G., Chiti, A., et al. (2008). Vertebral artery dissection onset mimics migraine with aura in a graphic designer. *Headache, 48*(4), 621–624.

Nedeltchev, K., Arnold, M., Schwerzmann, M., Nirkko, A., Lagger, F., Mattle, H. P., et al. (2004). Cerebrovascular response to repetitive visual stimulation in interictal migraine with aura. *Cephalalgia, 24*(9), 700–706.

Newman, D. S., Levine, S. R., Curtis, V. L., & Welch, K. M. (1989). Migraine-like visual phenomena associated with cerebral venous thrombosis. *Headache, 29*(2), 82–85.

Panayiotopoulos, C. P. (1999). Visual phenomena and headache in occipital epilepsy: A review, a systematic study and differentiation from migraine. *Epileptic Disorders, 1*(4), 205–216.

Panayiotopoulos, C. P. (2010). Migraine, migralepsy, basilar migraine with EEG occipital paroxysms and diagnostic errors. In: C. Panayiotopoulos (Ed.), *A clinical guide to epileptic syndromes and their treatment* (pp. 125–130). Springer Healthcare Ltd.

Prescot, A., Becerra, L., Pendse, G., Tully, S., Jensen, E., Hargreaves, R., et al. (2009). Excitatory neurotransmitters in brain regions in interictal migraine patients. *Molecular Pain, 5*, 34.

Ramadan, N. M., Tietjen, G. E., Levine, S. R., & Welch, K. M. (1991). Scintillating scotomata associated with internal carotid artery dissection: Report of three cases. *Neurology, 41*(7), 1084–1087.

Reyngoudt, H., Paemeleire, K., Descamps, B., De Deene, Y., & Achten, E. (2011). 31P-MRS demonstrates a reduction in high-energy phosphates in the occipital lobe of migraine without aura patients. *Cephalalgia, 31*(12), 1243–1253.

Riederer, F., Baumgartner, H., Sándor, P., Wessely, P., & Wöber, C. (2011). Headache in 25 consecutive patients with atrial septal defects before and after percutaneous closure—a prospective case series. *Headache, 51*(8), 1297–1304.

Riederer, F., Luft A. R., & Sandor, P. S. (2010) Atrial myxoma as a trigger of migraine with aura—pathophysiological considerations. *Cepahalalgia, 30*(9), 1149–1150.

Rist, P. M., Diener, H. C., Kurth, T., & Schurks, M. (2011). Migraine, migraine aura, and cervical artery dissection: A systematic review and meta-analysis. *Cephalalgia, 31*(8), 886–896.

Sandor, P. S., Afra, J., Ambrosini, A., & Schoenen, J. (2000). Prophylactic treatment of migraine with beta-blockers and riboflavin: Differential effects on the intensity dependence of auditory evoked cortical potentials. *Headache, 40*(1), 30–35.

Sandor, P. S., Afra, J., Proietti-Cecchini, A., Albert, A., & Schoenen, J. (1999). Familial influences on cortical evoked potentials in migraine. *Neuroreport, 10*(6), 1235–1238.

Sandor, P. S., Mascia, A., Seidel, L., de Pasqua, V., & Schoenen, J. (2001). Subclinical cerebellar impairment in the common types of migraine: A three-dimensional analysis of reaching movements. *Annals of Neurology, 49*(5), 668–672.

Sandrini, G., Friberg, L., Coppola, G., Janig, W., Jensen, R., Kruit, M., et al. (2011). Neurophysiological tests and neuroimaging procedures in non-acute headache (2nd edition). *European Journal of Neurology, 18*(3), 373–381.

Schoenen, J. (1994). Pathogenesis of migraine: The biobehavioural and hypoxia theories reconciled. *Acta Neurologica Belgium, 94*(2), 79–86.

Schoenen, J. (1996). Deficient habituation of evoked cortical potentials in migraine: A link between brain biology, behavior and trigeminovascular activation? *Biomedical Pharmacotherapy, 50*(2), 71–78.

Schoenen, J. (1998). Cortical electrophysiology in migraine and possible pathogenetic implications. *Clinical Neuroscience, 5*(1), 10–17.

Schoenen, J., Ambrosini, A., Sandor, P. S., & Maertens de Noordhout, A. (2003). Evoked potentials and transcranial magnetic stimulation in migraine: Published data and viewpoint on their pathophysiologic significance. *Clinical Neurophysiology, 114*(6), 955–972.

Schoenen, J., Jamart, B., & Delwaide, P. J. (1987). [Electroencephalographic mapping in migraine during the critical and intercritical periods]. *Revue d'Electroencéphalographie et de Neurophysiologie Clinique, 17*(3), 289–299.

Schoenen, J., & Timsit-Berthier, M. (1993). Contingent negative variation: methods and potential interest in headache. *Cephalalgia, 13*(1), 28–32.

Sharif, M., Trinick, T., & Khan, K. H. (2010). Identification of internal carotid artery dissection in patients with migraine—case report and literature review. *Journal of the Pakistan Medical Association, 60*(2), 131–133.

Siniatchkin, M., Gerber, W. D., Kropp, P., & Vein, A. (1999). How the brain anticipates an attack: A study of neurophysiological periodicity in migraine [In Process Citation]. *Functional Neurology, 14*(2), 69–77.

Siniatchkin, M., Kirsch, E., Kropp, P., Stephani, U., & Gerber, W. D. (2000). Slow cortical potentials in migraine families. *Cephalalgia, 20*(10), 881–892.

Siniatchkin, M., Kropp, P., & Gerber, W. D. (2003). What kind of habituation is impaired in migraine patients? *Cephalalgia, 23*(7), 511–518.

Siniatchkin, M., Kropp, P., Neumann, M., Gerber, W., & Stephani, U. (2000). Intensity dependence of auditory evoked cortical potentials in migraine families. *Pain, 85*(1–2), 247–254.

Soriano-Mas, C., Pujol, J., Alonso, P., Cardoner, N., Menchon, J. M., Harrison, B. J., et al. (2007). Identifying patients with obsessive-compulsive disorder using whole-brain anatomy. *Neuroimage, 35*(3), 1028–1037.

Spence, J. D., Wong, D. G., Melendez, L. J., Nichol, P. M., & Brown, J. D. (1984). Increased prevalence of mitral valve prolapse in patients with migraine. *Canadian Medical Association Journal, 131*(12), 1457–1460.

Stankewitz, A., & May, A. (2009). The phenomenon of changes in cortical excitability in migraine is not migraine-specific—a unifying thesis. *Pain, 145*(1–2), 14–17.

Tsounis, S., Milonas, J., & Gilliam, F. (1993). Hemi-field pattern reversal visual evoked potentials in migraine. *Cephalalgia, 13*(4), 267–271.

Walpurger, V., Hebing-Lennartz, G., Denecke, H., & Pietrowsky, R. (2003). Habituation deficit in auditory event-related potentials in tinnitus complainers. *Hearing Research, 181*(1–2), 57–64.

Wang, W., & Schoenen, J. (1998). Interictal potentiation of passive "oddball" auditory event-related potentials in migraine. *Cephalalgia, 18*(5), 261–265; discussion 41.

Wang, W., Timsit-Berthier, M., & Schoenen, J. (1996). Intensity dependence of auditory evoked potentials is pronounced in migraine: An indication of cortical potentiation and low serotonergic neurotransmission? *Neurology, 46*(5), 1404–1409.

Weiller, C., May, A., Limmroth, V., Juptner, M., Kaube, H., Schayck, R. V., et al. (1995). Brain stem activation in spontaneous human migraine attacks. *Nature Medicine, 1*(7), 658–660.

Wolf, M. E., Szabo, K., Griebe, M., Forster, A., Gass, A., Hennerici, M. G., et al. (2011). Clinical and MRI characteristics of acute migrainous infarction. *Neurology, 76*(22), 1911–1917.

Young, G., & Humphrey, P. (1995). Vertebral artery dissection mimicking migraine. *Journal of Neurology, Neurosurgery, and Psychiatry, 59*(3), 340–341.

13 Migraine Genes—Clinical and Preclinical Perspectives

CLAUDIA M. WELLER, BOUKJE DE VRIES, GISELA M. TERWINDT,

MICHEL D. FERRARI, JOOST HAAN, AND

ARN M.J.M. VAN DEN MAAGDENBERG

INTRODUCTION

Migraine is an episodic neurovascular disorder with a largely unknown etiology. This highly prevalent and debilitating disorder affects up to 15% of the adult population; approximately 10% of patients have weekly attacks (Launer et al., 1999; Stewart et al., 1994; Stovner et al., 2006.) Acute treatment with simple analgesics, nonsteroidal anti-inflammatory drugs, or serotonin agonists (triptans) is effective in many but not all patients. Recent trials with newly developed calcitonin gene–related peptide (CGRP) antagonists show promising results (Monteith & Goadsby, 2011). Current prophylactic treatment is not very effective either. Clearly, improved insight into the pathophysiology of migraine is needed, which hopefully will lead to better treatment options. This chapter will address findings in genetic research and their preclinical (scientific) and clinical implications.

CLINICAL ASPECTS OF MIGRAINE

Migraine attacks are characterized by recurrent, throbbing, unilateral headaches of moderate to severe intensity, which are aggravated by physical exercise, last 4 to 72 hours, and are accompanied by nausea, vomiting, photophobia, and/or phonophobia. To make a migraine diagnosis, a questionnaire and/or interview using criteria of the International Classification of Headache Disorders (ICHD-II) from the International Headache Society (IHS; Table 13–1) (Headache Classification Subcommittee of the International Headache Society, 2004) are needed, as no reliable biomarker for migraine currently is available. Approximately one third of migraine patients experience transient focal neurological symptoms, known as a migraine aura, preceding the headache phase. Aura symptoms typically have a duration between 5 and 60 minutes and almost always include visual symptoms. Sensory,

aphasic, and motor symptoms are less often part of the migraine aura (Russell & Olesen, 1996). Based on the presence or absence of an aura phase, two main migraine subtypes are distinguished: migraine with aura (MA) and migraine without aura (MO). Notably, migraine attacks with and without aura can co-occur in the same patient (Ferrari, 1998; Goadsby et al., 2002). The migraine aura is caused by cortical spreading depression (CSD), a wave of neuronal and glial depolarization that moves slowly over the cortex (Lauritzen, 1994). Unlike in humans, CSD can be easily investigated in experimental animals. Still, using functional magnetic resonance imaging (fMRI) to study the aura in MA patients, Hadjikhani and colleagues (2001) were able to detect local increases in blood oxygen level–dependent (BOLD) signals that spread through the visual cortex at a rate of 3.5 mm/min, a speed similar to what is seen when a CSD is evoked in an experimental animal. The headache itself is caused by activation of the trigeminovascular system, which consists of the meningeal and superficial cortical blood vessels that are innervated by the trigeminal nerve and that project into the trigeminal nucleus caudalis in the brainstem, which in turn projects into higher order pain centers, leading to pain (Ferrari & Goadsby, 2007).

GENETIC EPIDEMIOLOGY OF MIGRAINE

Migraine shows strong familial aggregation and is a multifactorial (i.e., complex) genetic disorder (Russell & Olesen, 1995; Stewart et al., 2006, 1997). Such complex disorders are likely caused by a combination of environmental factors and multiple genetic factors, each with a small effect size. Population-based family studies revealed that the relative risk of migraine for a first-degree relative of the index patient is 1.5 to 4 times higher compared to the general population, the risk being highest for patients with MA, an early age of onset, and a high attack severity

TABLE 13–1 *International Headache Criteria for Migraine without Aura and Migraine with Aura (IHS 2004)*

Migraine without aura

A. At least five attacks fulfilling criteria B–D

B. Headache attacks lasting 4–72 hours (untreated or unsuccessfully treated)

C. Headache has at least two of the following characteristics:

   1. Unilateral location

   2. Pulsating quality

   3. Moderate or severe pain intensity

   4. Aggravated by or causing avoidance of routine physical activity (e.g., walking or climbing stairs)

D. During headache at least one of the following;

   1. Nausea and/or vomiting

   2. Photophobia and phonophobia

E. Not attributed to another disorder

Migraine with aura

A. At least two attacks fulfilling criteria B–D

B. Aura consisting of at least one of the following, but no motor weakness:

   1. Fully reversible visual symptoms including positive features (e.g., flickering lights, spots, or lines) and/or negative features (e.g., loss of vision)

   2. Fully reversible sensory symptoms including positive features (e.g., pins and needles) and/or negative features (e.g., numbness)

   3. Fully reversible dysphasic speech disturbance

D. Headache fulfilling criteria B–D for migraine without aura begins during the aura or follows aura within 60 minutes

E. Not attributed to another disorder

From Headache Classification Subcommittee of the International Hedache Society. (2004). The international classification of headache disorders: 2nd edition. *Cephalalgia, 24*(Suppl 1), 9–160.

and disease disability (Stewart et al., 1997; Stewart et al., 2006). Studies of twins, which allow comparison of concordance rates in monozygotic versus dizygotic twins, also revealed a higher genetic load in MA than in MO (Gervil et al., 1999; Ulrich et al., 1999). A large study of approximately 30,000 twins from six different countries showed that genetic and environmental factors play an almost equal role in migraine susceptibility (Mulder et al., 2003). Heritability, which is defined as the contribution of genetic factors to susceptibility for a disease, was estimated to range from 34 to 57% in that study. Shared environmental factors seemed to play a minor role as shown by studies comparing twins that were raised together and apart (Svensson et al., 2003; Ziegler et al., 1998).

There is debate whether MA and MO are two separate disease entities or merely different expressions of the same disease. The first view is supported by observations that there is no increased co-occurrence of MA and MO in Danish twins (Russell et al., 2002) and the general Danish population (Russell & Olesen, 1995, 1996). In contrast, a study of 210 Finnish migraine families suggested the existence of a migraine continuum with pure MA and pure MO on both ends of the spectrum and a combination of

both types of attacks in between (Kallela et al., 2001). The idea that migraine indeed is a continuum is supported by other studies (Ligthart et al., 2006; Nyholt et al., 2004) as well as by clinical observations that headache characteristics are identical in MA and MO and that a large number of patients experience both types of attacks.

APPROACHES TO DISCOVER MIGRAINE GENES

To identify genetic factors that confer migraine susceptibility, several approaches have been used, which are discussed in more detail below. Most successes come from genetic studies investigating monogenic familial hemiplegic migraine (FHM), a subtype of migraine with aura. In addition, several genes were identified for monogenic diseases in which migraine was *part* of the phenotype. The assumption here is that the identified genes also may shed light on migraine pathophysiology itself. A third, more challenging but more direct approach is to perform genetic studies of common forms of migraine. Finally, genetic studies were performed taking advantage of the fact that certain diseases such as depression and bipolar disorders are comorbid in migraine patients. The rationale here is that investigating migraine patients who also have, for instance, depression will homogenize the patient population, which should make the gene hunt easier, although this still needs to be proven. In the section on preclinical perspectives, strategies and results from investigating the consequences of gene mutations will be discussed.

Investigating Monogenic Familial Hemiplegic Migraine

Identifying genes and biological pathways of a monogenic subtype of a disease is likely to provide useful insight into the pathophysiology also of the complex disease form, although there are, of course, differences between them. This strategy is worthwhile also because it is much harder to functionally characterize genetic factors that are involved in complex forms of the disease. This is because gene variants (i.e., polymorphisms) of a complex disease are expected to have only a small effect size; that is, multiple variants are needed to cause disease. As a consequence, it is more difficult, if not impossible in many cases, to investigate the true functional consequences of such variants in cellular and animal models. In contrast, gene mutations underlying a monogenic disease will have a large effect size; that is, the presence of such a mutation in almost all cases will be sufficient to cause disease in a patient. Consequently, such mutations must have clear consequences on either the level or the amino acid sequence of the affected protein, which can be investigated in cellular and animal disease model systems. With respect

to genetic migraine research, FHM is a monogenic subtype of MA and may therefore serve to help unravel part of the pathophysiology of common migraine as well.

Familial hemiplegic migraine is characterized by a transient hemiparesis during the aura phase, which may last several days. Diagnostic criteria for FHM were determined by the International Headache Society (Table 13–2) (Headache Classification Subcommittee of the International Headache Society, 2004). Because of its severity and symptoms, a significant number of patients initially are diagnosed with stroke or epilepsy. Notably, except for the hemiparesis, the visual and sensory aura symptoms are identical to those seen in MA, although the duration often is significantly longer than in MA patients (Thomsen et al., 2002). Notably, the headache characteristics in FHM patients and patients with the common forms of migraine are identical. Moreover, the majority of FHM patients experience attacks of MA or MO in addition to their hemiplegic attacks (Ducros et al., 2001; Terwindt et al., 1998). Thus, from a clinical perspective, FHM seems to be a valid model for both MO and MA (Ferrari, 1998).

Genetic studies in FHM resulted in the discovery of three FHM genes that are discussed in separate sections below. As several FHM families do not have a mutation in one of the known genes, more FHM genes must exist.

FAMILIAL HEMIPLEGIC MIGRAINE TYPE 1 IS CAUSED BY MUTATIONS IN THE CACNA1A GENE

CACNA1A, the first FHM gene (FHM type 1; FHM1) is located on chromosome 19p13 and encodes the α1

TABLE 13–2 *International Headache Society Criteria for Familial Hemiplegic Migraine*

A. At least two attacks fulfilling criteria B and C

B. Aura consisting of fully reversible motor weakness and at least one of the following:
  1. Fully reversible visual symptoms including positive features (e.g., flickering lights, spots, or lines) and/or negative features (e.g., loss of vision)
  2. Fully reversible sensory symptoms including positive features (e.g., pins and needles) and/or negative features (e.g., numbness)
  3. Fully reversible dysphasic speech disturbance

C. At least two of the following:
  1. At least one aura symptom develops gradually over ≥5 minutes, and/or different aura symptoms occur in succession over ≥5 minutes
  2. Each symptom lasts ≥5 and ≤24 hours
  3. Headache fulfilling criteria B–D for migraine without aura begins during the aura or follows aura within 60 minutes

D. At least one first- or second-degree relative has had attacks fulfilling criteria A–E

E. Not attributed to another disorder

From Headache Classification Subcommittee of the International Hedache Society. (2004). The international classification of headache disorders: 2nd edition. *Cephalalgia, 24*(Suppl 1), 9–160.

pore-forming subunit of $Ca_v2.1$ calcium channels (Ophoff et al., 1996). Certain *CACNA1A* mutations cause episodic ataxia type 2 (EA2) (Ophoff et al., 1996), spinocerebellar ataxia type 6 (SCA6) (Zhuchenko et al., 1997), or even a phenotype of absence epilepsy and generalized tonic-clonic seizures (Imbrici et al., 2004; Jouvenceau et al., 2001). To date, 29 FHM1 mutations were reported that are all missense mutations (Fig. 13–1). Several mutations (i.e., S218L, R583Q, T666M, I1710T, R1347Q) have been identified in multiple families. The fact that different genetic backgrounds were found indicates that they are recurrent mutations. An intriguing clinical heterogeneity was observed between and within FHM1 families (Ducros et al., 2001; Kors et al., 2003). Some FHM1 mutations lead to pure hemiplegic migraine, whereas other mutations are associated with additional clinical symptoms such as cerebellar ataxia or epilepsy. The phenotype of some of these mutations can be particularly severe. For instance, mutation S218L can be associated with hemiplegic migraine, ataxia, seizures, and even fatal cerebral edema, provoked by mild head trauma (Chan et al., 2008; Curtain et al., 2006; Debiais et al., 2009; Kors et al., 2001; Stam et al., 2009; Zangaladze et al., 2010). In a recent review of 13 S218L cases, the complexity of the occurrence of clinical symptoms was described in detail and led to a novel clinical entity coined ESCEATHT (which is the acronym for early seizures and cerebral edema after trivial head trauma) that was present in three patients with this mutation (Stam et al., 2009). Some 92% of S218L mutation carriers had cerebellar ataxia, 54% had seizures, and 69% had hemiplegic migraine that could be triggered by trivial head trauma. The study clearly shows the importance of performing extensive clinical-genetic research of cases with known gene mutations, not only to get a more complete picture of the clinical phenotype, but also to assess the mutation carriers' risk for particularly severe but rare complications. Another striking example of such research came from the observation that one carrier of the R1347Q mutation experienced recurrent childhood strokes (Knierim et al., 2011), a severe complication that had never been described for the R1347Q mutation, or any other FHM1 mutation, but that has important implications for physicians treating FHM1 patients. In addition, the observed link between ataxia, epilepsy, and stroke with FHM provides opportunities to study the shared underlying mechanisms, for instance, in animal models.

FAMILIAL HEMIPLEGIC MIGRAINE TYPE 2 IS CAUSED BY MUTATIONS IN THE ATP1A2 GENE

The second FHM gene (FHM2), *ATP1A2*, is located on chromosome 1q23 (De Fusco et al., 2003) and encodes the α2 subunit of sodium-potassium pumps. Over 30 FHM2 mutations are known (Fig. 13–2). In contrast to FHM1 mutations, hardly any recurrent mutations were reported for *ATP1A2* (Castro et al., 2007; Riant et al., 2010). Another striking difference with FHM1 mutations is that almost all *ATP1A2* mutations are associated with pure hemiplegic migraine, that is, without any additional clinical symptoms (De Fusco et al., 2003; Jurkat-Rott et al., 2004; Kaunisto et al., 2004; Pierelli et al., 2006; Riant et al., 2005), although some mutations are associated with epileptic seizures (Deprez et al., 2008; Jurkat-Rott et al., 2004), benign familial childhood convulsions (Vanmolkot et al., 2003), febrile seizures (de Vries, Stam, et al., 2009), and mental retardation (Jurkat-Rott et al., 2004). In addition, *ATP1A2* mutations were also reported in basilar migraine (Ambrosini et al., 2005) and, interestingly, two families with common migraine (Todt et al., 2005). Of these associations, the latter one is most debatable, although it is not a completely isolated observation: Several studies investigated the involvement of the *CACNA1A* and *ATP1A2* regions in the common forms of migraine, and some reported some evidence for their involvement (May et al., 1995; Nyholt, Dawkins, et al., 1998; Serra et al., 2010; Terwindt et al., 2001; Todt et al., 2005), whereas others did not find such evidence (Hovatta et al., 1994; Jen et al., 2004; Jones et al., 2001).

FAMILIAL HEMIPLEGIC MIGRAINE TYPE 3 IS CAUSED BY MUTATIONS IN THE SCN1A GENE

The FHM3 *SCN1A* gene is located on chromosome 2q24 and encodes the α1 subunit of neuronal $Na_v1.1$ sodium channels (Dichgans et al., 2005). *SCN1A* mutations seem to account for only a small proportion of FHM families. Interestingly, the *SCN1A* gene is a well-known epilepsy gene with many mutations causing monogenic forms of childhood epilepsy—that is, Dravet syndrome (also known as severe myoclonic epilepsy of infancy [SMEI]) or generalized epilepsy with febrile seizures (GEFS+) (Escayg & Goldin, 2010). Notably, whereas epilepsy is specifically mentioned in mutation reports describing hemiplegic migraine phenotypes, the opposite is not the case. The lack of reported migraine in patients with SMEI and GEFS+ who have *SCN1A* mutations possibly is due to the young age of the epileptic patients and/or the fact that migraine is not dominating the phenotype, and thereby is underreported in epilepsy patients.

To date, five FHM3 mutations have been reported (Castro et al., 2009; Dichgans et al., 2005; Gargus & Tournay, 2007; Vahedi et al., 2009; Vanmolkot, Babini, et al., 2007), as from the clinical description of the patients with the possible sixth mutation (T1174S) it is far from certain that they have hemiplegic migraine (Gargus & Tournay, 2007).

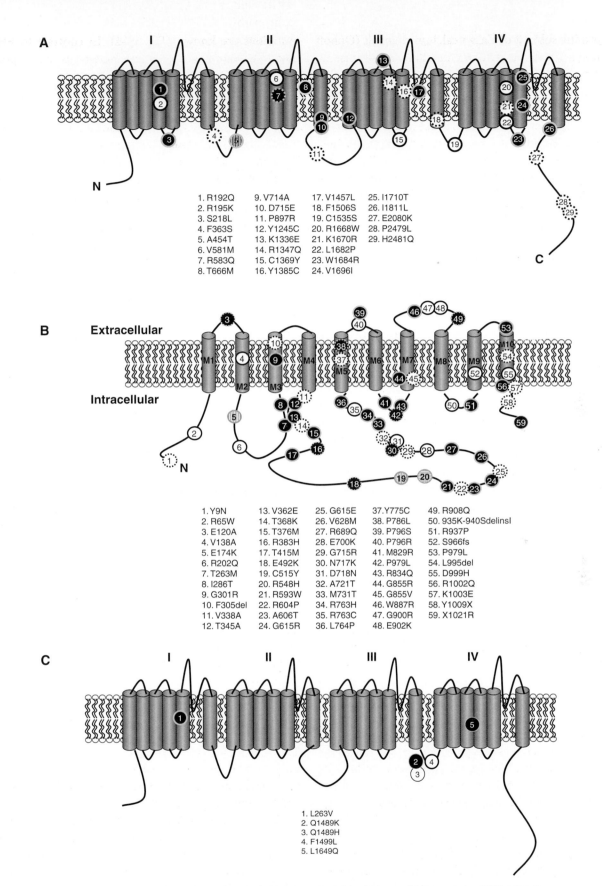

A

I   II   III   IV

1. R192Q	9. V714A	17. V1457L	25. I1710T
2. R195K	10. D715E	18. F1506S	26. I1811L
3. S218L	11. P897R	19. C1535S	27. E2080K
4. F363S	12. Y1245C	20. R1668W	28. P2479L
5. A454T	13. K1336E	21. K1670R	29. H2481Q
6. V581M	14. R1347Q	22. L1682P	
7. R583Q	15. C1369Y	23. W1684R	
8. T666M	16. Y1385C	24. V1696I	

B

Extracellular

Intracellular

N

1. Y9N	13. V362E	25. G615E	37. Y775C	49. R908Q
2. R65W	14. T368K	26. V628M	38. P786L	50. 935K-940Sdelinsl
3. E120A	15. T376M	27. R689Q	39. P796S	51. R937P
4. V138A	16. R383H	28. E700K	40. P796R	52. S966fs
5. E174L	17. T415M	29. G715R	41. M829R	53. P979L
6. R202Q	18. E492K	30. N717K	42. P979L	54. L995del
7. T263M	19. C515Y	31. D718N	43. R834Q	55. D999H
8. I286T	20. R548H	32. A721T	44. G855R	56. R1002Q
9. G301R	21. R593W	33. M731T	45. G855V	57. K1003E
10. F305del	22. R604P	34. R763H	46. W887R	58. Y1009X
11. V338A	23. A606T	35. R763C	47. G900R	59. X1021R
12. T345A	24. G615R	36. L764P	48. E902K	

C

I   II   III   IV

1. L263V
2. Q1489K
3. Q1489H
4. F1499L
5. L1649Q

FIGURE 13–1 *Mutations in the familial hemiplegic migraine (FHM) genes: (A) CACNA1A, (B) ATP1A2, and (C) SCN1A.*
Symbols: circle with solid line = FHM; circle with dotted line = sporadic hemiplegic migraine (SHM). Black circle = mutation was tested for functional consequences; white circle = mutation was not tested for functional consequences.

Mutations L1649Q and Q1489K are associated with pure familial hemiplegic migraine (Vanmolkot, Babini, et al., 2007), whereas mutations Q1489H and L263V have been associated with childhood epilepsy and generalized tonic-clonic seizures (Castro et al., 2009; Dichgans et al., 2005; Vahedi et al., 2009) in addition to FHM, at least in some of the mutation carriers. Some patients with FHM3 mutations Q1489H and F1499L were also reported to suffer from "elicited repetitive daily blindness" (ERDB), which occurred apart from their hemiplegic migraine attacks (Le Fort et al., 2004; Vahedi et al., 2009).

A ROLE FOR FAMILIAL HEMIPLEGIC MIGRAINE GENES IN SPORADIC HEMIPLEGIC MIGRAINE?

If hemiplegic migraine occurs not in a family but in an isolated case, it is called sporadic hemiplegic migraine (SHM). Apart from the absence of an affected close relative, the diagnostic criteria and attacks are identical to those in FHM. The first screens of FHM genes in SHM patients revealed mutations, predominantly in *ATP1A2*, in only a small proportion of patients (de Vries et al., 2007; Terwindt et al., 2002; Thomsen et al., 2007). Recently, however, Riant and co-workers (2010) studied a group of 25 SHM patients with an age of onset before 16 years, of which 18 patients had additional symptoms such as epilepsy, learning difficulties, cerebellar ataxia, and/or coma. Surprisingly, in no less than 23 patients mutations in *CACNA1A* and *ATP1A2* were identified. Three quarters of the mutations had occurred de novo and mutation carriers thus represent the first patients of new FHM families. The most recently identified de novo G715R *ATP1A2* mutation was found in a 6-year-old SHM patient with prolonged hemiparesis, which resolved after 4 weeks and required rehabilitation (De Sanctis et al., 2011); this further supports the observation that particularly de novo mutations are present in severely affected patients. The question remains what is causing SHM in the patients who do not carry an FHM gene mutation, which is a rather large proportion of patients in most studies (de Vries et al., 2007; Terwindt et al., 2002; Thomsen et al., 2007). Possibilities are that either other FHM genes may cause hemiplegic migraine in those patients or that SHM (especially when the phenotype is not severe) is due to a combination of multiple low-risk genetic variants, similar to what is predicted to occur in common migraine. Support for the latter hypothesis comes from the observation that MA is frequent in families of SHM patients (Russell & Ducros, 2011). Also, it would fit a view of migraine being a spectrum of disorders. It certainly stresses the importance of taking a reliable family history in patients with suspected hemiplegic migraine and of

follow-up of these patients. This is also exemplified by a recent clinical follow-up study of 19 Dutch SHM patients that showed that in a proportion of SHM patients, the diagnosis *changed* over time to FHM (Stam et al., 2011).

Investigating Monogenic Disorders in Which Migraine Is a Prominent Part of the Clinical Phenotype

Migraine can also be part of non-FHM monogenic disorders, which may be a useful source for identifying genes that may shed light on the pathophysiological mechanisms involved in migraine. In fact, the number of examples of this strategy that are relevant to migraine is increasing (Table 13–3). Several examples concern genetic vasculopathies (e.g., CADASIL and RVCL) and will be discussed in more detail below. The most recent addition is families with proximal renal tubular acidosis in addition to (hemiplegic) migraine.

CEREBRAL AUTOSOMAL DOMINANT ARTERIOPATHY WITH SUBCORTICAL INFARCTS AND LEUKOENCEPHALOPATHY

Cerebral autosomal dominant arteriopathy with subcortical infarcts and leukoencephalopathy (CADASIL) is a monogenic syndrome characterized by recurrent stroke, cognitive deterioration, and psychiatric disease (Dichgans et al., 1998). About one third of CADASIL patients also suffer from migraine, often with migraine as the presenting clinical symptom. No less than 80% to 90% of them have MA, which is considerably higher than the one third in migraine patients without CADASIL (Liem et al., 2010). CADASIL is caused by mutations in the *NOTCH3* gene (Joutel et al., 1996), which encodes a cell surface receptor that is expressed in vascular smooth muscle cells. Whether there is a genetic link between migraine and Notch3 is still under debate because genetic association studies investigating *NOTCH3* polymorphisms gave conflicting results (Borroni et al., 2006; Schwaag et al., 2006).

RETINAL VASCULOPATHY WITH CEREBRAL LEUKODYSTROPHY

Retinal vasculopathy with cerebral leukodystrophy (RVCL; which previously was known as cerebroretinal vasculopathy [CRV], hereditary vascular retinopathy [HVR], and hereditary endotheliopathy or retinopathy, nephropathy, and stroke [HERNS]) is a monogenic neurovascular syndrome caused by mutations in the *TREX1* gene (Richards et al., 2007). *TREX1* encodes the major 3'-5'-mammalian exonuclease, an enzyme thought to be involved in DNA repair and apoptosis after DNA damage, although it is more and more evident that the Trex1 protein may have additional functions. The predominant

TABLE 13–3 *Monogenic Disorders Associated with Migraine*

Syndrome	Symptoms	Migraine subtype	Gene	References
MELAS (mitochondrial encephalopathy, lactic acidosis, and strokelike episodes)	Strokelike episodes Encephalopathy with seizures and/or dementia Myopathy (lactic acidosis and/or ragged red fibers [RRF] on muscle biopsy)	MA	Specific mutations in mitochondrial genes	Cevoli et al. (2010) Montagna et al. (1988)
HIHRATL (hereditary infantile hemiparesis, retinal arteriolar tortuosity, and leukoencephalopathy)	Porencephaly Cerebral and retinal microangiopathy	MA	*COL4A1* Encodes a collagen IV α chain in the basement membrane	Gould et al. (2006) Vahedi et al. (2003, 2007)
POLG-related disorders	Ataxia Ophthalmoplegia Epilepsy Liver failure	MA and MO	*POLG* Encodes the mitochondrial DNA polymerase γ that is important for ATP homeostasis and normal cellular function	Hudson & Chinnery (2006) Tzoulis et al. (2006) Winterthun et al. (2005)
TGFR2-related disorder	Aortic dissection Joint hypermobility Skin abnormalities Arthralgia	Unspecified	*TGFR2* Encodes the transforming growth factor-β receptor 2, which is involved in regulation of cellular processes and formation of extracellular matrix	Law et al. (2006)
Proximal renal tubular acidosis (pRTA)	Renal dysfunction Ocular abnormalities	Hemiplegic migraine, MA, MO	*SLC4A4* Encodes a sodium bicarbonate cotransporter involved in regulating intracellular pH	Suzuki et al. (2010)

Note: MA = migraine with aura; MO = migraine without aura.

symptom in RVCL is a pronounced retinopathy, but cognitive disturbances, depression, focal neurological symptoms, Raynaud phenomenon, kidney and liver dysfunction, and gastrointestinal bleeding are also part of the clinical spectrum (Grand et al., 1988; Jen et al., 1997; Terwindt et al., 1998). In advanced stages of the disease, MRI shows characteristic contrast-enhancing white matter lesions (Terwindt et al., 1998). Particularly in a large Dutch RVCL family, a high prevalence of migraine was found, with 14 of the 20 TREX1 mutation carriers suffering from MO (Terwindt et al., 1998). A small genetic family-based study seemed to suggest a potential role for the RVCL gene as a susceptibility gene in both migraine and Raynaud phenomenon (Hottenga et al., 2005).

It is still unknown which mechanisms underlie the occurrence of migraine in these vasculopathies. In particular, it needs to be further investigated whether endothelial dysfunction, which was also observed for migraine (Tietjen et al., 2007; Vanmolkot, Van Bortel, et al., 2007), may underlie the extensive vasculopathy seen with CADASIL and RVCL. Given the high occurrence of MA in CADASIL patients, increased susceptibility for CSD may well explain the link with migraine. For RVCL this explanation seems unlikely, since the disease seems to be linked with MO, not MA.

OTHER VASCULOPATHIES WITH MIGRAINE AS
PART OF THE PHENOTYPE

An increased prevalence of MA was reported in a rare angiopathy that can be described as heriditary infantile hemiparesis, retinal arteriolar tortuosity, and leucoencephalopathy (HIHRATL) with clinical symptoms of porencephaly and cerebral and retinal microangiopathy, hemiparesis, and stroke (Vahedi et al., 2003). The causal gene is COL4A1, which encodes type IV collagen, an integral component of the vascular basement membrane (Gould et al., 2006). The association adds to growing evidence for a link between migraine and early-onset cerebral angiopathies that is remarkable, but the mechanisms underlying this association are still poorly understood (Dichgans & Hegele, 2007). An additional piece of information that links affected blood vessels with migraine comes from a genetic study in a large pedigree in which patients suffer from familial aortic dissection and several other blood vessel abnormalities (Law et al., 2006). Ten of 14 carriers of the R460H mutation in the transforming growth factor-β receptor 2 (TGFβR2) gene also suffer from migraine.

OTHER MONOGENIC SYNDROMES WITH
MIGRAINE AS PART OF THE PHENOTYPE

A monogenic disorder of a complex phenotype of episodic ataxia, hemiplegic migraine, and seizures was reported for a 10-year-old boy (Jen et al., 2005). His phenotype is caused by a P290R mutation in SLC1A3 that encodes the excitatory amino acid transporter 1 (EAAT1), which removes glutamate from the synaptic cleft. The missense mutation causes a dramatic loss in glutamate uptake in a cellular assay. Another monogenic syndrome associated with strokelike events is MELAS (mitochondrial encephalomyopathy, lactic acidosis, and strokelike syndrome); which is caused by a mitochondrial DNA (mtDNA) 3243 A>G tRNALeu point mutation (Montagna et al., 1988); and in which migraine was reported as a frequent clinical feature. Finally, many carriers of mutations in the POLG gene, which encodes the nuclear polymerase-γ that is essential for the maintenance of mitochondrial DNA, suffer from migraine as well (Hudson & Chinnery, 2006; Tzoulis et al., 2006; Winterthun et al., 2005). These findings support the hypothesis that mitochondrial dysfunction may occur in migraine, but additional research is needed to more firmly establish such a link.

Recently, Suzuki and co-workers (2010) were the first to report a homozygous 65-base-pair deletion resulting in an S982NfsX4 truncating mutation in the $Na^+ $-$HCO_3^-$ cotransporter NBCe1 in two sisters with reported hemiplegic migraine. Other homozygous mutations (i.e., Δ2311A, R510H, R881C, L522P) were found in patients with diverse clinical presentations (i.e., MA, MO, or hemiplegic migraine with episodic ataxia). These patients also suffered from proximal renal tubular acidosis and ocular anomalies, which are known to be caused by homozygous mutations in this gene. It was hypothesized that mutations in the NBCe1 cotransporter may lead to migraine by disturbing synaptic pH in astrocytes, thus providing an interesting new pathophysiological mechanism implicated in migraine. Although the mutations themselves clearly are pathogenic in the sense that they are the cause of the renal and ocular problems, it is less obvious why they would cause the migraine and hemiplegia phenotypes that are very common and sometimes hard to diagnose, respectively. Already, the observation that few of the heterozygous carriers of an NBCe1 mutation also suffer from migraine (and glaucoma) should cast reasonable doubt on the causality of the association with migraine. The authors seem to explain the disease association in heterozygous patients by dominant-negative effects of the mutation, but why, then, would essentially the same functional molecular phenotype (i.e., a defective protein) cause hemiplegic migraine in homozygous mutation carriers and common migraine in some heterozygous mutation carriers? The present scenario seems rather unlikely, but certainly deserves further investigation.

Genetic Studies in Common Forms of Migraine

LINKAGE STUDIES IN COMMON MIGRAINE

Identifying genes involved in complex disorders has proven difficult. Two main hypotheses are used to explain the genetic origin of complex diseases (Manolio et al., 2009). One hypothesis proposes that common disease is caused by common variants (i.e., CD-CV). Relatively frequent genetic variants only cause a slight increase in disease risk in isolation. It is the cumulative effect of multiple frequent genetic variants which leads to common diseases. In contrast, the common disease—rare variant (CD-RV) hypothesis assumes that multiple, relatively rare variants with a larger effect size may explain susceptibility to disease. To date, most findings in complex diseases confirm the first hypothesis only, although a few rare variants with a moderate effect have been detected, for example, factor V Leiden in deep venous thrombosis (Bertina et al., 1994) or rare protective variants in *IFIH1* for type 1 diabetes (Ionita-Laza et al., 2011). Apart from genetic heterogeneity, the gene hunt in common migraine is also complicated by extensive clinical heterogeneity regarding, for instance, presenting symptoms or age of onset in addition to the lack of reliable biomarkers to establish a migraine diagnosis. After all, diagnostic criteria of the International Headache Society that are useful to diagnose attacks in the clinic are less suited for genetic research, for instance, because multiple combinations of symptoms (e.g., pulsating headache, nausea, vomiting) lead to the same end-diagnosis, but not necessarily through the same pathophysiological mechanism.

Initially, *family-based linkage analysis* was used and led to the identification of many chromosomal regions, but did not result in the discovery of migraine genes (Table 13–4). With such a strategy, one looks for chromosomal regions that are shared by affected family members more than can be expected by chance. Instead of using a migraine end-diagnosis of MA or MO, Anttila and coworkers (2006) used *trait component analysis* (TCA) (i.e., the individual symptoms instead of IHS diagnosis as traits in the analysis) to reduce clinical heterogeneity among

TABLE 13–4 *Summary of Significant Linkage Results Performed for Migraine Using Either the International Headache Classification (IHC) Guidelines, Trait Component Analysis (TCA), or Latent Class Analysis (LCA)*

Chromosomal Locus	Phenotype	Applied Diagnostic Criteria	Reference
1q31[a]	MO and MA	IHC	Lea et al. (2002)
4q21	MO	IHC	Bjornsson et al. (2003)
4q24	MA	IHC	Wessman et al. (2002)
4q24	Age at onset, photophobia, phonophobia, photo- and phonophobia, pain intensity, unilaterality, pulsation, nausea and vomiting	TCA	Anttila et al. (2006)
5q21	Pulsation	LCA	Nyholt et al. (2005)
6p12.2-p21.1	MO and MA	IHC	Carlsson et al. (2002)
7q31-q33	Migraine	LCA	Chen et al. (2009)
10q22-q23	MA	IHC	Anttila et al. (2008)
10q22-23	Migrainous headache	LCA	Anttila et al. (2008)
10q22-23	Unilaterality, pulsation, pain intensity, nausea/vomiting, photophobia, phonophobia	TCA	Anttila et al. (2008)
11q24	MA	IHC	Cader et al. (2003)
14q21.2-q22.3	MO	IHC	Soragna et al. (2003)
15q11-q13	MA	IHC	Russo et al. (2005)
19p13	MA	IHC	Jones et al. (2001)
Xp22	MO and MA	IHC	Wieser et al. (2010)
Xq25-q28	MO and MA	IHC	Nyholt, Lea, et al. (1998)

Notes: MO = migraine without aura; MA = migraine with aura.

[a] Suggestive linkage for MA and MO combined.

patients. From studies of other complex disorders (e.g., schizophrenia and attention-deficit/hyperactivity disorder [ADHD]) it is apparent that individual traits may have a higher heritability than the end-diagnosis itself (Rommelse et al., 2008; Tuulio-Henriksson et al., 2002). Using the TCA approach, several chromosomal regions (e.g., 4q24, 10q22-q23, and 17p13) associated with one or more individual migraine symptoms were identified (Anttila et al., 2006, 2008). An alternative approach to migraine end-diagnosis or TCA is *latent class analysis* (LCA), which was first used for migraine by Nyholt and co-workers (2004, 2005). LCA subdivides migraine patients into separate classes according to the clustering of symptoms based on the severity of the disease. LCA does not address migraine with and without aura separately, but regards them as different expressions of the same underlying etiological entity. LCA was shown to be less specific, but equally sensitive compared to the IHS criteria. The LCA approach led to the discovery of novel regions on, for instance, chromosomes 5q21 and 7q31-q33 that harbor migraine susceptibility genes (Chen et al., 2009; Lea et al., 2005; Nyholt et al., 2005).

ASSOCIATION STUDIES IN COMMON MIGRAINE

A frequently used alternative to family-based linkage studies is the approach of *gene association studies* that search for significant differences in allele frequencies between migraine cases and controls. Initially, gene association studies tested only one or a few DNA polymorphisms in candidate genes that emerged from other knowledge of migraine pathophysiology. Candidate gene–based association studies in theory are a powerful tool, if carefully designed to overcome methodological issues regarding sample size, selection of cases and controls, selection of variants, correction for multiple testing, and replication of findings in independent populations. Among the selected candidate genes that were most often tested were genes in the dopaminergic and serotonergic systems, hormone receptors, and inflammatory pathways (for review see de Vries, Frants, et al., 2009). The best replicated finding is the association with the C677T polymorphism in the 5,-10-methylenetetrahydrofolate reductase (*MTHFR*) gene that increases the risk of migraine in carriers of the T-allele (Kara et al., 2003; Kowa et al., 2000; Lea et al., 2004; Oterino et al., 2004, 2005; Scher et al., 2006), although other, large, well-designed studies could not find such association (Kaunisto et al., 2006; Todt et al., 2006). Two meta-analyses showed an association of this polymorphism with MA, but not with MO (Rubino et al., 2009; Schurks et al., 2010). *MTHFR* codes for an enzyme that has an important role in homocysteine and folate metabolism (Goyette et al., 1994), with carriers of the T-allele having an increased homocysteine concentration. It is hypothesized that high homocysteine levels may induce vascular endothelial dysfunction and thereby increase migraine risk.

Although ion transporter genes clearly surfaced in genetic studies of monogenic FHM, there is little evidence that the same genes also play a major role in common migraine. For instance, a large association study of 900 MA patients that were tested for several thousands of DNA polymorphisms in 155 ion transporter genes did not produce convincing results for an association (Nyholt et al., 2008). Although in the discovery cohort 66 significantly associated variants were identified in 12 ion transporter genes, none could be replicated in a substantial set of 2,835 cases and 2,740 controls. Based on current knowledge of effect sizes of variants for many complex diseases, it is quite possible that even this particular study did not have sufficient power to detect an effect that realistically should be expected for a common disorder such as migraine. Notably, a similar case-control association study investigating 2,717 *epilepsy* patients also did not detect a meaningful association with an ion transporter gene (Cavalleri et al., 2007), although certain ion channels play an important role in monogenic forms of epilepsy, and it would be surprising that given the known action of drugs that are effective in common epilepsy (and migraine), ion channels and neurotransmitters do not play a role.

SEQUENCING OF CANDIDATE GENE TRESK IN COMMON MIGRAINE

A special but rather unexpected finding came from a study by Lafrenière and co-workers, who, according to the description in their paper, solely based on gene function, chose to sequence only the ion channel gene *KCNK18* (which plays a role in pain pathways) in a set of 150 migraine families and identified one truncating F139WfsX24 *KCNK18* mutation that fully explains migraine in a single MA family (Lafrenière et al., 2010). No TRESK mutations were identified in 620 additional migraine families. Functional studies showed a dominant-negative effect of the mutant protein on wild-type protein resulting in a complete loss of TRESK function by the mutation. If confirmed in another migraine family, this finding will certainly add potassium channels to the short list of interesting migraine targets for further investigations. At the moment, however, it is an isolated finding, which in itself is not definite proof of causality. For instance, the scenario that disease in this family may be caused by a mutation in close proximity (i.e., linkage disequilibrium) is still possible. Although this may seem at first a rather unlikely scenario, it needs to be proven whether loss of a functional copy of TRESK results in a disease phenotype. Therefore, studies proving that a dominant-negative effect of this particular TRESK mutation also occurs in vivo would certainly add important weight to the conclusion that *KCNK18* is a migraine gene. Without additional support, it seems somewhat premature to definitely label TRESK as a good therapeutic target for migraine patients, as was suggested by the authors.

GENOME-WIDE ASSOCIATION STUDIES IN COMMON MIGRAINE

Because of recent advances in genomic technologies, it has become feasible to perform genome-wide association (GWA) studies that now test hundreds of thousands of genetic DNA markers in several thousand cases and controls in a hypothesis-free manner. Such large sample sizes are needed to correct for the many tests performed. The first GWA study in migraine identified the first-ever genetic risk factor for migraine: a single nucleotide polymorphism (SNP) named rs1835740 that resides on chromosome 8q22.1 and that has an odds ratio (OR) of 1.18 (Anttila et al., 2010). Although the initial cohorts consisted of only pure MA patients of Finnish, German, and Dutch origin, robust replication was observed for both MA and MO. SNP rs1835740 is located between two genes: the *MTDH/AEG1* (metadherin/astrocyte elevated) gene and the *PGCP* (plasma glutamate carboxypeptidase) gene. Expression quantitative trait (eQTL) data showed that increased *MTDH* expression levels are correlated with the migraine-associated minor allele of SNP rs1835740. MTDH is located on astrocytes and was extensively studied in glioblastoma research (Boycott et al., 2008; Dallas et al., 2007; Emdad et al., 2009; Noch & Khalili, 2009). From these studies it is apparent that increased MTDH levels down-regulate EAAT2, a major glutamate transporter in the brain that is important for removal of glutamate from the synaptic cleft. As a consequence, the associated SNP that causes reduced EAAT2 expression will result in increased glutamate levels in the brain, which fits the molecular pathway of FHM gene mutations that also predicts an increase in glutamate levels.

More GWA studies with additional migraine gene variants are expected in the coming years. Although a recently published GWA study of six population-based cohorts of Dutch and Icelandic origin did not yield genome-wide significant findings, it did give some additional genetic support for the *MTDH* gene as a possible migraine gene. Despite the fact that SNP rs1835740 did not show any signal, no less than 19 of 28 SNPs in the *MTDH* gene showed nominal evidence for association and a gene-based *p* value of .002.

From a clinical perspective, such gene variants with low relative risks may seem of limited interest, but one has to keep in mind that their identification will shed important light on novel mechanisms that are relevant for migraine pathophysiology. From that perspective, genetic research certainly has the potential to highlight many yet unknown migraine pathways. Experience from genetic studies of other complex disorders is that *common variants* will at best explain only a small portion of the genetic variance (Manolio et al., 2009), and this likely applies also to migraine. Either there are common variants with even smaller effect sizes, which would require study populations of easily more than 5,000 or even 10,000 cases, or migraine is caused by variants with a low frequency in the population that are not covered by commercial array chips. Even more recent technical developments that are known as *next-generation sequencing* now allow the identification of such rare variants with a medium effect size either by *exome sequencing* (i.e., sequencing all coding exons of an individual) or—in the more distant future—*whole genome sequencing* (Teer & Mullikin, 2010). Other possibilities why current gene hunts capture only little of the variance in complex diseases may be that one has to take into account gene–gene interactions (epistasis) or even different genetic mechanisms such as epigenetic mechanisms, in which gene expression is modified by heritable changes in packaging of DNA.

Genetic Studies that Combine Migraine and Comorbid Disorders

Some studies took advantage of the fact that certain disorders are comorbid with migraine. Although the observation can be spurious due to selection bias or reflect a unidirectional causal relationship (i.e., migraine causes [or is caused by] the comorbid disorder), it may also be that shared genetic and/or environmental factors underlie both migraine *and* the comorbid disorder (Bigal et al., 2008). Taking advantage of comorbid disorders can be an attractive strategy for genetic migraine studies, as it will reduce genetic heterogeneity by selecting those migraine patients who also suffer from the comorbid disorder. Several recent studies that used this approach are discussed below.

INVESTIGATING COMORBID DEPRESSION IN MIGRAINE GENETICS

Depression is one of the psychiatric disorders comorbid with migraine. A recent meta-analysis estimated the OR for depression in a migraine patient at 2.2. The risk appears highest for MA patients (Antonaci et al., 2011). Conversely, depression also increases the risk of migraine (OR = 2.8–3.4), reflecting the well-established bidirectional relationship between both disorders that suggests shared pathophysiological mechanisms. Three recent studies investigated whether shared genetic factors for both disorders exist, although a direct comparison of the studies is complicated by methodological differences (Ligthart et al., 2010; Schur et al., 2009; Stam et al., 2010). Two of the studies investigated twins (Ligthart et al., 2010)—in fact, one of them included only male twin pairs (Schur et al., 2009)—whereas the third study was performed in a genetically isolated population (Stam et al., 2010). A decrease in heritability of migraine upon correction for the co-occurrence of depression was interpreted as evidence that part of the variance in migraine must be explained by genetic factors that play a role in both migraine and depression (Ligthart et al., 2010; Stam et al., 2010). Of these two studies, the one by Stam and co-workers found the largest prevalence of depression and the biggest drop in heritability in MA. The third study by Schur and co-workers (2009) concluded that the genetic architecture of migraine and depression is best described by a model that incorporated both genetic and environmental factors and estimated that shared genetic factors account for approximately 20% of the variance in migraine and depression. Preliminary data from a genome-wide linkage scan taking advantage of the comorbidity revealed some candidate chromosome regions with nominal evidence, but no susceptibility genes (Ligthart et al., 2008).

INVESTIGATING COMORBID BIPOLAR DISORDER IN MIGRAINE GENETICS

Bipolar disorder is another psychiatric disorder with an increased prevalence in migraine. Recently, the large Canadian Community Health Survey with 36,984 participants estimated the OR in patients with physician-diagnosed migraine at 3.7 (Jette et al., 2008). Oedegaard and co-workers performed a linkage analysis in a set of 31 families with both bipolar disorder and migraine (Oedegaard, Greenwood, Lunde, et al., 2010) and a GWA study in a very small sample of only 56 migraine cases with bipolar disorder and 699 controls with bipolar disorder but no migraine (Oedegaard, Greenwood, Johansson, et al., 2010); they reported two potential regions on chromosomes 13 and 20 that may harbor susceptibility genes for migraine and bipolar disorder.

PRECLINICAL PERSPECTIVE: SCIENTIFIC INSIGHTS FROM GENETIC STUDIES IN MIGRAINE

The identification of genes involved in disease should be considered only the first step in elucidating the mechanisms

involved. The following section highlights insights that came from in vitro and in vivo studies to better understand migraine pathophysiology.

Insights From Functional Studies in Familial Hemiplegic Migraine

CELLULAR AND ANIMAL MODELS TO STUDY FUNCTIONAL CONSEQUENCES OF FAMILIAL HEMIPLEGIC MIGRAINE TYPE 1 MUTATIONS

P/Q-type calcium channels that contain the pore-forming α1 subunit, which is encoded by *CACNA1A*, are widely expressed at the plasma membrane of neurons in the central and peripheral nervous systems, where they control the flow of calcium across membranes and thereby release of neurotransmitters into the synaptic cleft (Catterall, 1998; Westenbroek et al., 1995). The consequences of 12 FHM1 mutations were tested on calcium channel function at the whole-cell level, and eight of these were also tested at the single-channel level. All FHM1 mutations showed gain-of-function effects, implying that mutated channels open more readily than normal channels (Hans et al., 1999; Tottene et al., 2002, 2005). To investigate the in vivo functional consequences of FHM1 mutations, two knock-in mouse models were generated using a gene-targeting approach by which embryonic stem cells are modified in such a way that the genome carries either missense mutation R192Q or S218L in the mouse *Cacna1a* gene. In line with the clinical phenotype seen in patients with the same mutations, only the S218L mice exhibited a complex phenotype of cerebellar ataxia, susceptibility to seizures, and delayed cerebral edema after minor head trauma (Stam, Luijckx, et al., 2009; van den Maagdenberg et al., 2010). At the molecular level, both R192Q and S218L mice revealed increased neuronal calcium influx and neurotransmitter release and an increased susceptibility to CSD upon topical cortical application of KCl or current injection into the cortex (Eikermann-Haerter et al., 2009; van den Maagdenberg et al., 2004, 2010). These neurobiological phenotypes were more prominent in the more severe S218L mutant. Experimental CSD also caused a temporary hemiparesis, but only in mutant mice. Pharmacological blocking of excess cortical glutamate in slices was capable of preventing the increased susceptibility to CSD (Tottene et al., 2009). In the same study it was shown that inhibitory neurotransmission seemed not affected by the FHM1 mutation.

Some studies of FHM1 mice revealed gender differences that seem relevant in line with the female preponderance in migraine patients. For instance, CSD susceptibility was more pronounced in *female* than *male* mutant mice, whereas no such gender difference was observed in wild-type mice. Ovariectomy (and senescence) abrogated the increased female CSD susceptibility, suggesting that circulating female hormones (i.e., estrogen) are important in determining gender effects. However, the observation that estrogen replacement could only partially restore CSD susceptibility suggests that estrogen levels themselves are not the sole determinant of the gender differences.

CELLULAR AND ANIMAL MODELS TO STUDY FUNCTIONAL CONSEQUENCES OF FAMILIAL HEMIPLEGIC MIGRAINE TYPE 2 MUTATIONS

The $ATP1A2$ gene codes for the α2 subunit of sodium-potassium pumps (Na,K-ATPase) that catalyze the exchange of Na^+ and K^+ across the cell membrane and provide the steep sodium gradient that is essential for the transport of calcium and glutamate (De Fusco et al., 2003). The functional consequences of FHM2 mutations were mainly studied using cell survival assays, which test the capability of mutant Na,K-ATPase (that was rendered insensitive to blocker ouabain) to result in cell survival after a challenge. Most FHM2 mutations showed reduced cell survival, implying loss-of-function effects. Although the survival assay is a rapid and valuable tool to determine the pathogenicity of a potential mutation, it is not very helpful in determining the exact molecular consequences of the mutations. Additional, more detailed studies of the kinetics of certain FHM2 $ATP1A2$ mutations pointed to a decreased Na,K-ATPase function (Capendeguy & Horisberger, 2004; Koenderink et al., 2005; Segall et al., 2004, 2005; Tavraz et al., 2008, 2009). Since an FHM2 knock-in mouse model is not available, there may be validity in analyzing $Atp1a2$ knock-out mice to investigate the in vivo consequences of lack of Na,K-ATPase function. The $Atp1a2$ knock-out mice are severely affected and die immediately after birth due to severe motor and respiratory problems (Ikeda et al., 2003; James et al., 1999).

CELLULAR AND ANIMAL MODELS TO STUDY FUNCTIONAL CONSEQUENCES OF FAMILIAL HEMIPLEGIC MIGRAINE TYPE 3 MUTATIONS

The $SCN1A$ gene codes for a subunit of voltage-gated $Na_V1.1$ sodium channels that are mainly—but not exclusively—expressed on inhibitory neurons, where they are essential for generation and propagation of action potentials. Thus far, FHM3 mutations Q1489K, L1649Q, and L263V have been studied at the functional level. Despite initial gain-of-function effects for the first two FHM3 mutations, when testing the mutations in the closely related $Na_V1.5$ channel subunit protein (Dichgans et al., 2005; Kahlig et al., 2008; Vanmolkot, Babini, et al., 2007),

more recent experiments showed clear loss-of-function effects for these mutations when they were introduced in the proper $Na_V1.1$ channel subunit protein (Dichgans et al., 2005; Kahlig et al., 2008; Vanmolkot, Babini, et al., 2007). The third FHM3 mutation L263V that in patients causes FHM and in the majority of mutation carriers also causes generalized tonic-clonic epilepsy essentially had gain-of-function effects (Kahlig et al., 2008). It was hypothesized that loss of sodium channel activity primarily disturbs the functioning of inhibitory neurons, where the $Na_V1.1$ protein is expressed normally (Ogiwara et al., 2007; Yu et al., 2006), whereas gain of activity had a predominant effect on excitatory neurons. From a recent in vitro study expressing FHM3 mutation Q1489K in cultured neurons, it is clear that the functional consequences of FHM3 mutations can be very complex. Depending on the test paradigm, the mutation had functional consequences fitting either hyperexcitability or hypoexcitability (self-limiting hyperexcitability capacity) (Cestele et al., 2008), but this has not been tested in, for instance, knock-in mice with FHM3 mutations as they are not available. Instead, studies in a $Scn1a$ knock-out mouse model showed severe ataxia and death in homozygous mice, whereas heterozygous mice showed reduced sodium currents in inhibitory neurons leading to hyperexcitability (Ogiwara et al., 2007).

FROM FAMILIAL HEMIPLEGIC MIGRAINE MUTATIONS TO UNDERSTANDING DISEASE PATHOLOGY

From studies investigating functional consequences of gene mutations in the three FHM genes, a common pathway seems to emerge that points to FHM being caused by a state of hyperexcitability as a consequence of disturbed ion homeostasis (Fig. 13–2) (Barrett et al., 2008). Mutant $Ca_V2.1$ calcium channels from FHM1 knock-in mice reveal increased neuronal calcium influx and increased glutamate release from cortical neurons. FHM2 mutations in the sodium–potassium pump predict in vivo reduced glial uptake of K^+ and glutamate from the synaptic cleft. FHM3 mutations in the $Na_V1.1$ sodium channel predict in vivo hyperexcitability of excitatory neurons because of a reduced action of inhibitory neurons. Therefore, the predicted functional consequence for FHM1, FHM2, and FHM3 mutations is that they all seem to lead to increased levels of glutamate and K^+ in the synaptic cleft and, since both are considered facilitators of CSD, result in an increased propensity for CSD, which can well explain the aura in patients. It remains uncertain if this also leads to a lower threshold for activation of the trigeminovascular system implicated in the headache phase.

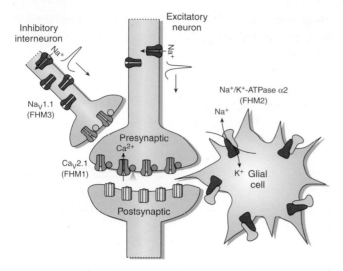

FIGURE 13–2 *Schematic overview of an excitatory (glutamatergic) synapse with its inhibitory neuron and a glial cell as well as the proteins encoded by the three familial hemiplegic migraine (FHM) genes. $Ca_V2.1$ calcium channels (encoded by CACNA1A) are located in the presynaptic terminal of excitatory and inhibitory neurons. In response to an invading action potential, Ca^{2+} enters via these channels, triggering glutamate release into the synaptic cleft. K^+ in the synaptic cleft is removed in part by the action of the Na^+/K^+-ATPase (encoded by ATP1A2) located on the membrane of glial cells (astrocytes). Removing extracellular K^+ generates a Na^+ gradient, which drives uptake of glutamate from the cleft. $Na_V1.1$ voltage-gated sodium channels (encoded by SCN1A) are expressed mainly—but not exclusively—on inhibitory interneurons, where they serve to initiate and propagate action potentials. Gain-of-function mutations in $Ca_V2.1$ channels and loss-of-function mutations in Na,K-ATPases and $Na_V1.1$ channels will each result in a net effect of increased excitability. Adapted from Barrett, C. F., van den Maagdenberg, A. M., Frants, R. R., & Ferrari, M. D. (2008). Familial hemiplegic migraine.* Advances in Genetics, 63, 57–83.

Molecular Insights from Other Genes with Relevance to Migraine Pathophysiology

In this section some key mechanisms are discussed that came from investigating CADASIL and RVCL as well as transgenic mice that overexpress RAMP1, which has relevance for understanding the role of CGRP receptor function.

MOLECULAR INSIGHTS FROM INVESTIGATING CADASIL

As a high number of CADASIL patients suffer from MA, one may expect that increased susceptibility to CSD may also act through the action of *NOTCH3* mutations that cause CADASIL. Enhanced CSD susceptibility was shown in *Notch3* knock-out mice as well as transgenic mice with an archetypical R90C missense mutation that overexpress smooth muscle cell promoter–driven Notch3

(Eikermann-Haerter & Moskowitz, 2008; Ruchoux et al., 2003), providing a reasonable explanation why CADASIL patients are at increased risk for MA. Liem et al. (2010) discuss four different hypotheses in their review. First, episodic ischemia may cause the migraine aura. An animal study showed that CSD-related flow changes become more pronounced and prolonged if the brain is in a preexistent state of hypoxia. Second, it could be that CADASIL increases susceptibility to CSD due to chronic brain damage caused by infarcts and white matter hyperintensities or that the onset of CSD is triggered by the occurrence of transient ischemia. Third, a direct or indirect relation could exist between the migraine aura and the pontine white matter lesions that are observed frequently in CADASIL patients and are more prevalent in migraine patients, especially with aura, than in the normal population. Last, *NOTCH3* mutations may increase migraine susceptibility via other pathways than those that cause microangiopathy.

MOLECULAR INSIGHTS FROM INVESTIGATING RETINAL VASCULOPATHY WITH CEREBRAL LEUKODYSTROPHY

Recently, truncating *TREX1* mutations were identified as the cause of RVCL (Richards et al., 2007). Trex1 functions as a $3'$-$5'$-exonuclease, and whereas it was proposed to play a role in DNA repair and drug resistance, current evidence suggests it plays a role in autoimmunity. Evidence from *Trex1* knock-out mice (Morita et al., 2004) revealed an accumulation of single-stranded DNA (which could activate the NF-κB pathway and the downstream inflammatory genes such as IFN-α via toll-like receptors) and endogenous retroelement-derived DNA, causing a dysregulation of the IFN-stimulatory DNA pathway, by which Trex1 deficiency may cause autoimmunity (Stetson et al., 2008). Whereas RVCL *TREX1* mutations still exhibit exonuclease function, the cellular localization of the protein is changed: Trex1 no longer resides at the endoplasmic reticulum, but now has a diffuse cellular localization (Richards et al., 2007). It is hypothesized that Trex1 protein when acting in the wrong cellular context will lead to accumulation of DNA intermediates that evoke an immune response and cause disease, but it needs to be investigated how this leads to the widespread vasculopathy seen in RVCL patients (Stam, Haan, et al., 2009). No knock-in mouse model carrying a human RVCL mutation is available to address these questions.

MOLECULAR INSIGHTS FROM INVESTIGATING RAMP1-OVEREXPRESSING MICE

CGRP antagonists were shown to be effective as acute treatment of migraine attacks (Monteith & Goadsby, 2011).

As CGRP levels rise during attacks (Goadsby et al., 1990; Juhasz et al., 2003), it therefore is interesting to study the in vivo consequences of elevated levels of CGRP in an animal model. To this end, nonmutated, human, receptor activity–modifying protein (RAMP1) cDNA was overexpressed in mice by introducing DNA copies of the transgene at a random position in the mouse genome using a technique of pronuclear injection combined with a Cre-mediated activation strategy (Zhang et al., 2007). RAMP1 is a transmembrane subunit necessary for functioning of the CGRP receptor (McLatchie et al., 1998). Increased expression of human RAMP1 (hRAMP1) sensitizes the mice to the action of CGRP. As a consequence, these mice exhibit increased CGRP-induced plasma extravasation in the trigeminal ganglion (Zhang et al., 2007). Signs of central sensitization were reported after induction of mechanical allodynia (Marquez de Prado et al., 2009). In addition, the hRAMP1 transgenic mice exhibit an enhanced light-aversive behavior that is further increased by direct CGRP administration and blocked by treatment with CGRP receptor antagonists (Recober et al., 2009, 2010), which are in agreement with migraine symptoms such as photophobia.

CLINICAL PERSPECTIVES: RELEVANCE OF GENETIC FINDINGS IN CLINICAL PRACTICE

The relevance to clinical practice of recent findings from GWA studies in common diseases such as migraine is low. Because of the low OR associated with individual gene variants, only combinations of multiple low-risk gene variants together with environmental factors will be sufficient to cause migraine. Still, these variants will highlight molecular pathways that likely will shed important new light on migraine pathophysiology. It will be challenging, though, to establish useful cellular and animal models for such variants, whereas the model systems harboring monogenic gene mutations (e.g., FHM1 knock-in mice) already have shown their potential.

The relevance for clinical practice of genetic findings from monogenic migraine diseases is much clearer. Information on high-risk mutations will help a physician to make a definite diagnosis in a patient. Increased awareness of syndromes such as CADASIL and RVCL and their relation with migraine is also beneficial for the physician. For instance, a diagnosis of CADASIL must be considered when a patient presents with MA and a history of strokes and cognitive decline at a young age, whereas a combination of retinopathy and migraine should remind a clinician of RVCL. Screening for mutations in NOTCH3 and TREX1, respectively, is indicated in these patients.

Moreover, once a diagnosis of hemiplegic migraine has been established in a patient, it is important to determine also the affected status of first-degree relatives. If an affected first-degree relative is present, it concerns an FHM family and mutation screening of CACNA1A, ATP1A2, and SCN1A is indicated. The presence of additional clinical symptoms can help prioritize which gene to test first: for instance, CACNA1A in families with ataxia or coma after minor head trauma, and ATP1A2 in families with pure FHM. Of the three FHM genes, ATP1A2 is the gene with the highest mutation detection rate, except perhaps for the very frequent T666M mutation in CACNA1A. In SHM, mutation scanning for CACNA1A and ATP1A2 is indicated, especially in severely affected patients with early onset of disease.

FUTURE PERSPECTIVES

Recent developments in the field of genetics enabled large-scale GWA studies in common migraine and recently led to the identification of the first genetic risk factor for common migraine (Anttila et al., 2010). In the near future several additional migraine genes are expected to be discovered as several GWA studies are currently being analyzed. Also, for gene identification of monogenic disorders new technology has become available. The availability of new high-throughput *next-generation sequencing* exome technology recently led to the identification of the first gene for the rare Miller syndrome (Ng et al., 2010), but since then the number of genes for monogenic diseases has rapidly increased. In the near future it will be feasible to apply the same technology to sequence rare variants for complex disorders on a large scale at the whole genome level. In conclusion, many new developments in the field of genetics will likely lead to the identification of a substantial number of migraine susceptibility genes in the near future. It will be a major challenge for the coming years to establish functional assays to investigate these novel migraine genes and thereby advance our knowledge of migraine pathophysiology and develop novel molecular targets for drug discovery.

REFERENCES

Ambrosini, A., D'Onofrio, M., Grieco, G. S., Di Mambro, A., Montagna, G., Fortini, D., et al. (2005). Familial basilar migraine associated with a new mutation in the ATP1A2 gene. *Neurology, 65,* 1826–1828.

Antonaci, F., Nappi, G., Galli, F., Manzoni, G. C., Calabresi, P., & Costa, A. (2011). Migraine and psychiatric comorbidity: A review of clinical findings. *Journal of Headache and Pain, 12,* 115–125.

Anttila, V., Kallela, M., Oswell, G., Kaunisto, M. A., Nyholt, D. R., Hamalainen, E., et al. (2006). Trait components provide tools to dissect the genetic susceptibility of migraine. *American Journal of Human Genetics, 79,* 85–99.

Anttila, V., Nyholt, D. R., Kallela, M., Artto, V., Vepsalainen, S., Jakkula, E., et al. (2008). Consistently replicating locus linked to migraine on 10q22-q23. *American Journal of Human Genetics, 82,* 1051–1063.

Anttila, V., Stefansson, H., Kallela, M., Todt, U., Terwindt, G. M., Calafato, M. S., et al. (2010). Genome-wide association study of migraine implicates a common susceptibility variant on 8q22.1. *Nature Genetics, 42,* 869–873.

Barrett, C. F., van den Maagdenberg, A. M., Frants, R. R., & Ferrari, M. D. (2008). Familial hemiplegic migraine. *Advances in Genetics, 63,* 57–83.

Bertina, R. M., Koeleman, B. P., Koster, T., Rosendaal, F. R., Dirven, R. J., de Ronde, H., et al. (1994). Mutation in blood coagulation factor V associated with resistance to activated protein C. *Nature, 369,* 64–67.

Bigal, M. E., Serrano, D., Buse, D., Scher, A., Stewart, W. F., & Lipton, R. B. (2008). Acute migraine medications and evolution from episodic to chronic migraine: A longitudinal population-based study. *Headache, 48,* 1157–1168.

Bjornsson, A., Gudmundsson, G., Gudfinnsson, E., Hrafnsdottir, M., Benedikz, J., Skuladottir, S., et al. (2003). Localization of a gene for migraine without aura to chromosome 4q21. *American Journal of Human Genetics, 73,* 986–993.

Borroni, B., Brambilla, C., Liberini, P., Rao, R., Archetti, S., Venturelli, E., et al. (2006). Investigating the association between Notch3 polymorphism and migraine. *Headache, 46,* 317–321.

Boycott, H. E., Wilkinson, J. A., Boyle, J. P., Pearson, H. A., & Peers, C. (2008). Differential involvement of TNF alpha in hypoxic suppression of astrocyte glutamate transporters. *Glia, 56,* 998–1004.

Cader, Z. M., Noble-Topham, S., Dyment, D. A., Cherny, S. S., Brown, J. D., Rice, G. P., et al. (2003). Significant linkage to migraine with aura on chromosome 11q24. *Human Molecular Genetics, 12,* 2511–2517.

Capendeguy, O., & Horisberger, J. D. (2004). Functional effects of Na+,K+-ATPase gene mutations linked to familial hemiplegic migraine. *Neuromolecular Medicine, 6,* 105–116.

Carlsson, A., Forsgren, L., Nylander, P. O., Hellman, U., Forsman-Semb, K., Holmgren, G., et al. (2002). Identification of a susceptibility locus for migraine with and without aura on 6p12.2-p21.1. *Neurology, 59,* 1804–1807.

Castro, M. J., Stam, A. H., Lemos, C., Barros, J., Gouveia, R. G., Martins, I. P., et al. (2007). Recurrent ATP1A2 mutations in Portuguese families with familial hemiplegic migraine. *Journal of Human Genetics, 52,* 990–998.

Castro, M. J., Stam, A. H., Lemos, C., de Vries, B., Vanmolkot, K. R., Barros, J., et al. (2009). First mutation in the voltage-gated Nav1.1 subunit gene SCN1A with co-occurring familial hemiplegic migraine and epilepsy. *Cephalalgia, 29,* 308–313.

Catterall, W. A. (1998). Structure and function of neuronal Ca2+ channels and their role in neurotransmitter release. *Cell Calcium, 24,* 307–323.

Cavalleri, G. L., Weale, M. E., Shianna, K. V., Singh, R., Lynch, J. M., Grinton, B., et al. (2007). Multicentre search for genetic susceptibility loci in sporadic epilepsy syndrome and seizure types: A case-control study. *Lancet Neurology, 6,* 970–980.

Cestele, S., Scalmani, P., Rusconi, R., Terragni, B., Franceschetti, S., & Mantegazza, M. (2008). Self-limited hyperexcitability: Functional effect of a familial hemiplegic migraine mutation of the Nav1.1 (SCN1A) Na+ channel. *Journal of Neuroscience, 28,* 7273–7283.

Cevoli, S., Pallotti, F., La Morgia, C., Valentino, M. L., Pierangeli, G., Cortelli, P., et al. (2010). High frequency of migraine-only patients negative for the 3243 A>G tRNALeu mtDNA mutation in two MELAS families. *Cephalalgia, 30,* 919–927.

Chan, Y. C., Burgunder, J. M., Wilder-Smith, E., Chew, S. E., Lam-Mok-Sing, K. M., Sharma, V., et al. (2008). Electroencephalographic changes and seizures in familial hemiplegic migraine patients with the CACNA1A gene S218L mutation. *Journal of Clinical Neuroscience, 15,* 891–894.

Chen, C. C., Keith, J. M., Nyholt, D. R., Martin, N. G., & Mengersen, K. L. (2009). Bayesian latent trait modeling of migraine symptom data. *Human Genetics, 126,* 277–288.

Curtain, R. P., Smith, R. L., Ovcaric, M., & Griffiths, L. R. (2006). Minor head trauma-induced sporadic hemiplegic migraine coma. *Pediatric Neurology, 34,* 329–332.

Dallas, M., Boycott, H. E., Atkinson, L., Miller, A., Boyle, J. P., Pearson, H. A., et al. (2007). Hypoxia suppresses glutamate transport in astrocytes. *Journal of Neuroscience, 27,* 3946–3955.

De Fusco, M., Marconi, R., Silvestri, L., Atorino, L., Rampoldi, L., Morgante, L., et al. (2003). Haploinsufficiency of ATP1A2 encoding the Na+/K+pump alpha2 subunit associated with familial hemiplegic migraine type 2. *Nature Genetics, 33,* 192–196.

De Sanctis, S., Grieco, G. S., Breda, L., Casali, C., Nozzi, M., Del Torto, M., et al. (2011). Prolonged sporadic hemiplegic migraine associated with a novel de novo missense ATP1A2 gene mutation. *Headache, 51,* 447–450.

de Vries, B., Frants, R. R., Ferrari, M. D., & van den Maagdenberg, A. M. (2009). Molecular genetics of migraine. *Human Genetics, 126,* 115–132.

de Vries, B., Freilinger, T., Vanmolkot, K. R., Koenderink, J. B., Stam, A. H., Terwindt, G. M., et al. (2007). Systematic analysis of three FHM genes in 39 sporadic patients with hemiplegic migraine. *Neurology, 69,* 2170–2176.

de Vries, B., Stam, A. H., Kirkpatrick, M., Vanmolkot, K. R., Koenderink, J. B., van den Heuvel, J. J., et al. (2009). Familial hemiplegic migraine is associated with febrile seizures in an FHM2 family with a novel de novo ATP1A2 mutation. *Epilepsia, 50,* 2503–2504.

Debiais, S., Hommet, C., Bonnaud, I., Barthez, M. A., Rimbaux, S., Riant, F., et al. (2009). The FHM1 mutation S218L: A severe clinical phenotype? A case report and review of the literature. *Cephalalgia, 29,* 1337–1339.

Deprez, L., Weckhuysen, S., Peeters, K., Deconinck, T., Claeys, K. G., Claes, L. R., et al. (2008). Epilepsy as part of the phenotype associated with ATP1A2 mutations. *Epilepsia, 49,* 500–508.

Dichgans, M., Freilinger, T., Eckstein, G., Babini, E., Lorenz-Depiereux, B., Biskup, S., et al. (2005). Mutation in the neuronal voltage-gated sodium channel SCN1A in familial hemiplegic migraine. *Lancet, 366,* 371–377.

Dichgans, M., & Hegele, R. A. (2007). Update on the genetics of stroke and cerebrovascular disease 2006. *Stroke, 38,* 216–218.

Dichgans, M., Mayer, M., Uttner, I., Bruning, R., Muller-Hocker, J., Rungger, G., et al. (1998). The phenotypic spectrum of CADASIL: Clinical findings in 102 cases. *Annals of Neurology, 44,* 731–739.

Ducros, A., Denier, C., Joutel, A., Cecillon, M., Lescoat, C., Vahedi, K., et al. (2001). The clinical spectrum of familial hemiplegic migraine associated with mutations in a neuronal calcium channel. *New England Journal of Medicine, 345,* 17–24.

Eikermann-Haerter, K., Dilekoz, E., Kudo, C., Savitz, S. I., Waeber, C., Baum, M. J., et al. (2009). Genetic and hormonal factors modulate spreading depression and transient hemiparesis in mouse models of familial hemiplegic migraine type 1. *Journal of Clinical Investigation, 119,* 99–109.

Eikermann-Haerter, K., & Moskowitz, M. A. (2008). Animal models of migraine headache and aura. *Current Opinion in Neurology, 21,* 294–300.

Emdad, L., Lee, S. G., Su, Z. Z., Jeon, H. Y., Boukerche, H., Sarkar, D., et al. (2009). Astrocyte elevated gene-1 (AEG-1) functions as an oncogene and regulates angiogenesis. *Proceedings of the National Academy of Sciences of the United States of America, 106,* 21300–21305.

Escayg, A., & Goldin, A. L. (2010). Sodium channel SCN1A and epilepsy: Mutations and mechanisms. *Epilepsia, 51,* 1650–1658.

Ferrari, M. D. (1998). Migraine. *Lancet, 351,* 1043–1051.

Ferrari, M. D., & Goadsby, P. J. (2007). Migraine as a cerebral ionopathy with abnormal central sensory processing. In S. Gilman (Ed.), *Neurobiology of disease* (pp. 333–348). Elsevier Academic Press: San Diego, CA.

Gargus, J. J., & Tournay, A. (2007). Novel mutation confirms seizure locus SCN1A is also familial hemiplegic migraine locus FHM3. *Pediatric Neurology, 37,* 407–410.

Gervil, M., Ulrich, V., Kyvik, K. O., Olesen, J., & Russell, M. B. (1999). Migraine without aura: A population-based twin study. *Annals of Neurology, 46,* 606–611.

Goadsby, P. J., Edvinsson, L., & Ekman, R. (1990). Vasoactive peptide release in the extracerebral circulation of humans during migraine headache. *Annals of Neurology, 28,* 183–187.

Goadsby, P. J., Lipton, R. B., & Ferrari, M. D. (2002). Migraine—current understanding and treatment. *New England Journal of Medicine, 346,* 257–270.

Gould, D. B., Phalan, F. C., van Mil, S. E., Sundberg, J. P., Vahedi, K., Massin, P., et al. (2006). Role of COL4A1 in small-vessel disease and hemorrhagic stroke. *New England Journal of Medicine, 354,* 1489–1496.

Goyette, P., Sumner, J. S., Milos, R., Duncan, A. M., Rosenblatt, D. S., Matthews, R. G., et al. (1994). Human methylenetetrahydrofolate reductase: Isolation of cDNA, mapping and mutation identification. *Nature Genetics, 7,* 195–200.

Grand, M. G., Kaine, J., Fulling, K., Atkinson, J., Dowton, S. B., Farber, M., et al. (1988). Cerebroretinal vasculopathy. A new hereditary syndrome. *Ophthalmology, 95,* 649–659.

Hadjikhani, N., Sanchez Del Rio, M., Wu, O., Schwartz, D., Bakker, D., Fischl, B., et al. (2001). Mechanisms of migraine aura revealed by functional MRI in human visual cortex. *Proceedings of the National Academy of Sciences of the United States of America, 98,* 4687–4692.

Hans, M., Luvisetto, S., Williams, M. E., Spagnolo, M., Urrutia, A., Tottene, A., et al. (1999). Functional consequences of mutations in the human alpha1A calcium channel subunit linked to familial hemiplegic migraine. *Journal of Neuroscience, 19,* 1610–1619.

Headache Classification Subcommittee of the International Hedache Society. (2004). The international classification of headache disorders: 2nd edition. *Cephalalgia, 24*(Suppl 1), 9–160.

Hottenga, J. J., Vanmolkot, K. R., Kors, E. E., Kheradmand Kia, S., de Jong, P. T., Haan, J., et al. (2005). The 3p.21.1-p21.3 hereditary vascular retinopathy locus increases the risk for Raynaud's phenomenon and migraine. *Cephalalgia, 25,* 1168–1172.

Hovatta, I., Kallela, M., Farkkila, M., & Peltonen, L. (1994). Familial migraine: Exclusion of the susceptibility gene from the reported locus of familial hemiplegic migraine on 19p. *Genomics, 23,* 707–709.

Hudson, G., & Chinnery, P. F. (2006). Mitochondrial DNA polymerase-gamma and human disease. *Human Molecular Genetics, 15*(Spec No 2), R244–R252.

Ikeda, K., Onaka, T., Yamakado, M., Nakai, J., Ishikawa, T. O., Taketo, M. M., et al. (2003). Degeneration of the amygdala/piriform cortex and enhanced fear/anxiety behaviors in sodium pump alpha2 subunit (Atp1a2)-deficient mice. *Journal of Neuroscience, 23,* 4667–4676.

Imbrici, P., Jaffe, S. L., Eunson, L. H., Davies, N. P., Herd, C., Robertson, R., et al. (2004). Dysfunction of the brain calcium channel CaV2.1 in absence epilepsy and episodic ataxia. *Brain, 127,* 2682–2692.

Ionita-Laza, I., Buxbaum, J. D., Laird, N. M., & Lange, C. (2011). A new testing strategy to identify rare variants with either risk or protective effect on disease. *PLoS Genetics, 7,* e1001289.

James, P. F., Grupp, I. L., Grupp, G., Woo, A. L., Askew, G. R., Croyle, M. L., et al. (1999). Identification of a specific role for the Na,K-ATPase alpha 2 isoform as a regulator of calcium in the heart. *Molecular Cell, 3,* 555–563.

Jen, J., Cohen, A. H., Yue, Q., Stout, J. T., Vinters, H. V., Nelson, S., et al. (1997). Hereditary endotheliopathy with retinopathy, nephropathy, and stroke (HERNS). *Neurology, 49,* 1322–1330.

Jen, J. C., Kim, G. W., Dudding, K. A., & Baloh, R. W. (2004). No mutations in CACNA1A and ATP1A2 in probands with common types of migraine. *Archives of Neurology, 61,* 926–928.

Jen, J. C., Wan, J., Palos, T. P., Howard, B. D., & Baloh, R. W. (2005). Mutation in the glutamate transporter EAAT1 causes episodic ataxia, hemiplegia, and seizures. *Neurology, 65,* 529–534.

Jette, N., Patten, S., Williams, J., Becker, W., & Wiebe, S. (2008). Comorbidity of migraine and psychiatric disorders—a national population-based study. *Headache, 48,* 501–516.

Jones, K. W., Ehm, M. G., Pericak-Vance, M. A., Haines, J. L., Boyd, P. R., & Peroutka, S. J. (2001). Migraine with aura susceptibility locus on chromosome 19p.13 is distinct from the familial hemiplegic migraine locus. *Genomics, 78,* 150–154.

Joutel, A., Corpechot, C., Ducros, A., Vahedi, K., Chabriat, H., Mouton, P., et al. (1996). Notch3 mutations in CADASIL, a hereditary adult-onset condition causing stroke and dementia. *Nature, 383,* 707–710.

Jouvenceau, A., Eunson, L. H., Spauschus, A., Ramesh, V., Zuberi, S. M., Kullmann, D. M., et al. (2001). Human epilepsy associated with dysfunction of the brain P./Q-type calcium channel. *Lancet, 358,* 801–807.

Juhasz, G., Zsombok, T., Modos, E. A., Olajos, S., Jakab, B., Nemeth, J., et al. (2003). NO-induced migraine attack: Strong increase in plasma calcitonin gene-related peptide (CGRP) concentration and negative correlation with platelet serotonin release. *Pain, 106,* 461–470.

Jurkat-Rott, K., Freilinger, T., Dreier, J. P., Herzog, J., Gobel, H., Petzold, G. C., et al. (2004). Variability of familial hemiplegic migraine with novel A1A2 Na+/K+-ATPase variants. *Neurology, 62,* 1857–1861.

Kahlig, K. M., Rhodes, T. H., Pusch, M., Freilinger, T., Pereira-Monteiro, J. M., Ferrari, M. D., et al. (2008). Divergent sodium channel defects in familial hemiplegic migraine. *Proceedings of the National Academy of Sciences of the United States of America, 105,* 9799–9804.

Kallela, M., Wessman, M., Havanka, H., Palotie, A., & Farkkila, M. (2001). Familial migraine with and without aura: Clinical characteristics and co-occurrence. *European Journal of Neurology, 8,* 441–449.

Kara, I., Sazci, A., Ergul, E., Kaya, G., & Kilic, G. (2003). Association of the C677T and A1298C polymorphisms in the 5,10 methylenetetrahydrofolate reductase gene in patients with migraine risk. *Brain Research: Molecular Brain Research, 111*, 84–90.

Kaunisto, M. A., Harno, H., Vanmolkot, K. R., Gargus, J. J., Sun, G., Hamalainen, E., et al. (2004). A novel missense ATP1A2 mutation in a Finnish family with familial hemiplegic migraine type 2. *Neurogenetics, 5*, 141–146.

Kaunisto, M. A., Kallela, M., Hamalainen, E., Kilpikari, R., Havanka, H., Harno, H., et al. (2006). Testing of variants of the MTHFR and ESR1 genes in 1798 Finnish individuals fails to confirm the association with migraine with aura. *Cephalalgia, 26*, 1462–1472.

Knierim, E., Leisle, L., Wagner, C., Weschke, B., Lucke, B., Bohner, G., et al. (2011). Recurrent stroke due to a novel voltage sensor mutation in Cav2.1 responds to verapamil. *Stroke, 42*, e14–e17.

Koenderink, J. B., Zifarelli, G., Qiu, L. Y., Schwarz, W., De Pont, J. J., Bamberg, E., et al. (2005). Na,K-ATPase mutations in familial hemiplegic migraine lead to functional inactivation. *Biochimica et Biophysica Acta, 1669*, 61–68.

Kors, E. E., Haan, J., Giffin, N. J., Pazdera, L., Schnittger, C., Lennox, G. G., et al. (2003). Expanding the phenotypic spectrum of the CACNA1A gene T666M mutation: A description of 5 families with familial hemiplegic migraine. *Archives of Neurology, 60*, 684–688.

Kors, E. E., Terwindt, G. M., Vermeulen, F. L., Fitzsimons, R. B., Jardine, P. E., Heywood, P., et al. (2001). Delayed cerebral edema and fatal coma after minor head trauma: Role of the CACNA1A calcium channel subunit gene and relationship with familial hemiplegic migraine. *Annals of Neurology, 49*, 753–760.

Kowa, H., Yasui, K., Takeshima, T., Urakami, K., Sakai, F., & Nakashima, K. (2000). The homozygous C677T mutation in the methylenetetrahydrofolate reductase gene is a genetic risk factor for migraine. *American Journal of Medical Genetics, 96*, 762–764.

Lafrenière, R. G., Cader, M. Z., Poulin, J. F., Andres-Enguix, I., Simoneau, M., Gupta N., et al. (2010). A dominant-negative mutation in the TRESK potassium channel is linked to familial migraine with aura. *Nature Medicine, 16*, 1157–1160.

Launer, L. J., Terwindt, G. M., & Ferrari, M. D. (1999). The prevalence and characteristics of migraine in a population-based cohort: The GEM study. *Neurology, 53*, 537–542.

Lauritzen, M. (1994). Pathophysiology of the migraine aura. The spreading depression theory. *Brain, 117*, 199–210.

Law, C., Bunyan, D., Castle, B., Day, L., Simpson, I., Westwood, G., et al. (2006). Clinical features in a family with an R460H mutation in transforming growth factor beta receptor 2 gene. *Journal of Medical Genetics, 43*, 908–916.

Le Fort, D., Safran, A. B., Picard, F., Bouchardy, I., & Morris, M. A. (2004). Elicited repetitive daily blindness: A new familial disorder related to migraine and epilepsy. *Neurology, 63*, 348–350.

Lea, R. A., Nyholt, D. R., Curtain, R. P., Ovcaric, M., Sciascia, R., Bellis, C., et al. (2005). A genome-wide scan provides evidence for loci influencing a severe heritable form of common migraine. *Neurogenetics, 6*, 67–72.

Lea, R. A., Ovcaric, M., Sundholm, J., MacMillan, J., & Griffiths, L. R. (2004). The methylenetetrahydrofolate reductase gene variant C677T influences susceptibility to migraine with aura. *BMC Medicine, 2*, 3.

Lea, R. A., Shepherd, A. G., Curtain, R. P., Nyholt, D. R., Quinlan, S., Brimage, P. J., et al. (2002). A typical migraine susceptibility region localizes to chromosome 1q31. *Neurogenetics, 4*, 17–22.

Liem, M. K., Lesnik Oberstein, S. A. J., Van der Grond, J., Ferrari, M. D., & Haan, J. (2010). CADASIL and migraine: A narrative review. *Cephalalgia.* 11, 1284-1289

Ligthart, L., Boomsma, D. I., Martin, N. G., Stubbe, J. H., & Nyholt, D. R. (2006). Migraine with aura and migraine without aura are not distinct entities: Further evidence from a large Dutch population study. *Twin Research Human Genetics, 9*, 54–63.

Ligthart, L., Nyholt, D. R., Hottenga, J. J., Distel, M. A., Willemsen, G., & Boomsma, D. I. (2008). A genome-wide linkage scan provides evidence for both new and previously reported loci influencing common migraine. *American Journal of Medical Genetics Series B Neuropsychiatric Genetics, 147B*, 1186–1195.

Ligthart, L., Nyholt, D. R., Penninx, B. W., & Boomsma, D. I. (2010). The shared genetics of migraine and anxious depression. *Headache, 50*, 1549–1560.

Manolio, T. A., Collins, F. S., Cox, N. J., Goldstein, D. B., Hindorff, L. A., Hunter, D. J., et al. (2009). Finding the missing heritability of complex diseases. *Nature, 461*, 747–753.

Marquez de Prado, B., Hammond, D. L., & Russo, A. F. (2009). Genetic enhancement of calcitonin gene-related peptide-induced central sensitization to mechanical stimuli in mice. *Journal of Pain, 10*, 992–1000.

May, A., Ophoff, R. A., Terwindt, G. M., Urban, C., van Eijk, R., Haan, J., et al. (1995). Familial hemiplegic migraine locus on 19p.13 is involved in the common forms of migraine with and without aura. *Human Genetics, 96*, 604–608.

McLatchie, L. M., Fraser, N. J., Main, M. J., Wise, A., Brown, J., Thompson, N., et al. (1998). RAMPs regulate the transport and ligand specificity of the calcitonin-receptor-like receptor. *Nature, 393*, 333–339.

Montagna, P., Gallassi, R., Medori, R., Govoni, E., Zeviani, M., Di Mauro, S., et al. (1988). MELAS syndrome: Characteristic migrainous and epileptic features and maternal transmission. *Neurology, 38*, 751–754.

Monteith, T. S., & Goadsby, P. J. (2011). Acute migraine therapy: New drugs and new approaches. *Current Treatment Options in Neurology, 13*, 1–14.

Morita, M., Stamp, G., Robins, P., Dulic, A., Rosewell, I., Hrivnak, G., et al. (2004). Gene-targeted mice lacking the Trex1 (DNase III) 3'→5' DNA exonuclease develop inflammatory myocarditis. *Molecular and Cellular Biology, 24*, 6719–6727.

Mulder, E. J., Van Baal, C., Gaist, D., Kallela, M., Kaprio, J., Svensson, D. A., et al. (2003). Genetic and environmental influences on migraine: A twin study across six countries. *Twin Research, 6*, 422–431.

Ng, S. B., Buckingham, K. J., Lee, C., Bigham, A. W., Tabor, H. K., Dent, K. M., et al. (2010). Exome sequencing identifies the cause of a mendelian disorder. *Nature Genetics, 42*, 30–35.

Noch, E., & Khalili, K. (2009). Molecular mechanisms of necrosis in glioblastoma: The role of glutamate excitotoxicity. *Cancer Biology and Therapy, 8*, 1791–1797.

Nyholt, D. R., Dawkins, J. L., Brimage, P. J., Goadsby, P. J., Nicholson, G. A., & Griffiths, L. R. (1998). Evidence for an X-linked genetic component in familial typical migraine. *Human Molecular Genetics, 7*, 459–463.

Nyholt, D. R., Gillespie, N. G., Heath, A. C., Merikangas, K. R., Duffy, D. L., & Martin, N. G. (2004). Latent class and genetic analysis does not support migraine with aura and migraine without aura as separate entities. *Genetic Epidemiology, 26*, 231–244.

Nyholt, D. R., LaForge, K. S., Kallela, M., Alakurtti, K., Anttila, V., Farkkila, M., et al. (2008). A high-density association screen of

155 ion transport genes for involvement with common migraine. *Human Molecular Genetics, 17*, 3318–3331.

Nyholt, D. R., Lea, R. A., Goadsby, P. J., Brimage, P. J., & Griffiths, L. R. (1998). Familial typical migraine: Linkage to chromosome 19p.13 and evidence for genetic heterogeneity. *Neurology, 50*, 1428–1432.

Nyholt, D. R., Morley, K. I., Ferreira, M. A., Medland, S. E., Boomsma, D. I., Heath, A. C., et al. (2005). Genomewide significant linkage to migrainous headache on chromosome 5q21. *American Journal of Human Genetics, 77*, 500–512.

Oedegaard, K. J., Greenwood, T. A., Johansson, S., Jacobsen, K. K., Halmoy, A., Fasmer, O. B., et al. (2010). A genome-wide association study of bipolar disorder and comorbid migraine. *Genes and Brain Behavior, 7*, 673–680.

Oedegaard, K. J., Greenwood, T. A., Lunde, A., Fasmer, O. B., Akiskal, H. S., & Kelsoe, J. R. (2010). A genome-wide linkage study of bipolar disorder and co-morbid migraine: Replication of migraine linkage on chromosome 4q24, and suggestion of an overlapping susceptibility region for both disorders on chromosome 20p. 11. *Journal of Affective Disorders, 122*, 14–26.

Ogiwara, I., Miyamoto, H., Morita, N., Atapour, N., Mazaki, E., Inoue, I., et al. (2007). Na(v)1.1 localizes to axons of parvalbumin-positive inhibitory interneurons: A circuit basis for epileptic seizures in mice carrying an Scn1a gene mutation. *Journal of Neuroscience, 27*, 5903–5914.

Ophoff, R. A., Terwindt, G. M., Vergouwe, M. N., van Eijk, R., Oefner, P. J., Hoffman, S. M., et al. (1996). Familial hemiplegic migraine and episodic ataxia type-2 are caused by mutations in the Ca2+ channel gene CACNL1A4. *Cell, 87*, 543–552.

Oterino, A., Valle, N., Bravo, Y., Munoz, P., Sanchez-Velasco, P., Ruiz-Alegria, C., et al. (2004). MTHFR T677 homozygosis influences the presence of aura in migraineurs. *Cephalalgia, 24*, 491–494.

Oterino, A., Valle, N., Pascual, J., Bravo, Y., Munoz, P., Castillo, J., et al. (2005). Thymidylate synthase promoter tandem repeat and MTHFD1 R653Q polymorphisms modulate the risk for migraine conferred by the MTHFR T677 allele. *Brain Research: Molecular Brain Research, 139*, 163–168.

Pierelli, F., Grieco, G. S., Pauri, F., Pirro, C., Fiermonte, G., Ambrosini, A., et al. (2006). A novel ATP1A2 mutation in a family with FHM type II. *Cephalalgia, 26*, 324–328.

Recober, A., Kaiser, E. A., Kuburas, A., & Russo, A. F. (2010). Induction of multiple photophobic behaviors in a transgenic mouse sensitized to CGRP. *Neuropharmacology, 58*, 156–165.

Recober, A., Kuburas, A., Zhang, Z., Wemmie, J. A., Anderson, M. G., & Russo, A. F. (2009). Role of calcitonin gene-related peptide in light-aversive behavior: implications for migraine. *Journal of Neuroscience, 29*, 8798–8804.

Riant, F., De Fusco, M., Aridon, P., Ducros, A., Ploton, C., Marchelli, F., et al. (2005). ATP1A2 mutations in 11 families with familial hemiplegic migraine. *Human Mutation, 26*, 281.

Riant, F., Ducros, A., Ploton, C., Barbance, C., Depienne, C., & Tournier-Lasserve, E. (2010). De novo mutations in ATP1A2 and CACNA1A are frequent in early-onset sporadic hemiplegic migraine. *Neurology, 75*, 967–972.

Richards, A., van den Maagdenberg, A. M., Jen, J. C., Kavanagh, D., Bertram, P., Spitzer, D., et al. (2007). C-terminal truncations in human 3'-5' DNA exonuclease TREX1 cause autosomal dominant retinal vasculopathy with cerebral leukodystrophy. *Nature Genetics, 39*, 1068–1070.

Rommelse, N. N., Altink, M. E., Martin, N. C., Buschgens, C. J., Buitelaar, J. K., Sergeant, J. A., et al. (2008). Neuropsychological measures probably facilitate heritability research of ADHD. *Archives of Clinical Neuropsychology, 23*, 579–591.

Rubino, E., Ferrero, M., Rainero, I., Binello, E., Vaula, G., & Pinessi, L. (2009). Association of the C677T polymorphism in the MTHFR gene with migraine: A meta-analysis. *Cephalalgia, 29*, 818–825.

Ruchoux, M. M., Domenga, V., Brulin, P., Maciazek, J., Limol, S., Tournier-Lasserve, E., et al. (2003). Transgenic mice expressing mutant Notch3 develop vascular alterations characteristic of cerebral autosomal dominant arteriopathy with subcortical infarcts and leukoencephalopathy. *American Journal of Pathology, 162*, 329–342.

Russell, M. B., & Ducros, A. (2011). Sporadic and familial hemiplegic migraine: Pathophysiological mechanisms, clinical characteristics, diagnosis, and management. *Lancet Neurology, 10*, 457–470.

Russell, M. B., & Olesen, J. (1995). Increased familial risk and evidence of genetic factor in migraine. *BMJ, 311*, 541–544.

Russell, M. B., & Olesen, J. (1996). A nosographic analysis of the migraine aura in a general population. *Brain, 119*, 355–361.

Russell, M. B., Ulrich, V., Gervil, M., & Olesen, J. (2002). Migraine without aura and migraine with aura are distinct disorders. A population-based twin survey. *Headache, 42*, 332–336.

Russo, L., Mariotti, P., Sangiorgi, E., Giordano, T., Ricci, I., Lupi, F., et al. (2007). A new susceptibility locus for migraine with aura in the 15q11-q13 genomic region containing three GABA-A receptor genes. *American Journal of Human Genetics, 76*, 327–333.

Scher, A. I., Terwindt, G. M., Verschuren, W. M., Kruit, M. C., Blom, H. J., Kowa, H., et al. (2006). Migraine and MTHFR C677T genotype in a population-based sample. *Annals of Neurology, 59*, 372–375.

Schur, E. A., Noonan, C., Buchwald, D., Goldberg, J., & Afari, N. (2009). A twin study of depression and migraine: Evidence for a shared genetic vulnerability. *Headache, 49*, 1493–1502.

Schurks, M., Rist, P. M., & Kurth, T. (2010). MTHFR 677C>T and ACE D/I polymorphisms in migraine: A systematic review and meta-analysis. *Headache, 50*, 588–599.

Schwaag, S., Evers, S., Schirmacher, A., Stogbauer, F., Ringelstein, E. B., & Kuhlenbaumer, G. (2006). Genetic variants of the NOTCH3 gene in migraine—a mutation analysis and association study. *Cephalalgia, 26*, 158–161.

Segall, L., Mezzetti, A., Scanzano, R., Gargus, J. J., Purisima, E., & Blostein, R. (2005). Alterations in the alpha2 isoform of Na,K-ATPase associated with familial hemiplegic migraine type 2. *Proceedings of the National Academy of Sciences of the United States of America, 102*, 11106–11111.

Segall, L., Scanzano, R., Kaunisto, M. A., Wessman, M., Palotie, A., Gargus, J. J., et al. (2004). Kinetic alterations due to a missense mutation in the Na,K-ATPase alpha2 subunit cause familial hemiplegic migraine type 2. *Journal of Biological Chemistry, 279*, 43692–43696.

Serra, S. A., Cuenca-Leon, E., Llobet, A., Rubio-Moscardo, F., Plata, C., Carreno, O., et al. (2010). A mutation in the first intracellular loop of CACNA1A prevents P./Q channel modulation by SNARE proteins and lowers exocytosis. *Proceedings of the National Academy of Sciences of the United States of America, 107*, 1672–1677.

Soragna, D., Vettori, A., Carraro, G., Marchioni, E., Vazza, G., Bellini, S., et al. (2003). A locus for migraine without aura maps on chromosome 14q21.2-q22.3. *American Journal of Human Genetics, 72*, 161–167.

Stam, A. H., Haan, J., van den Maagdenberg, A. M., Ferrari, M. D., & Terwindt, G. M. (2009). Migraine and genetic and acquired vasculopathies. *Cephalalgia, 29*, 1006–1017.

Stam, A. H., Louter, M. A., Haan, J., de Vries, B., van den Maagdenberg, A. M., Frants, R. R., et al. (2011). A long-term follow-up study of 18 patients with sporadic hemiplegic migraine. *Cephalalgia, 31*, 199–205.

Stam, A. H., Luijckx, G. J., Poll-The, B. T., Ginjaar, I. B., Frants, R. R., Haan, J., et al. (2009). Early seizures and cerebral oedema after trivial head trauma associated with the CACNA1A S218L mutation. *Journal of Neurology, Neurosurgery, and Psychiatry, 80*, 1125–1129.

Stam, A. H., de Vries, B., Janssens, A. C., Vanmolkot, K. R., Aulchenko, Y. S., Henneman, P., et al. (2010). Shared genetic factors in migraine and depression: Evidence from a genetic isolate. *Neurology, 74*, 288–294.

Stetson, D. B., Ko, J. S., Heidmann, T., & Medzhitov, R. (2008). Trex1 prevents cell-intrinsic initiation of autoimmunity. *Cell, 134*, 587–598.

Stewart, W. F., Bigal, M. E., Kolodner, K., Dowson, A., Liberman, J. N., & Lipton, R. B. (2006). Familial risk of migraine: Variation by proband age at onset and headache severity. *Neurology, 66*, 344–348.

Stewart, W. F., Shechter, A., & Rasmussen, B. K. (1994). Migraine prevalence. A review of population-based studies. *Neurology, 44*, S17–S23.

Stewart, W. F., Staffa, J., Lipton, R. B., & Ottman, R. (1997). Familial risk of migraine: A population-based study. *Annals of Neurology, 41*, 166–172.

Stovner, L. J., Zwart, J. A., Hagen, K., Terwindt, G. M., & Pascual, J. (2006). Epidemiology of headache in Europe. *European Journal of Neurology, 13*, 333–345.

Suzuki, M., Van Paesschen, W., Stalmans, I., Horita, S., Yamada, H., Bergmans, B. A., et al. (2010). Defective membrane expression of the Na(+)-HCO(3)(-) cotransporter NBCe1 is associated with familial migraine. *Proceedings of the National Academy of Sciences of the United States of America, 107*, 15963–15968.

Svensson, D. A., Larsson, B., Waldenlind, E., & Pedersen, N. L. (2003). Shared rearing environment in migraine: Results from twins reared apart and twins reared together. *Headache, 43*, 235–244.

Tavraz, N. N., Durr, K. L., Koenderink, J. B., Freilinger, T., Bamberg, E., Dichgans, M., et al. (2009). Impaired plasma membrane targeting or protein stability by certain ATP1A2 mutations identified in sporadic or familial hemiplegic migraine. *Channels (Austin), 3*, 82–87.

Tavraz, N. N., Friedrich, T., Durr, K. L., Koenderink, J. B., Bamberg, E., Freilinger, T., et al. (2008). Diverse functional consequences of mutations in the Na+/K+-ATPase alpha2-subunit causing familial hemiplegic migraine type 2. *Journal of Biological Chemistry, 283*, 31097–31106.

Teer, J. K., & Mullikin, J. C. (2010). Exome sequencing: The sweet spot before whole genomes. *Human Molecular Genetics, 19*, R145–R151.

Terwindt, G., Kors, E., Haan, J., Vermeulen, F., Van den Maagdenberg, A., Frants, R., et al. (2002). Mutation analysis of the CACNA1A calcium channel subunit gene in 27 patients with sporadic hemiplegic migraine. *Archives of Neurology, 59*, 1016–1018.

Terwindt, G. M., Haan, J., Ophoff, R. A., Groenen, S. M., Storimans, C. W., Lanser, J. B., et al. (1998). Clinical and genetic analysis of a large Dutch family with autosomal dominant vascular retinopathy, migraine and Raynaud's phenomenon. *Brain, 121*, 303–316.

Terwindt, G. M., Ophoff, R. A., van Eijk, R., Vergouwe, M. N., Haan, J., Frants, R. R., et al. (2001). Involvement of the CACNA1A gene containing region on 19p.13 in migraine with and without aura. *Neurology, 56*, 1028–1032.

Thomsen, L. L., Eriksen, M. K., Roemer, S. F., Andersen, I., Olesen, J., & Russell, M. B. (2002). A population-based study of familial hemiplegic migraine suggests revised diagnostic criteria. *Brain, 125*, 1379–1391.

Thomsen, L. L., Kirchmann, M., Bjornsson, A., Stefansson, H., Jensen, R. M., Fasquel, A. C., et al. (2007). The genetic spectrum of a population-based sample of familial hemiplegic migraine. *Brain, 130*, 346–356.

Tietjen, G. E., Al-Qasmi, M. M., Athanas, K., Utley, C., & Herial, N. A. (2007). Altered hemostasis in migraineurs studied with a dynamic flow system. *Thrombosis Research, 119*, 217–222.

Todt, U., Dichgans, M., Jurkat-Rott, K., Heinze, A., Zifarelli, G., Koenderink, J. B., et al. (2005). Rare missense variants in ATP1A2 in families with clustering of common forms of migraine. *Human Mutation, 26*, 315–321.

Todt, U., Freudenberg, J., Goebel, I., Netzer, C., Heinze, A., Heinze-Kuhn, K., et al. (2006). MTHFR C677T polymorphism and migraine with aura. *Annals of Neurology, 60*, 621–622; author reply 622–623.

Tottene, A., Conti, R., Fabbro, A., Vecchia, D., Shapovalova, M., Santello, M., et al. (2009). Enhanced excitatory transmission at cortical synapses as the basis for facilitated spreading depression in Ca(v)2.1 knockin migraine mice. *Neuron, 61*, 762–773.

Tottene, A., Fellin, T., Pagnutti, S., Luvisetto, S., Striessnig, J., Fletcher, C., et al. (2002). Familial hemiplegic migraine mutations increase Ca(2+) influx through single human CaV2.1 channels and decrease maximal CaV2.1 current density in neurons. *Proceedings of the National Academy of Sciences of the United States of America, 99*, 13284–13289.

Tottene, A., Pivotto, F., Fellin, T., Cesetti, T., van den Maagdenberg, A. M., & Pietrobon, D. (2005). Specific kinetic alterations of human CaV2.1 calcium channels produced by mutation S218L causing familial hemiplegic migraine and delayed cerebral edema and coma after minor head trauma. *Journal of Biological Chemistry, 280*, 17678–17686.

Tuulio-Henriksson, A., Haukka, J., Partonen, T., Varilo, T., Paunio, T., Ekelund, J., et al. (2002). Heritability and number of quantitative trait loci of neurocognitive functions in families with schizophrenia. *American Journal of Medical Genetics, 114*, 483–490.

Tzoulis, C., Engelsen, B. A., Telstad, W., Aasly, J., Zeviani, M., Winterthun, S., et al. (2006). The spectrum of clinical disease caused by the A467T and W748S POLG mutations: A study of 26 cases. *Brain, 129*, 1685–1692.

Ulrich, V., Gervil, M., Kyvik, K. O., Olesen, J., & Russell, M. B. (1999). Evidence of a genetic factor in migraine with aura: A population-based Danish twin study. *Annals of Neurology, 45*, 242–246.

Vahedi, K., Boukobza, M., Massin, P., Gould, D. B., Tournier-Lasserve, E., & Bousser, M. G. (2007). Clinical and brain MRI follow-up study of a family with COL4A1 mutation. *Neurology, 69*, 1564–1568.

Vahedi, K., Depienne, C., Le Fort, D., Riant, F., Chaine, P., Trouillard, O., et al. (2009). Elicited repetitive daily blindness: A new phenotype associated with hemiplegic migraine and SCN1A mutations. *Neurology, 72*, 1178–1183.

Vahedi, K., Massin, P., Guichard, J. P., Miocque, S., Polivka, M., Goutieres, F., et al. (2003). Hereditary infantile hemiparesis, retinal arteriolar tortuosity, and leukoencephalopathy. *Neurology, 60*, 57–63.

van den Maagdenberg, A. M., Pietrobon, D., Pizzorusso, T., Kaja, S., Broos, L. A., Cesetti, T., et al. (2004). A Cacna1a knockin migraine mouse model with increased susceptibility to cortical spreading depression. *Neuron, 41*, 701–710.

van den Maagdenberg, A. M., Pizzorusso, T., Kaja, S., Terpolilli, N., Shapovalova, M., Hoebeek, F. E., et al. (2010). High cortical spreading depression susceptibility and migraine-associated symptoms in Ca(v)2.1 S218L mice. *Annals of Neurology, 67*, 85–98.

Vanmolkot, F. H., Van Bortel, L. M., de Hoon, J. N. (2007). Altered arterial function in migraine of recent onset. *Neurology, 68*, 1563–1570.

Vanmolkot, K. R., Babini, E., de Vries, B., Stam, A. H., Freilinger, T., Terwindt, G. M., et al. (2007). The novel p.L1649Q mutation in the SCN1A epilepsy gene is associated with familial hemiplegic migraine: Genetic and functional studies. Mutation in brief #957. Online. *Human Mutation, 28*, 522.

Vanmolkot, K. R., Kors, E. E., Hottenga, J. J., Terwindt, G. M., Haan, J., Hoefnagels, W. A., et al. (2003). Novel mutations in the Na+, K+-ATPase pump gene ATP1A2 associated with familial hemiplegic migraine and benign familial infantile convulsions. *Annals of Neurology, 54*, 360–366.

Wessman, M., Kallela, M., Kaunisto, M. A., Marttila, P., Sobel, E., Hartiala, J., et al. (2002). A susceptibility locus for migraine with aura, on chromosome 4q24. *American Journal of Human Genetics, 70*, 652–662.

Westenbroek, R. E., Sakurai, T., Elliott, E. M., Hell, J. W., Starr, T. V., Snutch, T. P., et al. (1995). Immunochemical identification and subcellular distribution of the alpha 1A subunits of brain calcium channels. *Journal of Neuroscience, 15*, 6403–6418.

Wieser, T., Pascual, J., Oterino, A., Soso, M., Barmada, M., & Gardner, K. L. (2010). A novel locus for familial migraine on Xp22. *Headache, 50*, 955–962.

Winterthun, S., Ferrari, G., He, L., Taylor, R. W., Zeviani, M., Turnbull, D. M., et al. (2005). Autosomal recessive mitochondrial ataxic syndrome due to mitochondrial polymerase gamma mutations. *Neurology, 64*, 1204–1208.

Yu, F. H., Mantegazza, M., Westenbroek, R. E., Robbins, C. A., Kalume, F., Burton, K. A., et al. (2006). Reduced sodium current in GABAergic interneurons in a mouse model of severe myoclonic epilepsy in infancy. *Nature Neuroscience, 9*, 1142–1149.

Zangaladze, A., Asadi-Pooya, A. A., Ashkenazi, A., & Sperling, M. R. (2010). Sporadic hemiplegic migraine and epilepsy associated with CACNA1A gene mutation. *Epilepsy Behavior, 17*, 293–295.

Zhang, Z., Winborn, C. S., Marquez de Prado, B., & Russo, A. F. (2007). Sensitization of calcitonin gene-related peptide receptors by receptor activity-modifying protein-1 in the trigeminal ganglion. *Journal of Neuroscience, 27*, 2693–2703.

Zhuchenko, O., Bailey, J., Bonnen, P., Ashizawa, T., Stockton, D. W., Amos, C., et al. (1997). Autosomal dominant cerebellar ataxia (SCA6) associated with small polyglutamine expansions in the alpha 1A-voltage-dependent calcium channel. *Nature Genetics, 15*, 62–69.

Ziegler, D. K., Hur, Y. M., Bouchard, T. J. J., Hassanein, R. S., & Barter, R. (1998). Migraine in twins raised together and apart. *Headache, 38*, 417–422.

Part 4

Imaging Migraine

14 Imaging Migraine
A History

JES OLESEN AND PEER TFELT-HANSEN

INTRODUCTION

The history of migraine imaging may be divided into four epochs. The first epoch is the period until 1980, when thoughts about cerebral blood flow (CBF) in migraine were dominated by the so-called ischemic or vasospastic theory. In the second epoch from 1981 until 1990, most of our current knowledge about brain blood flow in migraine was gathered (Tfelt-Hansen, 2010). The third epoch lasted from 1991 until 2003. It confirmed and extended many of the findings from the 1980s using positron emission tomography (PET) or magnetic resonance imaging (MRI), and new important observations were made. The last and most recent epoch from 2004 onward is characterized by the application of advanced high-resolution imaging methods to the migraine problem. Determining CBF per se has diminished in importance, as imaging brain function and metabolism has became the focus of attention. This fourth epoch is the period to which most of the present volume is dedicated and so it will not be considered in this chapter, which focuses on the history of imaging migraine.

THE FIRST EPOCH: INVENTIVE, BUT FLAWED BY POOR METHODS

For centuries, migraine was considered a vascular headache because of the pulsating nature of migraine pain. In the late 19th century a neurogenic theory (Gowers, 1886–1888; Liveing 1873) was developed, which since then has competed with the vascular theory. Here we concentrate on the vascular changes observed in migraine and leave a discussion of the relative merits of these competing, but not mutually exclusive, hypotheses on migraine pathogenesis for others.

It was not until the early to mid-20th century that scientific evidence gave support to the vascular hypothesis The open cranial window animal experimental model with microscopic determination of pial arterial diameter.

Histamine, known to cause headache, proved in this model to be a dilator of pial arteries (Forbes et al., 1929). The next phase was the era of Harold G. Wolff (Wolff, 1963). He and his school devised many ingenious experiments with simple methods aimed at analyzing the relationship between migraine and vasodilatation. They measured pulsations of the spinal fluid, the effect of spinal fluid pressure increases on headache, and the pulsation of the superficial temporal artery (Graham & Wolff, 1938) and demonstrated the sensitivity of cranial blood vessels and other intracranial structures to painful stimuli in studies that are still valid today (Ray & Wolff, 1940). The conclusion of this era was that the migraine aura is caused by vasoconstriction and reduced brain blood flow. The relative cerebral ischemia would lead to reactive hyperemia, thought by some to explain the headache. Wolff, however, thought that the headache phase was caused by secondary vasodilation in the extracranial territory (Wolff, 1963). Increased intracranial pressure caused by injection of saline did not ameliorate migraine headache (Wolff, 1963), whereas headache induced by histamine infusion was improved by this procedure and hence was considered to be of intracranial origin (Wolff, 1963). The ischemic hypothesis was readily accepted in the medical community, often in a simplified or exaggerated form, forgetting that Wolff considered the pain to be extracranial and only indirectly due to reactive hyperemia of brain tissue. He anticipated some sort of intracranial/extracranial reflexes and anticipated the liberation of algogenic substances in the perivascular space of extracranial arteries (Wolff, 1963).

The Danish physiologist Niels A. Lassen developed the method of intracarotid injection of 133-Xenon for measuring regional cerebral blood flow (rCBF) during the 1960s. An atraumatic modification of his method used intravenous injection or inhalation of radioactive Xenon. This method was, however, fraught with methodological problems. Michael O'Brien found decreased blood flow during the aura and slightly increased blood flow after the aura but, typical of the poor sensitivity of the method, no difference between the hemispheres (O'Brien, 1971).

His findings were taken to support the vasospastic theory. Using the intracarotid 133-Xenon technique with 16 detectors, Skinhøj and Paulson (1969) investigated two patients. Blood flow was reduced during aura in the posterior part of the hemisphere in one patient and was increased in the other patient during the headache phase. Skinhøj (1973) further studied four patients during the aura, and all showed a severely reduced perfusion, while six patients examined during headache showed significant hyperperfusion and spinal fluid lactic acidosis. Their results were thought to support the ischemic hypothesis. Similar conclusions were drawn for studies by Simard and Paulson (1973), who demonstrated the lack of a vasodilator response to inhalation of 7% CO_2 during a migraine aura, and Norris (1975), who studied a patient before and after treatment of the headache with ergotamine and noted that rCBF was not reduced as ergotamine cured the headache.

THE SECOND EPOCH: CORTICAL SPREADING DEPRESSION CAUSES MIGRAINE WITH AURA BUT NOT MIGRAINE WITHOUT AURA

During the 1960s, Niels A. Lassen developed equipment to detect cerebral blood flow with an ever-increasing number of detectors (16 to 35) covering one hemisphere. This development made it possible for the first time to demonstrate localized changes in blood flow. In these studies Lassen pinpointed which brain regions had changes in blood flow during migraine with aura and how these changes progressed during a migraine attack. The development of imaging equipment with 254 detectors (Sveinsdottir et al., 1997) finally made it possible to give a highly detailed description of rCBF changes during migraine. In early single-patient studies with this equipment, Hachinski et al. (1977) described an individual with an atypical and very severe attack causing confusion and obtundation and very low blood flow. Conversely, in a patient without aura there were no changes in rCBF during attack (Hachinski et al., 1977). Subsequent to these case reports, it was the use of this equipment in larger patient groups, repeating measurements at short time intervals from the very beginning of the aura and into the headache phase, that led to the modern concepts of how brain blood flow changes in migraine.

The seminal breakthrough came in 1981 when Olesen and co-workers (1981) studied six patients with the 254-channel apparatus before and during the development of the aura and in some cases into the headache phase. The observations from these six patients were interpreted cautiously, because of their iconoclastic nature and the low number of subjects. In three cases the initial finding was a focal hyperemia. During the aura phase all six patients developed rCBF reduction, which in only one case approached ischemic values. The reduced blood flow started posteriorly and spread anteriorly in the course of 15 to 45 minutes. In four cases severe headache was present concomitantly with the low blood flow. The low-blood-flow area expanded gradually without respecting the territory of supply of the major cerebral arteries. Finally, functional activation by, for example, moving the hand or opening the eyes was abolished in the area of low blood flow. It was concluded that "The results indicate that the vasospastic model of the migraine attack is too simplistic. Alteration in neuronal function, in the blood-brain barrier, or in some other brain process is more likely to be the primary event of the attack" (Olesen, Lassen et al., 1981). The idea of cortical spreading depression was in the minds of the authors and was actually mentioned in a previous version of the manuscript but eliminated in the review process.

The observations in these six patients were unexpected and so were followed up by a prospective study designed to probe the new findings still further (Lauritzen et al., 1983a). rCBF measurements were repeated at shorter time intervals, allowing a more precise estimation of the spread of low blood flow. The rate of spread across the cortex was calculated to 3 mm/min. In the same series of patients the effect of changing blood pressure and carbon dioxide tension and the effect of functional activation were also studied (Lauritzen et al., 1983b). Functional activation by moving the hand or visual activation was almost abolished, while the reactivity to change in CO_2 was reduced to approximately half of normal. In contrast, the autoregulation to changes in blood pressure was normal in the low-flow area. In parallel with these studies, Olesen, Tfelt-Hansen et al. (1981) showed that brain blood flow remained normal during attacks of migraine without aura induced by red wine. There had already been observations of normal blood flow during migraine without aura, but this particular experiment was designed to pick up a hypothetical early asymptomatic reduction in brain blood flow similar to the findings in migraine with aura. Patients were hence studied before and at the very onset of an attack of migraine without aura. No changes were observed and this clearly distinguished migraine without aura from migraine with aura.

In the mid-1980s, Niels A. Lassen developed yet another revolutionary approach for the study of rCBF, single-photon computed emission tomography (SPECT) using inhalation of radioactive 133-Xenon (Stokely et al., 1980). This method allowed three-dimensional determination of rCBF and was atraumatic. Applying it to the study of acute migraine attacks, Lauritzen and Olesen (1984) demonstrated reduction in brain blood flow and in some cases spread of reduced blood flow in migraine with aura. During attacks of migraine without aura, rCBF remained completely normal. The particular value of this study was that the migraine attacks were spontaneous. Previous studies using the intracarotid Xenon method might be criticized for being induced by a carotid angiography. Subsequently, the SPECT technique was used to describe the longitudinal changes in brain blood flow during attacks of migraine with aura (Fig. 14–1). rCBF during or right after the aura showed the well-known reduction (Andersen et al., 1988). In an intermediate phase blood flow was normal, and in a later phase rCBF in the affected area was increased above normal. Finally, rCBF was normalized after 24 hours. Thus, the postulated hyperperfusion of Wolff was demonstrated, but it came at a late time, when headache was often cured and thus could not be responsible for the headache. What still remains to be done to this day is a study of the functional activation, CO_2 response, and blood flow autoregulation during attacks of migraine without aura.

In 1990, Olesen et al. analyzed 10 years of studies of rCBF in migraine (Olesen et al., 1990). Twenty patients had been investigated with the intracarotid technique

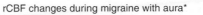
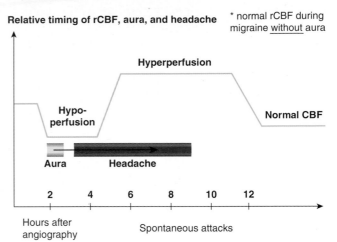

FIGURE 14–2 *Relation between regional cerebral blood flood (rCBF) and the different phases of attacks of migraine with aura. rCBF may be reduced before the onset of aura symptoms or at their very onset. This continues throughout the aura and into the headache phase. Subsequently and without a change in the headache, rCBF increases through normalization into an increase. This hyperperfusion continues even after headache has disappeared spontaneously or after treatment and then finally normalizes after many hours. Modified from Olesen, J., Friberg, L., Olesen, T. S., Iversen, H. K., Lassen, N. A., Andersen, A. R., et al. (1990). Timing and topography of cerebral blood flow, aura and headache during migraine attacks. Annals of Neurology, 28, 791–798.*

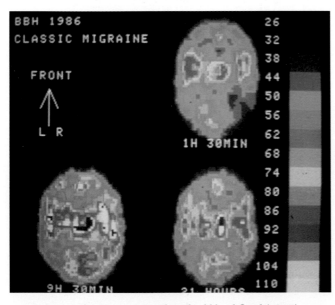

FIGURE 14–1 *Changes in regional cerebral blood flood (rCBF) over time during an attack of migraine with aura. At 1 hour and 30 minutes a low-flow area is observed in the right occipitotemporal area (blue color). At 9 hours and 30 minutes the same area shows an increased rCBF (red color). Finally, rCBF is symmetrical and normal at 21 hours. Reproduced from Andersen, A. R., Friberg, L., Olsen, T. S., & Olesen, J. (1988). Delayed hyperamia following hypoperfusion in classic migraine. Single photon emission tomographic demonstration. Archives of Neurology, 45, 154–159.*

providing results from the early phase of the attack, while 42 patients had been studied with SPECT providing data from the later phases of the attacks (Fig. 14–2). A number of conclusions could be drawn. Headache often started during the low-flow period and thus could not be caused by hyperemia. Furthermore, the low flow changed into high flow without any apparent change in headache, and the high flow often outlasted the headache. The great majority of patients had low flow on the side expected from their aura symptoms, while some had bilateral symptoms and very few had symptoms from the "wrong" hemisphere. On the basis of all this work, rCBF changes in migraine with aura were compared to findings during cortical spreading depression (Table 14–1). It was concluded that cortical spreading depression was the brain disturbance causing the migraine aura.

Unresolved Controversies

The first controversy in this epoch was whether rCBF is really different in migraine without aura and migraine with aura. While this was clearly so in the studies from the Copenhagen group as summarized above, there were

TABLE 14–1 *A Comparison of Cortical Spreading Depression (SD) and Regional Cerebral Blood Flow Findings during Attacks of Migraine with Aura*

	Migraine	SD
Site of origin	Primary visual cortex	High neurone density
Way of spread	Contiguous, cortical	Contiguous, cortical
Exitation/Depression	Yes	Yes
Rate of spread	2–6 mm/min	2–6 mm/min
Unilateral	Yes	Yes
Repeated waves	Yes	Yes
Initial hyperemia	Yes	Yes
Oligemia lasting	Hours	Hours
Degree of oligemia	Ischemic threshold	Less marked?
Cerebrovascular tone instability	Yes	?
Autoregulation	Preserved?	Preserved
CO_2 reactivity	Abolished?	Impaired
Provocation by arteriography	Yes	?

numerous reports of hyperemia in patients who had migraine without aura (common migraine at the time). In particular, the group of John Sterling Meyer in Houston, Texas, presented such data several times using inhalation of 133-Xenon (Mathew et al., 1976; Meyer et al., 1986; Sakai & Meyer, 1978) and also later using a stable Xenon method (Kobari et al., 1989). The issue was hotly debated at the first International Headache Research Seminar held in Copenhagen in 1991 (Olesen, 1991). The Copenhagen group had given a better patient description and used better rCBF methods, but the issue could not be definitively resolved at that time. Part of the problem was also that most groups did not distinguish sharply enough between migraine with and without aura, this being defined only in 1988 (Headache Classification Committee of the International Headache Society, 1988).

Just as it seemed clear that rCBF in migraine with aura was due to cortical spreading depression, a younger member of the Copenhagen group criticized the finding of previous studies by Olesen, Lauritzen, and others. Tom Skyhoej Olsen claimed that the changes observed in previous papers were actually indications of brain ischemia and that the ischemic hypothesis was still in force. He made elaborate corrections of scattered radiation (Compton scatter) and claimed that a slow reduction in rCBF caused by spasm of a major artery could explain previous findings of a slow spread of oligemia. Much international confusion ensued, not least because of the surname Olsen, which was confused with Jes Olesen. While Lauritzen and associates presented theoretical

arguments against Skyhoej Olsen, and Jes Olesen presented clinical arguments, the matter was again difficult to resolve completely at the time (Dalgaard et al., 1991; Kronborg et al., 1990).

A final controversy concerned the classification of migraine. On the basis of the findings of Olesen and others, the Copenhagen school maintained that there were major pathophysiological differences between migraine with aura and migraine without aura (classic migraine and common migraine). A clear distinction was first made in the first edition of the International Headache Classification (Headache Classification Committee of International Headache Society, 1988), where the terms *migraine with aura* and *migraine without aura* were coined and separate diagnostic criteria were developed for these two kinds of migraine. However, a critique of this subdivision was maintained from several quarters, most fiercely by Dr. Nathan Blau and associates (Blau, 1995). The dispute continues until this day, despite the fact that many differences in genetics, pathophysiology, and pharmacology have now been documented.

THE THIRD EPOCH: CONFIRMATION, RESOLUTION OF CONTROVERSIES, AND IMPORTANT NEW FINDINGS

In this epoch methods with better spatial resolution, no Compton scatter, and to some extent better time resolution were employed such as PET and perfusion-weighted

MRI (Cutrer et al., 1998; Hadjikhani et al., 2001; Woods et al., 1994). The vasospastic/ischemic theory was refuted in such studies that supported the gradual spread of low blood flow across arterial territories and showed that blood flow was reduced, but rarely to ischemic levels. In one of the most important studies, Hadjikhani et al. (2001) investigated three patients with visual aura using functional MRI. Changes in activity within the occipital cortex were mapped during the aura. In one patient with an exercise-induced aura, a perturbation in the blood oxygenation level–dependent (BOLD) signal progressed sequentially along the calcarine cortex beginning posteriorly and spreading anteriorly. It was concluded that the migraine aura was accompanied by a propagating brain event that was retinotopically related to the visual percept, probably a cortical spreading depression. Thus, the findings of the Copenhagen group in the 1980s were confirmed in finer detail and Skyhoej Olsen's revival of the ischemic hypothesis could finally be buried.

The differences between migraine with aura and migraine without aura were also largely confirmed in the 1990s and early 2000s. Thus, no change in perfusion-weighted MRI were found during attacks of migraine without aura (Sanchez Del Rio et al., 1999), Afridi et al. (2004, 2005), using $H_2{}^{15}O$-labled PET, studied 24 migraine patients in whom attacks of migraine without aura were induced by infusion of nitroglycerin and one patient during a spontaneous migraine attack. No mention was made of any hypoperfusion in the cerebral hemispheres during migraine attacks. While there is near consensus that cortical spreading depression–like changes in brain blood flow are only observed in migraine with aura, a single case who developed a migraine attack in the PET machine demonstrated bilateral cortical spreading oligemia and no definite aura symptoms were reported (Woods et al., 1994). This is the only patient found to have migraine without aura in whom such changes have ever been described. It is also the only case where changes were bilateral. More important, Denuelle et al. (2008) investigated seven patients with spontaneous migraine without aura using PET. Measurements were taken at a mean of 3 hours from the onset of attack and after headache relief by sumatriptan injection as well as in an attack-free period. A slight but significant posterior cortical hypoperfusion was shown that did not change after sumatriptan administration. The authors suggested that migraine with and without aura may have a common pathogenesis. This view was also supported by animal experiments demonstrating that prophylactic antimigraine drugs inhibit cortical spreading depression (Ayata et al., 2006). However, apart from the above-mentioned PET studies, no other study has shown reduced rCBF in migraine without aura and

no study has shown spreading oligemia in migraine without aura. Thus, it still seems overwhelmingly likely that no cortical spreading depression and no spreading hypoperfusion is present during attacks of migraine without aura.

The most important novel finding during this third migraine imaging epoch was perhaps the demonstration by Weiller et al. (1995) of a hyperemic area in the brainstem during attacks of migraine without aura. This increase persisted after alleviation of the attack by sumatriptan injection, but was not found outside of the migraine attack. It was hypothesized, therefore, that this activation might be a "driver" of the migraine attack. Subsequently, the term *migraine generator* was used to describe this regional response. This description might, however, be somewhat of an exaggeration since such brainstem changes of this nature have never been shown to precede a migraine attack. These imaging findings were partly reproduced by the Goadsby group (Afridi et al., 2005), but while the brainstem activation was contralateral to pain in one study, it was found to be ipsilateral in the other. These findings greatly stimulated the interest in brainstem activation as a possible driver of the migraine attack. In the cerebral cortex, the improved spatial resolution of PET demonstrated clear activation of the pain matrix during attacks of migraine without aura. Thus, the earlier findings of normal rCBF in the 1980s must be a result of the relatively poor spatial resolution and analytical methods used in the SPECT studies. However, the activation of the pain matrix was not specific to migraine but simply secondary to pain itself and therefore of little interest to the understanding of the pathological changes specific to migraine.

THE FOURTH EPOCH: MOVING FROM BLOOD FLOW TO CEREBRAL FUNCTION

While past studies allowed some inference about cerebral function because rCBF usually reflects metabolic need resulting from changes in cortical activity, the direct study of activation of the cerebral cortex and deeper cerebral structures became possible only relatively recently. This present book has its focuses on these investigations and so they will not be reviewed here. As reported by others in this book, the activation of different parts of the brain during migraine attacks is now being examined and, for the first time, the diameter of relatively small brain and dural arteries can now be measured directly using high-resolution magnetic resonance angiography. The combination of these high temporal and spatial resolution brain imaging methods with novel ways of inducing migraine attacks so that their evolution can be studied in the imaging laboratory is potentially a very rewarding future path forward. The new MRI and PET techniques hold great promise to shed more light on the old controversy of whether migraine with aura and migraine without aura are fundamentally different and to build on the discoveries made during the last 30 years by using the new imaging technologies to build new concepts and hypotheses that have to be solved in future investigations.

REFERENCES

Afridi, S. K., Kaube, H., & Goadsby, P. J. (2004). Glyceryl trinitrate triggers premonitory symptoms in migraineurs. *Pain, 110*, 675–680.

Afridi, S. K., Matharu, M. S., Lee, L., Kaube, H., Friston, K. J., Frackowiak, R. S., et al. (2005). A positron emission tomographic study in spontaneous migraine. *Archives of Neurology, 62*, 1270–1275.

Andersen, A. R., Friberg, L., Olsen, T. S., & Olesen, J. (1988). Delayed hyperamia following hypoperfusion in classic migraine. Single photon emission tomographic demonstration. *Archives of Neurology, 45*, 154–159.

Ayata, C., Hin, H., Kudo, C., Dalkara, T., & Moskowitz, M. A. (2006). Suppression of cortical spreading depression in migraine prophylaxis. *Annals of Neurology, 59*, 652–661.

Blau, J. N. (1995). Migraine with aura and migraine without aura are not different entities. *Cephalalgia, 15*, 186–190.

Cutrer, F. M., Sorensen, A. G., Weisskoff, R. M., Østergaard, L., Sanchez del Rio, M., Lee, J. E., et al. (1998). Perfusion-weighted imaging defects during spontaneous migrainous aura. *Annals of Neurology, 43*, 25–31.

Dalgaard, P., Kronborg, D., & Lauritzen, M. (1991). Migraine with aura, cerebral ischemia, spreading depression, and Compton scatter. *Headache, 31*, 49–53.

Denuelle, M., Fabre, N., Payoux, P., Chollet, F., & Geraud, G. (2008). Posterior cerebral hypoperfusion in migraine without aura. *Cephalalgia, 28*, 856–862.

Forbes, H. S., Wolff, H. G., & Cobb, S. (1929). The cerebral circulation. X. The action of histamine. *American Journal of Physiology, 89*, 266–272.

Gowers, W. (1886–1888). *A manual of diseases of the nervous system.* London: Churchill.

Graham, J. R., & Wolff, H. G. (1938). Mechanism of migraine headache and action of ergotamine tartrate. *Archives of Neurology and Psychiatry, 39*, 737–763.

Hachinski, V. C., Olesen, J., Norris, J. W., Larsen, B., Enevoldsen, E., & Lassen, N. A. (1977). Cerebral hemodynamics in migraine. *Canadian Journal of Neurological Science, 4*, 244–249.

Hajdikhani, N., Sanchez del Rio, M., Wu, O., Schwartz, D., Bakker, D., Fischl, B., et al. (2001). Mechanisms of migraine aura revealed by functional MRI in human visual cortex. *Proceedings of the National Academy of Sciences of the United States of American, 8*, 4687–4692.

Headache Classification Committee of the International Headache Society. (1988). Classification and diagnostic criteria for headache disorder, cranial neuralgias and facial pain. *Cephalalgia, 8*(Suppl 7), 1–96.

Kobari, M., Meyer, J. S., Ichijo, M., Imai, A., & Oravez, W. T. (1989). Hyperperfusion of cerebral cortex, thalamus and basal ganglia during spontaneously occurring migraine headaches. *Headache, 29*, 282–289.

Kronborg, D., Dalgaard, P., & Lauritzen, M. (1990). Ischemia may be the primary cause of neurological deficits in classic migraine. *Archives of Neurology, 47*, 124–127.

Lauritzen, M., & Olesen, J. (1984). Regional cerebral blood flow during migraine attacks by Xenon-133 inhalation and emission tomography. *Brain, 107*, 447–461.

Lauritzen, M., Olsen, T. S., Lassen, N. A., & Paulson, O. B. (1983a). Changes in regional cerebral blood flow during the course of classic migraine attacks. *Annals of Neurology, 13*, 633–641.

Lauritzen, M., Olsen, T. S., Lassen, N. A., & Paulson, O. B. (1983b). Regulation of regional cerebral blood flow during and between migraine attacks. *Annals of Neurology, 14*, 569–572.

Liveing, E. (1873). *On megrin, sick-headache, and related disorder. A contribution to the pathology of nerve-storms.* London: J. and A. Churchill.

Mathew, N. T., Hrastnik, F., & Meyer, J. S. (1976). Regional cerebral blood flow in the diagnosis of vascular headache. *Headache, 15*, 252–260.

Meyer, J. S., Zetusky, W., Jonsdottir, M., & Mortel, K. (1986). Cephalic hyperemia during migraine headaches. A prospective study. *Headache, 26*, 388–397.

Norris, J. W., Hachinski, V. C., & Cooper, P. W. (1975). Changes in cerebral blood flow during a migraine attack. *BMJ, 3*, 676–677.

O'Brien, M. D. (1971). Cerebral blood changes in migraine. *Headache, 10*, 139–143.

Olesen, J. (1991). *Migraine and other headaches: The vascular mechanisms* (pp. 1–358). New York: Raven Press.

Olesen, J., Friberg, L., Olesen, T. S., Iversen, H. K., Lassen, N. A., Andersen, A. R., et al. (1990). Timing and topography of cerebral blood flow, aura and headache during migraine attacks. *Annals of Neurology, 28*, 791–798.

Olesen, J., Larsen, B., & Lauritzen, M. (1981). Focal hyperemia followed by spreading oligemia and impaired activation of rCBF in classic migraine. *Annals of Neurology, 9*, 344–352.

Olesen, J., Tfelt-Hansen, P., Henriksen, L., & Larsen, B. (1981). Common migraine may not be initiated by cerebral ischemia. *Lancet, II*, 438–440.

Olsen, T. S., Friberg, L., & Lassen, N. A. (1987). Ischemia may be the primary cause of the neurological deficits in classic migraine. *Archives of Neurology, 44*, 156–161.

Ray, B. S., & Wolff, H. G. (1940). Experimental studies on headache: Pain sensitive structures of the brain and their significance in headache. *Archives of Surgery, 1*, 813–856.

Sakai, F., & Meyer, J. S. (1978). Regional cerebral hemodynamics during migraine and cluster headache measured by the 133Xe inhalation method. *Headache, 18*, 122–132.

Sanchez Del Rio, M., Bakker, D., Wu, O., Agosti, R., Mitsikostas, D. D., Ostergaard, L., et al. (1999). Perfusion weighted imaging during migraine: Spontaneous visual aura and headache. *Cephalalgia, 19*, 701–707.

Simard, D., & Paulson, O. B. (1973). Cerebral vasomotor paralysis during migraine attack. *Archives of Neurology, 29*, 207–209.

Skinhøj, E. (1973). Hemodynamic studies within the brain during migraine. *Archives of Neurology, 29*, 95–98.

Skinhøj, E., & Paulson, O. B. (1969). Regional blood flow in internal carotid distribution during migraine attack. *BMJ, 3*, 569–570.

Stokely, E. M., Sveinsdottir, E., Lassen N. A., & Rommer, P. (1980). A single photon dynamic computer assisted tomography

(DCAT) for imaging brain function in multiple cross sections. *Journal of Computer Assisted Tomography, 4,* 230–240.

Sveinsdottir, E., Larsen, B., Rommer, P., & Lassen, N. A. (1977). A multidetector scintillation camera with 254 channels. *Journal of Nuclear Medicine, 18,* 168–174.

Tfelt-Hansen, P. (2010). History of migraine with aura and cortical spreading depression from 1941 and onward. *Cephalalgia, 30,* 780–792.

Weiller, C., May, A., Limroth, V., Jüpter, M., Kaube, H., Schayck, R. V., et al. (1995). Brain stem activation in spontaneous human migraine attacks. *Nature Medicine, 1,* 658–660.

Wolff, H. G. (1963). *Headache and other head pain* (2nd ed.). New York: Oxford University Press.

Woods, R. P., Iacoboni, M., & Mazziotta, J. C. (1994). Brief report: Bilateral spreading hypoperfusion during spontaneous migraine headache. *New England Journal of Medicine, 331,* 1689–1692.

15 Focus on the Midbrain in Migraine

HANS-CHRISTOPH DIENER AND ARNE MAY

Migraine has a complex pathophysiology (Aurora & Nagesh, 2011; Goadsby et al., 2009). As shown in this chapter, the brainstem and midbrain play a crucial role in migraine. Functional and structural brain imaging was instrumental in elucidating the role of the midbrain in migraine (Cutrer & Black, 2006).

EARLY OBSERVATIONS

Raskin et al. (1987) reported on 15 of 175 patients, previously headache free, who underwent electrode implantation in the periaqueductal gray (PAG) and more specifically the dorsal raphe nucleus (DRN) for the treatment of intractable low-back pain. Either immediately or a few days after implantation, the patients reported severe continuous head pain with "migrainous" features, which persisted for 2 months to 10 years. These headaches were responsive to migraine treatment and some of the patients also developed aura symptoms. This observation was reproduced by Veloso et al. (1998) and was the first report indicating that the PAG or neighboring structures might have a role in the pathophysiology of headache and in particular migraine.

EARLY IMAGING DATA

Based on the above observations, Weiller et al. (1995) performed the first study with positron emission tomography (PET) in migraine patients during and outside of migraine attacks. In nine patients with right-sided headache, regional cerebral blood flow (rCBF) was measured using a ^{15}C-labeled O$_2$ inhalation technique during a spontaneous migraine attack. Each patient had three rCBF measurements:

1. During the attack
2. After relief from the headache by 6 mg sumatriptan given subcutaneously
3. During the headache-free interval

The authors observed a strong rCBF increase during the attack in several brain structures including the brainstem and midbrain compared to the headache-free interval (Fig. 15–1). This activation was slightly lateralized to the left. Attributing these activations to distinct anatomical nuclei was difficult at that time, given the poor spatial resolution of PET scanners. Moreover, these activations spanned brainstem structures over several planes. These structures were toward the midline but contralateral to the headache side and have most recently been refined in their localization to the dorsal pons (Bahra et al., 2001). The injection of sumatriptan relieved the patients from headache while they were still in the scanner. Another investigation immediately after patients became headache free due to sumatriptan administration showed that the activation of brainstem and midbrain structures persisted when compared to the headache-free interval. Therefore, it was considered unlikely that this activation was only due to increased activity of the endogenous antinociceptive system. The persistence of brainstem and midbrain activation after successful treatment with sumatriptan could also explain the phenomenon of headache recurrence after initial efficacy of a triptan (Pascual et al., 2007).

The results by Weiller et al. were replicated in a case study where the authors wanted to study a patient with cluster headache using H$_2$^{15}O-activation PET and triggering the attack using glyceryl titrate (Bahra et al., 2001). However, the patient developed a typical migraine attack and during this attack activation in the dorsal rostral brainstem was detected.

LATERALITY OF BRAINSTEM ACTIVATION IN MIGRAINE

A PET study performed by the Headache Group and the Wellcome Department of Imaging in London investigated in 24 migraineurs whether increased cerebral blood flow can be lateralized with respect to the side of the headache (Afridi et al., 2005). Migraine attacks were induced by infusion of glyceryl trinitrate (GTN). H$_2$^{15}O-labeled PET was used in 24 migraineurs and 8 healthy controls. The patients

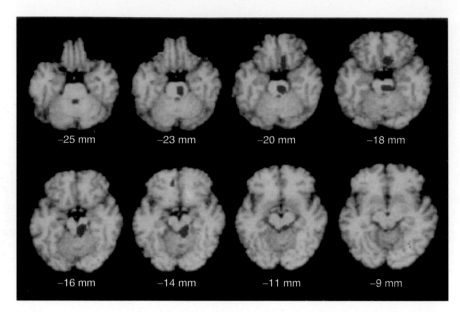

FIGURE 15–1 *Comparison of acute migraine attack and headache-free interval in nine patients with migraine without aura. The activations during the attack are shown as statistical parametric maps that show the areas of significant regional cerebral blood flow (rCBF) increases (p < .001) in red superimposed on an anatomical reference image derived from a T1-weighted magnetic resonance image. Numbers refer to the relative distance to the ACPC line (joining the anterior and posterior commissures), which is situated at 0 mm. The anterior part of the brain corresponds to the top of the image, the posterior parts to the bottom. The left side of each image is the right side of the brain. Significant increases in rCBF were detected over several planes in the brainstem slightly lateralized to the left, anterior to the aqueduct and posterior to the cranial nerve nuclei in the periaqueductal gray matter and midbrain reticular formation, as well as in the infero-antero-caudal part of the cingulated gyrus (Brodmann area 25). From Weiller, C., May, A., Limmroth, V., Jüptner, M., Kaube, H., Schayck, R. V., et al. (1995). Brain stem activation in spontaneous human migraine attacks.* Nature Medicine, 1, 658–660, Fig. 2.

were scanned four times: (a) preinfusion, (b) during GTN, (c) during migraine, and (d) after migraine. One could argue that GTN-induced migraine attacks are not comparable with spontaneous attacks of migraine. The Copenhagen group, however, showed in an elegant series of experiments that GTN-induced migraine attacks share many features with spontaneous attacks (Christiansen et al., 1999, 2000; Iversen et al., 1989; Thomsen et al., 1994).

Eight patients each had right- or left-sided headache and eight patients had bilateral migraine. Significant brainstem activation was seen in the dorsal lateral pons during migraine attacks compared to controls. Dorsal pontine activation was ipsilateral in lateralized headache and bilateral in patients with bilateral headache (Fig. 15–2). Consistent with the study of Weiller et al. (1995), the increase in rCBF persisted after headache was treated with 6 mg of sumatriptan subcutaneously. The authors concluded that unilateral headache in migraine results from asymmetrical brainstem dysfunction. In addition, eight patients with chronic migraine (>15 days per month of attacks of migraine without aura), who had shown a marked beneficial response to implanted bilateral suboccipital stimulators, were studied with PET. Comparison of

stimulation (improved headache) with no stimulation (headache) demonstrated significant changes in rCBF in the dorsal rostral pons, anterior cingulate cortex, and cuneus, which correlated with pain scores (Matharu et al., 2004). The localization and persistence of activity during stimulation was exactly consistent with the activity in the dorsal pontine region observed in episodic migraine and suggests a fundamental role for this structure in the pathophysiology of chronic migraine.

A French group investigated seven patients with migraine during spontaneous migraine attacks with $H_2^{15}O$ PET within 4 hours of onset, after headache relief by sumatriptan injection, and during the attack-free period (Denuelle et al., 2007). The authors reported significant activations not only in the midbrain and pons (Fig. 15–3) but also in the hypothalamus, which, just like the brainstem activation in the first study, persisted after headache relief with sumatriptan. Specific hypothalamic activation has been reported in the trigeminal autonomic cephalgias (May, 2009; May et al., 1998) but had not previously been observed in migraine. A major limitation of this study, however, is that it did not have a control group and is, therefore, potentially confounded by order and session effects.

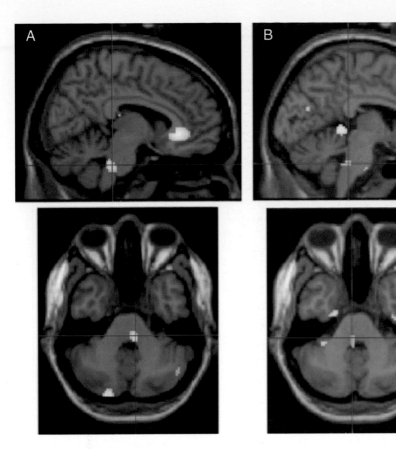

FIGURE 15–2 *Activation of the ipsilateral pons in patients with right-sided attacks (n = 8) and left-sided attacks (n = 8). The lower row shows right sided attacks (on the left side of the picture) and left sided attacks (on the right side of the picture). From Afridi, S. K., Matharu, M. S., Lee, L., Kaube, H., Friston, K. J., Frackowiak, R. S., et al. (2005). A PET study exploring the laterality of brainstem activation in migraine using glyceryl trinitrate.* Brain, 128, 932–939, Fig. 4.

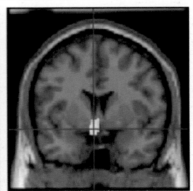

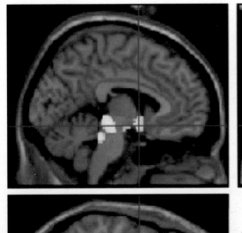

Activations during migraine attack, before sumatriptan, are shown as statistical parametric maps which show the areas of significant rCBF increases (p<0.001 uncorrected) in colour superimposed on an anatomical reference derived from a T1-weighted MRI. The hypothalamic activation is seen at the point of intersection.

FIGURE 15–3 *Hypothalamic activation during spontaneous migraine attacks in seven patients. Denuelle, M., Fabre, N., Payoux, P., Chollet, F., & Geraud, G. (2007). Hypothalamic activation in spontaneous migraine attacks.* Headache, 47, 1418–1426, Fig. 2.

Recently, the first imaging study using functional magnetic resonance imaging (fMRI) and an event-related paradigm reported that migraineurs showed a significant increase in activation of rostral parts of the pons (Stankewitz et al., 2011). Interestingly, this area only showed higher activation during the attack and not between attacks or shortly before an attack. This was unlike the activation in spinal trigeminal nuclei in response to nociceptive stimulation, which showed a cycling behavior over the migraine interval. While interictal (i.e., outside of attack) migraine patients revealed lower activations in the spinal trigeminal nuclei compared to controls, preictal (i.e., shortly before attack) patients showed activity similar to controls, which demonstrates that the trigeminal activation level increases over the pain-free migraine interval. Remarkably, the distance to the next headache attack was predictable by the height of the signal intensities in the spinal nuclei. Migraine patients scanned during the acute spontaneous migraine attack showed significantly lower signal intensities in the trigeminal nuclei compared with controls, demonstrating activity levels similar to interictal patients. The question arises whether other structures may operate as modulators of neuronal activity in the spinal trigeminal nuclei, namely, the endogenous pain control system, such as the PAG or the raphe nuclei (Wang & Nakai, 1994). The PAG modulates nociception via a descending pathway that relays in the rostral ventromedial medulla (RVM) and terminates in the spinal cord. The RVM has distinct cell classes that directly inhibit or facilitate nociception (Fields, 2004). Further evidence for deficient inhibition comes from a study reporting hypofunctional structures in the midbrain in migraineurs (Moulton et al., 2008).

Given that the brainstem was not specifically activated in the preictal state and given the clinical progression of the migraine cycle, it is tempting to consider oscillating impulse generators in the limbic system, perhaps including the hypothalamus, that may have (indirect) modulating effects on the activation level of the trigeminal nuclei toward an attack, which is succeeded by a specific activation of the rostral parts of the pons in the actual headache attack. Either way, the spinal trigeminal nuclei are key structures with rising excitability toward a migraine attack, whereas the increased activation in the rostral pons, the so-called migraine generator, occurs on a secondary level and only during the attack (Stankewitz et al., 2011).

BRAINSTEM LESIONS AND MIGRAINE

The assumption gained from PET imaging that the midbrain plays an important role in migraine spurred several case reports of de novo migraine in patients with lesions in this area. The first report was by Haas et al. (1993). They reported a case of multiple sclerosis with a lesion in the brainstem and severe migraine. This was also reported in two other cases of patients with multiple sclerosis (Fragoso & Brooks, 2007). Both patients developed severe treatment-refractory migraine in temporal relationship with an acute exacerbation of multiple sclerosis. Brain MRI showed lesions in the brainstem in the area of the PAG. Goadsby (2002) reported a patient who was headache free and developed severe chronic migraine after bleeding into a cavernoma in the midbrain. We observed a 38-year-old woman with symptomatic strictly right-sided migraine associated with a pontine cavernoma affecting the contralateral (left) nucleus raphe magnus (Katsarava et al., 2003). A persistent facilitation of the right-sided trigeminal nociception was detected interictally using the nociception-specific blink reflex, which was more pronounced during the acute attack. This case showed an impairment of the antinociceptive brainstem nuclei and the facilitation of the trigeminal nociception in the same subject, thus providing further evidence for the key role of the brainstem raphe nuclei in the pathophysiology of migraine. Of note, all the above lesions were quite large, taking into account the anatomical and functional complexity of the brainstem and that the brainstem is relatively small compared to the brain. Most lesions described above may have covered the migraine-specific area described in PET observations but have certainly spanned a region of up to 3 cm. Given that PET imaging has identified a region that is most certainly smaller than 10 mm, these clinical observations have to be interpreted with great caution.

BRAINSTEM AND MORPHOMETRIC IMAGING

Using morphometric imaging in migraine (see Chapter 18), Rocca et al. (2006), in a pioneering study, reported an increased density of the periaqueductal gray and of the dorsolateral pons in patients with migraine. The fact that four independent studies did not replicate this finding is difficult to interpret; one possible explanation for this discrepancy is that the latter studies used a 1.5-Tesla scanner, whereas Rocca et al. used a higher field strength (3 Tesla), which may enable the detection of more-subtle differences.

Welch et al. (2001) studied iron hemostasis in the PAG in patients with episodic migraine, daily chronic headache, and controls. The authors used sophisticated transverse relaxation rates R2, R2*, and R2' in a high-resolution magnetic resonance scanner. In the PAG there was a significant increase in iron deposits both in patients with episodic migraine and in patients with chronic daily headache. There was a clear correlation between duration of illness and R2'. These findings were replicated by a Dutch group (Kruit et al., 2009), and both reports underline at least the role of the PAG as a potential "generator" of migraine attacks.

In conclusion, dysfunction of the regulation of brainstem nuclei involved in antinociception and extra- and intracerebral vascular control provides a far-reaching explanation for many of the facets in migraine (Goadsby et al., 1991; Lance et al., 1983) The importance of the brainstem for the genesis of migraine is further underlined by the presence of binding sites for specific antimigraine compounds on these structures (Goadsby & Gundlach, 1991). The challenge now is to reveal the functional consequences of such findings as discussed above, to understand their implications, and to assess their therapeutic potential.

REFERENCES

Afridi, S. K., Matharu, M. S., Lee, L., Kaube, H., Friston, K. J., Frackowiak, R. S., et al. (2005). A PET study exploring the laterality of brainstem activation in migraine using glyceryl trinitrate. *Brain, 128*, 932–939.

Aurora, S. K., & Nagesh, V. (2011). Pathophysiology of migraine. *Handbook of Clinical Neurology, 97*, 267–273.

Bahra, A., Matharu, M. S., Büchel, C., Frackowiak, R. S. J., & Goadsby, P. J. (2001). Brainstem activation specific to migraine headache. *Lancet, 357*, 1016–1017.

Christiansen, I., Daugaard, D., Lykke Thomsen, L., & Olesen, J. (2000) Glyceryl trinitrate induced headache in migraineurs—relation to attack frequency. *European Journal of Neurology, 7*, 405–411.

Christiansen, I., Thomsen, L. L., Daugaard, D., Ulrich, V., & Olesen, J. (1999). Glyceryl trinitrate induces attacks of migraine without aura in sufferers of migraine with aura. *Cephalalgia, 19*, 660–667; discussion 626.

Cutrer, F. M., & Black, D. F. (2006). Imaging findings of migraine. *Headache, 46*, 1095–1107.

Denuelle, M., Fabre, N., Payoux, P., Chollet, F., & Geraud, G. (2007). Hypothalamic activation in spontaneous migraine attacks. *Headache, 47*, 1418–1426.

Fields, H. (2004). State-dependent opioid control of pain. *Nature Reviews Neuroscience, 5*, 565–575.

Fragoso, Y. D., & Brooks, J. B. (2007). Two cases of lesions in brainstem in multiple sclerosis and refractory migraine. *Headache, 47*, 852–854.

Goadsby, P. (2002). Neurovascular headache and a midbrain vascular malformation: Evidence for a role of the brainstem in chronic migraine. *Cephalalgia, 22*(2), 107–111.

Goadsby, P. J., Charbit, A. R., Andreou, A. P., Akerman, S., & Holland, P. R. (2009). Neurobiology of migraine. *Neuroscience, 161*, 327–341.

Goadsby, P. J., & Gundlach, A. L. (1991). Localization of 3H-hihydroergotamine-binding sites in the cat central nervous system: relevance to migraine. *Annals of Neurology, 29*, 91–94.

Goadsby, P. J., Zagami, A. S., & Lambert, G. A. (1991). Neural processing of craniovascular pain: A synthesis of the central structures involved in migraine. *Headache, 31*, 365–371.

Haas, D. C., Kent, P. F., & Friedman, D. I. (1993). Headache caused by a single lesion of multiple sclerosis in the periaqueductal gray area. *Headache, 33*, 452–455.

Iversen, H. K., Olesen, J., & Tfelt-Hansen, P. (1989). Intravenous nitroglycerin as an experimental headache model. Basic characteristics. *Pain, 38*, 17–24.

Katsarava, Z., Egelhof, T., Kaube, H., Diener, H., & Limmroth, V. (2003). Symptomatic migraine and sensitization of trigeminal nociception associated with contralateral pontine cavernoma. *Pain, 105*, 381–384.

Kruit, M. C., Launer, L. J., Overbosch, J., van Buchem, M. A., & Ferrari, M. D. (2009). Iron accumulation in deep brain nuclei in migraine: A population-based magnetic resonance imaging study. *Cephalalgia, 29*, 351–359.

Lance, J. W., Lambert, G. A., Goadsby, P. J., & Duckworth, J. W. (1983). Brainstem influences on cephalic circulation: Experimental data from cat and monkey of relevance to the mechanism of migraine. *Headache, 23*, 258–265.

Matharu, M. S., Bartsch, T., Ward, N., Frackowiak, R. S., Weiner, R., & Goadsby, P. J. (2004). Central neuromodulation in chronic migraine patients with suboccipital stimulators: A PET study. *Brain, 127*, 220–230.

May, A. (2009). New insights into headache: An update on functional and structural imaging findings. *Nature Reviews Neurology, 5*, 199–209.

May, A., Bahra, A., Buchel, C., Frackowiak, R. S., & Goadsby, P. J. (1998). Hypothalamic activation in cluster headache attacks. *Lancet, 352*, 275–278.

Moulton, E. A., Burstein, R., Tully, S., Hargreaves, R., Becerra, L., & Borsook, D. (2008). Interictal dysfunction of a brainstem descending modulatory center in migraine patients. *PLoS One, 3*, e3799.

Pascual, J., Mateos, V., Roig, C., Sanchez-Del-Rio, M., & Jimenez, D. (2007). Marketed oral triptans in the acute treatment of migraine: A systematic review on efficacy and tolerability. *Headache, 47*, 1152–1168.

Raskin, N. H., Hosobuchi, Y., & Lamb, S. (1987). Headache may arise from perturbation of brain. *Headache, 27*, 416–420.

Rocca, M. A., Ceccarelli, A., Falini, A., Colombo, B., Tortorella, P., Bernasconi, L., et al. (2006). Brain gray matter changes in migraine patients with T2-visible lesions: A 3-T MRI study. *Stroke, 37*, 1765–1770.

Stankewitz, A., Aderjan, D., Eippert, F., & May, A. (2011). Trigeminal nociceptive transmission in migraineurs predicts migraine attacks. *Journal of Neuroscience, 31*, 1937–1943.

Thomsen, S. S., Kruuse, H. K., & Olesen, J. (1994). A nitric oxide donor (nitroglycerin) triggers genuine migraine attacks. *European Journal of Neurology, 1*, 73–80.

Veloso, F., Kumar, K., & Toth, C. (1998). Headache secondary to deep brain implantation. *Headache, 38*, 507–515.

Wang, Q. P., & Nakai, Y. (1994). The dorsal raphe: An important nucleus in pain modulation. *Brain Research Bulletin, 34*, 575–585.

Weiller, C., May, A., Limmroth, V., Jüptner, M., Kaube, H., Schayck, R. V., et al. (1995). Brain stem activation in spontaneous human migraine attacks. *Nature Medicine, 1*, 658–660.

Welch, K. M., Nagesh, V., Aurora, S., & Gelman, N. (2001). Periaqueductal grey matter dysfunction in migraine: Cause or the burden of illness? *Headache, 41*, 629–637.

16 Diffusion-Weighted Imaging in Migraine

CHRISTOS SIDIROPOULOS AND PANAYIOTIS D. MITSIAS

Migraine is a common disorder with diverse clinical manifestations affecting approximately 18% of women and 6% of men in their lifetime (Lipton et al., 2001). Aura, one or more fully reversible symptoms indicating focal cerebral cortical or brainstem dysfunction, may be present in 15% to 20% of patients, but not necessarily during each attack. Cortical spreading depression, cerebrovascular tone dysregulation, and perineural inflammation are among the established inciting factors in migraine pathophysiology.

There is evidence to suggest a complex interaction between migraine and stroke (Etminan et al., 2005; Kurth et al., 2005; Stang et al., 2005). Migraine can be the direct cause of ischemic stroke, the so-called migrainous infarction (Bousser & Welch, 2005). Reversely, acute cerebral ischemia can induce clinical syndromes that mimic migraine (Nardi et al., 2008). In addition, migraine has been established as an independent risk factor for stroke (Buring et al., 1995), especially in patients with migraine with aura and even more so in women on oral contraceptive pills (Davis, 2008). On conventional magnetic resonance T2-weighted imaging (T2WI), 6% to 46% of patients with migraine exhibit increased signal in the periventricular and deep white matter (Osborn et al., 1991; Rocca et al., 2000). This frequency may vary according to migraine type (Fazekas et al., 2002). These changes are postulated to be the result of microvascular ischemic damage from repeated perturbations in cerebral blood flow, known to occur during a migrainous attack. However, it has been difficult to prove this point by pathology studies.

DWI has been extensively used in the setting of acute stroke because of its high sensitivity in detecting restricted diffusion of water molecules resulting in cytotoxic edema and cellular damage. By means of other advanced magnetic resonance imaging (MRI) techniques, such as magnetization transfer imaging and perfusion MRI, several cerebral tissue alterations can be detected (Jager et al., 2005; Oberndorfer et al., 2004; Rocca et al., 2000). The present chapter will focus on reviewing the findings from DWI studies in migraine patients, their clinical significance, and the light they shed on the understanding of migraine pathophysiology.

The theoretical foundation for DWI was laid in the 1960s. It was however only until 1990 when Moseley et al. (1990) showed that it can be used for early detection of cerebral ischemia in experimental ischemia, and in 1995, when Warach et al. (1995) demonstrated its significance in the early detection and prognosis of cerebral ischemia in patients with acute stroke. DWI utilizes inhomogeneous magnetic fields (i.e., gradients) to detect alterations in the propensity of water molecules to diffuse preferentially across boundaries of biological membranes. Water diffusion across cellular membranes is an energy-dependent process. The main measure of diffusivity of water molecules is the ADC. Acute cerebral ischemia results in cytotoxic edema and is accompanied by markedly reduced ADC values, which produces a bright signal on DWI (Fig. 16–1) lasting for several days to weeks, followed by elevated ADC values producing a dark signal on DWI. Vasogenic edema is associated with increased ADC (Schabitz & Fisher, 1995). Increased ADC values may also be seen in neurodegenerative conditions in regions with disturbed ultrastructural integrity (Nicoletti et al., 2006). Application of gradients in multiple intersecting directions allows for further information to be acquired, which, if appropriately processed, can lead to visual estimation of white matter fiber tracts, the so-called diffusion tensor imaging and tractography. A detailed description of the physics and methodology involved is beyond the scope of this chapter and the reader is referred to the pertinent literature (Bammer, 2003).

The reasons for potentially using DWI in patients with migraine are multiple. These include the following: (a) migraine can cause ischemic stroke, also called migrainous infarction (Bousser & Welch, 2005); (b) migraine is a risk factor for ischemic stroke (Etminan et al., 2005); (c) migraine has been suggested to be associated with a hypercoagulable state, further increasing the risk for ischemic damage (Tietjen et al., 2001); and (d) the well-known perturbations of cerebral blood flow during the ictal and interictal phases of migraine (Viola et al., 2010). Until now, however, there has been no large systematic study addressing the DWI findings at distinct time points in various types of migraine.

It seems most appealing, however, to apply DWI in the study of the migraine aura. During this phase of migraine, there are well-documented alterations in cerebral blood

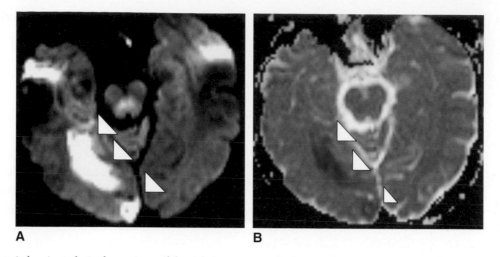

FIGURE 16–1 *Acute ischemic stroke in the territory of the right posterior cerebral artery demonstrating increased signal on diffusion-weighted image (arrows) (A) and decreased signal on the apparent diffusion coefficient map (arrows) (B).*

flow dynamics, revealed by the use of imaging techniques such as perfusion MRI, Xenon-133 computed tomography (CT), positron emission tomography (PET), and single-photon emission computed tomography (SPECT). These changes include an initial phase of spreading oligemia followed by hyperperfusion (Cutrer et al., 1998; Olesen et al., 1981; Seto et al., 1994; Woods et al., 1994). This has been correlated with the phenomenon of spreading neuronal depolarization, also called cortical spreading depression (Barkley et al., 1990; Leao, 1947). Experimental work in cats demonstrated DWI changes at the onset of cortical spreading depression (James et al., 1999). However, the literature pertaining to the application of DWI in migraine patients is rather limited and restricted to case reports or small series. Certainly, a major confounding factor is the time interval from symptom onset to MRI scan, as changes in water diffusion are time-sensitive phenomena and the cerebral blood flow changes are very dynamic and volatile.

One of the first reports of reversible diffusion changes was by Chabriat et al. (2000), who studied a patient with familial hemiplegic migraine (FHM) in whom the T1- and T2-weighted images were normal. Butteriss et al. (2003) followed another patient with FHM with serial MRI scans and reported reversible ischemic changes on DWI, which did not respect vascular boundaries, strongly suggesting a primary neuronal dysfunction as the underlying cause of neurological deficits, rather than cerebral vasoconstriction. However, the opposite pattern has also been described in an FHM patient with marked hyperperfusion without associated diffusion changes (Lindahl et al., 2002).

In a study of four women with FHM type 2 (Grimaldi et al., 2010), statistically significant increases in the ADC values in the vermis, superior and middle cerebellar peduncles, and cerebellar hemispheres as well as optic radiations compared with healthy controls were observed. In two subjects those changes preceded the expression of cerebellar dysfunction. In another patient with reversible hemiparesis lasting more than 9 days, DWI revealed no deficits, whereas perfusion-weighted imaging (PWI) prolonged hyperperfusion and hexamethylpropylene amine oxime (HMPAO) SPECT showed increased tracer uptake in the ipsilateral to the hemiparesis hemisphere (Oberndorfer et al., 2004).

In a very elegant case report, Arai et al. (2008) followed a patient with prolonged visual aura resulting in the development of migrainous infarction using serial DWI and PWI studies. They studied this patient at 5, 9, and 50 days after symptom onset. At 5 days, there were increased signal lesions in the right occipital and temporal lobes on both DWI and fluid attenuation inversion recovery (FLAIR) sequences, while the ADC map showed increased, instead of decreased, diffusion of the lesion. At 9 days, FLAIR and DWI showed higher signal intensity of the lesion, and the ADC increased diffusion. At 50 days, while there was mild residual hemianopsia, FLAIR and DWI showed high signal intensity, and the ADC revealed pseudonormalization of the lesion (Arai et al., 2008). This is an uncharacteristic imaging behavior for a typical ischemic lesion, suggesting early vasogenic edema (elevated ADC) in the presence of an acute ischemic lesion (high signal on DWI and FLAIR) and late pseudonormalization of the ADC. It may be an indication that the events of a prolonged aura culminating in the development of infarction are different than those occurring during a typical ischemic infarction.

In a study of four patients with persistent migrainous visual disturbances, Jager et al. (2005) focused on the primary visual, frontal, insular, and temporal cortices. They found no changes in water diffusion or blood perfusion, inferring that those factors are unlikely to play a role in the pathophysiology of persistent migraine aura. On the other hand, Belvis et al. (2010) described a patient with prolonged visual aura, in whom there was increased signal in the left occipital lobe on the ADC map but not on DWI, implying some form of cerebral edema.

Degirmenci et al. (2007) recruited 22 migraineurs and 18 age- and sex-matched controls. MRI was done within 3 hours of the attack onset. Although patients with migraine exhibited more T2 hyperintense lesions than controls, consistent with previous observations, there was no statistical difference in the regional ADC values among patients with and without aura or controls. However, the authors acknowledge the fact that they did not perform a mean diffusivity histogram analysis, which represents a pixel-by-pixel evaluation of the mean diffusivity of normal-appearing brain tissue, thought to correspond to truly normal tissue. This technique has been applied before to other disorders such as multiple sclerosis (Cercignani et al., 2001). It has also been shown that subtle changes apparent on DWI, undetected by conventional MRI, may correlate with clinical and neuropsychological measures (O'Sullivan et al., 2001).

Rocca et al. were among the first to apply mean diffusivity (MD) and fractional anisotropy (FA) histogram analysis in patients with migraine and healthy controls. Those two metrics represent a quantitative measure of the ability of water molecules to diffuse freely. In two elegant studies they initially evaluated normal-appearing white matter (NAWM) in both healthy subjects and migraineurs and were able to demonstrate a lower height in the peak of the mean diffusivity histogram for patients with migraine (Rocca, Colombo, Inglese, et al., 2003; Rocca, Colombo, Pagani, et al., 2003). Maximum height is thought to represent the residual amount of truly normal tissue (Nusbaum et al., 2000). They also measured MD in T2 lesions in their migraine group and found that it was 3.4% higher than the NAWM, significantly less than for other T2 changes seen in conditions such as CADASIL (Chabriat et al., 1999) or leukoaraiosis (O'Sullivan et al., 2001). They proposed that the increase in MD in NAWM may be either the result of subtle ischemic changes or secondary wallerian degeneration. The same group extended their studies to the gray matter (GM) of patients with migraine using a 3-T magnet.

There was a statistically significant reduction in the peak height of MD in the GM of migraineurs compared to healthy controls, although they could not reproduce the previously demonstrated differences in NAWM (Rocca et al., 2006). Moving a further step ahead, Rocca et al. (2008) performed tractography of the optic radiations (ORs) in patients with and without aura and healthy controls at 3 T and detected reduced OR fractional anisotropy and increased mean diffusivity in patients with aura compared to controls, without, however, correlation to disease severity or T2 lesion load. Table 16–1 summarizes all case studies and reports on diffusion-weighted imaging in migraine.

The overriding theme in almost all studies on DWI and migraine aura is that despite the prolonged duration of the transient focal neurological events of migraine, DWI is typically negative for acute lesions, or that in the rare case of positivity, the lesions typically reverse without leaving a permanent T2WI lesion behind. This is in contrast with what is observed in transient ischemic attacks, where a high proportion of the patients demonstrate DWI lesion after the attacks, and almost half of those end up becoming permanent ischemic lesions on T2WI (Kidwell et al., 1999). These findings point against the possibility of cerebral ischemia as the reason for the focal deficits of migraine aura, but cannot confirm the exact etiology. Other MRI sequences are expected to shed more light on this issue.

Based on the above findings, it is evident that the field of DWI application in migraine is still evolving, but offers a whole new perspective in understanding the pathophysiology of a disorder that affects millions of patients worldwide. One of its major advantages is the noninvasiveness and the wide availability of MRI. On the other hand, most of the data acquired so far come from case reports and small-sized samples with questionable power. Furthermore, since DWI is a relatively new technique, there is no uniformity in imaging protocols, and some of them are subject to improvement due to inadequate accuracy. Even more interesting is the fact that we are just now beginning to grasp the anatomical/physiological substrate of many DWI metrics and thus a clear interpretation is still elusive. In any case, the future prospects and applications of DWI in deciphering the mysteries of migraine remain very promising. I summary, DWI has been extensively studied in the context of acute stroke because of its high sensitivity in detecting acute cerebral ischemia. Migraine is associated with cerebral blood flow perturbations, especially during the aura phase, and also with an increased risk for cerebral ischemia. However, there has been no large systematic study of DWI findings in various

TABLE 16–1 *Summary of Case Studies/Reports on Diffusion-Weighted Imaging (DWI) in Patients with Migraine*

Reference	Number of Cases	Age	Migraine Type	Attack Onset–Imaging Time Interval	DWI-ADC Findings
Belvis et al. (2010)	22	17–49 years	Without and with aura	1–3 hours	Normal DWI (except one patient)
Lindahl et al. (2002)	4	15–51 years	FHM	24 hours	Increased ADC in CWM, SCP, MCP, OR
Arai et al. (2008)	1	41 years	BM	4 days	Increased ADC in left occipital lobe
Oberndorfer et al. (2004)	1	21 years	FHM	48 hours	Normal DWI
Jager et al. (2005)	4	27–46 years	Visual aura and visual "snow"	Not specified	Normal DWI and ADC

Notes. ADC = apparent diffusion coefficient; FHM = familial hemiplegic migraine; CWM = cerebellar white matter; SCP = superior cerebellar peduncle; MCP = middle cerebellar peduncle; OR = optic radiation; BM = basilar migraine.

types of migraine. Case reports and small series indicate that three patterns of DWI findings in migraine with aura are observed: (a) usually normal, despite the persistence of the focal neurological deficit and extensive blood flow changes during migraine attacks; (b) reversible DWI hyperintensities not respecting vascular territories and corresponding with the localization of the aura; and (c) elevated ADC values typically in regions related to the aura phase. In contrast, in transient cerebral ischemia, DWI frequently reveals acute ischemic changes. More extensive systematic studies are needed to clarify the DWI findings in migraine and allow conclusions to be reached. Newer DWI methodologies, such as diffusion tensor imaging, are expected to shed more light on the functional but also the structural integrity of the migrainous brain.

ACKNOWLEDGMENTS

Dr. Panayiotis Mitsias is supported by NIH/NINDS grant RO1 NS070922.

REFERENCES

Arai, S., Utsunomiya, H., Arihiro, S., & Arakawa, S. (2008). Migrainous infarction in an adult: Evaluation with serial diffusion-weighted images and cerebral blood flow studies. *Radiation Medicine, 26*(5), 313–317.

Bammer, R. (2003). Basic principles of diffusion-weighted imaging. *European Journal of Radiology, 45*(3), 169–184.

Barkley, G. L., Tepley, N., Nagel-Leiby, S., Moran, J. E., Simkins, R. T., & Welch, K. M. (1990). Magnetoencephalographic studies of migraine. *Headache, 30*(7), 428–434.

Belvis, R., Ramos, R., Villa, C., Segura, C., Pagonabarraga, J., Ormazabal, I., et al. (2010). Brain apparent water diffusion coefficient magnetic resonance image during a prolonged visual aura. *Headache, 50*(6), 1045–1049.

Bousser, M. G., & Welch, K. M. (2005). Relation between migraine and stroke. *Lancet Neurology, 4*(9), 533–542.

Buring, J. E., Hebert, P., Romero, J., Kittross, A., Cook, N., Manson, J., et al. (1995). Migraine and subsequent risk of stroke in the Physicians' Health Study. *Archives of Neurology, 52*(2), 129–134.

Butteriss, D. J., Ramesh, V., & Birchall, D. (2003). Serial MRI in a case of familial hemiplegic migraine. *Neuroradiology, 45*(5), 300–303.

Cercignani, M., Inglese, M., Pagani, E., Comi, G., & Filippi, M. (2001). Mean diffusivity and fractional anisotropy histograms of patients with multiple sclerosis. *AJNR American Journal of Neuroradiology, 22*(5), 952–958.

Chabriat, H., Pappata, S., Poupon, C., Clark, C. A., Vahedi, K., Poupon, F., et al. (1999). Clinical severity in CADASIL related to ultrastructural damage in white matter: In vivo study with diffusion tensor MRI. *Stroke, 30*(12), 2637–2643.

Chabriat, H., Vahedi, K., Clark, C. A., Poupon, C., Ducros, A., Denier, C., et al. (2000). Decreased hemispheric water mobility in hemiplegic migraine related to mutation of CACNA1A gene. *Neurology, 54*(2), 510–512.

Cutrer, F. M., Sorensen, A. G., Weisskoff, R. M., Ostergaard, L., Sanchez del Rio, M., Lee, E. J., et al. (1998). Perfusion-weighted imaging defects during spontaneous migrainous aura. *Annals of Neurology, 43*(1), 25–31.

Davis, P. H. (2008). Use of oral contraceptives and postmenopausal hormone replacement: Evidence on risk of stroke. *Current Treatments Options in Neurology, 10*(6), 468–474.

Degirmenci, B., Yaman, M., Haktanir, A., Albayrak, R., Acar, M., & Yucel, A. (2007). Cerebral and cerebellar ADC values during a migraine attack. *Neuroradiology, 49*(5), 419–426.

Etminan, M., Takkouche, B., Isorna, F. C., & Samii, A. (2005). Risk of ischaemic stroke in people with migraine: Systematic review and meta-analysis of observational studies. *BMJ, 330*(7482), 63.

Fazekas, F., Koch, M., Schmidt, R., Offenbacher, H., Payer, F., Freidl, W., et al. (1992). The prevalence of cerebral damage varies with migraine type: A MRI study. *Headache, 32*(6), 287–291.

Grimaldi, D., Tonon, C., Cevoli, S., Pierangeli, G., Malucelli, E., Rizzo, G., et al. (2010). Clinical and neuroimaging evidence of interictal cerebellar dysfunction in FHM2. *Cephalalgia, 30*(5), 552–559.

Jager, H. R., Giffin, N. J., & Goadsby, P. J. (2005). Diffusion- and perfusion-weighted MR imaging in persistent migrainous visual disturbances. *Cephalalgia, 25*(5), 323–332.

James, M. F., Smith, M. I., Bockhorst, K. H., Hall, L. D., Houston, G. C., Papadakis, N. G., et al. (1999). Cortical spreading depression in the gyrencephalic feline brain studied by magnetic resonance imaging. *Journal of Physiology, 519*(Pt 2), 415–425.

Kidwell, C. S., Alger, J. R., Di Salle, F., Starkman, S., Villablanca, P., Bentson, J., et al. (1999). Diffusion MRI in patients with transient ischemic attacks. *Stroke, 30*(6), 1174–1180.

Kurth, T., Slomke, M. A., Kase, C. S., Cook, N. R., Lee, I. M., Gaziano, J. M., et al. (2005). Migraine, headache, and the risk of stroke in women: A prospective study. *Neurology, 64*(6), 1020–1026.

Leao, A. A. (1947). Further observations on the spreading depression of activity in the cerebral cortex. *Journal of Neurophysiology, 10*(6), 409–414.

Lindahl, A. J., Allder, S., Jefferson, D., Moody, A., & Martel, A. (2002). Prolonged hemiplegic migraine associated with unilateral hyperperfusion on perfusion weighted magnetic resonance imaging. *Journal of Neurology, Neurosurgery, and Psychiatry, 73*(2), 202–203.

Lipton, R. B., Stewart, W. F., Diamond, S., Diamond, M. L., & Reed, M. (2001). Prevalence and burden of migraine in the United States: Data from the American Migraine Study II. *Headache, 41*(7), 646–657.

Moseley, M. E., Cohen, Y., Mintorovitch, J., Chileuitt, L., Shimizu, H., Kucharczyk, J., et al. (1990). Early detection of regional cerebral ischemia in cats: Comparison of diffusion- and T2-weighted MRI and spectroscopy. *Magnetic Resonance Medicine, 14*(2), 330–346.

Nardi, K., Parnetti, L., Pieri, M. L., Eusebi, P., Calabresi, P., & Sarchielli, P. (2008). Association between migraine and headache attributed to stroke: A case-control study. *Headache, 48*(10), 1468–1475.

Nicoletti, G., Lodi, R., Condino, F., Tonon, C., Fera, F., Malucelli, E., et al. (2006). Apparent diffusion coefficient measurements of the middle cerebellar peduncle differentiate the Parkinson variant of MSA from Parkinson's disease and progressive supranuclear palsy. *Brain, 129*(Pt 10), 2679–2687.

Nusbaum, A. O., Tang, C. Y., Wei, T., Buchsbaum, M. S., & Atlas, S. W. (2000). Whole-brain diffusion MR histograms differ between MS subtypes. *Neurology, 54*(7), 1421–1427.

Oberndorfer, S., Wober, C., Nasel, C., Asenbaum, S., Lahrmann, H., Fueger, B., et al. (2004). Familial hemiplegic migraine: Follow-up findings of diffusion-weighted magnetic resonance imaging (MRI), perfusion-MRI and [99mTc] HMPAO-SPECT in a patient with prolonged hemiplegic aura. *Cephalalgia, 24*(7), 533–539.

Olesen, J., Larsen, B., & Lauritzen, M. (1981). Focal hyperemia followed by spreading oligemia and impaired activation of rCBF in classic migraine. *Annals of Neurology, 9*(4), 344–352.

Osborn, R. E., Alder, D. C., & Mitchell, C. S. (1991). MR imaging of the brain in patients with migraine headaches. *AJNR American Journal of Neuroradiology, 12*(3), 521–524.

O'Sullivan, M., Summers, P. E., Jones, D. K., Jarosz, J. M., Williams, S. C., & Markus, H. S. (2001). Normal-appearing white matter in ischemic leukoaraiosis: A diffusion tensor MRI study. *Neurology, 57*(12), 2307–2310.

Rocca, M. A., Ceccarelli, A., Falini, A., Tortorella, P., Colombo, B., Pagani, E., et al. (2006). Diffusion tensor magnetic resonance imaging at 3.0 tesla shows subtle cerebral grey matter abnormalities in patients with migraine. *Journal of Neurology, Neurosurgery, and Psychiatry, 77*(5), 686–689.

Rocca, M. A., Colombo, B., Inglese, M., Codella, M., Comi, G., & Filippi, M. (2003). A diffusion tensor magnetic resonance imaging study of brain tissue from patients with migraine. *Journal of Neurology, Neurosurgery, and Psychiatry, 74*(4), 501–503.

Rocca, M. A., Colombo, B., Pagani, E., Falini, A., Codella, M., Scotti, G., et al. (2003). Evidence for cortical functional changes in patients with migraine and white matter abnormalities on conventional and diffusion tensor magnetic resonance imaging. *Stroke, 34*(3), 665–670.

Rocca, M. A., Colombo, B., Pratesi, A., Comi, G., & Filippi, M. (2000). A magnetization transfer imaging study of the brain in patients with migraine. *Neurology, 54*(2), 507–509.

Rocca, M. A., Pagani, E., Colombo, B., Tortorella, P., Falini, A., Comi, G., et al. (2008). Selective diffusion changes of the visual pathways in patients with migraine: A 3-T tractography study. *Cephalalgia, 28*(10), 1061–1068.

Schabitz, W. R., & Fisher, M. (1995). Diffusion weighted imaging for acute cerebral infarction. *Neurological Research, 17*(4), 270–274.

Seto, H., Shimizu, M., Futatsuya, R., Kageyama, M., Wu, Y., Kamei, T., et al. (1994). Basilar artery migraine. Reversible ischemia demonstrated by Tc-99m HMPAO brain SPECT. *Clinical Nuclear Medicine, 19*(3), 215–218.

Stang, P. E., Carson, A. P., Rose, K. M., Mo, J., Ephross, S. A., Shahar, E., et al. (2005). Headache, cerebrovascular symptoms, and stroke: The Atherosclerosis Risk in Communities Study. *Neurology, 64*(9), 1573–1577.

Tietjen, G. E., Al-Qasmi, M. M., Athanas, K., Dafer, R. M., & Khuder, S. A. (2001). Increased von Willebrand factor in migraine. *Neurology, 57*(2), 334–336.

Viola, S., Viola, P., Litterio, P., Buongarzone, M. P., & Fiorelli, L. (2010). Pathophysiology of migraine attack with prolonged aura revealed by transcranial Doppler and near infrared spectroscopy. *Neurological Science, 31*(Suppl 1), S165–S166.

Warach, S., Gaa, J., Siewert, B., Wielopolski, P., & Edelman, R. R. (1995). Acute human stroke studied by whole brain echo planar diffusion-weighted magnetic resonance imaging. *Annals of Neurology, 37*(2), 231–241.

Woods, R. P., Iacoboni, M., & Mazziotta, J. C. (1994). Brief report: Bilateral spreading cerebral hypoperfusion during spontaneous migraine headache. *New England Journal of Medicine, 331*(25), 1689–1692.

17 Diffusion Tensor Imaging Abnormalities in Migraine

MARIA A. ROCCA AND MASSIMO FILIPPI

INTRODUCTION

Diffusion is the microscopic random translational motion of molecules in a fluid system. In the central nervous system (CNS), diffusion is influenced by the microstructural components of tissue, including cell membranes and organelles. The diffusion coefficients of biological tissues (which can be measured in vivo by diffusion weighted [DW] magnetic resonance imaging [MRI]) is, therefore, lower than the diffusion coefficient in free water and for this reason is named apparent diffusion coefficient (ADC) (Le Bihan et al., 1986). Pathological processes, such as inflammatory demyelination and ischemia, which can modify tissue integrity, result in a loss or increased permeability of "restricting" barriers and can determine an increase of the ADC. The measurement of diffusion is also dependent on the direction in which diffusion is measured, since within the time scale of the diffusion experiment water may diffuse unevenly in different directions, depending on the size and shape of the cellular structures. As a consequence, diffusion measurements can give information about integrity, orientation, and geometry of tissues (Le Bihan et al., 1991), which can be altered by pathology. A full characterization of diffusion can be obtained in terms of a tensor (Basser et al., 1994), a 3×3 matrix that accounts for the correlation existing between molecular displacement along orthogonal directions. From the tensor, it is possible to derive mean diffusivity (MD), a measure of diffusion, which is independent of the orientation of structures (since it results from an average of the ADCs measured in the three orthogonal directions) and is equal to one third of its trace and some other dimensionless indexes of anisotropy. One of the most used of these indices is named fractional anisotropy (FA) (Basser & Pierpaoli, 1996; Pierpaoli & Basser, 1996).

Given its potential to provide a more accurate picture of the pathological changes associated with neurological diseases than conventional T2-weighted imaging, diffusion tensor (DT) MRI has been applied extensively to quantify the extent of tissue damage in several neurological conditions, including migraine. Seminal studies in patients with this condition used histogram-based methods of analysis and provided a global estimation of CNS damage. More recently several approaches have been developed to investigate damage to selected white matter (WM) fiber bundles, with the ultimate aim of improving our understanding of the pathophysiology of the disease. These approaches include DT MRI tractography and the quantification of abnormalities at a voxel level (voxel-based analysis). DT MRI tractography exploits the fact that axonal structures constitute a barrier to water diffusion, making it freer along the axis of the fibers than perpendicular to them (Mori et al., 2002). By tracking the principal diffusion direction (i.e., the direction of the primary eigenvector of the DT), fiber bundle pathways can be reconstructed and their intrinsic damage measured (Mori et al., 2002). Voxelwise approaches to the analysis of DT MRI data allow us to assess the presence and quantify the extent of brain damage at a regional level. As a consequence, they also hold promise to improve our ability to study the structural features of migraine damage, too.

The present chapter outlines the major contributions given by DW and DT MRI to the study of CNS involvement in patients with migraine, as well as the role of newer acquisition schemes and postprocessing methods in the assessment of this condition.

DIFFUSIVITY ABNORMALITIES IN THE ICTAL PHASE

Neurological symptoms, usually defined as "aura," occur in approximately one third of migraine patients and may precede the migraine attack. The progression of aura has been shown to have similarities with cortical spreading depression (CSD), a neurophysiological event characterized by a redistribution of ions between intracellular and extracellular compartments, increased cellular water uptake, and cell swelling (James et al., 2001). DT MRI is sensitive to the transient disturbances of cerebral water distribution occurring during CSD (Bradley et al., 2001) and, as a consequence, its application to image patients with aura during the migraine attack might contribute to improving our understanding of aura pathophysiology.

Nevertheless, several studies of migraine patients with and without aura found no ADC abnormalities during the migraine attack (Cutrer et al., 1998; Degirmenci et al., 2007; Jager et al., 2005). These results are partially in contrast with those of single-case studies, which reported reversible signal abnormalities in DW images during the phase of aura. In particular, a reversible increase of signal intensity on DW images, not associated with ADC abnormalities, has been detected in a patient with a 30-year history of migraine with an acute onset of headache associated with a typical aura lasting several hours and characterized by hemianopsia and a parietal syndrome (Resnick et al., 2006). Another study in a patient with persistent (more than 2 weeks) visual migraine aura (Bereczki et al., 2008) showed increased signal on DW maps and decreased ADC in the left occipital cortex at day 2, with a shift of ADC decrease to the temporoparietal cortex between day 2 and day 17. The ADC abnormality was limited to the cortex and was associated with a decreased local glucose metabolism and cortical edema. A subsequent MRI scan performed 8 weeks after the attack (when the clinical symptomatology had resolved completely) revealed no MRI abnormalities (Fig. 17–1). Reversible changes, possibly secondary to cytotoxic edema, have also been detected in the occipital region of the ADC map from a patient during persistent visual aura and bilateral paresthesias in the extremities, which lasted 4 days (Belvis et al., 2010).

The prolonged duration of the aura attack in these single-case studies with respect to those of the previous cohort studies (Cutrer et al., 1998; Degirmenci et al., 2007) is likely to be the reason for their discrepant results. This hypothesis is supported by studies in patients with sporadic or familial hemiplegic migraine, which is an autosomal dominant subtype of migraine with aura associated with transient hemiparesis, as well as visual, somatosensory, and dysphasic symptoms and cerebellar signs. Reduced ADC values in the right temporo-occipital regions, which resolved after 3 months, have been found in a patient with a prolonged hemiparesis during the course of a migraine attack (Jacob et al., 2006). Reversible DW abnormalities have been described by Chabriat et al. (2000) in a woman with familial hemiplegic migraine. Such abnormalities were characterized by an approximately 25% decrease in ADC in the affected hemisphere at day 21, which persisted for 5 weeks and resolved after 3 months. Noteworthy, the observed 25% reduction of ADC is much less than the 40% to 50% decrease described in the core of acute cerebral ischemia (Warach et al., 1995). That the ischemic threshold is not reached in migraine patients might contribute to explain the reversibility of ADC abnormalities. Unilateral cortical swelling, reduced ADC, and vascular dilatation on the side contralateral to the aura have been observed in a child with familial hemiplegic migraine during two different episodes. Clinical and MRI abnormalities resolved completely at 6-month follow-up (Butteriss et al., 2003). An increase in cortical swelling of the left hemisphere associated with a hyperintensity on DW images and a reduction of ADC have been described in an 8-year-old child 9 hours after the onset of hemiplegia (Toldo et al., 2010). Also in this case, DW abnormalities were not detectable on a scan obtained 6 months later.

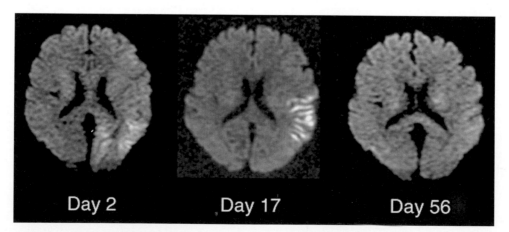

FIGURE 17–1 *Increased signal intensity on diffusion weighted scans from a 58-year-old man with persistent visual migraine aura. Signal abnormality shifted from the occipital to the temporo-parietal cortex between days 2 and 17. No signal abnormalities are clearly visible at day 56. From Bereczli et al. (Bereczki et al., 2008), with permission.*

DIFFUSIVITY ABNORMALITIES DURING THE INTERICTAL PHASE

Several studies have applied DT MRI in an attempt to quantify the presence and extent of tissue abnormalities of the CNS and its compartments in patients with migraine outside an acute attack.

Diffusion Tensor Magnetic Resonance Imaging Features of Normal-Appearing Brain Tissues

Using a histogram-based approach, Rocca et al. (2003) detected abnormal MD values in the normal-appearing brain tissue (NABT) of patients with migraine in comparison with healthy controls, whereas no FA abnormalities were found (Fig. 2). In this study, no difference in the severity of NABT damage was shown between patients with and without aura, or between those with or without focal brain T2 lesions. However, in patients with focal WM lesions, a correlation was found between MD increase of T2 lesions and MD abnormalities of the NABT, suggesting that secondary wallerian degeneration of fibers traversing macroscopic lesions might be one of the mechanisms responsible for the observed NABT abnormalities in these patients.

To define whether the normal-appearing white matter (NAWM) and gray matter (GM) are equally affected by the disease, DT MRI histograms from these two brain compartments, separately, were derived in another study, performed using a 3.0-tesla scanner (Rocca et al., 2006b). This study revealed that DT MRI abnormalities, as reflected by an increased MD, involved mainly the GM, with a relative sparing of the NAWM. The notion that the

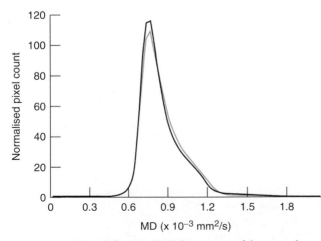

FIGURE 17-2 *Mean diffusivity (MD) histograms of the normal appearing brain tissue from healthy subjects (black line) and patients with migraine (grey line). Compared to healthy subjects, migraine patients had a significant reduction of MD histogram peak height. From Rocca et al. (Rocca et al., 2003), with permission.*

GM is damaged in patients with migraine fits with the results of several voxel-based morphometry studies, which have shown regional GM abnormalities, in terms of both decreased and increased volumes, not only in patients with migraine (Rocca et al., 2006a), but also in those suffering from different painful conditions (Apkarian et al., 2004).

Voxel-based methods have been applied in an attempt to map the regional distribution of DT MRI abnormalities in the WM of migraine patients. Using this approach, reduced FA values have been detected in the frontal lobes, brainstem, and cerebellum in 28 patients with migraine (Schmitz, Admiraal-Behloul, et al., 2008). Again, the detected frontal lobe diffusivity abnormalities of migraineurs are in line with the results of voxel-based morphometry studies, which showed atrophy of these regions (Rocca et al., 2006a). DaSilva et al. (DaSilva, Granziera, Tuch, et al., 2007) found a decreased FA along the thalamocortical tracts in migraineurs. In this study, migraineurs with aura had lower FA in the ventral trigeminothalamic tract, and migraineurs without aura had lower FA in the ventrolateral periaqueductal GM, indicating an involvement of the trigeminal somatosensory and pain modulatory systems. Using a similar approach, FA abnormalities in WM areas in the vicinity of regions that are part of the motion-processing visual network, including V3A, MT/V5, the superior colliculus, and the lateral geniculate nucleus, were found in migraine patients both with and without aura (Fig. 17-3) (Granziera et al., 2006). These WM FA abnormalities might be due to a chronic dysfunction of these GM areas, which in turn might be the consequence of repetitive migraine attacks.

Using DT tractography, an FA reduction in both the optic radiations, and an MD increase in the right optic radiation have been shown in migraine patients with aura in comparison to healthy controls and to those without aura (Rocca et al., 2008). No DT MRI abnormalities were found in the corpus callosum (CC) and corticospinal tracts. Conversely, using a regions of interest (ROI)–based analysis to assess damage to the CC, decreased FA values in this structure were found in migraine patients when compared to healthy controls (Li et al., 2010). Interestingly, such FA abnormalities were significantly more pronounced in migraine patients with depression (Li et al., 2010).

Clinical Correlations

Several studies assessed the possible clinical relevance of DT MRI abnormalities in migraine patients. In the study by Rocca et al. (2006b), GM MD abnormalities were correlated with patients' age, while no relation was found with disease duration and the number of yearly episodes.

Similarly, no difference in FA values was found in the study of Schmitz et al. (Schmitz, Admiraal-Behloul, et al., 2008) between patients with high (more than three attacks per month) or low attack frequencies. Remarkably, in this latter study (Schmitz, Admiraal-Behloul, et al., 2008), FA values in the right frontal lobe were lower in patients with disease duration longer than 15 years in comparison with those with a shorter disease duration.

With the exception of the study of Schmitz et al. (Schmitz, Admiraal-Behloul, et al., 2008), all studies performed in patients with migraine confirmed our findings (Rocca et al., 2006b) and no correlation between the presence and extent of DT MRI abnormalities and the number of attacks and disease duration has been reported (DaSilva, Granziera, Tuch, et al., 2007; Rocca et al., 2003, 2006b, 2008). This suggests that one of the mechanisms that has been considered by several authors to explain MRI findings in migraine, that is, the repetition of episodes of oligemia (Wolff, 1963), is unlikely to be important. Conversely, the lack of a clinical/magnetic resonance correlation suggests that the observed DT MRI changes might represent a phenotypic biomarker of the disease, reflecting a congenital condition rather than a process related to disease progression over time. This hypothesis is supported by the results of another study (DaSilva, Granziera, Snyder, et al., 2007), which found no correlation between changes of cortical thickness of the somatosensory cortex and disease duration, age at onset, and attack frequency. This notion also agrees with the previously proposed theory of an intrinsic increased susceptibility to spontaneous depolarization in migraine patients, which might reflect abnormal presynaptic P/Q-type calcium channels (Ophoff et al., 1996), low brain magnesium levels (Ramadan et al., 1989), and a disorder of mitochondrial energy metabolism (Barbiroli et al., 1992; Welch et al., 1989).

The application of DT MRI technology in patients with migraine might help to explain some of the other clinical manifestations usually described in this condition, including cognitive impairment (Schmitz, Arkink, et al., 2008) and depression (Breslau et al., 1994). In this context, age-related GM abnormalities in migraineurs might contribute to the impairment of their executive functions, which is known to occur not only during the acute attacks but also in attack-free stages (Rocca et al., 2006b; Schmitz, Arkink, et al., 2008). FA abnormalities in the CC have been correlated with the severity of depression (Li et al., 2010).

DT MRI has also been used to characterize some genetic-determined variants of migraine. In patients with familial hemiplegic migraine (Grimaldi et al., 2010), both ROI- and histogram-based analysis showed increased ADC values in several regions of the cerebellum (i.e., the cerebellar peduncles, vermis, and cerebellar hemispheres) in patients in the interictal phase of the disease in comparison to healthy controls. Remarkably, such diffusivity abnormalities in the cerebellum were detected 4 years before the development of cerebellar signs.

CONCLUSION

DW and DT MRI are valuable tools to detect and quantify tissue damage in patients with migraine, both in the course of an acute attack and during the interictal phases. This should, therefore, be the focus of future research. At present, little is known about the pathological features underlying diffusivity changes in these patients. The contribution of newer and more sophisticated methods of acquisition and postprocessing of DT MRI data also needs to be further evaluated in patients with migraine. Finally, the utility of DT MRI scans in detecting longitudinal disease-related changes warrant being investigated in ad hoc

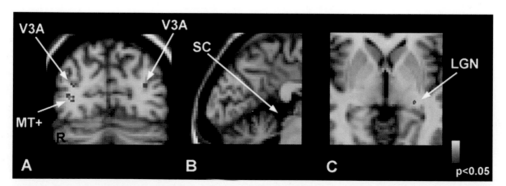

FIGURE 17–3 *Fractional anisotropy (FA) differences between patients with migraine and healthy controls. Coronal (A) and sagittal (B) sections show areas exhibiting statistically significant lower FA values in migraineurs compared to healthy controls: (A) white matter underneath MT/V5 and V3A areas, (B) superior colliculus (SC), and (C) left lateral geniculate nucleus (LGN). From Granziera et al. (Granziera et al., 2006), with permission [Open Access Journal, no permission needed].*

large-scale, prospective studies. All of this is critical not only to improve the understanding of disease pathophysiology but also to characterize better its heterogeneous clinical manifestations and to develop imaging biomarkers to be applied in treatment trials of new experimental drugs.

REFERENCES

Apkarian, A. V., Sosa, Y., Sonty, S., Levy, R. M., Harden, R. N., Parrish, T. B., et al. (2004). Chronic back pain is associated with decreased prefrontal and thalamic gray matter density. *Journal of Neuroscience, 24*, 10410–10415.

Barbiroli, B., Montagna, P., Cortelli, P., Funicello, R., Iotti, S., Monari, L., et al. (1992). Abnormal brain and muscle energy metabolism shown by 31P magnetic resonance spectroscopy in patients affected by migraine with aura. *Neurology, 42*, 1209–1214.

Basser, P. J., Mattiello, J., & LeBihan, D. (1994). Estimation of the effective self-diffusion tensor from the NMR spin echo. *Journal of Magnetic Resonance Series B, 103*, 247–254.

Basser, P. J., & Pierpaoli, C. (1996). Microstructural and physiological features of tissues elucidated by quantitative-diffusion-tensor MRI. *Journal of Magnetic Resonance Series B, 111*, 209–219.

Belvis, R., Ramos, R., Villa, C., Segura, C., Pagonabarraga, J., Ormazabal, I., et al. (2010). Brain apparent water diffusion coefficient magnetic resonance image during a prolonged visual aura. *Headache, 50*, 1045–1049.

Bereczki, D., Kollar, J., Kozak, N., Viszokay, K., Barta, Z., Sikula, J., et al. (2008). Cortical spreading edema in persistent visual migraine aura. *Headache, 48*, 1226–1229.

Bradley, D. P., Smith, M. I., Netsiri, C., Smith, J. M., Bockhorst, K. H., Hall, L. D., et al. (2001). Diffusion-weighted MRI used to detect in vivo modulation of cortical spreading depression: comparison of sumatriptan and tonabersat. *Experimental Neurology, 172*, 342–353.

Breslau, N., Merikangas, K., & Bowden, C. L. (1994). Comorbidity of migraine and major affective disorders. *Neurology, 44*, S17–S22.

Butteriss, D. J., Ramesh, V., & Birchall, D. (2003). Serial MRI in a case of familial hemiplegic migraine. *Neuroradiology, 45*, 300–303.

Chabriat, H., Vahedi, K., Clark, C. A., Poupon, C., Ducros, A., Denier, C., et al. (2000). Decreased hemispheric water mobility in hemiplegic migraine related to mutation of CACNA1A gene. *Neurology, 54*, 510–512.

Cutrer, F. M., Sorensen, A. G., Weisskoff, R. M., Ostergaard, L., Sanchez del Rio, M., Lee, E. J., et al. (1998). Perfusion-weighted imaging defects during spontaneous migrainous aura. *Annals of Neurology, 43*, 25–31.

DaSilva, A. F., Granziera, C., Snyder, J., & Hadjikhani, N. (2007). Thickening in the somatosensory cortex of patients with migraine. *Neurology, 69*, 1990–1995.

DaSilva, A. F., Granziera, C., Tuch, D. S., Snyder, J., Vincent, M., & Hadjikhani, N. (2007). Interictal alterations of the trigeminal somatosensory pathway and periaqueductal gray matter in migraine. *Neuroreport, 18*, 301–305.

Degirmenci, B., Yaman, M., Haktanir, A., Albayrak, R., Acar, M., Yucel, A. (2007). Cerebral and cerebellar ADC values during a migraine attack. *Neuroradiology, 49*, 419–426.

Granziera, C., DaSilva, A. F., Snyder, J., Tuch, D. S., & Hadjikhani, N. (2006). Anatomical alterations of the visual motion processing network in migraine with and without aura. *PLoS Medicine, 3*, e402.

Grimaldi, D., Tonon, C., Cevoli, S., Pierangeli, G., Malucelli, E., Rizzo, G., et al. (2010). Clinical and neuroimaging evidence of interictal cerebellar dysfunction in FHM2. *Cephalalgia, 30*, 552–559.

Jacob, A., Mahavish, K., Bowden, A., Smith, E. T., Enevoldson, P., & White, R. P.(2006). Imaging abnormalities in sporadic hemiplegic migraine on conventional MRI, diffusion and perfusion MRI and MRS. *Cephalalgia, 26*, 1004–1009.

Jager, H. R., Giffin, N. J., & Goadsby, P. J. (2005). Diffusion- and perfusion-weighted MR imaging in persistent migrainous visual disturbances. *Cephalalgia, 25*, 323–332.

James, M. F., Smith, J. M., Boniface, S. J., Huang, C. L., & Leslie, R. A. (2001). Cortical spreading depression and migraine: New insights from imaging? *Trends in Neuroscience, 24*, 266–271.

Le Bihan, D., Breton, E., Lallemand, D., Grenier, P., Cabanis, E., & Laval-Jeantet, M. (1986). MR imaging of intravoxel incoherent motions: Application to diffusion and perfusion in neurologic disorders. *Radiology, 161*, 401–407.

Le Bihan, D., Turner, R., Moonen, C. T., & Pekar, J. (1991). Imaging of diffusion and microcirculation with gradient sensitization: Design, strategy, and significance. *Journal of Magnetic Resonance Imaging, 1*, 7–28.

Li, X. L., Fang, Y. N., Gao, Q. C., Lin, E. J., Hu, S. H., Ren, L., et al. (2010). A diffusion tensor magnetic resonance imaging study of corpus callosum from adult patients with migraine complicated with depressive/anxious disorder. *Headache, 51*, 237–245.

Mori, S., Kaufmann, W. E., Davatzikos, C., Stieltjes, B., Amodei, L., Fredericksen, K., et al. (2002). Imaging cortical association tracts in the human brain using diffusion-tensor-based axonal tracking. *Magnetic Resonance Medicine, 47*, 215–223.

Ophoff, R. A., Terwindt, G. M., Vergouwe, M. N., van Eijk, R., Oefner, P. J., Hoffman, S. M., et al. (1996). Familial hemiplegic migraine and episodic ataxia type-2 are caused by mutations in the Ca2+ channel gene CACNL1A4. *Cell, 87*, 543–552.

Pierpaoli, C., & Basser, P. J. (1996). Toward a quantitative assessment of diffusion anisotropy. *Magnetic Resonance Medicine, 36*, 893–906.

Ramadan, N. M., Halvorson, H., Vande-Linde, A., Levine, S. R., Helpern, J. A., & Welch, K. M. (1989). Low brain magnesium in migraine. *Headache, 29*, 416–419.

Resnick, S., Reyes-Iglesias, Y., Carreras, R., & Villalobos, E. (2006). Migraine with aura associated with reversible MRI abnormalities. *Neurology, 66*, 946–947.

Rocca, M. A., Ceccarelli, A., Falini, A., Colombo, B., Tortorella, P., Bernasconi, L., et al. (2006a). Brain gray matter changes in migraine patients with T2-visible lesions: A 3-T MRI study. *Stroke, 37*, 1765–1770.

Rocca, M. A., Ceccarelli, A., Falini, A., Tortorella, P., Colombo, B., Pagani, E., et al. (2006b). Diffusion tensor magnetic resonance imaging at 3.0 tesla shows subtle cerebral grey matter abnormalities in patients with migraine. *Journal of Neurology, Neurosurgery, and Psychiatry, 77*, 686–689.

Rocca, M. A., Colombo, B., Inglese, M., Codella, M., Comi, G., & Filippi, M. (2003). A diffusion tensor magnetic resonance imaging study of brain tissue from patients with migraine. *Journal of Neurology, Neurosurgery, and Psychiatry, 74*, 501–503.

Rocca, M. A., Pagani, E., Colombo, B., Tortorella, P., Falini, A., Comi, G., et al. (2008). Selective diffusion changes of the visual pathways in patients with migraine: A 3-T tractography study. *Cephalalgia, 28*, 1061–1068.

Schmitz, N., Admiraal-Behloul, F., Arkink, E. B., Kruit, M. C., Schoonman, G. G., Ferrari, M. D., et al. (2008). Attack frequency and disease duration as indicators for brain damage in migraine. *Headache, 48*, 1044–1055.

Schmitz, N., Arkink, E. B., Mulder, M., Admiraal-Behloul, F., Schoonman, G. G., Kruit, M. C., et al. (2008). Frontal lobe structure and executive function in migraine patients. *Neuroscience Letters, 440*, 92–96.

Toldo, I., Cecchin, D., Sartori, S., Calderone, M., Mardari, R., Cattelan, F., et al. (2010). Multimodal neuroimaging in a child with sporadic hemiplegic migraine: A contribution to understanding pathogenesis. *Cephalalgia, 31*, 751–756.

Warach, S., Gaa, J., Siewert, B., Wielopolski, P., & Edelman, R. R. (1995). Acute human stroke studied by whole brain echo planar diffusion-weighted magnetic resonance imaging. *Annals of Neurology, 37*, 231–241.

Welch, K. M., Levine, S. R., D'Andrea, G., Schultz, L. R., & Helpern, J. A. (1989). Preliminary observations on brain energy metabolism in migraine studied by in vivo phosphorus 31 NMR spectroscopy. *Neurology, 39*, 538–541.

Wolff, H. G. (1963). *Headache and other head pain.* New York: Oxford University Press.

18 Morphometric Changes and Voxel-Based Morphometry in Migraine

ARNE MAY

INTRODUCTION

While early imaging studies of the brain provided a qualitative description of normal brain morphology and its deviations in disease states, more recently developed magnetic resonance (MR)–based methods allow a quantitative evaluation of brain morphology (Draganski & May, 2008). The whole assortment of these MR-based methods comes under the heading of MR morphometry of the brain. One of the immense advantages is the in vivo observation of temporal changes in brain morphology and the correlation of brain morphology with brain function (Ashburner et al., 2003). Normally, three-dimensional, high-resolution, T1-weighted MR images acquired with conventional 1.5-tesla MR scanners and 1-mm³ voxels provide sufficient detail and contrast. One of the most widespread and validated morphometric techniques used to capture structural alterations in the brain is voxel-based morphometry (VBM). VBM is a whole-brain method for analysis of automatically preprocessed structural high-resolution magnetic resonance imaging (MRI) data treating images as continuous scalar measurements (Draganski & May, 2008). VBM is relatively simple to use, has moderate demands on computational resources, and is available in common software packages like FSL or SPM. This technique relies on the segmentation of MR images into different tissue types (gray matter, white matter, and cerebrospinal fluid [CSF]) using information derived from image intensity. The gray matter map as a result of this segmentation thus describes the spatial distribution for each individual at the level of every voxel. Additional a priori knowledge about the spatial distribution of different tissue types can be applied to refine this segmentation process. To take advantage of this approach, MR data have to be registered to the same stereotactic space as the a priori images—making the segmentation accuracy sensitive to registration errors. Because of this dependency of registration errors, several approaches have been developed to improve registration accuracy, such as the use of segmented images for registration rather than MR images

(Good et al., 2001b); a combined model of image registration, tissue classification, and bias correction (Ashburner & Friston, 2005); and the application of high-resolution registration methods (Shen & Davatzikos, 2003). These solutions have been implemented in advanced VBM protocols, which then allow voxel-wise statistical testing of gray matter volume in each voxel.

MORPHOMETRIC STUDIES IN HEADACHE SYNDROMES

Cluster Headache

The pioneering study using VBM to find possible brain differences between headache patients and healthy volunteers found a significant structural difference in gray matter density, a "lesion" coinciding with the inferior posterior hypothalamus, which showed a colocalization of morphometric alterations and functional activation in cluster headache patients (May et al., 1999). These studies prompted the use of stereotactic stimulation (deep brain stimulation [DBS]) of this target point identified by functional and structural neuroimaging (May, 2008b). Up until now, nearly 50 successfully operated intractable chronic cluster headache patients have been reported (Fontaine et al., 2010; Leone et al., 2008). However, the method of hypothalamic DBS is not without risk (Schoenen et al., 2005), and it only works in about 50% of patients (Bartsch et al., 2008; Leone et al., 2008). One of the reasons why it only works in some patients could be the fact that the target point is not defined exactly enough in patients in whom higher voltage is needed, or that the target point is simply wrong in those patients in whom hypothalamic DBS does not work (Fontaine et al., 2010). The target point for hypothalamic DBS was directly taken from the structural and functional studies mentioned above. It needs to be pointed out that these studies are the result of group studies done with positron emission tomography (PET) and that the original data needed to be normalized into a stereotactic space and additionally were smoothed with a filter kernel of at least 10 mm (May et al., 1998). It is more than questionable to use this point as a definite answer to the source of the headache in cluster, and even more so when it is uncritically used in individuals. Each individual's brain anatomy is different (the simple reason why normalization is used in functional neuroimaging) and these subtle differences are corrected in the normalization process (Ashburner & Friston, 1999, 2000). The original work by Franzini and Leone (Leone et al., 2001) is ingenious in that it is the first and only time that functional imaging was directly translated into a treatment that proved to be effective, and it definitely opened new avenues in cluster headache treatment. However, the more we learned about this method in the last 8 years, the more we have had to ask ourselves whether the discussion about the target region should be exhausted by discussing the correct name (e.g., hypothalamic gray versus ventral tegmentum, etc.) of this anatomical point, which is undoubtedly crucial for the pathogenesis of the trigeminal autonomic syndromes (May, 2005). We need more and better studies and above all we need to address the question of individual anatomy and possible anomalies. We need a way to study each patient individually using the functional imaging method with the highest spatial and temporal resolution available to enable us to target the seed point for deep brain stimulation on this individual basis.

Chronic Tension-Type Headache

Recently, 20 patients with chronic tension-type headache (CTTH) were compared to healthy volunteers and showed a significant decrease in gray matter in the dorsal rostral and ventral pons, the perigenual cingulate cortex, the middle cingulate cortex and the right posterior cingulate cortex, the anterior and posterior insulae bilaterally, the right posterior temporal lobe, the orbitofrontal cortex and parahippocampus bilaterally, and the right cerebellum. Interestingly, this decrease in gray matter correlated positively with increasing headache duration in years; that is, patients with a longer history had less gray matter in these regions (Schmidt-Wilcke et al., 2005). In the same paper, patients with medication overuse showed a nonsignificant decrease in the left orbitofrontal cortex and the right midbrain. As the change in gray matter in CTTH patients was restricted to structures involved in pain processing, the authors concluded that these data may be interpreted as the consequence of central sensitization, generated by prolonged nociceptive input from the pericranial myofascial tissues (Schmidt-Wilcke et al., 2005).

Migraine

Regarding migraine, a pioneering study by Matharu et al. (2003) did not find any significant morphometric changes in gray or white matter in patients suffering from episodic migraine. However, five more recent studies question this negative finding. The first one was published by Rocca et al. (2006), who investigated 16 migraine patients with T2-visible abnormalities and 15 matched controls using VBM and reported an increased density of the periaqueductal gray and of the dorsolateral pons in migraine patients. The authors also found a decrease in gray matter in the anterior cingulate cortex (ACC) and both insulae in migraine patients. One possibility why this study found structural changes in migraine, whereas an earlier study did not, may be the fact that Rocca et al. used a scanner with higher field strength (3 T), whereas the former studies were done on a 1.5-T scanner. However, the migraine cohort was rather small (16 patients) and comprised only patients with T2-visible brain lesions, a finding that is not part of the International Headache Society criteria (Headache Classification Committee of the International Headache Society, 2004).

Population-based findings suggest that some patients with migraine (with and without aura) are at an increased risk for subclinical lesions in certain brain areas (Kruit et al., 2004; Tietjen, 2004), which was also suggested by a meta-analysis (Swartz & Kern, 2004). Although it is more than questionable that these white matter changes are true vascular infarcts, given that they can vanish spontaneously (Agarwal et al., 2008; Rozen, 2007), it has been shown that they are independent of right-to-left shunts (Adami et al., 2008) and therefore cannot simply be attributed to the occurrence of a patent foramen ovale (PFO) (Dowson et al., 2008), as has been discussed before (Wilmshurst et al., 2000, 2006). In any case, studying only migraine patients with visible MR lesions may imply a significant bias. Nevertheless, the findings of this study were, in essence, replicated by four independent other studies so far (Kim et al., 2008; Schmidt-Wilcke et al., 2008; Schmitz et al., 2008; Valfre et al., 2008). All of these studies reported a decrease in gray matter in the frontal and temporal cortex. The first one was published by Valfre et al. (2008), who investigated 27 migraine patients and 27 healthy controls. In comparison with controls, migraineurs presented a significant focal gray matter reduction in the right superior temporal gyrus, right inferior frontal gyrus, and left precentral gyrus. The patients were divided into episodic and chronic migraine (n = 11), and chronic migraine patients showed additionally a focal gray matter decrease in the bilateral anterior cingulate cortex. Other clusters were found in the amygdala, parietal operculum, frontal gyrus, and bilateral insula. Comparing all the migraine patients with controls, a significant correlation between gray matter reduction in the anterior cingulate cortex and the frequency of migraine attacks was found (Valfre et al., 2008). The authors concluded that their study supports the concept that migraine is a progressive disorder (Valfre et al., 2008). The same conclusion was drawn by another study investigating 28 patients and demonstrating less gray matter in migraineurs in the frontal lobes, brainstem, and cerebellum. In this study, both the attack frequency and the disease duration correlated with the extent of gray matter reduction, and the authors interpreted this finding as an indicator for "brain damage" in migraine. The third study was published by Kim et al. (2008), who compared gray matter volume between 20 migraine patients (5 with aura and 15 without aura) with 33 healthy controls matched for age and sex. Although the statistics have to be seen with caution, given the different sample size per cohort, the findings are remarkably similar to the ones above: Migraine patients had significant gray matter reductions in the bilateral insula, motor/premotor cortex, prefrontal cortex, cingulate cortex, right posterior parietal cortex, and orbitofrontal cortex. Moreover, all of these regions were negatively correlated with headache duration and lifetime headache frequency. The authors interpret their findings as suggesting "that repeated migraine attacks over time result in selective damage to several brain regions involved in central pain processing"(Kim et al., 2008).

The biggest study so far was published by Schmidt-Wilcke et al. (2008), who compared 35 patients suffering from migraine with 31 healthy controls with no headache history. They found a decrease in gray matter in the anterior and middle cingulate cortex in migraineurs. The authors discussed their findings in context with recent findings in chronic pain states, such as chronic phantom pain (Draganski et al., 2006) and chronic back pain (Apkarian et al., 2004), and suggested that the gray matter change in migraine patients is the consequence of frequent nociceptive input and should thus be reversible when migraine attacks cease (Schmidt-Wilcke et al., 2008). In summary, the authors of all but the last study in migraine interpreted their finding—a focal reduction in gray matter—as damage of the brain or as an indicator that migraine is a progressive disease. This argumentation disregards the point that migraine is a self-remitting disease that usually resolves with age. Until longitudinal studies have been conducted that assess whether these changes also recede, we should not overinterpret these data as "brain damage." In this context it is interesting that CTTH does not always resolve with age and that morphometric changes seen in these patients may theoretically be more functionally relevant.

MORPHOMETRIC CHANGES IN CHRONIC PAIN

Any morphometric findings in headache patients have to be seen in the light of a wealth of morphometric studies on chronic pain (May, 2008a) and exercise-dependent plasticity (Duerden and Laverdure-Dupont, 2008). In the last 2 or 3 years, several studies were published that demonstrated structural brain changes in chronic pain syndromes. A striking feature of all of these studies is the fact that the gray matter changes were not randomly distributed, but concerned defined and functionally highly specific brain areas—namely, involvement in supraspinal nociceptive processing. The most prominent findings were different for each pain syndrome, but overlapped in the cingulate cortex, the orbitofrontal cortex, the insula, and the dorsal pons (May, 2008a). Further structures included the thalamus, basal ganglia, and parahippocampus bilaterally. All of the studies conducted so far in chronic pain syndromes, including fibromyalgia (Kuchinad et al., 2007), irritable bowel syndrome (Davis et al., 2008), phantom pain (Draganski et al., 2006), chronic back pain (Apkarian et al., 2004; Schmidt-Wilcke et al., 2006), and thoracic spinal cord injury (Wrigley et al., 2008), showed a decrease in some of the above-mentioned areas. Nevertheless, all available clinical MR morphometric studies have their limitations. One of the major drawbacks is the poor comparability of studies from different research centers. In addition, many studies were done in small patient samples and did not analyze the temporal dynamics and the determinants of brain morphological changes. Consequently, routine clinical application of MR-based morphometry is currently not feasible. However, the fact that the above-mentioned findings in migraine and tension-type headache (Figure 8-1). have been replicated by nearly all studies investigating brain changes in patients suffering from all sorts of chronic pain suggests that these findings are not specific to head pain but to the chronicity of pain If it is true that chronic pain patients have a common "brain signature" in areas known to be involved in pain control, the question arises whether the central reorganization processes in chronic pain syndromes could involve a "degeneration" of specific brain areas. Most recently two studies questioned the concept of irreversible atrophy and clearly showed that a gray matter decrease is at least partly reversible when pain is successfully treated (Obermann et al., 2009; Rodriguez-Raecke et al., 2009). This question is not redundant, as a degenerative process is irreversible. Although some of these studies in chronic pain also fall for the assumption that a decrease in brain gray matter must mean damage to the brain (Apkarian et al., 2004; Kuchinad et al., 2007), the crucial question is, What do we measure when we measure gray matter?

The neurobiological basis of structural alterations (increase or decrease in gray matter demonstrated by VBM) on a microscopic level is not well defined. VBM

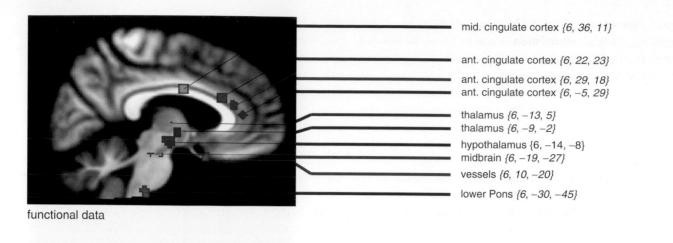

functional data

mid. cingulate cortex {6, 36, 11}

ant. cingulate cortex {6, 22, 23}

ant. cingulate cortex {6, 29, 18}
ant. cingulate cortex {6, −5, 29}

thalamus {6, −13, 5}
thalamus {6, −9, −2}
hypothalamus {6, −14, −8}
midbrain {6, −19, −27}
vessels {6, 10, −20}

lower Pons {6, −30, −45}

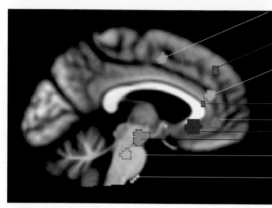

structural data

left mid. cingulate cortex {−3, 0, 48}

middle frontal gyrus {−3, 38, 39}

ant. cingulate cortex {−3, 35, 21}

ant. cingulate cortex {−3, 29, 14}
ant. cingulate cortex {−3, 40, 0}
ant. cingulate cortex, rostral part {−3, 22, −3}
hypothalamus {−3, −17, −12}
dorsal rostral pons {−3, −27, −25}

ventral pons {−3, −21, −42}

FIGURE 18–1. *Summary of the functional (positron emission tomography) and structural (voxel-based morphometry) data of all studies cited in the text. For each paper all available stereotactic coordinates were included in a meta-analysis (http://www.brainmap.org/index.html) using GingerALE via the activation likelihood estimation (ALE) method. We used a 10-mm full width at half-maximum filter and 5,000 permutations to determine the null distribution of the ALE statistic at each voxel. We used a normalized template as the anatomical underlay and the threshold ALE results as the overlay. The colors code the different headache types investigated so far and show the finding for each headache type in Talairach space. Papers showing significant activations that form the results of this analysis are cited in the text.*

detects changes in gray matter concentration per voxel as well as changes in the classification of individual voxels, for example, from white to gray matter (Good et al., 2001a), and probably a combination of both. In general, a decrease in gray matter could be due to a simple decrease in cell size, atrophy of neurons or glia, inactivation of spine density, or even changes in blood flow or interstitial fluid. Unfortunately, all available studies compared cohorts of patients and therefore no statement regarding dynamic changes can be made. In some respects, this situation resembles that in the functional MRI field some years ago, when its use for our understanding of brain function was undebated, yet the long-supposed physiological correlate of the blood oxygenation level–dependent (BOLD) signal was not yet proven (Logothetis & Pfeuffer, 2004). As long as the causes of these changes on a histological-anatomical

level remain unresolved, the clinical relevance of MR morphometric results is limited.

THE BRAIN IN PAIN: DYNAMIC
ALTERATIONS AND NEURONAL
PLASTICITY

Considering that activation-dependent brain plasticity in humans on a structural level has already been demonstrated in adults (Boyke et al., 2008; Draganski et al., 2004), it is an interesting question whether repeated painful stimulation may lead to structural changes of the brain. In a very recent study, 14 healthy subjects were stimulated daily with a 20-minute pain paradigm for 8 consecutive days, and structural MRI was performed on days 1, 8, and 22 and again after 1 year. Using VBM, it was demonstrated that repeated painful stimulation resulted in a substantial increase of gray matter in classical somatosensory areas, including the midcingulate and somatosensory cortex (Teutsch et al., 2008). These data are in line with most morphometric studies investigating structural brain plasticity as a result of exercise and learning (Draganski et al., 2004; Gaser & Schlaug, 2003; May et al., 2007). The changes in brain structure are usually exclusively demonstrated in brain areas that are ascribable to the task (May, 2011). Moreover, the finding of structural changes follows the previously described functional pattern (Bingel et al., 2007) precisely, that is, a significant change during the protocol that reverses to prestimulation levels at the fourth time point (i.e., after 1 year). It is an intriguing fact that chronic pain patients suffer constant pain but seem not to develop an increase in gray matter in somatosensory areas, although several studies showed that exercise is accompanied by an increase in gray matter in the regions that are specific for the respective task (for review see May & Gaser, 2006).

It is not understood why only a relatively small proportion of humans develop a chronic pain syndrome, considering that pain is a universal experience. The question arises whether in some humans a structural difference in central pain-transmitting systems may act as a diathesis for chronic pain. In the course of chronicity, numerous modulatory mechanisms have been postulated and altogether addressed as "neuronal plasticity" (Woolf & Salter, 2000), and structural changes of the brain may be added to this list (May, 2008a). There are no conclusive data regarding the cause or the consequence of the different cortical and subcortical morphological changes that have been observed in chronic pain states, although the correlation of pain duration and degree of gray matter decrease in most studies suggests that the morphological changes are, at least in part, secondary to constant pain.

WHICH STRUCTURAL CHANGES ARE SPECIFIC FOR HEADACHE?

Given that nearly all studies investigating structural changes in different headache syndromes found similar results (May, 2009), and given that these results have been found in most studies of chronic pain as well (May, 2011), one has to address these changes, namely, a decrease of gray matter in pain-transmitting structures, as unspecific for a given headache or pain syndrome and further studies will be required to definitively address this issue. As most changes correlate to pain duration, it seems plausible to argue that the alteration of this region is a consequence, rather than a cause, of frequent nociceptive input.

The nature of chronic pain makes it difficult to prove this point. Regarding headache, however, it is not known why migraine usually remits with age. It is a very interesting question for future studies whether the morphological changes reverse when migraine and hence the disproportionate amount of nociceptive stimulation stops.

Two studies reported structural changes that may be specific for the respective disease: the hypothalamus in cluster headache (May et al., 1999) and the brainstem in migraine (Rocca et al., 2006). The data in cluster headache describe an increase in gray matter that follows the functional pattern during the acute headache attack (May et al., 1998). The study in migraine patients reported an increased density of gray matter in the dorsal pontine region at virtually the same location as the activation reported in the migraine PET studies. The anatomical colocalization of functional and structural changes raises the possibility that the observed changes may be causal rather than a consequence of the pain. In both cases the question arises whether these changes (an increase of regional gray matter rather than a decrease) reflect the above-mentioned morphometric studies investigating structural brain plasticity as a result of exercise and learning. Further studies need to be done, and as migraine has a strong genetic component, the ideal inclusion criteria for future studies to render groups as homogenous as possible could be based on genotype (cohort study) or response to treatment (longitudinal study including controls). However, any data showing a decrease in gray matter in headache syndromes need to be seen in the light of all the information that has been gathered in the last 10 years and probably do not justify discussion of brain damage or whether or not the disease is progressive.

LIMITATIONS OF VOXEL-BASED MORPHOMETRY

As a noninvasive procedure, MR morphometry has the potential to be the ideal tool for the quest to find the morphological substrates of diseases, deepening our understanding of the relationship between brain structure and function, and even to monitor therapeutic interventions. VBM is for research purposes only and requires groups of at least 20 subjects per group to produce stable results (May & Gaser, 2006). However, headache and pain studies so far suffer relatively often from small sample sizes and selected patient samples (e.g., cases from specialized centers rather than population cases). Given that the groups that are to be compared need to be highly homogenous, an excellent and scrupulous matching of cases and controls is mandatory. However, who is the proper control for a migraine study, volunteers who claim to never have experienced a headache in their life or volunteers who just have no migraine and no first-degree family member with migraine? Both choices make this very challenging due to recall issues and the long-term nature of the disorder. Perhaps structural studies of a condition that is potentially genetically heterogenous, such as migraine, miss subtle changes that might segregate with a more homogenous genotype (Matharu et al., 2003). The advantage of VBM is that it is fully automated and allows for changes elsewhere in the brain and thus avoids observer bias, and moreover, it incorporates a voxel-wise estimation of variance. However, differences in imaging modalities, equipment, analysis, and above all image preprocessing steps such as smoothing, registration, choice of small-volume correction, etc., may well account for differences in VBM findings. Until there is a better standardization between different studies and centers (Magis et al., 2007; May & Gaser, 2006), we need to be cautious not to overinterpret morphometric data in headache patients.

ACKNOWLEDGMENTS

This work was supported by grants from the DFG (MA 1862/2–3) and BMBF (371 57 01 & NeuroImageNord).

REFERENCES

Adami, A., Rossato, G., Cerini, R., Thijs, V. N., Pozzi-Mucelli, R., Anzola, G. P., et al. (2008). Right-to-left shunt does not increase white matter lesion load in migraine with aura patients. *Neurology, 71*, 101–107.

Agarwal, S., Magu, S., & Kamal, K. (2008). Reversible white matter abnormalities in a patient with migraine. *Neurology India, 56*, 182–185.

Apkarian, A. V., Sosa, Y., Sonty, S., Levy, R. M., Harden, R. N., Parrish, T. B., et al. (2004). Chronic back pain is associated with decreased prefrontal and thalamic gray matter density. *Journal of Neuroscience, 24*, 10410–10415.

Ashburner, J., Csernansky, J. G., Davatzikos, C., Fox, N. C., Frisoni, G. B., & Thompson, P. M. (2003). Computer-assisted imaging to assess brain structure in healthy and diseased brains. *Lancet Neurology, 2*, 79–88.

Ashburner, J., & Friston, K. J. (1999). Nonlinear spatial normalization using basis functions. *Human Brain Mapping, 7*, 254–266.

Ashburner, J., & Friston, K. J. (2000). Voxel-based morphometry—the methods. *Neuroimage, 11*, 805–821.

Ashburner, J., & Friston, K. J. (2005). Unified segmentation. *Neuroimage, 26*, 839–851.

Bartsch, T., Pinsker, M. O., Rasche, D., Kinfe, T., Hertel, F., Diener, H. C., et al. (2008). Hypothalamic deep brain stimulation for cluster headache: Experience from a new multicase series. *Cephalalgia, 28*, 285–295.

Bingel, U., Schoell, E., Herken, W., Buchel, C., & May, A. (2007). Habituation to painful stimulation involves the antinociceptive system. *Pain, 131*, 21–30.

Boyke, J., Driemeyer, J., Gaser, C., Büchel, C., & May, A. (2008). Training induced brain structure changes in the elderly. *Journal of Neuroscience, 28*, 7031–7035.

Davis, K. D., Pope, G., Chen, J., Kwan, C. L., Crawley, A. P., & Diamant, N. E. (2008). Cortical thinning in IBS: Implications for homeostatic, attention, and pain processing. *Neurology, 70*, 153–154.

Dowson, A., Mullen, M. J., Peatfield, R., Muir, K., Khan, A. A., Wells, C., et al. (2008). Migraine Intervention With STARFlex Technology (MIST) trial: A prospective, multicenter, double-blind, sham-controlled trial to evaluate the effectiveness of patent foramen ovale closure with STARFlex septal repair implant to resolve refractory migraine headache. *Circulation, 117*, 1397–1404.

Draganski, B., Gaser, C., Busch, V., Schuierer, G., Bogdahn, U., & May, A. (2004). Neuroplasticity: Changes in grey matter induced by training. *Nature, 427*, 311–312.

Draganski, B., & May, A. (2008). Training-induced structural changes in the adult human brain. *Behavioural Brain Research, 192*, 137–142.

Draganski, B., Moser, T., Lummel, N., Ganssbauer, S., Bogdahn, U., Haas, F., et al. (2006). Decrease of thalamic gray matter following limb amputation. *Neuroimage, 31*, 951–957.

Duerden, E. G., & Laverdure-Dupont, D. (2008). Practice makes cortex. *Journal of Neuroscience, 28*, 8655–8657.

Fontaine, D., Lanteri-Minet, M., Ouchchane, L., Lazorthes, Y., Mertens, P., Blond, S., et al. (2010). Anatomical location of effective deep brain stimulation electrodes in chronic cluster headache. *Brain, 133*, 1214–1223.

Gaser, C., & Schlaug, G. (2003). Brain structures differ between musicians and non-musicians. *Journal of Neuroscience, 23*, 9240–9245.

Good, C. D., Johnsrude, I., Ashburner, J., Henson, R. N., Friston, K. J., & Frackowiak, R. S. (2001a). Cerebral asymmetry and the effects of sex and handedness on brain structure: A voxel-based morphometric analysis of 465 normal adult human brains. *Neuroimage, 14*, 685–700.

Good, C. D., Johnsrude, I. S., Ashburner, J., Henson, R. N., Friston, K. J., & Frackowiak, R. S. (2001b). A voxel-based morphometric study of ageing in 465 normal adult human brains. *Neuroimage, 14*, 21–36.

Headache Classification Committee of the International Headache Society. (2004). The international classification of headache disorders, 2nd edition. *Cephalalgia, 24*, 1–160.

Kim, J. H., Suh, S. I., Seol, H. Y., Oh, K., Seo, W. K., Yu, S. W., et al. (2008). Regional grey matter changes in patients with migraine: a voxel-based morphometry study. *Cephalalgia, 28*, 598–604.

Kruit, M. C., van Buchem, M. A., Hofman, P. A., Bakkers, J. T., Terwindt, G. M., Ferrari, M. D., et al. (2004). Migraine as a risk factor for subclinical brain lesions. *Journal of the American Medical Association, 291*, 427–434.

Kuchinad, A., Schweinhardt, P., Seminowicz, D. A., Wood, P. B., Chizh, B. A., & Bushnell, M. C. (2007). Accelerated brain gray matter loss in fibromyalgia patients: Premature aging of the brain? *Journal of Neuroscience, 27*, 4004–4007.

Leone, M., Franzini, A., & Bussone, G. (2001). Stereotactic stimulation of posterior hypothalamic gray matter in a patient with intractable cluster headache. *New England Journal of Medicine, 345*, 1428–1429.

Leone, M., Proietti Cecchini, A., Franzini, A., Broggi, G., Cortelli, P., Montagna, P., et al. (2008). Lessons from 8 years' experience of hypothalamic stimulation in cluster headache. *Cephalalgia, 28*, 787–797; discussion 798.

Logothetis, N. K., & Pfeuffer, J. (2004). On the nature of the BOLD fMRI contrast mechanism. *Magnetic Resonance Imaging, 22*, 1517–1531.

Magis, D., Bendtsen, L., Goadsby, P. J., May, A., Sanchez del Rio, M., Sandor, P. S., et al. (2007). Evaluation and proposal for optimization of neurophysiological tests in migraine: Part 2—neuroimaging and the nitroglycerin test. *Cephalalgia, 27*, 1339–1359.

Matharu, M. S., Good, C. D., May, A., Bahra, A., & Goadsby, P. J. (2003). No change in the structure of the brain in migraine: a voxel-based morphometric study. *European Journal of Neurology, 10*, 53–57.

May, A. (2005). Cluster headache: Pathogenesis, diagnosis, and management. *Lancet, 366*, 843–855.

May, A. (2008a). Chronic pain may change the structure of the brain. *Pain, 137*, 7–15.

May, A. (2008b). Hypothalamic deep-brain stimulation: Target and potential mechanism for the treatment of cluster headache. *Cephalalgia, 28*, 799–803.

May, A. (2009). Morphing voxels: the hype around structural imaging of headache patients. *Brain, 132*(Pt 6), 1419–1425.

May, A. (2011). Structural brain imaging: A window into chronic pain. *Neuroscientist, 17*, 209–220.

May, A., Ashburner, J., Buchel, C., McGonigle, D. J., Friston, K. J., Frackowiak, R. S., et al. (1999). Correlation between structural and functional changes in brain in an idiopathic headache syndrome. *Nature Medicine, 5*, 836–838.

May, A., Bahra, A., Büchel, C., Frackowiak, R. S. J., & Goadsby, P. J. (1998). Hypothalamic activation in cluster headache attacks. *Lancet, 352*, 275–278.

May, A., & Gaser, C. (2006). Magnetic resonance-based morphometry: A window into structural plasticity of the brain. *Current Opinion in Neurology, 19*, 407–411.

May, A., Hajak, G., Ganssbauer, S., Steffens, T., Langguth, B., Kleinjung, T., et al. (2007). Structural brain alterations following 5 days of intervention: Dynamic aspects of neuroplasticity. *Cerebral Cortex, 17*, 205–210.

Obermann, M., Nebel, K., Schumann, C., Holle, D., Gizewski, E. R., Maschke, M., et al. (2009). Gray matter changes related to chronic posttraumatic headache. *Neurology, 73*, 978–983.

Rocca, M. A., Ceccarelli, A., Falini, A., Colombo, B., Tortorella, P., Bernasconi, L., et al. (2006). Brain gray matter changes in migraine patients with T2-visible lesions: A 3-T MRI study. *Stroke, 37*, 1765–1770.

Rodriguez-Raecke, R., Niemeier, A., Ihle, K., Ruether, W., & May, A. (2009). Brain gray matter decrease in chronic pain is the consequence and not the cause of pain. *Journal of Neuroscience, 29*, 13746–750.

Rozen, T. D. (2007). Vanishing cerebellar infarcts in a migraine patient. *Cephalalgia, 27*, 557–560.

Schmidt-Wilcke, T., Ganssbauer, S., Neuner, T., Bogdahn, U., & May, A. (2008). Subtle grey matter changes between migraine patients and healthy controls. *Cephalalgia, 28*, 1–4.

Schmidt-Wilcke, T., Leinisch, E., Ganssbauer, S., Draganski, B., Bogdahn, U., Altmeppen, J., et al. (2006). Affective components and intensity of pain correlate with structural differences in gray matter in chronic back pain patients. *Pain, 125*, 89–97.

Schmidt-Wilcke, T., Leinisch, E., Straube, A., Kampfe, N., Draganski, B., Diener, H. C., et al. (2005). Gray matter decrease in patients with chronic tension type headache. *Neurology, 65*, 1483–1486.

Schmitz, N., Admiraal-Behloul, F., Arkink, E. B., Kruit, M. C., Schoonman, G. G., Ferrari, M. D., et al. (2008). Attack frequency and disease duration as indicators for brain damage in migraine. *Headache, 48*, 1044–1055.

Schoenen, J., Di Clemente, L., Vandenheede, M., Fumal, A., De Pasqua, V., Mouchamps, M., et al. (2005). Hypothalamic stimulation in chronic cluster headache: A pilot study of efficacy and mode of action. *Brain, 128*, 940–947.

Shen, D., & Davatzikos, C. (2003). Very high-resolution morphometry using mass-preserving deformations and HAMMER elastic registration. *Neuroimage, 18*, 28–41.

Swartz, R. H., & Kern, R. Z. (2004). Migraine is associated with magnetic resonance imaging white matter abnormalities: A meta-analysis. *Archives of Neurology, 61*, 1366–1368.

Teutsch, S., Herken, W., Bingel, U., Schoell, E., & May, A. (2008). Changes in brain gray matter due to repetitive painful stimulation. *Neuroimage, 42*, 845–849.

Tietjen, G. E. (2004). Stroke and migraine linked by silent lesions. *Lancet Neurology, 3*, 267.

Valfre, W., Rainero, I., Bergui, M., & Pinessi, L. (2008). Voxel-based morphometry reveals gray matter abnormalities in migraine. *Headache, 48*, 109–117.

Wilmshurst, P., Nightingale, S., Pearson, M., Morrison, L., & Walsh, K. (2006). Relation of atrial shunts to migraine in patients with ischemic stroke and peripheral emboli. *American Journal of Cardiology, 98*, 831–833.

Wilmshurst, P. T., Nightingale, S., Walsh, K. P., & Morrison, W. L. (2000). Effect on migraine of closure of cardiac right-to-left shunts to prevent recurrence of decompression illness or stroke or for haemodynamic reasons. *Lancet, 356*, 1648–1651.

Woolf, C. J., & Salter, M. W. (2000). Neuronal plasticity: Increasing the gain in pain. *Science, 288*, 1765–1769.

Wrigley, P. J., Gustin, S. M., Macey, P. M., Nash, P. G., Gandevia, S. C., Macefield, V. G., et al. (2008). Anatomical changes in human motor cortex and motor pathways following complete thoracic spinal cord injury. *Cerebral Cortex, 19*, 224–232.

19 Surface-Based Structural Changes in Migraine

CRISTINA GRANZIERA AND NOUCHINE HADJIKHANI

INTRODUCTION

The human cortex is a convoluted structure consisting of layers of neuronal cells, glial cells, and blood vessels. The neocortex is differentiated into six horizontal layers, whereas the archicortex (hippocampus) is mostly organized into three cellular layers (Morrison, 1992).

During development, the cortical folding process begins at around 10 weeks of fetal life (A. Fees-Higgins, 1987) and is influenced by distinct genetic factors (Panizzon et al., 2009). During the third trimester of fetal life, the cerebral cortex acquires the complex folded structure that resembles the morphology of the adult cortex.

The cortical thickness varies considerably across different regions of the brain (Fischl & Dale, 2000; Jones et al., 2000). In healthy subjects, the cortex has an average thickness of 3 mm. It tends to be thinnest in the calcarine cortex (2 mm) and thickest in the precentral gyrus (4 mm) (Morrison, 1992).

Changes in the thickness of the human cerebral cortex have been described in physiological processes (aging), brain neurodegenerative diseases (Alzheimer disease, Huntington disease), psychiatric pathologies (autism and schizophrenia), and migraine.

MAGNETIC RESONANCE IMAGING VISUALIZATION AND QUANTIFICATION OF THE HUMAN CEREBRAL CORTEX

Visualizing and, more important, quantifying the properties of the cerebral cortex and of its layers is an exciting and challenging research field. In this context, magnetic resonance imaging (MRI) may provide an important contribution at both the acquisition and image processing levels to obtain more information of the brain in migraine.

Ultra-high magnetic fields for MRI have become particularly promising as the improved signal-to-noise ratio (SNR) allows a better visualization of details in the anatomy such as the fine substructure of the cerebral cortex (Fukunaga et al., 2010; Marques, van der Zwaag, et al., 2010).

Various postprocessing techniques propose ways to extract the cortical surface from MRI brain scans and calculate parameters such as cortical thickness (Fjell et al., 2006; Toro & Burnod, 2003; Van Essen et al., 2001) or complexity (Thompson et al., 2005). Moreover, recently, this has also allowed the local three-dimensional computation of the gyrification index as a measure of the degree of folding of a given cortical area (Luders et al., 2006).

The study of cortical folding by means of MRI is known as surface-based morphometry (SBM) and is presumably particularly sensitive to detect subtle changes in the cortical brain morphometry. However, it provides two specific challenges. The first is how to measure the properties of a curved structure; the second is accurately determining the boundaries of the gray matter gyri (gyrification), a structure only a few millimeters thick.

In a recent work, Aganj et al. (2009) summarized some of the techniques currently used in the research that deal with these problems. It is worth noting, however, that none of the techniques reported below can currently be considered as "the" established method to study the features of the cortex.

According to the work by Aganj et al. (2009), the various existing methods fall under five main categories:

1. *Coupled-surface methods* (Fischl & Dale, 2000; MacDonald et al., 2000), which define the cortical thickness as the mean of the distances between corresponding point pairs on the gray–white matter boundaries and the pial surfaces (Fig. 19–1A). The method of Fischl et al. is freely available at http://surfer.nmr.mgh.harvard.edu and for this reason is probably the most commonly applied.
2. *Closest point methods*, which compute and measure for each point on one of the two surfaces the closest point on the other surface (Fig. 19–1B)
3. The *regional histogram of thickness* (Scott & Thacker, 2005), where a measure is performed of the length of the line segments connecting the inner and outer surfaces of the gray matter (GM) layer, normal to one of the surfaces

4. *"Laplace" methods* (Haidar & Soul, 2006; Jones et al., 2000; Yezzi & Prince, 2003), which apply the Laplace approach to GM regions (Fig. 19–1C)
5. *Largest enclosed spheres methods* (Pizer et al., 1998), where a central axis of the GM layer is defined and the cortical thickness is estimated as the diameter of the largest enclosed sphere with the diameter centered on a point on the central axis (Fig. 1D)

The vast majority of the methods reported in the literature propagate segmentation errors to later steps, and segmentation remains a challenging problem in brain imaging. Considering that the GM layer spans only a few voxels at the commonly used 1- to 2-mm resolutions, these errors can be significant and measuring tissue thickness avoiding this hard segmentation step may be very beneficial.

A method dealing with this problem has been recently published by Aganj et al. (2009) and is based on *minimization of the line integrals* over the probability map of GM in the MRI volume. The cortical thickness measure is therefore defined for each voxel as the minimum line integral of the probability map along a line centered at the point of interest. This method has been validated on artificial values and real three-dimensional brain MRIs from healthy subjects and Alzheimer disease patients (Aganj et al., 2009).

All the measures relative to the cortical mantle can be applied globally, at the lobar level, at the sulcus level, or locally using a normalization-based coordinate system mentioned above (coupled surface methods).

Applying these methods, simple features can be calculated such as the length, the area, and the depth (Mangin et al., 2004). However, more complex parameters have also been proposed to quantify the complete three-dimensional shape: (a) the three-dimensional gyrification index (Thompson et al., 2005), (b) multishapes clustering (Sun et al., 2009), and (c) the central sulcus surface area (Kloppel et al., 2010).

VALUE OF SURFACE-BASED MORPHOMETRY IN MEASURING CORTICAL THICKNESS

There are a number of *advantages* of SBM methods compared to other morphometric techniques.

Compared to voxel-based morphometry (VBM) techniques, SBM can take into account the complex and highly variable folding pattern of the cortical sheet. In addition, while VBM compares only regional cortical volume, SBM can decompose the volume of the cortical sheet into two properties as cortical thickness and surface area (SA).

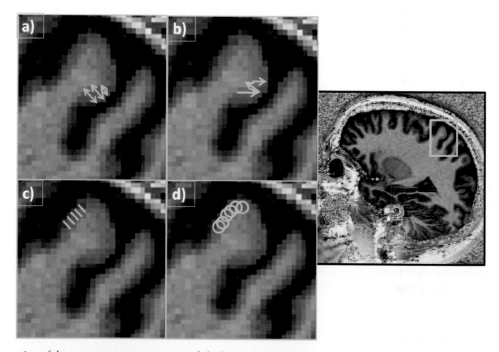

FIGURE 19–1 *Illustration of the concepts to measure cortical thickness: (A) coupled-surface methods, (B) closest point methods, (C) Laplace methods, and (D) largest enclosed sphere methods. The underlying T1-weighted image has been acquired at 7 T using the MP2RAGE approach. From Marques, J. P., Kober, T., Krueger, G., van der Zwaag, W., Van de Moortele, P. F., & Gruetter, R. (2010). MP2RAGE, a self bias-field corrected sequence for improved segmentation and T1-mapping at high field.* Neuroimage, 49(2), 1271–1281.

This may become important for interpretation of the results, since cortical thickness and SA capture very different sets of biological processes as evidenced by their differing evolutionary histories (Rakic, 1995) and genetic determinants (Panizzon et al., 2009). Furthermore, SA is determined by overall brain size and the degree of cortical folding (gyrification), which are shaped by distinct influences.

Moreover, a vertex-based rather than a VBM-based assessment of cortical thickness after surface-based registration provides a more sensitive and informative marker of cortical differences between clinical groups (Park et al., 2009).

By interrelating measures of the cortical thickness at different vertices, it is possible to describe patterns of structural covariance across the cortex. The extent to which cortical regions are structurally similar to each other (as indexed by cortical thickness covariance) may appear neurobiologically meaningful because in typical development (a) cortical regions that show high cortical thickness covariance also show strong shared genetic influences on cortical thickness (Schmitt et al., 2009), and (b) maps of cortical thickness covariance between cortical regions have been found to strongly resemble maps of corticocortical connectivity derived from other techniques such as diffusion tensor imaging (DTI) of white matter tracts (Lerch et al., 2006) and functional MRI (fMRI) studies of "functional connectivity" (Chen et al., 2008; Toro et al., 2008). Maps of cortical thickness covariance also vary as a function of disease processes (He & Liu, 2008), developmental stage, cognitive ability, and skill proficiency (Lerch et al., 2006).

Less favorable for SBM, however, is that it generally imposes a high demand on computational resources and requires a long computational time; the results highly depend on the quality of the segmentation and/or surface extraction, which may require manual adaptations and corrections; and last but not least, results are sensitive to appropriate MRI quality. In addition, at present SBM allows studying exclusively the hemispheric cortical layer and compared to VBM does not provide any information about the cerebellum, the subcortical white matter, and deep gray matter nuclei, structures that have been hypothesized to be involved in migraine (Kruit et al., 2009, 2010; Vincent & Hadjikhani, 2007).

OVERVIEW OF SURFACE-BASED TECHNIQUES APPLICATIONS

Changes in properties of the cortical layer of the brain have been measured by SBM in physiological processes such as aging and in a number of neurodegenerative, psychiatric, and genetic diseases.

Various measures of cortical structure, such as thickness, exhibit linear decrease with aging (Fjell, Westlye, et al., 2009; Kochunov et al., 2008; Salat et al., 2004). Cortical thinning showed consistent age effects across samples in the superior, middle, and inferior frontal gyri; superior and middle temporal gyri; precuneus, inferior, and superior parietal cortices; fusiform and lingual gyri; and the temporoparietal junction. The strongest effects were seen in the superior and inferior frontal gyri, as well as superior parts of the temporal lobe. The inferior temporal lobe and anterior cingulate cortices were less affected by age (Fjell, Westlye, et al., 2009).

Cortical thinning in the temporal lobe has been observed in mild cognitive impairment (MCI) and Alzheimer disease (AD) (Dickerson et al., 2009; Fjell, Walhovd, et al., 2009). In addition to the findings in the temporal lobes, Lerch et al. (2005) observed significant cortical thickness decline in orbitofrontal and parietal regions in AD patients compared to healthy controls. Moreover, the cortical thinning pattern observed in MCI and AD allowed prediction of evolution to Alzheimer disease for 76% of amnestic MCI subjects, pointing out a possible role of cortical thickness measures for early AD diagnosis (Lerch et al., 2005).

In chronic neurological disorders such as multiple sclerosis (MS), global and focal cortical thinning (frontal and temporal lobe) has also been shown with surface-based techniques (Sailer et al., 2003). Cortical thinning in the cingulum, insula, and associative cortical regions correlated with total lesion load and disability (Charil et al., 2007).

In presymptomatic individuals with the Huntington disease (HD) mutation, Rosas et al. (2005) showed that cortical thinning was regionally selective (in precentral, superior and middle frontal, parietal, temporal, and occipital areas) and correlated with cognitive performance.

Increases in total cerebral sulcal and gyral thickness as well as in the temporal and parietal lobes were observed in children with autism relative to healthy age- and gender-matched subjects (Hardan et al., 2006). However, more recently, it was shown that cortical thickness in patients with autism increases early in development and thins in adolescence (Shaw et al., 2008). This may explain controversial results reported by other studies investigating cortical thickness in autism. For example, Chung et al. (2005) showed mostly thinner cortex in a group of male autistic subjects with an age range between 12 and 15 years; similarly, Hadjikhani et al. (2006) as well as Wallace et al. (2009) found thinner temporal, parietal, and frontal cortices in high-functioning autism spectrum disorders and an adult male savant with Asperger syndrome. In addition to this, Wallace et al. (2010) confirmed the age-related changes in cortical thickness showing that participants with autism spectrum disorders had thinner cortex in the temporal lobe with increasing age and that this process was more pronounced in patients than in an age- and gender-matched group of healthy controls.

Studies investigating the cortical thickness have also been conducted in schizophrenic patients. In first-episode schizophrenia, cortical thinning was demonstrated in prefrontal, frontal, cingulate, temporal, occipital, and parietal cortices (Narr, Bilder, et al., 2005; Narr, Toga, et al., 2005; Venkatasubramanian et al., 2008). In patients with multiple episodes, decreased cortical thickness was found mainly in prefronto-temporal areas (Kuperberg et al., 2003; Nesvag et al., 2008). However, these studies showed some heterogeneity regarding the affected anatomical regions. Finally, in patients with short- to medium-term disease, a significant reduction of cortical thickness was found in a spatially complex pattern of focal anatomical regions making up the dorsolateral prefrontal cortex, medial prefrontal cortex, lateral temporal cortices, left entorhinal cortex, posterior cingulate cortex, and precuneus and lingual cortex, bilaterally.

Other genetic diseases such as Turner disease and Williams disease have been examined using the SBM method. They have been shown to result in diffuse cortical thinning. Specific patterns of abnormal folding have been reported after performing group averaging of surface-based analysis results (Van Essen et al., 2006).

SURFACE-BASED MEASUREMENTS IN MIGRAINE

Migraine attacks are characterized by a series of neurovascular and electric events involving both subcortical and cortical structures and pathways.

There are only two studies addressing the question of the presence of abnormalities of the cortical surface in migraineurs (DaSilva, Granziera, Snyder et al., 2007; Granziera et al., 2006). Both studies applied a *coupled-surface method* described by Fischl and Dale (2000) for surface reconstruction and cortical thickness estimation.

To measure cortical thickness, first a reconstruction of the gray–white matter boundary is performed and subsequently the cortical surface is computed (Fischl & Dale, 2000). The distance between these two surfaces serves then to calculate maps of cortical thickness. These maps are not based on single-voxel intensities but are based on spatial intensity gradients across tissue classes (Fischl &

Dale, 2000). The thickness measures are then reported onto the inflated surfaces of each subject's brain, which are mapped into a common spherical system (Fischl & Dale, 2000). Cortical surface data are smoothed on the surface using an iterative nearest-neighbor procedure. No averaging of data is normally performed across sulci or outside the gray matter. A mean measure of the cortical thickness at each point on the cortical surface is then computed. The interindividual standard deviation (SD) of the thickness measure is less than 0.5 mm, implying the ability to detect measureable focal atrophy in small populations or even individual participants. The reliability and accuracy of this method have been assessed by Fischl and Dale (2000) with test–retest studies and by comparison with published values. In addition, it has been validated with histological and manual measurements (Kuperberg et al., 2003; Rosas et al., 2005).

Using this technique, Da Silva et al. (DaSilva, Granziera, Snyder et al., 2007) showed that patients with migraine with aura (MWA) and without aura (MWoA) have on average thicker somatosensory cortices (SSCs) than the group of healthy controls (HCs, Fig. 19–2). The most significant thickness changes were noticed in the caudal SSC, where the trigeminal area, including the head and face, is somatotopically represented (Fig. 19–2). In this migraine cohort the average group thickening magnitude in the SSC reached 21% (MWA vs. HCs: right side). The area of cortical thickening was larger in the MWoA compared to the MWA group.

Da Silva et al. (DaSilva, Granziera, Snyder et al., 2007) hypothesized that the observed structural changes in migraineurs' SSCs are due to the fact that most patients suffered from migraine since childhood (age at onset, mean ± SD: 14.6 ± 5.9 years), with consequent long-term overstimulation of the sensory cortex by the frequent headache attacks.

However, it is unclear why the increased thickness in the MWoA group extended to anterosuperior regions in the SSC compared with the MWA group. The anterosuperior region of the SSC contains, in fact, sensory receptors from somatotopic regions of the body other than the face and head, which had to be equally stimulated if the "hyperstimulation" theory were true. This could indeed be the case if we consider that the descending pain modulatory system was altered in this MWoA cohort. This hypothesis is supported by the results reported in another work of Da Silva et al. (DaSilva, Granziera, Tuch et al., 2007), where lower fractional anisotropy (FA) values were observed in the ventrolateral periaqueductal gray of the MWoA group compared with the MWA and control cohorts. A dysfunction of the pain modulatory system could lead to a lack of inhibition of all sensory inputs (from both the trigeminal

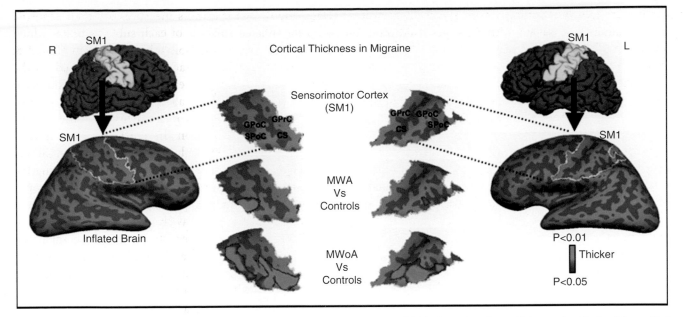

FIGURE 19-2 *Lateral views of the folded and inflated brain hemispheres exposing sulci (dark gray) and gyri (light gray) with the right and left sensorimotor cortices (SMCs) delineated in yellow (lateral columns). CS, central sulcus; GPoC, gyrus postcentralis; GprC, gyrus precentralis; MWA, migraine with aura; MWoA, migraine without aura; SPoC, sulcus postcentralis. From DaSilva, A. F., Granziera, C., Snyder, J., & Hadjikhani, N. (2007). Thickening in the somatosensory cortex of patients with migraine.* Neurology, *69(21), 1990–1995.*

and nontrigeminal areas of the body) and to a lower pain threshold. Supporting this theory are the presence of allodynia in migraine patients (Burstein et al., 2000) and the fact that migraine patients are often suffering from other pain disorders such as back pain (Hagen et al., 2006) temporomandibular disorders (Liljestrom et al., 2005), and fibromyalgia (Ifergane et al., 2006).

Another possible explanation could be that the SSC of migraine patients is originally thicker than the one of subjects without migraine and that the SSC of some patients with migraine undergoes progressive thinning in certain regions due to more frequent stimulation of the "non-image-forming retinal pathway." This pathway, according to a very recent and elegant study from Noseda et al. (2010), is responsible for the photophobia experienced by migraine patients. Anatomically, it is constituted by projections from the photosensitive ganglion cells of the retina that, converging to the dorsocaudal posterior thalamus, modulate the activity of dura-sensitive pain neurons and stimulate thalamic neurons projecting to several regions in the cortex, including the primary SSC (Noseda et al., 2010).

Future work could investigate if migraineurs with thicker SSC only in its caudal part (trigeminal region) experience more photophobia than others.

Previous animal work has demonstrated that changes of the sensory experience in rats cause functional and structural plasticity (dendritic reorganization) in their

SSC (Hickmott & Steen, 2005). In humans, abnormal variations of the cortical thickness in chronic pain disorders have been reported using VBM in migraine (Rocca et al., 2006) and back pain patients (Apkarian et al., 2004). Both studies showed altered thickness in the frontal and temporal cortices but not in the SCC.

The other study using SBM to study the properties of the cortical mantle in migraine was performed by the same group (Granziera et al., 2006) and also used the most often applied method for surface-based analysis (Fischl & Dale, 2000). In this study, the motion-processing network in 24 migraine patients (12 MWA, 12 MWoA) was examined and compared with 15 age-matched healthy controls (Granziera et al., 2006). Measures of cortical thickness in these three cohorts showed thicker motion-processing visual areas MT+ and V3A in migraineurs compared to the HCs (Fig. 19–3). The thicker V3A area corresponded to the location of the source of a cortical spreading depression (CSD) event in a single individual described in a previous work of Hadjikhani et al. (2001) (Fig. 19–4). In addition, the same study revealed that diffusion tensor imaging (DTI) showed a decreased anisotropy index (FA) in the white matter subjacent the motion-sensitive areas. Moreover, DTI revealed that migraineurs have FA alterations in the superior colliculus and lateral geniculate nucleus, structures that are also part of the visual processing stream.

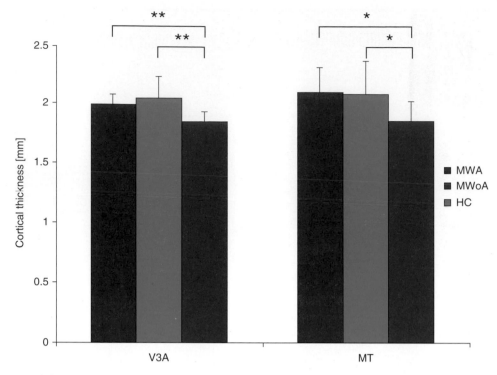

FIGURE 19–3 *The cortical thickness in migraineurs is increased in motion-processing areas. MWA, migraine with aura; MWoA, migraine without aura; HC, healthy control. * p < .05; ** p < .01. From Granziera, C., DaSilva, A. F., Snyder, J., Tuch, D. S., & Hadjikhani, N. (2006). Anatomical alterations of the visual motion processing network in migraine with and without aura. PloS Med, 3(10), e402.*

Motion perception deficits and altered functions of areas MT+ and V3A have been described in both the acute and the interictal periods of patients with MWA and MWoA (Aurora et al., 2003; Battelli et al., 2002; McKendrick & Badcock, 2004). Furthermore, psychophysical studies suggested that migraineurs are impaired in detecting coherent motion between attacks (McKendrick & Badcock, 2004).

Transcranial magnetic stimulation (TMS) studies have shown that MWA and MWoA patients have a lower phosphene threshold than HCs in experiments when transcranial magnetic stimulation is delivered over V1 and over area MT+ (Aurora et al., 2003; Battelli et al., 2002). More recently, a functional MRI study performed on 12 MWA patients, 12 MWoA patients, and 12 HCs demonstrated that migraineurs had significantly stronger activation in the superior anterior portion of the MT complex after exposure to visual stimulation (medial superior temporal area) (Antal et al., 2011).

Flattened maps of the right occipital cortex, gyri, and sulci are indicated as a grayscale image in Figure 19–4 that has been generated using the FreeSurfer software (http://surfer.nmr.mgh.harvard.edu). The borders of retinotopic areas are illustrated in white (horizontal meridians, solid lines; upper vertical meridians, dotted lines; lower vertical meridians, dashed lines). The image on the left shows the progression of CSD during a visual aura, starting in area V3A, in a single participant. The image on the right shows the average map of the mean thickness difference of 24 migraineurs compared with 15 matched controls, projected on the same brain, with the superimposed retinotopy for one participant.

As mentioned above, area V3A has been previously suggested to be the source of CSD during the aura phase (Hadjikhani et al., 2001). The study from Granziera et al. (2006) showed that this brain region is characterized by thickened cortex in both migraineur groups (MWA and MWoA) compared to healthy subjects. Moreover, interictal FA abnormalities were found using DTI in the white matter underlying the cortical area V3A. Together, these results suggest that the V3A area plays a role in both MWA and MWoA.

Nevertheless, a number of questions still need to be answered: Is the abnormality of area V3A in MWoA patients responsible for CSD in this group of migraineurs? If yes, why do MWoA patients not experience any obvious neurological symptoms? If CSD is a common phenomenon in both MWoA and MWA patients, why do only some migraine patients experience aura?

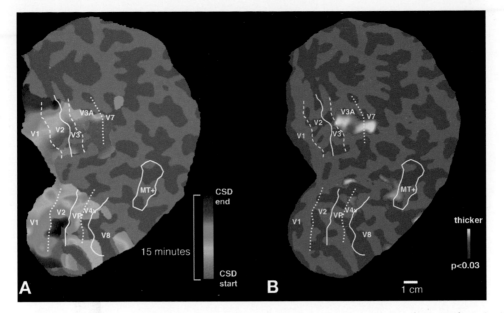

FIGURE 19–4 *Retinotopic localization of cortical thickness changes. From Granziera, C., DaSilva, A. F., Snyder, J., Tuch, D. S., & Hadjikhani, N. (2006). Anatomical alterations of the visual motion processing network in migraine with and without aura. PLoS Med, 3(10), e402.*

CSD-like events in migraine have been suggested in two imaging studies: Woods et al. (1994) used positron emission tomography (PET) to show bilateral cortical spreading hypoperfusion in MWoA during an aura episode (Woods et al., 1994), and Cao et al. (1999) reported that visually triggered headache and visual changes in patients with migraine are accompanied by spreading suppression of initial neuronal activation and increased occipital cortex oxygenation. These data suggest that CSD can occur without being symptomatic and that it could be common to both MWA and MWoA.

POTENTIAL IMPLICATIONS OF CORTICAL THICKNESS MEASUREMENTS IN MIGRAINE

Summarizing, the recent literature suggests that migraine in humans is linked to increased cortical thickness of some dedicated brain regions. Increases in the cortical thickness, however, could be either the cause or the consequence of migraine.

If the observed increase in cortical thickness is a *cause* of migraine, a possible explanation could be that the brain of migraineurs is structurally different from the brain of people without migraine. Migraineurs have in fact a peculiar genetic background (de Vries et al., 2009; Kors et al., 2004), which could influence the anatomy of the SSC and the MT area. And this is not only for a specific category of migraine called familial hemiplegic migraine (Ophoff et al., 1996; Vanmolkot et al., 2006).

Recently, a locus for migraine with visual aura was identified, which maps on chromosome 9q21-q22 (Tikka-Kleemola et al., 2010). This gene overlaps with another newly discovered gene for occipitotemporal lobe epilepsy, suggesting a potential involvement in abnormalities in ion channels implicated in neuronal excitability.

Thus, it could be speculated that increases in cortical thickness could be due to a focal increased number and/or density of neuronal and glial cells that may be responsible for the hyperexcitability observed in migraineurs' brains (Aurora et al., 2003; Battelli et al., 2002; Welch, 2003).

Similarly, hyperexcitability in motion-sensitive regions could explain why CSD has been found to originate in these areas (Hadjikhani et al., 2001), why children who will develop migraine experience motion sickness, and why migraineurs are sensitive to moving visual stimuli. The brain hyperexcitability in migraine could also be the cause of the underlying sensitivity of migraineurs to specific foods, drinks, and hormonal changes that are harmless for healthy subjects. Moreover, this could also explain why antiepileptic drugs are satisfactorily used as preventive medication for migraine.

On the other hand, if the cortical thickness abnormality is a *consequence* of migraine, it could result from plastic changes due to repetitive pain and motion processing.

Similar to the observations of Draganski et al. (2004), who found that people who learned to juggle developed increased thickness in the involved brain areas, we could think that migraineurs' brains have been trained to process pain and motion and that, therefore, the respective brain areas became thicker.

Another possible explanation may be that gliotic processes had been stimulated by the underlying brain pathology leading to increased cortical thickness. Supporting this explanation, glial proliferation has been previously described after repetitive CSD in rats (Kraig et al., 1991) and ischemia (Petito et al., 1991).

Neurogenesis also could be responsible for increased cortical thickness in certain brain areas. In fact, it has been described in rats that CDS could stimulate neurogenesis in cortical layers V to VI and the proliferation of astrocytic cells in the subpial zone, which may be potent neural progenitors (Xue et al., 2009).

Finally, a further scenario could be that increased cortical thickness is both a cause and a consequence of migraine. Future studies with bigger cohorts could aim at correlating clinical characteristics with MRI findings to better understand the origin and the mechanism of the discussed structural differences between the brains of migraineurs and healthy subjects.

REFERENCES

A. Fees-Higgins, L. J. (Ed.). (1987). *Development of the human fetal brain, an anatomical atlas.* Paris: Masson.

Aganj, I., Sapiro, G., Parikshak, N., Madsen, S. K., & Thompson, P. M. (2009). Measurement of cortical thickness from MRI by minimum line integrals on soft-classified tissue. *Human Brain Mapping, 30*(10), 3188–3199.

Antal, A., Polania, R., Saller, K., Morawetz, C., Schmidt-Samoa, C., Baudewig, J., et al. (2011). Differential activation of the middle-temporal complex to visual stimulation in migraineurs. *Cephalalgia, 31*(3), 338–345.

Apkarian, A. V., Sosa, Y., Sonty, S., Levy, R. M., Harden, R. N., Parrish, T. B., et al. (2004). Chronic back pain is associated with decreased prefrontal and thalamic gray matter density. *The Journal of Neuroscience, 24*(46), 10410–10415.

Aurora, S. K., Welch, K. M., & Al-Sayed, F. (2003). The threshold for phosphenes is lower in migraine. *Cephalalgia, 23*(4), 258–263.

Battelli, L., Black, K. R., & Wray, S. H. (2002). Transcranial magnetic stimulation of visual area V5 in migraine. *Neurology, 58*(7), 1066–1069.

Burstein, R., Yarnitsky, D., Goor-Aryeh, I., Ransil, B. J., & Bajwa, Z. H. (2000). An association between migraine and cutaneous allodynia. *Annals of Neurology, 47*(5), 614–624.

Cao, Y., Welch, K. M., Aurora, S., & Vikingstad, E. M. (1999). Functional MRI-BOLD of visually triggered headache in patients with migraine. *Archives of Neurology, 56*(5), 548–554.

Charil, A., Dagher, A., Lerch, J. P., Zijdenbos, A. P., Worsley, K. J., & Evans, A. C. (2007). Focal cortical atrophy in multiple sclerosis: relation to lesion load and disability. *Neuroimage, 34*(2), 509–517.

Chen, Z. J., He, Y., Rosa-Neto, P., Germann, J., & Evans, A. C. (2008). Revealing modular architecture of human brain structural networks by using cortical thickness from MRI. *Cerebral Cortex, 18*(10), 2374–2381.

Chung, M. K., Robbins, S. M., Dalton, K. M., Davidson, R. J., Alexander, A. L., & Evans, A. C. (2005). Cortical thickness analysis in autism with heat kernel smoothing. *Neuroimage, 25*(4), 1256–1265.

DaSilva, A. F., Granziera, C., Snyder, J., & Hadjikhani, N. (2007). Thickening in the somatosensory cortex of patients with migraine. *Neurology, 69*(21), 1990–1995.

DaSilva, A. F., Granziera, C., Tuch, D. S., Snyder, J., Vincent, M., & Hadjikhani, N. (2007). Interictal alterations of the trigeminal somatosensory pathway and periaqueductal gray matter in migraine. *Neuroreport, 18*(4), 301–305.

de Vries, B., Frants, R. R., Ferrari, M. D., & van den Maagdenberg, A. M. (2009). Molecular genetics of migraine. *Human Genetics, 126*(1), 115–132.

Dickerson, B. C., Bakkour, A., Salat, D. H., Feczko, E., Pacheco, J., Greve, D. N., et al. (2009). The cortical signature of Alzheimer's disease: regionally specific cortical thinning relates to symptom severity in very mild to mild AD dementia and is detectable in asymptomatic amyloid-positive individuals. *Cerebral Cortex, 19*(3), 497–510.

Draganski, B., Gaser, C., Busch, V., Schuierer, G., Bogdahn, U., & May, A. (2004). Neuroplasticity: changes in grey matter induced by training. *Nature, 427*(6972), 311–312.

Fischl, B., & Dale, A. M. (2000). Measuring the thickness of the human cerebral cortex from magnetic resonance images. *Proceedings of the National Academy of Sciences of the United States of America, 97*(20), 11050–11055.

Fjell, A. M., Walhovd, K. B., Fennema-Notestine, C., McEvoy, L. K., Hagler, D. J., Holland, D., et al. (2009). One-year brain atrophy evident in healthy aging. *The Journal of Neuroscience, 29*(48), 15223–15231.

Fjell, A. M., Walhovd, K. B., Reinvang, I., Lundervold, A., Salat, D., Quinn, B. T., et al. (2006). Selective increase of cortical thickness in high-performing elderly—structural indices of optimal cognitive aging. *Neuroimage, 29*(3), 984–994.

Fjell, A. M., Westlye, L. T., Amlien, I., Espeseth, T., Reinvang, I., Raz, N., et al. (2009). High consistency of regional cortical thinning in aging across multiple samples. *Cerebral Cortex, 19*(9), 2001–2012.

Fukunaga, M., Li, T. Q., van Gelderen, P., de Zwart, J. A., Shmueli, K., Yao, B., et al. (2010). Layer-specific variation of iron content in cerebral cortex as a source of MRI contrast. *Proceedings of the National Academy of Sciences of the United States of America, 107*(8), 3834–3839.

Granziera, C., DaSilva, A. F., Snyder, J., Tuch, D. S., & Hadjikhani, N. (2006). Anatomical alterations of the visual motion processing network in migraine with and without aura. *PLoS Med, 3*(10), e402.

Hadjikhani, N., Joseph, R. M., Snyder, J., & Tager-Flusberg, H. (2006). Anatomical differences in the mirror neuron system and social cognition network in autism. *Cerebral Cortex, 16*(9), 1276–1282.

Hadjikhani, N., Sanchez Del Rio, M., Wu, O., Schwartz, D., Bakker, D., Fischl, B., et al. (2001). Mechanisms of migraine aura revealed by functional MRI in human visual cortex. *Proceedings of the National Academy of Sciences of the United States of America, 98*(8), 4687–4692.

Hagen, E. M., Svensen, E., Eriksen, H. R., Ihlebaek, C. M., & Ursin, H. (2006). Comorbid subjective health complaints in low back pain. *Spine (Phila Pa 1976), 31*(13), 1491–1495.

Haidar, H., & Soul, J. S. (2006). Measurement of cortical thickness in 3D brain MRI data: validation of the Laplacian method. *J Neuroimaging, 16*(2), 146–153.

Hardan, A. Y., Muddasani, S., Vemulapalli, M., Keshavan, M. S., & Minshew, N. J. (2006). An MRI study of increased cortical thickness in autism. *American Journal of Psychiatry, 163*(7), 1290–1292.

He, B., & Liu, Z. (2008). Multimodal Functional Neuroimaging: Integrating Functional MRI and EEG/MEG. *IEEE Rev Biomed Eng, 1*(2008), 23–40.

Hickmott, P. W., & Steen, P. A. (2005). Large-scale changes in dendritic structure during reorganization of adult somatosensory cortex. *Nature Neuroscience, 8*(2), 140–142.

Ifergane, G., Buskila, D., Simiseshvely, N., Zeev, K., & Cohen, H. (2006). Prevalence of fibromyalgia syndrome in migraine patients. *Cephalalgia, 26*(4), 451–456.

Jones, S. E., Buchbinder, B. R., & Aharon, I. (2000). Three-dimensional mapping of cortical thickness using Laplace's equation. *Human Brain Mapping, 11*(1), 12–32.

Kloppel, S., Mangin, J. F., Vongerichten, A., Frackowiak, R. S., & Siebner, H. R. (2010). Nurture versus nature: long-term impact of forced right-handedness on structure of pericentral cortex and basal ganglia. *The Journal of Neuroscience, 30*(9), 3271–3275.

Kochunov, P., Thompson, P. M., Coyle, T. R., Lancaster, J. L., Kochunov, V., Royall, D., et al. (2008). Relationship among neuroimaging indices of cerebral health during normal aging. *Human Brain Mapping, 29*(1), 36–45.

Kors, E. E., Melberg, A., Vanmolkot, K. R., Kumlien, E., Haan, J., Raininko, R., et al. (2004). Childhood epilepsy, familial hemiplegic migraine, cerebellar ataxia, and a new CACNA1A mutation. *Neurology, 63*(6), 1136–1137.

Kraig, R. P., Dong, L. M., Thisted, R., & Jaeger, C. B. (1991). Spreading depression increases immunohistochemical staining of glial fibrillary acidic protein. *The Journal of Neuroscience, 11*(7), 2187–2198.

Kruit, M. C., Launer, L. J., Overbosch, J., van Buchem, M. A., & Ferrari, M. D. (2009). Iron accumulation in deep brain nuclei in migraine: a population-based magnetic resonance imaging study. *Cephalalgia, 29*(3), 351–359.

Kruit, M. C., van Buchem, M. A., Launer, L. J., Terwindt, G. M., & Ferrari, M. D. (2010). Migraine is associated with an increased risk of deep white matter lesions, subclinical posterior circulation infarcts and brain iron accumulation: the population-based MRI CAMERA study. *Cephalalgia, 30*(2), 129–136.

Kuperberg, G. R., Broome, M. R., McGuire, P. K., David, A. S., Eddy, M., Ozawa, F., et al. (2003). Regionally localized thinning of the cerebral cortex in schizophrenia. *Archives of General Psychiatry, 60*(9), 878–888.

Lerch, J. P., Pruessner, J. C., Zijdenbos, A., Hampel, H., Teipel, S. J., & Evans, A. C. (2005). Focal decline of cortical thickness in Alzheimer's disease identified by computational neuroanatomy. *Cerebral Cortex, 15*(7), 995–1001.

Lerch, J. P., Worsley, K., Shaw, W. P., Greenstein, D. K., Lenroot, R. K., Giedd, J., et al. (2006). Mapping anatomical correlations across cerebral cortex (MACACC) using cortical thickness from MRI. *Neuroimage, 31*(3), 993–1003.

Liljestrom, M., Kujala, J., Jensen, O., & Salmelin, R. (2005). Neuromagnetic localization of rhythmic activity in the human brain: a comparison of three methods. *Neuroimage, 25*(3), 734–745.

Luders, E., Thompson, P. M., Narr, K. L., Toga, A. W., Jancke, L., & Gaser, C. (2006). A curvature-based approach to estimate local gyrification on the cortical surface. *Neuroimage, 29*(4), 1224–1230.

MacDonald, D., Kabani, N., Avis, D., & Evans, A. C. (2000). Automated 3-D extraction of inner and outer surfaces of cerebral cortex from MRI. *Neuroimage, 12*(3), 340–356.

Mangin, J. F., Poupon, F., Duchesnay, E., Riviere, D., Cachia, A., Collins, D. L., et al. (2004). Brain morphometry using 3D moment invariants. *Medical Image Analysis, 8*(3), 187–196.

Marques, J. P., van der Zwaag, W., Granziera, C., Krueger, G., & Gruetter, R. (2010). Cerebellar cortical layers: in vivo visualization with structural high-field-strength MR imaging. *Radiology, 254*(3), 942–948.

McKendrick, A. M., & Badcock, D. R. (2004). Motion processing deficits in migraine. *Cephalalgia, 24*(5), 363–372.

Morrison JH, Hof PR (Ed.). (1992). *The organization of the cerebral cortex from molecules to circuits.* New York Elsevier in Amsterdam.

Narr, K. L., Bilder, R. M., Toga, A. W., Woods, R. P., Rex, D. E., Szeszko, P. R., et al. (2005). Mapping cortical thickness and gray matter concentration in first episode schizophrenia. *Cerebral Cortex, 15*(6), 708–719.

Narr, K. L., Toga, A. W., Szeszko, P., Thompson, P. M., Woods, R. P., Robinson, D., et al. (2005). Cortical thinning in cingulate and occipital cortices in first episode schizophrenia. *Biological Psychiatry, 58*(1), 32–40.

Nesvag, R., Lawyer, G., Varnas, K., Fjell, A. M., Walhovd, K. B., Frigessi, A., et al. (2008). Regional thinning of the cerebral cortex in schizophrenia: effects of diagnosis, age and antipsychotic medication. *Schizophrenia Research, 98*(1–3), 16–28.

Noseda, R., Kainz, V., Jakubowski, M., Gooley, J. J., Saper, C. B., Digre, K., et al. (2010). A neural mechanism for exacerbation of headache by light. *Nature Neuroscience, 13*(2), 239–245.

Ophoff, R. A., Terwindt, G. M., Vergouwe, M. N., van Eijk, R., Oefner, P. J., Hoffman, S. M., et al. (1996). Familial hemiplegic migraine and episodic ataxia type-2 are caused by mutations in the Ca2+ channel gene CACNL1A4. *Cell, 87*(3), 543–552.

Panizzon, M. S., Fennema-Notestine, C., Eyler, L. T., Jernigan, T. L., Prom-Wormley, E., Neale, M., et al. (2009). Distinct genetic influences on cortical surface area and cortical thickness. *Cerebral Cortex, 19*(11), 2728–2735.

Park, H. J., Lee, J. D., Kim, E. Y., Park, B., Oh, M. K., Lee, S., et al. (2009). Morphological alterations in the congenital blind based on the analysis of cortical thickness and surface area. *Neuroimage, 47*(1), 98–106.

Petito, C. K., Juurlink, B. H., & Hertz, L. (1991). In vitro models differentiating between direct and indirect effects of ischemia on astrocytes. *Experimental Neurology, 113*(3), 364–372.

Rakic, P. (1995). Radial versus tangential migration of neuronal clones in the developing cerebral cortex. *Proceedings of the National Academy of Sciences of the United States of America, 92*(25), 11323–11327.

Rocca, M. A., Ceccarelli, A., Falini, A., Colombo, B., Tortorella, P., Bernasconi, L., et al. (2006). Brain gray matter changes in migraine patients with T2-visible lesions: a 3-T MRI study. *Stroke, 37*(7), 1765–1770.

Rosas, H. D., Hevelone, N. D., Zaleta, A. K., Greve, D. N., Salat, D. H., & Fischl, B. (2005). Regional cortical thinning in preclinical Huntington disease and its relationship to cognition. *Neurology, 65*(5), 745–747.

Sailer, M., Fischl, B., Salat, D., Tempelmann, C., Schonfeld, M. A., Busa, E., et al. (2003). Focal thinning of the cerebral cortex in multiple sclerosis. *Brain, 126*(Pt 8), 1734–1744.

Salat, D. H., Buckner, R. L., Snyder, A. Z., Greve, D. N., Desikan, R. S., Busa, E., et al. (2004). Thinning of the cerebral cortex in aging. *Cerebral Cortex, 14*(7), 721–730.

Schmitt, J. E., Lenroot, R. K., Ordaz, S. E., Wallace, G. L., Lerch, J. P., Evans, A. C., et al. (2009). Variance decomposition of MRI-based covariance maps using genetically informative samples and structural equation modeling. *Neuroimage, 47*(1), 56–64.

Scott, M. L., & Thacker, N. A. (2005). Robust tissue boundary detection for cerebral cortical thickness estimation. *Medical Image Computing and Computer Assisted Intervention, 8*(Pt 2), 878–885.

Shaw, P., Kabani, N. J., Lerch, J. P., Eckstrand, K., Lenroot, R., Gogtay, N., et al. (2008). Neurodevelopmental trajectories of the human cerebral cortex. *The Journal of Neuroscience, 28*(14), 3586–3594.

Sun Z.Y., Perrot M., Tucholka A., Rivi`ere D. and Mangin JF. (2009). *Constructing a Dictionary of Human Brain Folding Patterns . Proceedings of the 12th International Conference on Medical Image Computing and Computer-Assisted Intervention: Part II.* 117–124

Thompson, P. M., Lee, A. D., Dutton, R. A., Geaga, J. A., Hayashi, K. M., Eckert, M. A., et al. (2005). Abnormal cortical complexity and thickness profiles mapped in Williams syndrome. *The Journal of Neuroscience, 25*(16), 4146–4158.

Tikka-Kleemola, P., Artto, V., Vepsalainen, S., Sobel, E. M., Raty, S., Kaunisto, M. A., et al. (2010). A visual migraine aura locus maps to 9q21-q22. *Neurology, 74*(15), 1171–1177.

Toro, R., & Burnod, Y. (2003). Geometric atlas: modeling the cortex as an organized surface. *Neuroimage, 20*(3), 1468–1484.

Toro, R., Fox, P. T., & Paus, T. (2008). Functional coactivation map of the human brain. *Cerebral Cortex, 18*(11), 2553–2559.

Van Essen, D. C., Dierker, D., Snyder, A. Z., Raichle, M. E., Reiss, A. L., & Korenberg, J. (2006). Symmetry of cortical folding abnormalities in Williams syndrome revealed by surface-based analyses. *The Journal of Neuroscience, 26*(20), 5470–5483.

Van Essen, D. C., Drury, H. A., Dickson, J., Harwell, J., Hanlon, D., & Anderson, C. H. (2001). An integrated software suite for surface-based analyses of cerebral cortex. *Journal of the American Medical Informatics Association, 8*(5), 443–459.

Vanmolkot, K. R., Kors, E. E., Turk, U., Turkdogan, D., Keyser, A., Broos, L. A., et al. (2006). Two de novo mutations in the Na,K-ATPase gene ATP1A2 associated with pure familial hemiplegic migraine. *European Journal of Human Genetics, 14*(5), 555–560.

Venkatasubramanian, G., Jayakumar, P. N., Gangadhar, B. N., & Keshavan, M. S. (2008). Automated MRI parcellation study of regional volume and thickness of prefrontal cortex (PFC) in antipsychotic-naive schizophrenia. *Acta Psychiatrica Scandinavica, 117*(6), 420–431.

Vincent, M., & Hadjikhani, N. (2007). The cerebellum and migraine. *Headache, 47*(6), 820–833.

Wallace, G. L., Dankner, N., Kenworthy, L., Giedd, J. N., & Martin, A. (2010). Age-related temporal and parietal cortical thinning in autism spectrum disorders. *Brain, 133*(Pt 12), 3745–3754.

Wallace, G. L., Happe, F., & Giedd, J. N. (2009). A case study of a multiply talented savant with an autism spectrum disorder: neuropsychological functioning and brain morphometry. *Philosophical Transactions of the Royal Society B, 364*(1522), 1425–1432.

Welch, K. M. (2003). Contemporary concepts of migraine pathogenesis. *Neurology, 61*(8 Suppl 4), S2–8.

Woods, R. P., Iacoboni, M., & Mazziotta, J. C. (1994). Brief report: bilateral spreading cerebral hypoperfusion during spontaneous migraine headache. *The New England Journal of Medicine, 331*(25), 1689–1692.

Xue, J. H., Yanamoto, H., Nakajo, Y., Tohnai, N., Nakano, Y., Hori, T., et al. (2009). Induced spreading depression evokes cell division of astrocytes in the subpial zone, generating neural precursor-like cells and new immature neurons in the adult cerebral cortex. *Stroke, 40*(11), e606–613.

Yezzi, A. J., Jr., & Prince, J. L. (2003). An Eulerian PDE approach for computing tissue thickness. *IEEE Transactions on Medical Imaging, 22*(10), 1332–1339.

20 Changing Receptors in Migraine State

GENEVIÈVE DEMARQUAY AND FRANÇOIS MAUGUIÈRE

INTRODUCTION

Migraine is one of the most common headache disorders and affects a large portion of the adult population. Attacks are characterized by recurrent throbbing headaches accompanied by nausea, vomiting, photophobia, and/or phonophobia and are aggravated by movements (Headache Classification Committee, 2004). In at least 20% of patients, the attack is preceded or accompanied by focal neurological disturbances, known as migraine aura. Converging lines of evidence support the role of the central nervous system (CNS) in migraine pathophysiology. It is generally thought that the development of migraine headache depends on the activation of the trigeminovascular system and a dysfunction of brainstem nuclei involved in the central control of pain. Based on the initial vascular inflammation theory of migraine, the first neurotransmitters studied were vasoactive inflammatory peptides released from the trigeminal nerve such as substance P (Moskowitz et al., 1979) and calcitonin gene–related peptide (CGRP) (Uddman et al., 1985). Recently pharmacological and neuroimaging investigations have focused on the receptor populations expressed in the anatomical structures involved in migraine pathophysiology including the trigeminovascular system and brainstem. In vivo imaging of receptors and identification of changes during migraine may help our understanding of migraine pathophysiology and guide the development of new antimigraine agents. This chapter reviews current knowledge on neurotransmission dysfunction and neuroreceptor abnormalities in migraine and then considers neuroreceptor imaging evidence for changes that could be specific to migraineurs.

WHAT DO WE KNOW ABOUT THE ROLE OF NEUROTRANSMISSION DISORDERS AND RECEPTOR CHANGES IN MIGRAINE?

Serotonin

SEROTONIN BIOSYNTHESIS AND RECEPTORS

Serotonin (5-hydroxytryptamine, 5-HT) regulates a broad range of behaviors including circadian activity, food intake (Leibowitz, 1990), sexual behavior (Metson & Gorzalka, 1992), and emotional states. Serotonin dysfunction has been associated with neurological and psychiatric disorders including anxiety (Gross et al., 2002), depression (Cowen, 2008), epilepsy (Chugani, 2004), and migraine (Hamel, 2007). Serotonin was isolated from serum in 1948, and its name reflects where it was first detected, in the serum ("sero"), and its pharmacological vasoconstrictor properties ("tonin") (Rapport et al., 1948). Further studies showed that 5-HT is located in the enterochromaffin cells of the intestine, which contain up to 90% of the total amount of the total body serotonin; in blood platelets; and in the brain, where it acts as a neurotransmitter and a neuromodulator.

Serotonin is synthesized from tryptophan, which crosses the blood-brain barrier. Transformation of tryptophan into serotonin involves two steps: (a) hydroxylation of tryptophan to 5-hydroxytryptophan by tryptophan hydroxylase (THP) and (b) decarboxylation of 5-hydroxytryptophan catalyzed by l-aromatic amino acid decarboxylase (AADC). After synthesis, 5-HT is transported by the vesicular monoamine transporter and stored in vesicles at neuronal presynaptic endings (Visser et al., 2011). When serotoninergic neurons fire, serotonin is released in the synaptic cleft and can bind to different receptors or be taken back up into neurons by the serotoninergic reuptake transporter (SERT). 5-HT is mainly degraded by monoamine oxidase (MAO) to 5-hydroxyindoleacetic acid (5-HIAA), which is excreted in urine.

The physiological effects of serotonin in the brain are mediated by a widespread family of 5-HT receptors. To date, 14 different mammalian serotonin receptors have been identified and these are grouped in seven families, namely, 5-HT_1 (subdivided into 5-HT_{1A}, 5-HT_{1B}, 5-HT_{1D}, 5-HT_{1E}, and 5-HT_{1F} subtypes), 5-HT_{2A} (subdivided into 5-HT_{2A} to 5-HT_{2C} subtypes), and 5-HT_3 to 5-HT_7 families (Barnes & Sharp, 1999; Daubert & Condron, 2010). With the exception of the 5-HT_3 receptor, a ligand-gated ion channel that belongs, as do nicotinic acetylcholine and γ-aminobutyric acid A ($GABA_A$) receptors, to the Cys-loop family, all other serotonin receptors are G-protein-coupled receptors.

WHAT DO WE KNOW ABOUT SEROTONIN TRANSMISSION AND RECEPTORS IN MIGRAINE?

Evidence for a Role of Serotonin in the Periphery

The serotoninergic system is thought to play an important role in migraine pathophysiology. Early studies showed that the urinary excretion of 5-HIAA, the main metabolite of 5-HT, increases during attacks (Curran et al., 1965; Sicuteri et al., 1961). A number of studies have also evaluated the distribution of systemic 5-HT in whole blood, platelets/platelet-rich plasma, and blood/plasma. Some papers suggested that between attacks, migraine patients have chronically low systemic serotonin concentration redundant with "between attacks" associated with an increase in 5-HT release during attacks (Ferrari & Saxena, 1993). Other authors have found that plasma 5-HT decreases only in migraineurs with aura (Nagata et al., 2006). Overall, however, the majority of data show normal platelet and plasma serotonin concentration during and between migraine attacks (for review see Panconesi, 2008). One possible explanation for these contradictory findings might be that blood serotonin levels, including platelets levels (Visser et al., 2011), do not exactly reflect brain 5-HT turnover.

Evaluation of Central Brain Serotonin

Many studies have supported the hypothesis that chronically low serotonin levels may represent one of the biochemical features of migraine pathogenesis and that a sudden increase in 5-HT release could be part of the triggering events that culminate in migraine attacks (Hamel, 2007).

First, the administration of a 5-HT-releasing agent such as m-chlorophenylpiperazine (mCPP) induces migraine-like headache (Leone et al., 2000), but the exact mechanism is unknown. Second, in a rat model, the effect of 5-HT depletion induced by administration of para-chlorophenylalanine, a tryptophan hydroxylase inhibitor, enhances cortical spreading depression (CSD) induced by topical application of KCl on the cortical surface (Supornsilpchai et al., 2006). The number of CSD waves and the area under the curve of each CSD wave were greater in the low-5-HT rats. CSD-induced trigeminal activation, which was evaluated in this study by counting Fos-immunoreactive (Fos-IR) neurons in the trigeminal nucleus caudalis, was greater in rats with 5-HT depletion than in the control group. Third, it has been shown that reducing brain 5-HT synthesis by giving a tryptophan-depleted diet induced more intense headache, nausea, and glare- and light-induced pain in migraine patients than in controls (Drummond, 2006). Moreover, glare- and light-induced pain was greater in the low-tryptophan than in

the balanced-amino-acid food intake condition, in both migraineurs and control subjects, suggesting that a reduction in brain 5-HT concentration might lead to a hyperexcitable brain state and thereby contribute to migraine attack pathogenesis in susceptible individuals. Fourth, 5-HT facilitates sensory and behavioral habituation, processes that are known to be altered in migraine patients. Indeed, one of the most reproducible electrophysiological features observed in migraine patients between attacks consists of a lack of habituation of evoked and event-related cortical potentials (for review see Giffin & Kaube, 2002, and Schoenen et al., 2003). Auditory processing in migraine was explored through the study of intensity dependence of auditory potentials (IDAP). An increased IDAP was reported in migraine sufferers that could reflect decreased 5-HT neurotransmission (Wang et al., 1996). In addition, administration of fluoxetine, a selective serotonin reuptake inhibitor, corrects interictal visual habituation deficits in migraineurs (Ozkul & Bozlar, 2002). Lastly, some positron emission tomography (PET) data support the possibility of an abnormal central serotonin turnover in migraineurs. As tryptophan is a precursor of 5-HT synthesis, PET imaging using α-[^{11}C]methyl-l-tryptophan (AMT), a radio-labeled analog of tryptophan, can be used to estimate brain 5-HT synthesis. A first PET study using [^{11}C]-AMT showed that brain uptake values were higher in migraineurs than those measured in control subjects throughout the whole brain, suggesting that the serotonin synthesis capacity of the brain was increased between attacks in migraine patients (Chugani et al., 1999). A single-photon emission computed tomography (SPECT) study used a ligand (^{123}I-ADAM, 2-((2-((dimethylamino) methyl)phenyl)thio)-5iodophenylamine) specific for the serotonin transport protein (SERT) responsible for the uptake of 5-HT from the synaptic cleft to estimate the presynaptic uptake of serotonin (Schuh-Hofer et al., 2007) in migraine patients. This study showed a significantly higher ^{123}I-ADAM uptake in the brainstem of migraineurs as compared to control subjects, with a mild positive statistical correlation between mean monthly migraine attacks and the uptake of ^{123}I-ADAM in the brainstem (Figs. 20–1 and 20–2). This SPECT study suggests a dysregulation of brainstem serotoninergic turnover, which could reflect either a constitutional up-regulation of SERT causing an increase of serotonin reuptake or a compensatory overexpression of this transporter due to changes in endogenous 5-HT levels (Schuh-Hofer et al., 2007). However, these results were not replicated in a third imaging study that used [^{11}C]-AMT (Sakai et al., 2008). In this third study, the global brain 5-HT synthetic rate appeared slightly, but not statistically significantly, lower in migraineurs than in controls between attacks. The seemingly discordant results observed between the two [^{11}C]-AMT PET studies performed during the interictal state might reflect a lack of statistical power due to the relatively small number of subjects in each of the studies (11 patients including 3 patients with migraine with aura in Chugani et al 1999. study; 5 patients in Sakai et al. study). The later study (Sakai et al., 2008) also suggested differences of endogenous 5-HT synthesis between the first 6 hours of a migraine attack and the interictal state by showing, in six migraine patients, that the highest [^{11}C]-AMT uptake occurred during attacks and the lowest occurred 2 hours after subcutaneous sumatriptan injection, with intermediate levels in the interictal state (Fig. 20–3). These latter findings suggest fluctuations in brain 5-HT synthetic rate during migraine attacks and emphasize a potential role for serotonin acting at 5-HT receptors.

Evaluation of Serotoninergic Receptors in Migraine Patients

5-HT$_{1A}$ Receptors 5-HT$_{1A}$ receptors are widely distributed in the central nervous system but with a higher density in the hippocampus, cingulate cortex, entorhinal cortex, and raphe nuclei. In the raphe nuclei, these receptors exist as autoreceptors exerting a negative feedback to inhibit serotoninergic neuron firing, thereby playing a key role in the regulation of central serotoninergic tone (Richer et al., 2002; Weissmann-Nanopoulos et al., 1985). The regionally specific location of auto-5-HT$_{1A}$ receptors in the raphe nuclei together with specific brainstem activation shown by [^{15}O]H$_2$O PET studies (Afridi, Giffin, et al., 2005; Afridi, Matharu, et al., 2005; Bahra et al., 2001; Denuelle et al., 2007; Weiller et al., 1995), suggesting the involvement of the locus coeruleus and/or the raphe nuclei in migraine attacks, provides a strong argument to

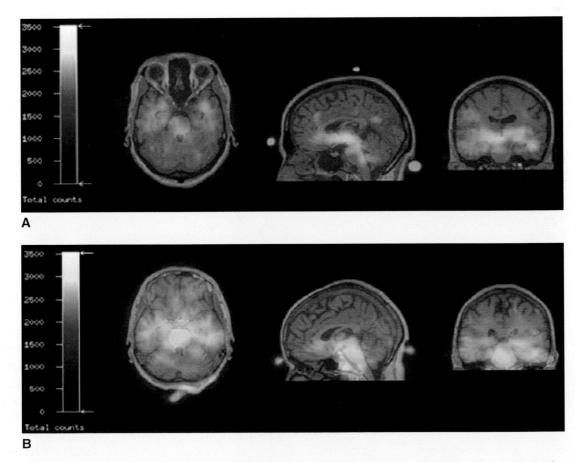

FIGURE 20–1 *Serotoninergic reuptake transporter (SERT) availability evaluated by 123I-ADAM single-photon emission computed tomography in migraine patients and healthy subjects. Migraineurs show a higher 123I-ADAM uptake in the mesopontine brainstem (B) when compared with healthy subjects (A). From Schuh-Hofer, S., Richter, M., Geworski, L., Villringer, A., Israel, H., Wenzel, R., et al. (2007). Increased serotonin transporter availability in the brainstem of migraineurs.* Journal of Neurology, 254, 789–796, Figure 3, with permission.

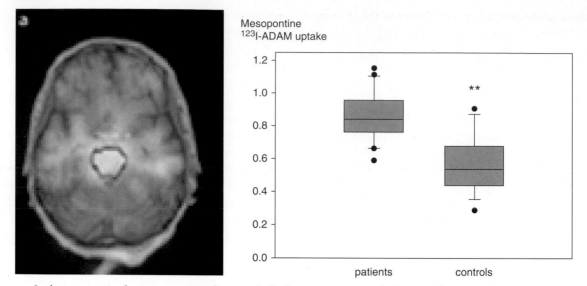

Mesopontine
^{123}I-ADAM uptake

FIGURE 20–2 *In the mesopontine brainstem region of interest (left), the 123I-ADAM uptake (presented as an outlier box plot) is higher in migraineurs than in healthy subjects (right). From Schuh-Hofer, S., Richter, M., Geworski, L., Villringer, A., Israel, H., Wenzel, R., et al. (2007). Increased serotonin transporter availability in the brainstem of migraineurs. Journal of Neurology, 254, 789–796, Figures 1 and 2, with permission.*

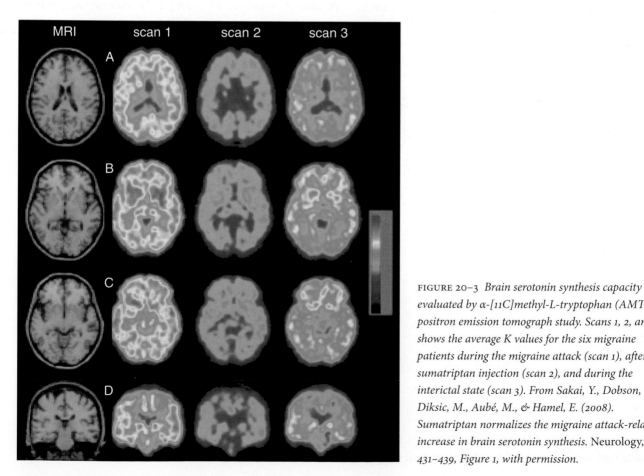

FIGURE 20–3 *Brain serotonin synthesis capacity evaluated by α-[11C]methyl-L-tryptophan (AMT) positron emission tomograph study. Scans 1, 2, and 3 shows the average K values for the six migraine patients during the migraine attack (scan 1), after sumatriptan injection (scan 2), and during the interictal state (scan 3). From Sakai, Y., Dobson, C., Diksic, M., Aubé, M., & Hamel, E. (2008). Sumatriptan normalizes the migraine attack-related increase in brain serotonin synthesis. Neurology, 70, 431–439, Figure 1, with permission.*

target these proteins as a key contributor to the abnormal brain 5-HT turnover suspected in migraine.

The raphe nuclei are interconnected with the periaqueductal gray (PAG) and the locus coeruleus and play an important role in endogenous pain control. Indeed, the dorsal raphe and raphe magnus nuclei that are interconnected by a descending projection (Hornung, 2003) are key to the central modulation of noxious stimuli. Animal experiments modeling migraine pain, by noxious stimulation of the superior sagittal venous sinus, suggest that the pain modulation resulting from concomitant stimulation of the PAG is mediated by the raphe magnus (Kaube et al., 1993; Knight & Goadsby, 2001; Knight et al., 2005). Interestingly, the neuronal activity of the raphe magnus is inhibited by migraine-triggering factors such as repetitive flashing lights, while stimulation of this nucleus suppresses responses of trigeminal neurons to noxious stimulation of the dura mater (Lambert et al., 2008). In humans, dysfunction of the pontine raphe was implicated in a migraine patient who presented with right-sided attacks associated with a pontine cavernoma affecting the left raphe magnus (Katsarava et al., 2003).

The specific involvement of 5-HT$_{1A}$ receptors in the trigeminovascular system modulation was evaluated by Boers et al. (2000) in an experimental preclinical model of headache. The authors showed that microiontophoretic injection of (+)8-OH-DPAT, a selective 5-HT$_{1A}$ agonist, suppressed the evoked activity of trigeminal neurons responding to electrical stimulation of the superior sagittal sinus.

In humans, 5-HT$_{1A}$ receptor sensitivity has been studied using a neuroendocrine challenge paradigm based on the observation that 5-HT modulates prolactin release (Cassidy, Tomkins, Dinan et al., 2003). The presence of a 5-HT$_{1A}$ receptor hypersensitivity was suggested in migraineurs by a heightened prolactin response to various 5-HT$_{1A}$ receptor agonists, such mCPP (Leone et al., 2000) and buspirone (Cassidy, Tomkins, Dinan, et al., 2003; Cassidy, Tomkins, Sharifi, et al., 2003).

5-HT$_{1B/D}$ Receptors 5-HT$_{1B/D}$ receptors are located in several brain areas, mainly in the basal ganglia (Filip & Bader, 2009; Varnäs et al., 2001). Autoradiographic mapping of these receptors in postmortem human brain shows that 5-HT$_{1B}$ receptors are much more abundant than 5-HT$_{1D}$ receptors (Varnäs et al., 2001). Both receptors have an important place in migraine therapy, through the use of triptans, which are potent serotonin 5-HT$_{1B/D}$ receptor agonists. 5-HT$_{1B}$ receptors are located within the smooth muscle wall of small cerebral arteries (Nilsson et al., 1999), whereas 5-HT$_{1D}$ receptors are mainly expressed by the trigeminal ganglion and free trigeminal nerve fibers (Longmore et al., 1997). However, both receptors are expressed in human trigeminal ganglion, and more specifically in medium-sized cells that contain CGRP, nitric oxide synthase (NOS), and substance P (Hou et al., 2001). 5-HT$_{1B/D}$ receptors are expressed (with 5-HT$_{1F}$ receptors) in the trigeminal ganglia but also in dorsal root ganglia at the cervical thoracic and lumbar levels (Classey et al., 2010). The spinal distribution is interesting as triptans treat migraine-specific pain and are not general analgesics. The exact site and antimigraine mode of action of the triptans have been extensively discussed in the literature and could involve a cranial vasoconstriction, a peripheral trigeminal neuronal inhibition inhibiting the release of neuroinflammatory peptides, and/or an inhibition of pain signal transmission through second-order sensory neurons of the trigeminocervical complex (Classey et al., 2010).

5-HT$_{1F}$ Receptors 5-HT$_{1F}$ receptors are distributed in several central nervous system areas including the dorsal raphe nucleus, hippocampus, cingulate and entorhinal cortices claustrum, and caudate nucleus (Filip & Bader, 2009). They are also expressed in the trigeminal ganglia (Classey et al., 2010). 5-HT$_{1F}$ receptor activation also inhibits trigeminal nucleus C-Fos activation and neuronal firing (Monteith & Goadsby, 2011). 5-HT$_{1F}$ receptor agonist lasmiditan (COL-144) may be a new treatment in acute migraine (Ferrari et al., 2010). Although the mechanisms of action of this molecule are not completely understood, preclinical models of migraine have shown that COL-144 is active without causing vasoconstriction (Nelson et al., 2010), enhancing the role of neuronal structures in migraine pathophysiology.

Dopamine

DOPAMINE BIOSYNTHESIS AND RECEPTORS

Dopamine is involved in many critical CNS functions including movement, cognition, reward, motivation, and memory. Dopamine is a member of the catecholaminergic group of neurotransmitters and was first identified in the brain in 1962 (Carlsson et al., 1962). Dopamine is biosynthesized via hydroxylation of tyrosine to l-dopa via the enzyme tyrosine hydroxylase (TH) followed by the decarboxylation of l-dopa by aromatic amino acid decarboxylase (AADC or dopa decarboxylase). In dopaminergic neurons, dopamine is transported from the cytoplasm to specialized storage vesicles. Several different processes terminate dopamine activity at the synapse. The primary mechanism consists of dopamine reuptake from the synaptic cleft by the dopamine transporter (DAT). In the second process, dopamine is metabolized by MAO and catechol-*O*-methyltransferase (COMT). The product of dopamine degradation is homovanillic acid.

The physiological actions of dopamine are mediated by five G-protein-coupled dopamine receptors named D_1 to D_5. Dopamine receptors are divided into two major groups: the D_1-class dopamine receptors (D_1 and D_5 receptors) and D_2-class dopamine receptors (D_2, D_3, D_4) (Beaulieu et al., 2011).

Interestingly, serotoninergic and dopaminergic systems are closely related in the central nervous system. More specifically, serotonergic cell bodies of the raphe nuclei send projections to dopaminergic cells both in the substantia nigra and ventral tegmental area and to their terminal fields in the nucleus accumbens, prefrontal cortex, and striatum (Di Giovanni et al., 2010).

WHAT DO WE KNOW ABOUT DOPAMINE RECEPTORS IN MIGRAINE?

Clinical and preclinical data implicate dopamine abnormalities in the pathophysiology of migraine.

Clinical Considerations

Before migraine attacks, some patients experience premonitory symptoms including yawning, nausea, mood changes, irritability, concentration difficulties, physical hyperactivity, and/or feeling cold (Quintela et al., 2006; Schoonman et al., 2006). Almost all of these premonitory symptoms are thought to be dopamine-driven processes (Barbanti & Fabbrini, 2002). In a double-blind placebo-controlled study, a dopamine agonist (0.25 mg of sublingual apomorphine) induced a significantly higher number of yawns in migraineurs than controls (Del Bene et al., 1994). Cerbo et al. (1997) showed that subcutaneous administration of apomorphine (10 mcg/kg) induced a higher incidence of dopaminergic symptoms (nausea, vomiting, drowsiness, yawning, dizziness, sweating) in headache-free migraineurs than in controls. Interestingly, symptoms reflecting postsynaptic dopamine receptor activation such as nausea and vomiting occurred only in migraine patients.

Pharmacological Data

Central and peripheral antiemetics (metoclopramide and domperidone) and some neuroleptics such as haloperidol or prochlorperazine, which are dopamine D_2 antagonists, are used in the acute treatment of attacks (Friedman et al., 2011; Honkaniemi et al., 2006; Miller al., 2009). The mechanism by which these D_2-like receptor blocking drugs are effective in migraine treatment remains to be determined (Charbit et al., 2010); these treatments could act via dopaminergic pathways that are activated in migraine or via other mechanisms in their pharmacology such as serotoninergic or adrenergic channels (Akerman & Goadsby, 2007).

Experimental Studies of the Trigeminocervical Complex

Animal studies have demonstrated the presence of dopamine receptors in the trigeminovascular system. Both D_1 and D_2 dopamine receptors were identified in the rat trigeminocervical complex (Bergerot et al., 2007), and animal experimental data support the argument that dopamine could play a role in trigeminal nociceptive processing. However, in contrast to clinical considerations suggesting a dopamine-driven mechanism of some migraine attack symptoms, dopamine was found to attenuate the spontaneous activity of trigeminal neurons (Bergerot et al., 2007). Moreover, dopamine D_2 receptor agonists that cross the blood-brain barrier inhibited neurons in the trigeminocervical complex with dural inputs, while D_2 receptor antagonists facilitated firing of these neurons (Charbit, Akerman, & Goadsby 2009). In contrast, it has been shown that central and peripheral D_1-like receptor agonists facilitate innocuous brush-evoked firing in the trigeminocervical complex. This later data suggest that D_1-like receptors may contribute to peripheral sensitization (Charbit, Akerman, & Goadsby 2009). Regarding brain dopaminergic nuclei, it has been shown that the A11 nucleus has an inhibitory effect on nociceptive processing at D_2-like receptors in the trigeminocervical complex (Charbit, Akerman, Goadsby, & Holland, 2009).

Calcitonin Gene–Related Peptide Receptor

CALCITONIN GENE–RELATED PEPTIDE AND CALCITONIN GENE–RELATED PEPTIDE RECEPTORS

CGRP is a 37-amino-acid neuropeptide (Arulmani et al., 2004) that belongs to the calcitonin family of peptides. Two forms of CGRP are expressed, α-CGRP, which is predominantly expressed in the nervous system, and β-CGRP, which is primarily localized in the enteric nervous system. The CGRP receptor is an atypical receptor. It is formed by the combination of the main functional unit of the receptor, the seven-transmembrane-spanning protein called calcitonin receptorlike receptor (CLR), and of a single transmembrane protein, the receptor activity–modifying protein (RAMP). An additional intracellular protein called receptor component protein (RCP) is also required for the functionality of the CGRP receptor (Walker et al., 2010). CGRP receptors are distributed in the smooth muscle layer of the middle meningeal, middle cerebral, pial, and superficial arteries (see Eftekhari & Edvinsson, 2010, for review). In the central nervous system, CGRP is expressed in several regions such as the striatum, amygdala, hypothalamus, cerebellum, brainstem, and trigeminal complex (Eftekhari & Edvinsson, 2010). Recently, it has been shown that 37% of the trigeminal ganglion neurons express CLR and 36% express RAMP (Eftekhari et al., 2010). CGRP is a potent vasodilator (Brain et al., 1985) and mediates vascular responses through interaction with G-protein-coupled receptors of the B type that are primarily coupled to the activation of adenylcyclase. In isolated human cerebral and middle meningeal arteries, CGRP induces vasodilatation (Edvinson et al., 2010). Recently, a double-blind, randomized, placebo-controlled, crossover magnetic resonance angiography study conducted in healthy volunteers showed that the infusion of 1.5 mcg/min human α-CGRP dilates extracranial vessels, causing a significant vasodilatation of the middle meningeal artery, but not of the middle cerebral artery (Asghar et al., 2010).

WHAT DO WE KNOW ABOUT CALCITONIN GENE–RELATED PEPTIDE TRANSMISSION AND RECEPTORS IN MIGRAINE?

Many studies support the role of CGRP in the pathophysiology of migraine. First, experimental studies show that CGRP is found in brain areas relevant to migraine pathophysiology such as the trigeminal neurons (see above). Moreover, stimulation of the trigeminal ganglion neurons in cats and in humans treated for trigeminal neuralgia by thermocoagulation leads to a CGRP increase in jugular venous blood (Goadsby et al., 1988). Second, external jugular CGRP levels increase during nitroglycerin-induced and during spontaneous migraine attacks (Goadsby et al., 1990; Juhasz et al., 2003), although a recent study found normal CGRP levels during migraine attacks (Tvedskov et al., 2005). Third, clinical studies show that the administration of human α-CGRP triggers a migrainelike headache in patients with migraine without aura (Lassen et al., 2002) as well as in patients with migraine with aura (Hansen et al., 2010). Interestingly, CGRP could be less involved in the pathophysiology of familial hemiplegic migraine (FHM), since CGRP infusion does induce migrainelike headache in patients with known FHM mutations (Hansen et al., 2008, 2011). Last, the development of CGRP receptor antagonists such as olcegepant and telcagepant that are effective in the treatment of migraine attacks also supports the role of CGRP in migraine pathophysiology (Ho et al., 2008).

Cannabinoid Receptors

Two cannabinoid receptors have been described, type 1 (CB_1) and type 2 (CB_2), which are members of the superfamily of G-protein-coupled receptors. CB_1 receptors are found mainly at the terminals of central and peripheral neurons, where they inhibit ongoing release of different excitatory and inhibitory neurotransmitters (for review see Pertwee et al., 2010). CB_2 receptors are mainly located in immune cells. Ligands activating cannabinoid receptors include endogenous compounds known as endocannabinoids, phytocannabinoid Δ^9-tetrahydrocannabinol (Δ^9-THC), and synthetic compounds. The best-studied endocannabinoids are arachidonoylethanolamine (anandamide or AEA) and 2-arachidonoylglycerol (2-AG). AEA is hydrolyzed by the enzyme fatty acid amide hydrolase (FAAH), whereas 2-AG is degraded by the enzyme monoacylglycerol lipase (MAGL).

The endocannabinoid system is thought to be involved in the modulation of pain and hyperalgesia (Guindon & Hohmann, 2009). In migraine pathophysiology, a role for the endocannabinoid system has been suggested by animal models of migraine. AEA inhibits dural blood vessel dilatation caused by nitric oxide (NO) and CGRP in the murine model of trigeminovascular activation (Akerman et al., 2004) and inhibits NTG-induced c-Fos expression in the nucleus trigeminal caudalis (Greco et al., 2010). Specifically, electrophysiological single-unit recording studies show that neurons in the trigeminocervical complex (TCC) with input from the ophthalmic division of the trigeminal nerve are inhibited by activation of the CB_1 receptors (Akerman et al., 2007). To date, the effectiveness of cannabinoids in the treatment of migraine is unknown.

Other Receptors in Migraine

TRANSIENT RECEPTOR POTENTIAL VANILLOID RECEPTORS

The transient receptor potential vanilloid receptors (TRPV1) belong to the transient receptor potential family receptors and are preferentially expressed in primary afferent neurons including nociceptive sensory nerves. They are activated by various stimuli such as capsaicin; anandamide (AEA), which also activates the cannabinoid receptors; inflammatory mediators; and nonselective stimuli such as high temperature ($>43°C$) and acidic pH (<5.3). The possible involvement of TRPV1 has been suggested in migraine pathophysiology (Meents et al., 2010). However, a recent study showed that TRPV1 receptor blockade by the TRPV1 antagonist A-993610 in animal models of migraine has no effect on trigeminal firing of Aδ- or C-fibers elicited by electrical stimulation of the middle meningeal artery, on neurogenic dural vasodilatation, and on mechanically induced cortical spreading depression (Summ et al., 2011). These data suggest that the TRPV1 receptor is unlikely to play a major role in migraine pathophysiology, although responses to inflammatory stimuli rather than electrical stimulation remain to be tested.

GLUTAMATE RECEPTORS

Glutamate receptors are divided into ionotropic (N-methyl-d-aspartate [NMDA], kainate, and α-amino-3-hydroxy-5-methyl-4-isoxazolepropionic acid [AMPA] receptors) and metabotropic glutamate receptors (mGluRs). CSD is associated with an increase in extracellular levels of glutamate and is thought to involve NMDA receptors. LY-293558, an AMPA and kainate receptor antagonist, may have a potential therapeutic role in treating migraine (Ramadan et al., 2003; Sang et al., 2004), but to date, the role of glutamate receptors in animal models of migraine (Andreou et al., 2009) and the therapeutic effect of glutamate receptor antagonists are still under evaluation (Monteith & Goadsby, 2011).

SUBSTANCE P

Although substance P was one of the first transmitters supposed to be involved in pain and migraine due to its anatomic distribution in the sensory nervous system, there is no evidence that neurokinin-1 receptor antagonists have any analgesic or antimigraine properties (May & Goadsby, 2001).

EP$_4$ PROSTANOID RECEPTOR

Prostanoids and thromboxanes are important mediators of pain. The role of the prostanoid receptor subtype (EP$_4$) receptor in migraine pathophysiology is suggested by experimental and pharmacological data. In vitro, prostaglandin E$_2$ mediates human cerebral vasodilatation via prostanoid receptor subtype (EP$_4$) (Davis et al., 2004). Recently, the therapeutic role of a selective EP$_4$ receptor antagonist (BGC20–1531) has been suggested in migraine (Maubach et al., 2009; Monteith & Goadsby, 2011).

IMAGING NEURORECEPTOR CHANGES IN MIGRAINE

Before describing the data issued from neuroimaging studies of receptor changes in migraine, we will briefly review the state of the art, limitations, and potential pitfalls of in vivo neuroreceptor imaging.

State of the Art, Limitations, and Pitfalls of In Vivo Neuroreceptor Imaging in Humans

PET and, to a lesser degree, SPECT are the two functional neuroimaging techniques that can be used to study neurotransmission and neuroreceptor changes in migraine. Based on the assumption that changes in neurotransmission could be one of the basic mechanisms of migraine, one of the most promising applications of PET is to image the distribution of receptors in the brain between and during migraine attacks. To do this effectively, the methods of quantification and functional interpretation of images are particularly important to optimize to obtain useful comparative data between migraine states.

Since the early days of PET neuroreceptor imaging, two analytical methods have most often been used to extract specific binding images from raw PET data of radiolabeled ligands bound to CNS receptors (Delforge et al., 1989). The first method consists of evaluating the nonspecific binding by studying the kinetics of radioactivity in a brain region known as deprived of specific receptors. The second consists of performing data acquisition in two conditions, one in which specific receptors are free for binding with the injected radiolabeled ligand and the other in which specific receptors are occupied by the nonlabeled ligand injected at a high and pharmacologically active dose, prior to radiolabeled ligand injection (saturation method). This second method requires that the injection of the cold nonlabeled ligand have no adverse pharmacological effects. This method often requires very long and intensive imaging protocols to quantify specific receptor binding, and these often cannot be implemented routinely in patients, especially under the changing conditions of a migraine attack.

It should be noted that in brain neuroreceptor imaging when the specific binding represents a high percentage of the activity detected in uptake images, the volume of distribution of the ligand (V$_d$) reflects receptor availability (B$_{max}$). Voxel-based images of the V$_d$ of the radiolabeled ligand can then be produced from the brain uptake and arterial plasma input functions. Importantly for use in patients, simplified protocols that do not necessitate arterial blood sampling have been proposed. These methods rely on correlations being demonstrated between late uptake and distribution volume images, or quantified parametric images to reflect receptor density, which can be assessed by the binding potential (BP; ratio of available receptor density to receptor affinity; BP = B$_{max}$/K$_d$, where K$_d$ is the dissociation constant).

Another practical limitation to the use of PET to study brain receptor populations in migraine patients is that any drug treatments including antimigraine molecules that could interfere with the specific binding of the radioligand must be interrupted for days or weeks before the study. Moreover, some comorbid disorders may also influence radioligand binding and so confound data interpretation; for instance, the availability of serotonin receptors may be altered by migraine but also by depression (Veltman et al., 2010).

The main concern in PET neuroreceptor imaging studies is making an unequivocal physiological interpretation of the data, even when the problems of mathematical modeling and correction for imaging artifacts such as the partial volume effect have been resolved. This uncertainty is because the same quantified image of a change in receptor binding in brain tissue may reflect different biological changes:

- Changes in receptor binding could simply reflect changes in the density of neurons per volume of cortex; this issue is at stake when the pathology under study can cause, or be associated with, a cell loss, a situation that is not a major concern in migraine.
- Changes in receptor binding can be the "net effect" of changes in neurotransmission and so can theoretically be caused by several, even opposite, abnormalities of neurotransmission. For instance, an increase of specific receptors binding could be due either to an up-regulation of receptors in response to increased synthesis and release of the endogenous ligand, or, when a ligand that is sensitive to endogenous neurotransmitters is used, to an increase in the proportion of receptors that are unoccupied as a consequence of decreased endogenous ligand release into the synaptic cleft.
- Changes in receptor binding can also reflect a change in receptor pharmacology that affects the affinity of the radioligand, such as internalization, or genetically determined changes that affect the molecular architecture of the ligand binding site.
- Even when receptor binding images are unequivocal, the challenge remains to interpret changes in binding in terms of function and neuronal firing. For instance, serotonin 5-HT$_{1A}$ neuronal receptors of raphe nuclei, which are supposed to be involved in the pathophysiology of migraine, are autoreceptors that decrease the neuronal firing (see below). As a consequence, an increase of 5-HT$_{1A}$ activation in the raphe nuclei causes a decrease of 5-HT transmission in the projection fields of these neurons, and vice versa; it remains then to be decided which of the two effects is relevant as a potential determinant of migraine.

Since several mechanisms can combine in the same individual to produce the binding changes, it is often not possible to distinguish between them without quantitative correlation studies between in vivo PET data and in vitro evaluations. Combining images of neurotransmitter synthesis and receptor binding, which is feasible, for instance, with ^{18}F-dopa and ^{11}C-raclopride for dopaminergic transmission or with ^{11}C-α-methyl-tryptophan and (2'-methoxyphenyl-[N-2'-pyridinyl]-p-^{18}F-fluoro-benzamidoethylpiperazine) ([^{18}F]MPPF) for serotoninergic transmission, partly resolves this issue, but unfortunately these images cannot be acquired simultaneously. Apart from the inconvenience of two separate acquisitions and the ensuing increase of the subject's levels of irradiation, this strategy is valid only when the expected changes can

be considered as markers of a pathology that is stable in time, a condition that is not met in diseases manifesting by transient ictal attacks such as migraine or epilepsy.

A further complication of neuroreceptor imaging in migraine is that we have no precise knowledge of the timing of changes in neuroreceptor population changes. These may already be present before the migraine attack, may be altered after the migraine attack, or may change during the ictal phase. Indeed, getting patients to the imaging centers in time to study the ictal phase of migraine represents a major difficulty of all functional neuroimaging investigations, including PET neuroreceptor binding studies. Migraine attacks can be provoked in a few patients by a natural stimulus to which they have developed a specific hypersensitivity (Demarquay et al., 2011), but in most cases triggering a migraine attack requires the use of a pharmacological agent influencing, for instance, nitric oxide (NO) levels and formation of cyclic guanosine monophosphate (cGMP) such as glyceryl trinitrate (GTN) (Afridi & Matharu, 2005) or production of cyclic adenosine monophosphate (cAMP) such as CGRP, or interfering with other neuroendocrine systems supposed to be involved in migraine attack triggering (see Schytz et al., 2010, for a review). However, to our knowledge, there have been no neuroreceptor binding studies using this approach to triggering a migraine attack. This use of pharmacological migraine triggers requires, as a prerequisite, knowledge of the effects of the migraine-triggering agents on neuroreceptor availability in normal subjects and thus is a long, but not impossible, road to take in migraine research.

What Have Neuroreceptor Imaging Studies in Migraine Patients Brought to Our Understanding of the Disease?

Human neuroimaging data on receptor availability in migraine patients are scarce, in contrast with the large number of preclinical studies in experimental models of migraine. Historically, dopamine D$_2$ receptors were the first studied with SPECT, followed by PET studies of the 5-HT$_2$ and 5-HT$_{1A}$ receptors. Very recently, a new CGRP receptor PET tracer, (^{11}C)MK-4232, has been developed (Borsook & Hargreaves, 2010; Sur et al., 2009), which could enhance our knowledge of CGRP receptor involvement in migraine but has not yet been validated for migraine studies.

DOPAMINE RECEPTORS

Relatively few and somewhat old imaging studies have evaluated dopamine receptor populations in migraine. In 1993, two migraine patients were evaluated by SPECT using the D_2-receptor radioligand ^{123}I-3-iodo-6-methoxy-benzamide (^{123}I-IBZM) during ergotamine abuse and after withdrawal (Verhoeff et al., 1993). This study hypothesized that dopamine D_2-receptor up-regulation might be an important causal factor of ergotamine withdrawal symptoms on the basis of a suspected interaction between ergotamine and dopamine receptors. D_2 receptor availability was thus expected to be different between migraineurs on and off ergotamine and normal subjects. Unfortunately, no difference in ^{123}I-IBZM uptake in the striatum was observed between healthy controls and migraineurs, either before or after ergotamine withdrawal.

In 1994, a SPECT study also using ^{123}I-IBZM radioligand aimed to evaluate the role of flunarizine on D_2 receptors (Wöber et al., 1994). Eleven migraine patients treated with flunarizine (10 mg/day) and 21 control subjects were included in this SPECT study. The authors showed that dopamine D_2 receptor binding potential (BP) was reduced in all migraine patients when compared to age-matched controls. However, there was no correlation between the D_2 receptor BP and the therapeutic efficacy of flunarizine. To our knowledge, no other study of dopamine receptors has been conducted in the field of migraine.

5-HT$_2$ RECEPTORS

The PET ligand ^{18}F-fluorosetoperone was used to visualize 5-HT$_2$ receptors in a study comparing 9 migraineurs (five suffering from migraine with and without aura and four from migraine without aura only) with 12 control subjects (Chabriat et al., 1995). The results showed that the specific distribution volume (SDV) of the ligand did not differ between migraineurs and control subjects, leading to the conclusion that cortical 5-HT$_2$ receptors were unaltered in migraine patients between attacks.

5-HT$_{1A}$ RECEPTORS

Although several carbonyl and fluoryl radioligands have been developed for in vivo quantification of 5-HT$_{1A}$ receptors (Table 20–1), only two ([^{11}C]WAY 100635 and [^{18}F]MPPF) have been used for clinical PET studies of 5-HT$_{1A}$ receptors. To our knowledge, only [^{18}F]MPPF, which is a specific antagonist of 5-HT$_{1A}$ receptors, has been applied to migraine studies. Importantly, unlike ^{11}C-WAY-100635, [^{18}F]MPPF has an affinity for 5-HT$_{1A}$ receptors similar to that of 5-HT, thus allowing displacement of the fraction bound to 5-HT$_{1A}$ receptors by endogenous 5-HT (Pleneveaux et al., 2000; Rbah et al. 2003; Zimmer et al., 2002).

5-HT$_{1A}$ Receptor Availability Between Attacks

5-HT$_{1A}$ receptor availability using [^{18}F]MPPFPET was first assessed in a study during the interictal period of migraine (Lothe et al., 2008). Ten female migraine patients and 24 female healthy volunteers were included. All patients suffered from migraine without aura and were headache free during the PET investigation. As illustrated in Figure 20–4, an increase of [^{18}F]MPPF BP, which measures the density of available 5-HT$_{1A}$ receptors, was revealed by SPM analysis in migraine patients compared to healthy controls, which was located mostly in posterior and limbic areas, including the lateral parieto-occipital junction, postcentral gyrus, and inferior parietal lobule in the left hemisphere; the junctional area between the superior and middle temporal gyri; and the mesial parieto-occipital junction in the right hemisphere and hippocampus bilaterally.

Region of interest (ROI) analysis showed a BP increase in the left medial occipitotemporal gyrus, right cuneus, right precuneus, and right superotemporal gyrus at $p < .05$.

The increase of [^{18}F]MPPF BP observed in migraine patients in the parieto-occipital, temporal, and limbic areas may theoretically reflect either an increase of 5-HT$_{1A}$ receptor density or a reduction in endogenous 5-HT. Even though an overexpression of 5-HT$_{1A}$ receptors cannot totally be ruled out, available data favor the interpretation that the concentration of 5-HT in the brain of migraineurs is reduced (see above), making it most likely that the imaging reflects a reduced occupancy of 5-HT$_{1A}$ receptors by endogenous 5-HT during the attack-free period.

TABLE 20–1 *Positron Emission Tomography Tracers Used for Serotoninergic Receptor Studies*

Serotoninergic Receptor	Radioligand
5-HT$_{1A}$ receptor	[^{11}C]NAD-195
	[^{18}F]MPPF
	[carbonyl-^{11}C]WAY-100635
	[carbonyl-^{11}C]desmethyl-WAY-100635
	[^{18}F]FCWAY
	[^{18}F]MEFWAY
	[^{11}C]RWAY
	[^{11}C]CUMI-101
5-HT$_{1B}$ receptor	[^{11}C]AZ10419369
	[^{11}C]P943
5-HT$_{2A}$ receptor	[^{18}F]setoperone
	[^{18}F]altanserin
5-HT$_4$	[^{11}C]SB207145

Adapted from Visser, A. K., van Waarde, A., Willemsen, A. T., Bosker, F. J., Luiten, P. G., den Boer, J. A., et al. (2011). Measuring serotonin synthesis: From conventional methods to PET tracers and their (pre)clinical implications. *European Journal of Nuclear Medicine and Molecular Imaging, 38,* 576–591.

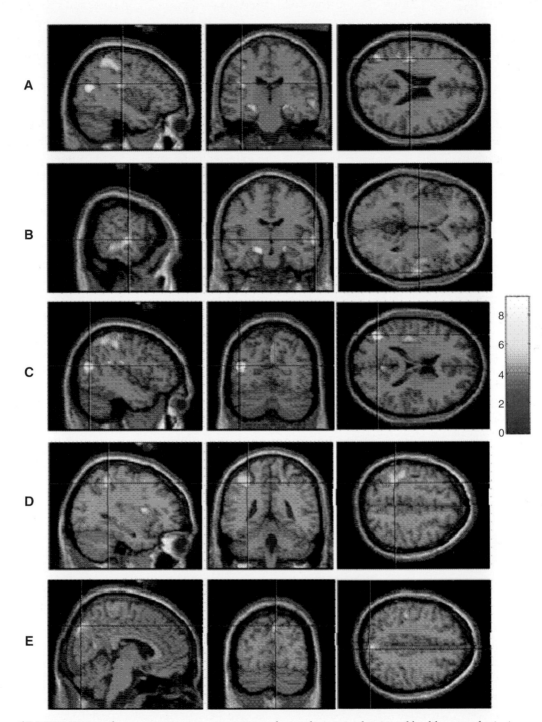

FIGURE 20–4 ^{18}F-MPPF SPM analysis contrasting migraine patients during the interictal state and healthy controls. An increase of 5-HT$_{1A}$ binding potential (BP) is observed in migraine patients in (A) the left inferior parietal lobule, (B) the left and right hippocampi and right superior temporal and middle temporal gyri, (C) the left lateral parieto-occipital junction, (D) the left postcentral gyrus, and (E) the right parieto-occipital junction. From Lothe, A., Merlet, I., Demarquay, G., Costes, N., Ryvlin, P., & Mauguière, F. (2008). Interictal brain 5-HT1A receptors binding in migraine without aura: A MPPF PET study. Cephalagia, 28, 1282–1291.

The localization of 5-HT$_{1A}$ receptor binding changes predominantly in the posterior areas was an unexpected finding. The increase of [^{18}F]MPPF binding observed in migraine patients could be associated with the reduced sensory habituation to external stimuli, which is mainly observed for the visual modality (see for review Giffin & Kaube, 2002, and Schoenen et al., 2003) and a decreased 5-HT neurotransmission (Wang et al., 1996).

5-HT$_{1A}$ Receptors Availability During Attacks

A single study has evaluated 5-HT$_{1A}$ receptor availability during migraine attacks (Demarquay et al., 2011). This [^{18}F]MPPF PET study was performed in 10 migraineurs suffering from interictal olfactory hypersensitivity (OHS) and odor-triggered migraine attacks and 10 age-matched control subjects. All subjects underwent prior calibrated olfactory stimulations in a [^{15}O]H$_2$O PET study conducted to investigate olfactory hypersensitivity in migraineurs (Demarquay et al., 2008). Four patients developed a migraine attack during the [^{18}F]MPPF PET study. In these patients, SPM and ROI analyses showed an increased [^{18}F]MPPF BP in the pontine raphe when compared to headache-free migraineurs and control subjects (Fig. 20–5). This ictal change was confirmed at the individual level in each of the four affected patients. This study emphasizes the involvement of 5-HT$_{1A}$ receptors in the pontine raphe nuclei at the early stage of migraine attacks (during the first hour of the attack), without changes in midbrain 5-HT$_{1A}$ receptor availability. The lack of detectable change in the mesencephalon argues against the involvement of the dorsal raphe nucleus, which extends from the level of the oculomotor nucleus to the middle of the pons (Hornung, 2003). Although this negative finding might just reflect a lack of sensitivity, it points to the possibility that the dorsal raphe nucleus might be less directly involved than pontine raphe nuclei in the pathophysiology of migraine. Due to the lack of resolution of PET images, it is not possible to precisely identify which specific nuclei of the pontine raphe were detected in the MPPF PET study. However the location of increased [^{18}F]MPPF BP observed in the pontine raphe is consistent with an involvement of the raphe magnus nucleus, which exerts an inhibitory effect on trigeminal neurons (see above).

The increase of [^{18}F]MPPF BP observed in the pontine raphe nuclei emphasizes the involvement of serotonin acting at 5-HT$_{1A}$ receptors during migraine attacks, but remains complex to interpret. Indeed, an increase in [^{18}F]MPPF BP can reflect either an up-regulation of 5-HT$_{1A}$ receptors, an increased affinity, a decreased extracellular concentration of endogenous 5-HT, or any combination of these. The hypothesis of a decreased endogenous 5-HT at the early stage of the attack is, however, consistent with previous studies, which showed that a decrease of endogenous 5-HT intensifies the development of migrainous symptoms in humans, while the reduction of brain 5-HT synthesis enhances CSD and the trigeminal response to CSD in rats (see section on evaluation of central brain serotonin). Moreover, a decrease in the occupancy of 5-HT$_{1A}$ inhibitory autoreceptors in the pontine raphe nuclei could secondarily increase neuronal firing in these structures and presumably increase liberation of 5-HT in structures with afferent innervation from the raphe, including the trigeminal nucleus caudalis. This interpretation of the [^{18}F]MPPF imaging data fits with the increase of 5-HT synthesis during the first 4 to 6 hours of the migraine attack shown by ^{11}C-AMT PET (Sakai et al., 2008, see above), but not with preclinical studies showing the suppressive effect of microiontophoretic injection of 5-HT$_{1A}$ receptor agonists on the activity of the trigeminal nucleus caudalis (Boers et al., 2000). Such discrepancies could reflect species differences in the receptor pharmacology of the raphe or, more likely, the fact that changes in 5-HT synthesis and 5-HT receptor binding are not the same when the migraine attack is triggered and when the crisis has fully developed a few hours later.

It is also noteworthy that, in comparison with the headache-free migraineurs, patients with a migraine attack also showed significantly increased [^{18}F]MPPF binding in the left orbitofrontal cortex, precentral gyrus, and temporal pole, which are targets for serotoninergic projections from the raphe nuclei (Mamounas et al., 1988; Wilson & Molliver, 1991) and are involved in pain and/or olfactory processing.

CONCLUSIONS

Searching for a holistic vision of migraine pathogenesis through the study of brain receptors is an ambitious challenge that has little chance, if any, to identify a single disorder of neurotransmission that might switch on the cascade of receptor changes hitherto reported in experimental and clinical literature. However, each of these receptor changes potentially offers a new track for developing innovative antimigraine pharmacological agents. Interictal studies converge to the conclusion that a decreased serotonin synthesis and release by raphe nuclei represents the main biological background underlying brain susceptibility to migraine attacks. Research into the ictal stage of migraine faces two main difficulties: The first is that the migraine attack is a sequence of events that

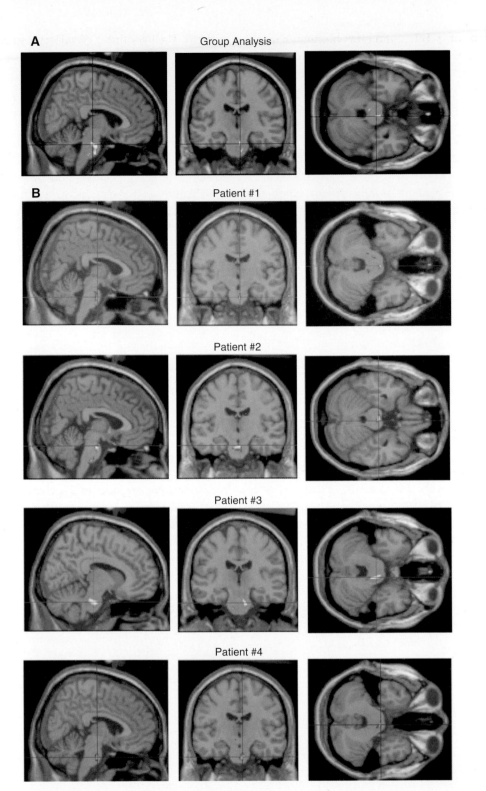

A Group Analysis

B Patient #1

Patient #2

Patient #3

Patient #4

FIGURE 20–5 *SPM analysis with a brainstem mask contrasting the four patients with a migraine attack during the positron emission tomography study with the six age-matched controls. (A) Group analysis shows significant increased ^{18}F-MPPF binding in three clusters. (B) Individual analyses show significant increased 18F-MPPF binding in the pons of each of the four patients. From Demarquay, G., Lothe, A., Royet, J. P., Costes, N., Mick, G., Mauguière, F., et al. (2011). Brainstem changes in 5-HT1A receptor availability during migraine attack. Cephalalgia, 31, 84–94.*

develops over several hours and very probably involves fluctuating changes in neurotransmission and neuroreceptor availability; the second is that current imaging techniques do not offer the possibility of linking neuroreceptor changes with neuronal activity. In the near future simultaneous acquisition of PET and functional magnetic resonance imaging (fMRI) data (Judenhofer et al., 2008) will represent a true breakthrough in migraine research by providing the opportunity to acquire synchronous information on neuronal activity as reflected by blood flow with fMRI/perfusion MRI and tracer kinetics with PET.

REFERENCES

Afridi, S. K., Giffin, N. J., Kaube, H., Friston, K. J., Ward, N. S., Frackowiak, R. S. J., et al. (2005). A PET study in spontaneous migraine. *Archives of Neurology, 62,* 1270–1275.

Afridi, S. K., Matharu, M. S., Lee, L., Kaube, H., Friston, K. J., Frackowiak, R. S. J., et al. (2005). A PET study exploring the laterality of brainstem activation in migraine using glyceryltrinitrate. *Brain, 128,* 932–939.

Akerman, S., & Goadsby, P. J. (2007). Dopamine and migraine: Biology and clinical implications. *Cephalalgia, 27,* 1308–1314.

Akerman, S., Holland, P. R., & Goadsby, P. J. (2007). Cannabinoid (CB1) receptor activation inhibits trigeminovascular neurons. *Journal of Pharmacology and Experimental Therapeutics, 320,* 64–71.

Akerman, S., Kaube, H., & Goadsby, P. J. (2004). Anandamide is able to inhibit trigeminal neurons using an in vivo model of trigeminovascular-mediated nociception. *Journal of Pharmacology and Experimental Therapeutics, 309,* 56–63.

Andreou, A. P., Holland, P. R., & Goadsby, P. J. (2009). Activation of iGluR5 kainate receptors inhibits neurogenic dural vasodilatation in an animal model of trigeminovascular activation. *British Journal of Pharmacology, 157,* 464–473.

Arulmani, U., Maassenvandenbrink, A., Villalón, C. M., & Saxena, P. R. (2004). Calcitonin gene-related peptide and its role in migraine pathophysiology. *European Journal of Pharmacology, 500,* 315–330.

Asghar, M. S., Hansen, A. E., Kapijimpanga, T., van der Geest, R. J., van der Koning, P., Larsson, H. B., et al. (2010). Dilation by CGRP of middle meningeal artery and reversal by sumatriptan in normal volunteers. *Neurology, 75,* 1520–1526.

Bahra, A., Matharu, M. S., Buchel, C., Frackowiak, R. S. J., & Goadsby, P. J. (2001). Brainstem activation specific to migraine headache. *Lancet, 357,* 1016–1017.

Barbanti, P., & Fabbrini, G. (2002). Migraine and the extrapyramidal system. *Cephalalgia, 22,* 2–11.

Barnes, N. M., & Sharp, T. (1999). A review of central 5-HT receptors and their function. *Neuropharmacology, 38,* 1083–1152.

Beaulieu, J. M., & Gainetdinov, R. R. (2011). The physiology, signaling, and pharmacology of dopamine receptors. *Pharmacological Reviews, 63,* 182–217.

Bergerot, A., Storer, R. J., & Goadsby, P. J. (2007). Dopamine inhibits trigeminovascular transmission in the rat. *Annals of Neurology, 61,* 251–262.

Boers, P. M., Donaldson, C., Zagami, A. S., & Lambert, G. A. (2000). 5-HT(1A) and 5-HT(1B/1D) receptors are involved in the modulation of the trigeminovascular system of the cat: A microiontophoretic study. *Neuropharmacology, 39,* 1833–1847.

Borsook, D., & Hargreaves, R. (2010). Brain imaging in migraine research. *Headache, 50,* 1523–1527.

Brain, S. D., Williams, T. J., Tippins, J. R., Morris, H. R., & MacIntyre, I. (1985). Calcitonin gene-related peptide is a potent vasodilator. *Nature, 313,* 54–56.

Carlsson, A., Falck, B., & Hillarp, N. A. (1962). Cellular localization of brain monoamines. *Acta Physiologica Scandinavica Supplementum, 56,* 1–28.

Cassidy, E. M., Tomkins, E., Dinan, T., Hardiman, O., & O'Keane, V. (2003). Central 5-HT receptor hypersensitivity in migraine without aura. *Cephalalgia, 23,* 29–34.

Cassidy, E. M., Tomkins, E., Sharifi, N., Dinan, T., Hardiman, O., & O'Keane, V. (2003). Differing central amine receptor sensitivity in different migraine subtypes? A neuroendocrine study using buspirone. *Pain, 101,* 283–290.

Cerbo, R., Barbanti, P., Buzzi, M. G., Fabbrini, G., Brusa, L., Roberti, C., et al. (1997). Dopamine hypersensitivity in migraine: role of the apomorphine test. *Clinical Neuropharmacology, 20,* 36–41.

Chabriat, H., Tehindrazanarivelo, A., Vera, P., Samson, Y., Pappata, S., Boullais, N., et al. (1995). 5HT2 receptors in cerebral cortex of migraineurs studied using PET and 18F-fluorosetoperone. *Cephalalgia, 15,* 104–108

Charbit, A. R., Akerman, S., & Goadsby, P. J. (2009). Comparison of the effects of central and peripheral dopamine receptor activation on evoked firing in the trigeminocervical complex. *Journal of Pharmacology and Experimental Therapeutics, 331,* 752–763.

Charbit, A. R., Akerman, S., & Goadsby, P. J. (2010). Dopamine: What's new in migraine? *Current Opinion in Neurology, 23,* 275–281.

Charbit, A. R., Akerman, S., Holland, P. R., & Goadsby, P. J. (2009). Neurons of the dopaminergic/calcitonin gene-related peptide A11 cell group modulate neuronal firing in the trigeminocervical complex: An electrophysiological and immunohistochemical study. *Journal of Neuroscience, 29,* 12532–12541.

Chugani, D. C. (2004). Serotonin in autism and pediatric epilepsies. *Mental Retardation and Developmental Disabilities Research Reviews, 10,* 112–116.

Chugani, D. C., Niimura, K., Chaturvedi, S., Muzik, O., Fakhouri, M., Lee, M. L., et al. (1999). Increased brain synthesis in migraine. *Neurology, 53,* 1473–1479.

Classey, J. D., Bartsch, T., & Goadsby, P. J. (2010). Distribution of 5-HT(1B), 5-HT(1D) and 5-HT(1F) receptor expression in rat trigeminal and dorsal root ganglia neurons: Relevance to the selective anti-migraine effect of triptans. *Brain Research, 1361,* 76–85.

Cowen, P. J. (2008). Serotonin and depression: Pathophysiological mechanism or marketing myth? *Trends in Pharmacological Sciences, 29,* 433–436.

Curran, D. A., Hinterberger, H., & Lance, J. W. (1965). Total plasma serotonin, 5-hydroxyindoleacetic acid and p-hydroxy-m-methoxymandelic acid excretion in normal and migrainous subjects. *Brain, 88,* 997–1010.

Daubert, E. A., & Condron, B. G. (2010). Serotonin: A regulator of neuronal morphology and circuitry. *Trends in Neuroscience, 33,* 424–434.

Davis, R. J., Murdoch, C. E., Ali, M., Purbrick, S., Ravid, R., Baxter, G. S., et al. (2004). EP4 prostanoid receptor-mediated vasodilatation of human middle cerebral arteries. *British Journal of Pharmacology, 141,* 580–585.

Del Bene, E., Poggioni, M., & De Tommasi, F. (1994). Video assessment of yawning induced by sublingual apomorphine in migraine. *Headache, 34*, 536–538.

Delforge, J., Syrota, A., & Mazoyer, B. M. (1989). Experimental design optimisation: Theory and application to estimation of receptor model parameters using dynamic positron emission tomography. *Physics in Medicine and Biology, 34*, 419–435.

Demarquay, G., Lothe, A., Royet, J. P., Costes, N., Mick, G., Mauguière, F., et al. (2011). Brainstem changes in 5-HT1A receptor availability during migraine attack. *Cephalalgia, 31*, 84–94.

Demarquay, G., Royet, J. P., Mick, G., & Ryvlin, P. (2008). Olfactory hypersensitivity in migraineurs: A H215O-PET study. *Cephalalgia, 28*, 1069–1080.

Denuelle, M., Fabre, N., Payoux, P., Chollet, F., & Geraud, G. (2007). Hypothalamic activation in spontaneous migraine attacks. *Headache, 47*, 1418–1426.

Di Giovanni, G., Esposito, E., & Di Matteo, V. (2010). Role of serotonin in central dopamine dysfunction. *CNS Neuroscience Therapy, 16*, 179–194.

Drummond, P. D. (2006). Tryptophan depletion increases nausea, headache and photophobia in migraine sufferers. *Cephalalgia, 26*, 1225–1233.

Edvinsson, L., Chan, K. Y., Eftekhari, S., Nilsson, E, de Vries, R., Säveland, H., et al. (2010). Effect of the calcitonin gene-related peptide (CGRP) receptor antagonist telcagepant in human cranial arteries. *Cephalalgia, 30*, 1233–1240.

Eftekhari, S., & Edvinsson, L. (2010). Possible sites of action of the new calcitonin gene-related peptide receptor antagonists. *Therapeutic Advances in Neurological Disorders, 3*, 369–378.

Eftekhari, S., Salvatore, C. A., Calamari, A., Kane, S. A., Tajti, J., & Edvinsson, L. (2010). Differential distribution of calcitonin gene-related peptide and its receptor components in the human trigeminal ganglion. *Neuroscience, 169*, 683–696.

Ferrari, M. D., Färkkilä, M., Reuter, U., Pilgrim, A., Davis, C., Krauss, M., et al.; European COL-144 Investigators. (2010). Acute treatment of migraine with the selective 5-HT1F receptor agonist lasmiditan—a randomised proof-of-concept trial. *Cephalalgia, 30*, 1170–1178.

Ferrari, M. D., & Saxena, P. R. (1993). On serotonin and migraine: A clinical and pharmacological review. *Cephalalgia, 13*, 151–165.

Filip, M., & Bader, M. (2009). Overview on 5-HT receptors and their role in physiology and pathology of the central nervous system. *Pharmacological Reports, 61*(5), 761–777.

Friedman, B. W., Mulvey, L., Esses, D., Solorzano, C., Paternoster, J., Lipton, R. B., et al. (2011). Metoclopramide for acute migraine: A dose-finding randomized clinical trial. *Annals of Emergency Medicine, 57*, 475–482.e1.

Giffin, N. J., & Kaube, H. (2002). The electrophysiology of migraine. *Current Opinion in Neurology, 15*, 303–309.

Goadsby, P. J., Edvinsson, L., & Ekman, R. (1988). Release of vasoactive peptides in the extracerebral circulation of humans and the cat during activation of the trigeminovascular system. *Annals of Neurology, 23*, 193–196.

Goadsby, P. J., Edvinsson, L., & Ekman, R. (1990). Vasoactive peptide release in the extracerebral circulation of humans during migraine headache. *Annals of Neurology, 28*, 183–187.

Greco, R., Gasperi, V., Sandrini, G., Bagetta, G., Nappi, G., Maccarrone, M., et al. (2010). Alterations of the endocannabinoid system in an animal model of migraine: Evaluation in cerebral areas of rat. *Cephalalgia, 30*, 296–302.

Gross, C., Zhuang, X., Stark, K., Ramboz, S., Oosting, R., Kirby, L., et al. (2002). Serotonin1A receptor acts during development to establish normal anxiety-like behaviour in the adult. *Nature, 416*, 396–400.

Guindon, J., & Hohmann, A. G. (2009). The endocannabinoid system and pain. *CNS and Neurological Disorders, Drug Targets, 8*, 403–421.

Hamel, E. (2007). Serotonin and migraine: Biology and clinical implications. *Cephalalgia, 27*, 1293–1300.

Hansen, J. M., Hauge, A. W., Olesen, J., & Ashina, M. (2010). Calcitonin gene-related peptide triggers migraine-like attacks in patients with migraine with aura. *Cephalalgia, 30*, 1179–1186.

Hansen, J. M., Thomsen, L. L., Olesen, J., & Ashina, M. (2008). Calcitonin gene-related peptide does not cause the familial hemiplegic migraine phenotype. *Neurology, 71*, 841–847.

Hansen, J. M., Thomsen, L. L., Olesen, J., & Ashina, M. (2011). Calcitonin gene-related peptide does not cause migraine attacks in patients with familial hemiplegic migraine. *Headache, 51*, 544–553.

Headache Classification Committee. (2004). The international classification of headache disorders, 2nd ed. *Cephalalgia, 1*(Suppl. 1), 1–160.

Ho, T. W., Ferrari, M. D., Dodick, D. W., Galet, V., Kost, J., Fan, X., et al. (2008). Efficacy and tolerability of MK-0974 (telcagepant), a new oral antagonist of calcitonin gene-related peptide receptor, compared with zolmitriptan for acute migraine: A randomised, placebo-controlled, parallel-treatment trial. *Lancet, 372*, 2115–2123.

Honkaniemi, J., Liimatainen, S., Rainesalo, S., & Sulavuori, S. (2006). Haloperidol in the acute treatment of migraine: A randomized, double-blind, placebo-controlled study. *Headache, 46*, 781–787.

Hornung, J. P. (2003). The human raphe nuclei and the serotonergic system. *Journal of Chemical Neuroanatomy, 26*, 331–343.

Hou, M., Kanje, M., Longmore, J., Tajti, J., Uddman, R., & Edvinsson, L. (2001). 5-HT(1B) and 5-HT(1D) receptors in the human trigeminal ganglion: Co-localization with calcitonin gene-related peptide, substance P and nitric oxide synthase. *Brain Research, 909*, 112–120.

Judenhofer, M. S., Wehrl, H. F., Newport, D. F., Catana, C., Siegel, S. B., Becker, M., et al. (2008). Simultaneous PET-MRI: a new approach for functional and morphological imaging. *Nature Medicine, 14*, 459–465.

Juhasz, G., Zsombok, T., Modos, E. A., Olajos, S., Jakab, B., Nemeth, J., et al. NO-induced migraine attack: Strong increase in plasma calcitonin gene-related peptide (CGRP) concentration and negative correlation with platelet serotonin release. *Pain, 106*, 461–470.

Katsarava, Z., Egelhof, T., Kaube, H., Diener, H. C., & Limmroth, V. (2003). Symptomatic migraine and sensitization of trigeminal nociception associated with contralateral pontine cavernoma. *Pain, 105*, 381–384.

Kaube, H., Keay, K. A., Hoskin, K. L., Bandler, R., & Goadsby, P. J. (1993). Expression of c-Fos-like immunoreactivity in the caudal medulla and upper cervical spinal cord following stimulation of the superior sagittal sinus in the cat. *Brain Research, 629*, 95–102.

Knight, Y. E., Classey, J. D., Lasalandra, M. P., Akerman, S., Kowacs, F., Hoskin, K. L., et al. (2005). Patterns of fos expression in the rostral medulla and caudal pons evoked by noxious craniovascular stimulation and periaqueductal gray stimulation in the cat. *Brain Research, 1045*, 1–11.

Knight, Y. E., & Goadsby, P. J. (2001). The periaqueductal grey matter modulates trigeminovascular input: A role in migraine? *Neuroscience, 106*, 793–800.

Lambert, G. A., Hoskin, K. L., & Zagami, A. S. (2008). Cortico-NRM influences on trigeminal neuronal sensation. *Cephalalgia, 28*, 640–652.

Lassen, L. H., Haderslev, P. A., Jacobsen, V. B., Iversen, H. K., Sperling, B., & Olesen, J. (2002). CGRP may play a causative role in migraine. *Cephalalgia, 22*, 54–61.

Leibowitz, S. F. (1990). The role of serotonin in eating disorders. *Drugs, 39*(Suppl 3), 33–48.

Leone, M., Attanasio, A., Croci, D., Filippini, G., D'Amico, D., Grazzi, L., et al. (2000). The serotonergic agent m-chlorophenylpiperazine induces migraine attacks: A controlled study. *Neurology, 55*, 136–139.

Longmore, J., Shaw, D., Smith, D., Hopkins, R., McAllister, G., Pickard, J. D., et al. (1997). Differential distribution of 5HT1D- and 5HT1B-immunoreactivity within the human trigemino-cerebrovascular system: Implications for the discovery of new antimigraine drugs. *Cephalalgia, 17*, 833–842.

Lothe, A., Merlet, I., Demarquay, G., Costes, N., Ryvlin, P., & Mauguière, F. (2008). Interictal Brain 5-HT1A receptors binding in migraine without aura: A MPPF PET study. *Cephalagia, 28*, 1282–1291.

Mamounas, L. A., & Molliver, M. E. (1988). Evidence for dual serotonergic projections to neocortex: Axons from the dorsal and median raphe nuclei are differentially vulnerable to the neurotoxin p-chloroamphetamine (PCA). *Experimental Neurology, 102*, 23–36.

Maubach, K. A., Davis, R. J., Clark, D. E., Fenton, G., Lockey, P. M., Clark, K. L., et al. (2009). BGC20-1531, a novel, potent and selective prostanoid EP receptor antagonist: A putative new treatment for migraine headache. *British Journal of Pharmacology, 156*, 316–327.

May, A., & Goadsby, P. J. (2001). Substance P receptor antagonists in the therapy of migraine. *Expert Opinion on Investigational Drugs, 10*, 673–678.

Meents, J. E., Neeb, L., & Reuter, U. (2010). TRPV1 in migraine pathophysiology. *Trends in Molecular Medicine, 16*, 153–159.

Meston, C. M., & Gorzalka, B. B. (1992). Psychoactive drugs and human sexual behavior: The role of serotonergic activity. *Journal of Psychoactive Drugs, 24*, 1–40.

Miller, M. A., Levsky, M. E., Enslow, W., & Rosin, A. (2009). Randomized evaluation of octreotidevsprochlorperazine for ED treatment of migraine headache. *American Journal of Emergency Medicine, 27*, 160–164.

Monteith, T. S., & Goadsby, P. J. (2011). Acute migraine therapy: New drugs and new approaches. *Current Treatment Options in Neurology, 13*, 1–14.

Moskowitz, M. A., Reinhard, J. F., Jr., Romero, J., Melamed, E., & Pettibone, D. J. (1979). Neurotransmitters and the fifth cranial nerve: is there a relation to the headache phase of migraine? *Lancet, 2*, 883–885.

Nagata, E., Shibata, M., Hamada, J., Shimizu, T., Katoh, Y., Gotoh, K., et al. (2006). Plasma 5-hydroxytryptamine (5-HT) in migraine during an attack-free period. *Headache, 46*, 592–596.

Nelson, D. L., Phebus, L. A., Johnson, K. W., Wainscott, D. B., Cohen, M. L., Calligaro, D. O., et al. (2010). Preclinical pharmacological profile of the selective 5-HT1F receptor agonist lasmiditan. *Cephalalgia, 30*, 1159–1169.

Nilsson, T., Longmore, J., Shaw, D., Olesen, I. J., & Edvinsson, L. (1999). Contractile 5-HT1B receptors in human cerebral arteries: Pharmacological characterization and localization with immunocytochemistry. *British Journal of Pharmacology, 128*, 1133–1140.

Ozkul, Y., & Bozlar, S. (2002). Effects of fluoxetine on habituation of pattern reversal visually evoked potentials in migraine prophylaxis. *Headache, 42*, 582–587.

Panconesi, A. (2008). Serotonin and migraine: A reconsideration of the central theory. *Journal of Headache and Pain, 9*, 267–276.

Pertwee, R. G., Howlett, A. C., Abood, M. E., Alexander, S. P., Di Marzo, V., Elphick, M. R., et al. International Union of Basic and Clinical Pharmacology. LXXIX. Cannabinoid receptors and their ligands: Beyond CB1 and CB2. *Pharmacological Reviews, 62*, 588–631.

Plenevaux, A., Lemaire, C., Aerts, J., Lacan, G., Rubins, D., Melega, W. P., et al. (2000). [(18)F]p-MPPF: A radiolabeled antagonist for the study of 5-HT(1A) receptors with PET. *Nuclear Medicine and Biology, 27*, 467–471.

Quintela, E., Castillo, J., Muñoz, P., & Pascual, J. (2006). Premonitory and resolution symptoms in migraine: A prospective study in 100 unselected patients. *Cephalalgia, 26*, 1051–1060.

Ramadan, N. M., Skljarevski, V., Phebus, L. A., & Johnson, K. W. (2003). 5-HT1F receptor agonists in acute migraine treatment: A hypothesis. *Cephalalgia, 23*, 776–785.

Rapport, M. M., Green A. A., & Page, I. H. (1948). Serum vasoconstrictor, serotonin; isolation and characterization. *Journal of Biological Chemistry, 176*, 1243–1251.

Rbah, L., Leviel, V., & Zimmer, L. (2003). Displacement of the PET ligand 18F-MPPF by the electrically evoked serotonin release in the rat hippocampus. *Synapse, 49*, 239–245.

Richer, M., Hen, R., & Blier, P. (2002). Modification of serotonin neuron properties in mice lacking 5-HT1A receptors. *European Journal of Pharmacology, 435*, 195–203.

Sakai, Y., Dobson, C., Diksic, M., Aubé, M., & Hamel, E. (2008). Sumatriptan normalizes the migraine attack-related increase in brain serotonin synthesis. *Neurology, 70*, 431–439.

Sang, C. N., Ramadan, N. M., Wallihan, R. G., Chappell, A. S., Freitag, F. G., Smith, T. R., et al. (2004). LY293558, a novel AMPA/GluR5 antagonist, is efficacious and well-tolerated in acute migraine. *Cephalalgia, 24*, 596–602.

Schoenen, J., Ambrosini, A., Sandor, P. S., & Maertens de Noordhout, A. (2003). Evoked potentials and transcranial magnetic stimulation in migraine: Published data and viewpoint on their pathophysiologic significance. *Clinical Neurophysiology, 114*, 955–972.

Schoonman, G. G., Evers, D. J., Terwindt, G. M., van Dijk, J. G., & Ferrari, M. D. (2006). The prevalence of premonitory symptoms in migraine: A questionnaire study in 461 patients. *Cephalalgia, 26*, 1209–1213.

Schuh-Hofer, S., Richter, M., Geworski, L., Villringer, A., Israel, H., Wenzel, R., et al. (2007). Increased serotonin transporter availability in the brainstem of migraineurs. *Journal of Neurology, 254*, 789–796.

Schytz, H. W., Schoonman, G. G., & Ashina, M. (2010). What have we learnt from triggering migraine? *Current Opinion in Neurology, 23*, 259–265.

Sicuteri, F., Testi, A., & Anselmi, B. (1961). Biochemical investigations in headache increase in hydroxyindoleacetic acid excretion during migraine attacks. *International Archives of Allergy, 19*, 55–58.

Summ, O., Holland, P. R., Akerman, S., & Goadsby, P. J. (2011). TRPV1 receptor blockade is ineffective in different in vivo models of migraine. *Cephalalgia, 31,* 172–180.

Supornsilpchai, W., Sanguanrangsirikul, S., Maneesri, S., & Srikiatkhachorn, A. (2006). Serotonin depletion, cortical spreading depression, and trigeminal nociception. *Headache, 46,* 34–39.

Sur, C., Hargreaves, R., Bell, I., Dancho, M., Graham, S., Hostetler, E., et al. (2009). CSF levels and binding pattern of novel CGRP receptor antagonists in rhesus monkey and human central nervous system: Toward the development of a PET tracer. *Cephalalgia, 26*(Suppl 1), 136–137.

Tvedskov, J. F., Lipka, K., Ashina, M., Iversen, H. K., Schifter, S., & Olesen, J. (2005). No increase of calcitonin gene-related peptide in jugular blood during migraine. *Annals of Neurology, 58,* 561–568.

Uddman, R., Edvinsson, L., Ekman, R., Kingman, T., & McCulloch, J. (1985). Innervation of the feline cerebral vasculature by nerve fibers containing calcitonin gene-related peptide: Trigeminal origin and co-existence with substance P. *Neuroscience Letters, 62,* 131–136.

Varnäs, K., Hall, H., Bonaventure, P., & Sedvall, G. (2001). Autoradiographic mapping of 5-HT(1B) and 5-HT(1D) receptors in the post mortem human brain using [(3)H]GR 125743. *Brain Research, 915,* 47–57.

Veltman, D. J., Ruhé, H. G., & Booij, J. (2010). Investigating serotonergic function using positron emission tomography: Overview and recent findings. *Current Pharmaceutical Design, 16,* 1979–1989.

Verhoeff, N. P., Visser, W. H., Ferrari, M. D., Saxena, P. R., & van Royen, E. A. (1993). Dopamine D2-receptor imaging with 123I-iodobenzamide SPECT in migraine patients abusing ergotamine: Does ergotamine cross the blood brain barrier? *Cephalalgia, 13,* 325–329.

Visser, A. K., van Waarde, A., Willemsen, A. T., Bosker, F. J., Luiten, P. G., den Boer, J. A., et al. (2011). Measuring serotonin synthesis: From conventional methods to PET tracers and their (pre)clinical implications. *European Journal of Nuclear Medicine and Molecular Imaging, 38,* 576–591.

Walker, C. S., Conner, A. C., Poyner, D. R., & Hay, D. L. (2010). Regulation of signal transduction by calcitonin gene-related peptide receptors. *Trends in Pharmacological Science, 31,* 476–483.

Wang, W., Timsit-Berthier, M., & Schoenen, J. (1996). Intensity dependence of auditory evoked potentials is pronounced in migraine: An indication of cortical potentiation and low serotonergic neurotransmission? *Neurology, 46,* 1404–1409.

Weiller, C., May, A., Limmroth, V., Juptner, M., Kaube, H., Schayck, R. V., et al. (1995). Brainstem activation in spontaneous human migraine attacks. *Nature Medicine, 1,* 568–660.

Weissmann-Nanopoulos, D., Mach, E., Magre, S., Demassay, Y., & Pujol, J. F. (1985). Evidence for the localization of 5HT1-A binding sites on serotonin containing neurons in the raphe dorsalis and raphe centralis nuclei of the rat brain. *Neurochemistry International, 7,* 1061–1072.

Wilson, M. A., & Molliver, M. E. (1991). The organization of serotonergic projections to cerebral cortex in primates: Regional distribution of axon terminals. *Neuroscience, 44,* 537–553.

Wöber, C., Brücke, T., Wöber-Bingöl, C., Asenbaum, S., Wessely, P., & Podreka, I. (1994). Dopamine D2 receptor blockade and antimigraine action of flunarizine. *Cephalalgia, 14,* 235–240.

Zimmer, L., Mauger, G., Le Bars, D., Bonmarchand, G., Luxen, A., & Pujol, J. F. (2002). Effect of endogenous serotonin on the binding of the 5-hT1A PET ligand 18F-MPPF in the rat hippocampus: Kinetic beta measurements combined with microdialysis. *Journal of Neurochemistry, 80,* 278–286.

21 ^{15}O Positron Emission Tomography Studies in Migraine

MARIE DENUELLE, PIERRE PAYOUX, NELLY FABRE,
AND GILLES GÉRAUD

INTRODUCTION

Although reports of migraine headache go back to antiquity, the understanding of the pathophysiology of migraine has shown major advances over the last 30 years thanks to functional neuroimaging. Throughout most of the 20th century, the dogma of headache pathogenesis was that migraine was caused by changes in the caliber of cerebral vessels. It was the vascular theory of migraine. The aura was thought to be caused by a vasoconstriction and a resulting relative decrease in cerebral blood flow to visual and/or sensory cortices. The headache was thought to be caused by a rebound vasodilatation, which resulted in mechanical activation of nociceptive neurons within the walls of the engorged vessels. Attempts to confirm this model by measuring cerebral blood flow (CBF) have produced a wide range of findings. In the early 1980s, many studies used external scintillation counters or single-photon emission computed tomography (SPECT) with ^{133}Xenon by inhalation or carotid injection. Even if the results were quite heterogeneous, most consistently a focal hypoperfusion in the posterior regions of the brain was found during the aura of induced attacks, whereas no regional CBF (rCBF) changes were reported during migraine without aura attacks. In the 1990s, the first two positron emission tomography (PET) studies in migraine gave new insight into migraine pathophysiology, demonstrating for the first time a spreading oligemia during a migraine without aura attack, and a brainstem activation persisting after headache relief during spontaneous migraine attacks (Weiller et al., 1995; Woods et al., 1994). PET offers a method for noninvasively measuring rCBF with a better spatial resolution than with SPECT. Nowadays functional neuroimaging, mainly represented by PET and functional magnetic resonance imaging (fMRI), is the main tool that allows the capture of neurovascular events during a migraine attack. High-resolution PET scanning allows the detection of subtle changes in rCBF during defined behavioral tasks and provides an index of synaptic activity relating a network of regions to the tested brain function. Therefore, regional blood flow changes are a useful surrogate to detect synaptic activity, without determining whether the underlying physiological event is excitation or inhibition, or any other energy-consuming process. All the results of functional imaging, including PET studies, need to be interpreted in the light of other studies such as neurobiology, electrophysiology, and animal studies.

In this chapter, first we will detail the techniques of PET study and its advantages and limitations, and second we will present and discuss the results of PET studies in migraine.

^{15}O POSITRON EMISSION TOMOGRAPHY IMAGING

PET is a nuclear medicine imaging procedure that produces a three-dimensional image of functional processes of the brain. From a physical point of view, the PET method is based on the detection of pairs of gamma photons emitted by a positron-emitting radionuclide (tracer), labeling a molecule of biological interest (vector). Three-dimensional images of tracer distribution within the brain are then reconstructed by software analysis.

In the past years, the development of PET allowed in vivo, noninvasive measurement of the absolute and relative concentration of positron-emitting nuclides. A variety of tracer kinetic models were formulated to obtain physiological measurements from tomographic images of the distribution of ^{15}O-labeled radiopharmaceuticals in the brain. ^{15}O is a positron emitter with a very short half-life, and it was widely used as rCBF tracer in vivo. Furthermore, this radionuclide was also developed to measure cerebral blood flow, blood volume, and oxygen metabolism.

In addition to the access to cyclotron PET radiopharmaceuticals, PET imaging requires a PET camera consisting of several full-ring detectors: BGO (bismuth germinate orthosilicate), lutetium orthosilicate, or gadolinium orthosilicate. In modern PET machines, three-dimensional imaging is usually accomplished with the aid of a computed tomography (CT) X-ray scan performed on the patient during the same session, in the same machine, in order to improve anatomical reference and correct attenuation of the tissue. These cameras are much faster and sensitive than the older generation of PET cameras and usually present acquisition software improvement to optimize spatial resolution (around 2.5 mm at the center of the view field). In the next decade, PET will be certainly coupled with MRI.

Whole-body radiation exposure by PET examination is usually 0.5 to 2.0 mSv per scan. The radiation dose may differ among institutions depending on the protocol or quality of the PET camera. The duration of the data acquisition depends on the selected method and tracer. It typically ranges from 5 to 9 minutes for one acquisition for a routine clinical PET.

In this chapter we focus on radionuclide ^{15}O methods used to explore migraine.

Oxygen 15

Oxygen 15 (^{15}O) is an isotope of oxygen positron-emitting radionuclide. It has eight protons, seven neutrons, and eight electrons and a short half-life of 122 seconds. The major consequence of such a short half-life is the absolute necessity to produce the isotope in a cyclotron close to the PET center in order to use the ^{15}O compound by injection or inhalation.

The introduction of oxygen into the vascular compartment of the body leads to a distribution of the labeled oxygen to the tissues, and especially in the cortex, where it is converted to oxygen-15-labeled water ($H_2^{15}O$). The labeled water then redistributes to all tissues by way of the same vascular compartment. Unmetabolized labeled molecular oxygen is ultimately removed by respiration.

These characteristics of the oxygen-15 tracer have been incorporated into an equilibrium model used to measure oxygen consumption in the human brain using data from the sequential inhalation to equilibrium of ^{15}O oxygen and carbon dioxide (Hamilton et al., 1948; Stewart, 1921).

^{15}O-labeled carbon monoxide, administered by inhalation, binds to hemoglobin in blood cells, and therefore can be used as an intravascular tracer to measure regional cerebral blood volume (rCBV). Several strategies have been developed to measure rCBF using ^{15}O-labeled water as an inert, diffusible flow tracer. Regional cerebral oxygen metabolism is measured using scan data obtained following the inhalation of ^{15}O-labeled oxygen; independent determinations of local blood flow and blood volume are also required for this measurement.

What Can Be Measured with O^{15} Positron Emission Tomography Imaging?

The most common PET tracers used for the measurement of CBF are ^{15}O$_2$, ^{15}CO$_2$, and $H_2^{15}O$:

- $H_2^{15}O$ is administered by intravenous injection and a short-duration scan (1 to 2 minutes) is performed just after injection. To obtain absolute quantification, PET measurements are combined with arterial blood sampling to obtain an input function and allow the application of the Kety-Schmidt model to this dataset for quantitative CBF maps (Herscovitch et al., 1983; Raichle et al., 1983).
- ^{15}CO$_2$ is inhaled continuously for 8 to 10 minutes, the catalytic action of carbonic anhydrase in the pulmonary vascularization resulting in rapid transfer of the ^{15}O label to $H_2^{15}O$. A 1- to 2-minute scan is performed once a steady state is reached; the same approach as that described above is used to calculate a quantitative CBF map (Jones et al., 1976).
- Successive inhalation of ^{15}O$_2$, C$_{15}$O$_2$, and C$_{15}$O over 60 minutes allows measurement of the rCBV, the regional cerebral metabolic rate of oxygen (rCMRO$_2$), and the fraction of the oxygen delivered to brain (rOEF). About 40% is extracted by the brain parenchyma and metabolized (Frackowiak et al., 1980; Grubb et al., 1978; Ibaraki et al., 2004; Kety & Schmidt, 1948).

More recently, with the diffusion of whole-body oncological exploration with ^{18}fluorodeoxyglucose (^{18}FDG) PET, neurologists could have easy access to the measure of the regional glucose consumption in the brain and so have a reliable method to detect a regional metabolic deficit or hypermetabolism in the brain. Unfortunately, as ^{18}FDG is trapped in neurons, this radiopharmaceutical doesn't allowed repetition of measurement and can't be used in complex activation studies (Phelps et al., 1979; Reivich et al., 1979).

PET measurements of CBF are mainly performed using the bolus injection of $H_2^{15}O$ or by the continuous inhalation of ^{15}CO$_2$. In both methods, CBF can be quantified based on the Kety-Schmidt equation (Frackowiak et al., 1980).

PET results consist of maps describing CBF and CBV. CBV is calculated from the ratio of the radioactivity in the brain to that in peripheral whole blood. PET results may present rOEF and rCMRO$_2$ values.

Data processing to obtain these maps typically takes 5 to 10 minutes. PET results can be visually interpreted. Correlation with structural information (CT, MRI) is highly recommended for accurate interpretation (Nariai et al., 1997).

Quantification is, of course, one key point for research study and completes the visual interpretation. Quantification allows objectively assessing changes in the inactivation paradigm (e.g., between basal state and pain state) or follow-up studies. The main advantage of the PET technique lies in this quantitative accuracy, even in pixels containing large vessels and in brain regions with altered brain perfusion or metabolism. PET results are very reproducible in the current standardized settings (Fox et al., 1984; Frackowiak et al., 1980; Raichle, 1979).

Correlation Between Regional Cerebral Blood Flow and Synaptic Activity

The energy metabolism of the adult human brain depends mainly on glucose consumption. The functional coupling of regional cerebral blood flow and local cerebral glucose metabolism has been clearly demonstrated in many preclinical studies and in humans using double markers or autoradiographic methods. Glucose utilization reflects neuronal activity and mainly presynaptic activity. PET and especially $H_2^{15}O$ PET monitor changes of synaptic activity in a population of cells. These changes may be due to cell excitation or inhibition. More than 85% of cerebral glucose is used by neurons, mainly presynaptic axon terminals, while the remainder is preferentially used for metabolic processes in glial cells. Monitoring of regional cerebral blood flow with PET thus mainly reflects neuronal and more specifically presynaptic activity (Jueptner & Weiller, 1995). The balance between inhibition and activation is assumed. However, model studies suggest that, in neuroimaging, activation is predominant upon inhibition (Almeida & Stetter, 2002; Tagamets & Horwitz, 2001).

In summary, $H_2^{15}O$ PET measures rCBF variation. rCBF is thought to be highly correlated to synaptic activity (Jueptner & Weiller, 1995), but can also reflect primary vascular events. So, it is important to notice that in this context the term *hypoperfusion* (decrease of the PET signal) is not a synonym of *deactivation* and *hyperperfusion* (increase of the signal) is not a synonym of *activation*.

Limits of Positron Emission Tomography Imaging

Theoretically, quantitative PET with ^{15}O provides absolute values for rCBF, CBV, $CMRO_2$, and OEF (Herscovitch et al., 1983; Jones et al., 1976; Raichle et al., 1983). Quantitative oxygen metabolic images cannot be obtained by other imaging modalities such as MRI, and this is one of the major advantages of PET with ^{15}O. Unfortunately, those quantitative PET techniques need an arterial catheter, mostly a radial arterial puncture, quite invasive and nowadays not used anymore. Classically "absolute" quantification has

been replaced by "relative" quantification using a ratio between two brain areas and using an analysis of covariance model implemented through the general linear model formulation after normalization for global effect by proportional scaling. Statistical parametric mapping (SPM) is one of the most widely programs for such analysis (Friston 2003, Wellcome Department of Cognitive Neurology, University College London). This voxel-based analysis software requires the images to be in the same anatomical space. For this reason, the data need to first be realigned. After realignment, the images are subject to nonlinear warping so that they match a template that already conforms to a standard anatomical space. After smoothing, the general linear model is employed to estimate the parameters of the model and derive the appropriate univariate statistic test at every voxel. The test statistics constitute the SPM. The final stage is to make statistical inferences on the basis of the SPM and random field theory and to characterize the responses observed using the fitted responses or parameter estimates. Such software cannot be used routinely in clinical conditions and is mainly encountered in research laboratories. Furthermore, realignment, normalization, and smoothing could introduce bias in analysis and must be carefully used.

One other major criticism about the PET method is the relatively poor spatial resolution. For the current clinical systems, spatial resolution in the center-of-view field is around 3 mm. This disadvantage should be corrected in the next decade with efforts focused on scintillator-based detectors and various solid-state devices in PET detector designs for very high spatial resolution applications (Lewellen, 2008). A poor spatial resolution is particularly damaging in the study of subcortical structures, including the thalamus or brainstem.

To conclude, the main drawback of the PET methodology is its use of radioactive substances and the relatively poor spatial and time resolution compared to fMRI. But fMRI has other disadvantages: for the patient, lying in a noisy and confined space (quite uncomfortable during migraine attack) and the magnetic restraint limiting material for activation tasks.

O^{15} POSITRON EMISSION TOMOGRAPHY STUDIES IN MIGRAINE

PET studies in migraine are scarce and the majority comprise a small number of subjects (see Table 21–1). The challenge of imaging a paroxysmal disorder of relatively short duration on the one hand and the difficulties of access to the PET camera on the other hand explain this scarcity. Imaging spontaneous migraine attacks is particularly difficult because the attack onset is unpredictable and scheduling PET examinations is impossible. Despite these difficulties, some authors succeeded in the challenge of capturing spontaneous migraine attacks (Afridi, Giffin, et al., 2005; Denuelle et al., 2007; Weiller et al., 1995). Some others used glyceryl trinitrate to induce migraine attacks and to enable the study of a migraine attack from its earliest point (Afridi et al., 2004; Bahra et al., 2001). Thanks to the glyceryl trinitrate induction of migraine, one case of migraine aura has been imaged with PET (Afridi, Kaube, et al., 2005).

These few ^{15}O PET studies have nevertheless provided important information about the pathophysiology of migraine. As explained above, functional activation of brain regions is thought to be indicated by increases in the rCBF in PET. Early functional imaging using PET has demonstrated a consistent increase in rCBF in the rostral brainstem in spontaneous migraine attacks, which persisted even after sumatriptan had induced complete relief from headache, nausea, phonophobia, and photophobia (Weiller et al., 1995). This rCBF increase in the rostral brainstem was significant when compared with the interictal state. This finding was confirmed by other studies, reinforcing the role of brainstem nuclei in the migraine attack (Afridi, Giffin, et al., 2005; Afridi, Matharu, et al., 2005; Bahra et al., 2001; Denuelle et al., 2007). Activation of brainstem nuclei involved in antinociception, extra- and intracerebral vascular control, and sensory gating could explain many migraine facets. These results are presented and discussed in detail in the next chapter, Imaging Activation in the Migraine State. In this chapter we will focus on the meaning of the posterior CBF decrease found during migraine attack without aura and on the PET studies dealing with photophobia and osmophobia in migraineurs.

Posterior Regional Cerebral Blood Flow Decrease During Migraine Attack Without Aura

In the 1980s, cerebral blood flow studies introduced the concept of a hemodynamic pattern different in migraine with and without aura: migraine without aura characterized by a lack of global hemodynamic modifications and migraine with aura characterized by a spreading oligemia. This fact has been denied by PET studies showing a CBF decrease during migraine without aura attacks (Andersson et al., 1997; Bednarczyk et al., 1998; Denuelle et al., 2009; Woods et al., 1994). The first study by Woods et al. (1994) was due to serendipity: A patient with migraine without aura was fortuitously caught at the onset of a spontaneous attack while undergoing a series of blood flow measurements with H$_2$^{15}O PET for another purpose. A bilateral decrease in rCBF in the visual associative cortex was

observed within a few minutes after the beginning of a bilateral occipital throbbing headache with nausea and photophobia. The hypoperfusion spread forward across vascular and anatomic boundaries at a relatively constant rate. This hypoperfusion in migraine without aura was afterward confirmed by other PET studies specially designed to investigate migraine without aura attacks, spontaneous or provoked. A PET study in nine patients studied within 13 hours of the onset of a spontaneous migraine without aura attack showed a global hypoperfusion (Bednarczyk et al., 1998). This hypoperfusion persisted for at least 6 hours. No relationship was observed between the time from onset of headache and change in blood flow. No significant changes were observed in oxygen metabolism or oxygen extraction. Another PET study included attacks provoked by red wine in migraineurs (Andersson et al., 1997). In a total of 10 headaches studied, including both migraine with aura and migraine without aura, the authors observed a 23% decrease in the blood flow and a 22.5% decrease in metabolism in the primary visual cortex. No significant differences in rCBF were detected during either the aura or the headache phase. More recently, seven patients with migraine without aura were studied within 4 hours after spontaneous attack onset and after headache relief by sumatriptan (Denuelle et al., 2008). Compared with the attack-free interval, a posterior cortical hypoperfusion was found during the headache phase and persisted after headache relief by sumatriptan (see Fig. 21-1).

In the Weiller et al. and Afridi et al. studies, there was no hypoperfusion found during migraine without aura attacks. This discrepancy between PET study results may be explained by methodological differences and by the time between PET acquisition and migraine attack onset (Denuelle et al., 2009).

IS THIS RELATIVE POSTERIOR HYPOPERFUSION SPECIFIC TO MIGRAINE?

Posterior hypoperfusion has been described in response to various activation tasks such as acute experimental pain (Coghill et al., 1999; Maihofner et al., 2006; Petrovic et al., 1999; Peyron et al., 1998) but also nonpainful stimulation (Peyron et al., 1998), vestibular stimulation (Deutschlander et al., 2002; Wenzel et al., 1996), or semantic tasks (Warburton et al., 1996). The concept of a default mode of brain function was proposed to explain the appearance of activity decreases in functional neuroimaging data when the control state was passive visual fixation or eyes closed resting (Raichle & Snyder, 2007). The default mode hypothesis is based on the repeated observation that certain brain areas show task-induced deactivations across a wide variety of task conditions, especially

	n	Timing of Recordings	Main Findings
Woods et al. (1994)	1 MO	During spontaneous attack	Bilateral spreading cerebral hypoperfusion
Weiller et al. (1995)	9 MO	During spontaneous attack, after pain relief by sumatriptan, and interictally	During attack, increased rCBF in brainstem, cingulate, auditory and visual association cortices After pain relief, persistence of an isolated brainstem activation
Andersson et al. (1997)	4 MO, 6 MWA	During red wine–provoked attack, after pain relief by sumatriptan, and interictally	Significant reduction in rCBF and rCMRO$_2$ in visual cortex but no change in rOER during the headache
Bednarczyk et al. (1998)	9 MO	During spontaneous attack and interictally	Reduced CBF and CBV during the headache
Bahra et al. (2001)	1 MO	During glyceryl trinitrate–induced attack	Increased rCBF in the dorsal rostral brainstem
Matharu et al. (2004)	8 chronic migraine	Suboccipital stimulator switch on and partially activated	Increased rCBF in the dorsal pons, anterior cingulate cortex, and cuneus correlated to stimulation-induced paresthesia scores
Afridi, Matharu et al. (2005)	24 MO	Before, during, and after glyceryl trinitrate–induced attack	Lateralized dorsal pontine increased rCBF ipsilateral to headache side
Afridi, Giffin et al. 2005	3 MO, 2 MWA	During spontaneous attack and interictally	Increased rCBF in left dorsal pons, anterior and posterior cingulate, cerebellum, thalamus, insula, prefrontal cortex, and temporal lobes Decreased rCBF in right dorsal pons
Afridi, Kaube et al. (2005)	1 MWA	During glyceryl trinitrate–induced attack	Increased rCBF in the primary visual cortex during the aura
Denuelle et al. (2007, 2008)	7 MO	During spontaneous attack, after pain relief by sumatriptan, and interictally	Increased rCBF in brainstem and hypothalamus persisting after headache relief Significant bilateral posterior hypoperfusion persisting after headache relief
Demarquay et al. (2008)	10 MO, 1 MWA compared with 12 controls	Interictally with and without olfactory stimulation	With olfactory stimulation, higher activation in migraineurs than in controls in piriform and temporal cortex, and lower activation in frontal, temporoparietal, posterior cingulated cortex, and dorsal pons

(Continued)

TABLE 21–1 *Summary of ^{15}O Positron Emission Tomography Studies in Migraine (Continued)*

	n	Timing of Recordings	Main Findings
Boulloche et al. (2010)	4 MWA, 3 MO compared with 7 controls	Interictally, with and without luminous stimulation, and with and without painful stimulation	With luminous stimulation, visual cortex bilaterally in migraineurs but not in controls Concomitant pain stimulation allowed visual cortex activation in control subjects and potentiated its activation in migraineurs
Denuelle et al. (2011)	8 MO	During spontaneous attack with and without luminous stimulation	Increased rCBF in visual cortex during migraine attacks and after headache relief but not during the attack-free interval

Note. MO = migraine without aura; CBF = cerebral blood flow (rCBF if regional); MWA = migraine with aura; rCMRO$_2$= regional oxygen metabolism; rOER = regional oxygen extraction; CBV = cerebral blood volume.

cognitive tasks. Analyses based on PET have revealed a highly stereotypic pattern of brain regions that manifest greater activity during passive (resting) states as compared to a variety of active task states (Binder et al., 1999; Mazoyer et al., 2001; Shulman et al., 1997). More recent analyses of the temporal dynamics of fMRI-measured activity during rest have further revealed that networks of regions spontaneously increase and decrease together in a correlated manner (Greicius & Menon, 2004; Greicius et al., 2003; Laufs et al., 2003). To date, five resting-state networks have been identified including distinct sensory, motor, and cognitive brain systems (De Luca et al., 2006). One of those involves predominantly the occipital cortex (Brodmann areas 18 and 19). According to the default

mode hypothesis, the posterior hypoperfusion found during migraine attack would not be specific for migraine but related to a baseline shift in this area attributable to attentional and arousal mechanisms in the pain state. However, the persistence of posterior hypoperfusion in a resting condition after total pain relief by sumatriptan compared to another resting condition during the headache-free interval (Denuelle et al., 2008) is not congruent with this hypothesis. The presence of posterior hypoperfusion in both the pain condition and the resting condition cannot be explained by a baseline shift. The posterior hypoperfusion during migraine headache persisting after pain relief seems more likely to be in relation to the migraine attack itself.

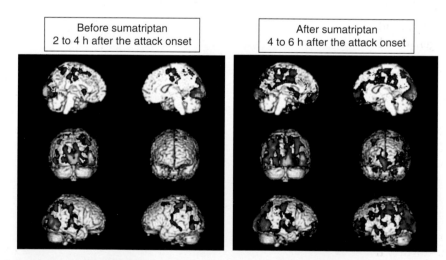

FIGURE 21–1 *Hypoperfusion during migraine without aura attacks in seven patients. Statistical parametric maps (SPMs) showing significant regional cerebral blood flow (rCBF) decreases during migraine without aura attacks. Blue plots correspond to rCBF decrease (p < .01 corrected FDR (False Discovery Rate), cluster >200 voxels) before and after sumatriptan compared with the attack-free interval. Posterior bilateral hypoperfusion can be seen. From Denuelle, M., Fabre, N., Payoux, P., Chollet, F., & Geraud, G. (2008). Posterior cerebral hypoperfusion in migraine without aura. Cephalalgia, 28, 856–862.*

IS HYPOPERFUSION A CONSEQUENCE OF A CORTICAL SPREADING DEPRESSION?

Posterior cortical hypoperfusion has been demonstrated repeatedly in migraine with aura (Andersen et al., 1988; Lauritzen & Olesen, 1984; Lauritzen et al., 1983; Olesen et al., 1981; Sakai & Meyer, 1978). In the early 1980s, Jes Olesen, using intracarotid Xenon blood flow in patients with migraine with aura, demonstrated that the attacks were initiated by focal hyperemia and that during aura, all patients displayed a posterior oligemia, which gradually spread anteriorly (Olesen et al., 1981). This finding refocused attention on the possible importance of cortical spreading depression (CSD) in migraine aura because of the congruence between cerebrovascular changes during migraine aura and CSD (Lauritzen, 1985). More than 60 years before, Aristides Leao coined the term *spreading depression*. Originally, Leao intended to study experimental epilepsy. He stimulated electrically cortical areas in rabbit. Unexpectedly, instead of seizurelike discharge, the stimulation was followed by a suppression of neuronal activity, which spread over the cortical surface. The recovery of neuronal activity occurred in the same sequence. Leao described CSD as a wave of cortical hyperexcitability followed by suppression, which migrated at a slow rate of 3 mm/min, associated with marked dilation of pial arteries, in some cases followed by a sustained smaller constriction (Leao, 1944). Based on the similarities between the symptomatology of migraine aura and the electrophysiological features of CSD, a causal relationship between the two was first hypothesized by Milner in 1958 (Milner, 1958). Arguably, the most striking evidence for the occurrence of CSD during migraine aura was obtained using high-field-strength fMRI (Hadjikhani et al., 2001). One patient with an exercise-induced aura showed a focal increase in blood oxygenation level–dependent (BOLD) signal (possibly reflecting vasodilation), developed within the visual cortex. Then the BOLD signal decreased (possibly reflecting vasoconstriction after the initial vasodilation). Two facts strongly suggest that the observed BOLD changes are CSD related: the same rate of progression (3.5 mm/min) as the CSD described by Leao, and the congruence of BOLD changes with the retinotopy of the visual percept, confirming the primary neural nature of the phenomenon. In migraine without aura, only the Woods case report of a nonexpected migraine attack shows the spreading character of the posterior hypoperfusion (Woods et al., 1994), and unfortunately the other studies were not designed to capture temporal rCBF modifications during migraine attack (Andersson et al., 1997; Denuelle et al., 2008).

Research in animals strongly suggests that CSD can activate nociceptive mechanisms directly consistent with the development of headache. First, up-regulation of c-Fos expression was detectable in brainstem trigeminal nucleus caudalis after a CSD (Kunkler & Kraig, 2003; Moskowitz et al., 1993). Moreover, CSD could induce a blood flow increase in the middle meningeal artery dependent upon trigeminal and parasympathetic activation (Bolay et al., 2002). Consistent with this fact, a recent study demonstrated that induction of CSD by focal stimulation of the rat visual cortex can lead to activation of meningeal nociceptors in the trigeminal ganglion (Zhang et al., 2010). These results suggest that if we can transpose these data in animals to migraine attacks in humans, a CSD supposedly being the primary event would be able to activate trigeminal nucleus caudalis and trigger headache.

If we consider CSD as the primary event in migraine attacks, in migraine with and without aura, we have to explain how a CSD can produce in one case the typical symptoms of visual aura and in another no visual symptoms. Besides, CSD must be predominantly asymptomatic, because the majority of migraine attacks are not preceded by aura, and even patients with migraine with aura commonly experience attacks without aura. Moreover, if the relationship between the aura symptoms and CSD seems to be clear, the temporal link between posterior hypoperfusion and CSD remains unclear. According to the Olesen et al. study, the oligemia starts before the onset of aura and extends into the headache phase, outlasting the aura symptoms (Olesen et al., 1990). This discrepancy between hemodynamics and symptoms of aura and headache has also been found in studies of visual triggered attacks using BOLD fMRI (Cao et al., 1999). In perfusion-weighted imaging during spontaneous migraine with aura, the rCBV decrease persisted up to 2.5 hours into the headache phase (Sanchez del Rio et al., 1999). In the Bednarczyk et al. (1998) PET study, global hypoperfusion was found within a mean time of 13.3 hours from the onset of headache. In the Denuelle et al. (2008) PET study, the posterior hypoperfusion persisted 6 hours after the attack onset. It is difficult to explain how CSD characterized by a sustained suppression of neuronal activity concerning such an extended cortical area, with such duration, would not induce more significant neurological deficits. The absence of symptoms of migraine aura is hard to reconcile with the extreme perturbations in cellular function that occur in large areas of the cortex with CSD.

Some authors propose that astrocytic calcium waves could be an alternative mechanism to explain the spreading hypoperfusion in migraine with and without aura. Recent studies indicate that astrocytes may be actively involved in the initiation and propagation of CSD, as well as the accompanying vascular response (Charles &

Brennan, 2009). Indeed, astrocytes play, in the neurovascular unit, a key role in coupling neuronal activity and vascular tone. Intercellular calcium waves occur in conjunction with CSD in multiple in vitro and in vivo models, but CSD and astrocyte calcium waves can also occur independently (Basarsky et al., 1998; Chuquet et al., 2007; Guthrie et al., 1999; Peters et al., 2003). Even if astrocyte calcium waves have temporal and spatial characteristics that are remarkably similar to those of CSD, they have been observed to travel faster and farther than concomitant CSD, and to modulate the propagation characteristics of CSD (Guthrie et al., 1999). Thus, astrocyte calcium waves and CSD appear to be two distinct but interrelated phenomena. More than five decades of experiments in animals have shown that vascular responses to CSD are complex and variable (Busija et al., 2008). Moreover the vasculature does not respond only passively to CSD, but might play an active role in CSD propagation. Leao in 1945 was the first to observe that vascular changes may precede a CSD (Leao & Morison, 1945). More recently, it has been found that vasodilation of cortical surface arterioles could travel ahead of the CSD wavefront with characteristics that are consistent with an intrinsic vascular mechanism of propagation, and that vasodilation could be propagated into areas beyond the spread of electrophysiological changes of the CSD wave (Brennan et al., 2007).

Therefore, astrocyte calcium waves and intrinsic vascular tone modifications spreading beyond a spatially limited CSD event or, even more, in the absence of CSD could explain hypoperfusion in a migraine without aura attack in the absence of the significant neurological symptoms that might be expected with CSD.

IS HYPOPERFUSION A PRIMARY NEUROVASCULAR EVENT FROM BRAINSTEM?

A breakthrough in migraine research has been the activation of brainstem nuclei shown in functional imaging during migraine attacks (Afridi, Kaube, et al., 2005; Afridi, Giffin, et al., 2005; Bahra et al., 2001; Denuelle et al., 2007; Weiller et al., 1995). Even if it is difficult to locate them precisely, these activations involve the dorsal midbrain and the dorsolateral pons areas that could correspond to the dorsal raphe nucleus, periaqueductal gray, locus coeruleus, and, as was most recently suggested, hypothalamic activation (Denuelle et al., 2007). The persistence of these activations after headache relief following treatment with sumatriptan has fueled a very animated controversy about a possible role of generators of migraine attacks. These nuclei play a complex role in the control of intra- and extracerebral vasculature. A primary activation of these nuclei could produce a vasoconstriction of intracerebral vasculature and then could explain the posterior hypoperfusion found by functional imaging during migraine attack.

Experimental works in animals have shown that stimulation of brainstem nuclei provoked vascular changes that can be transposed to migraine (Lance et al., 1983). Electrical stimulation of the locus ceruleus in monkeys at physiological frequencies reduces blood flow in the ipsilateral internal carotid artery by some 20% (Goadsby et al., 1982). Moreover, additional studies in cats have shown that the diminution in rCBF produced by such a stimulation is maximal in the occipital cortex (Goadsby & Duckworth, 1989), the area of the brain affected by hypoperfusion during migraine attack. A primary dysfunction of cerebrovascular control in relation to an abnormal discharge in the locus ceruleus and raphe nuclei could explain the occurrence of a posterior hypoperfusion during migraine attack. However, the action of brainstem nuclei cannot be reduced to a simple control of vascular tone. Their actions on the neurovascular unit are complex and only partly elucidated. Low-frequency discharge along the projection from the locus ceruleus could inhibit neuronal activity in the cortex directly and constrict microcirculation in the cat (Adams et al., 1989; Katayama et al., 1981). This cascade of events could eventually initiate a CSD or a similar phenomenon during migraine attack.

Some arguments from neuroimaging studies in migraineurs are in favor of a primary brainstem dysfunction responsible for posterior hypoperfusion. In the Cao et al. study, the brainstem activation appeared before the neuronal suppression in the occipital cortex or the onset of visually triggered symptoms (Cao et al., 2002). The persistence of both brainstem activation and posterior hypoperfusion after sumatriptan injection suggests that the hypoperfusion could be in relationship with the brainstem activation and then would persist as long as the brainstem activation does, independently of the migraine symptoms relieved by the action of the triptan on the peripheral trigeminovascular system (Denuelle et al., 2007, 2008).

If brainstem and hypothalamic activation is involved at the onset of a migraine attack, it could explain why in some patients their attack can be predicted by premonitory symptoms as yawning, fatigue, and polyuria, which occur up to several hours before the onset of headache (Giffin et al., 2003; Kelman, 2004). Indeed, in these patients, the brainstem and hypothalamus may be activated well before the onset of the cortical waves that occur with migraine with aura. Selecting migraineurs with clear premonitory symptoms and imaging the migraine attack at this premonitory phase could be the only way of establishing the chronological link between brainstem activation and occurrence of a posterior cortical hypoperfusion.

CONCLUSION

The identification of hypoperfusion in migraine with and without aura suggests that CSD could be a common physiological process that occurs at the onset of both migraine subtypes. But the most plausible explanation is that altered activity of brainstem nuclei that project diffusely to the cortex results in changes in glial activity, cortical neuronal activity, and cerebral blood flow in all patients with migraine, but that CSD, producing aura symptoms, would be triggered only in genetically predisposed migraineurs and depending on metabolic or hormonal factors at a given time, explaining why the same patient could present with migraine attacks with or without aura.

Photophobia and Osmophobia Studied with Positron Emission Tomography

Migraine is a complex brain disorder involving not only head pain but also modifications in perception of light, sound, and odor during and outside attacks. Photophobia and phonophobia are included as criteria for migraine diagnosis in the International Headache Society classification. Osmophobia seems also to be specific to migraine (Kelman, 2004, 2005; Vingen et al., 1999; Zanchin et al., 2005). The sensory sensitivity developed by migraineurs persists at a lower level between attacks (Main et al., 1997; Mulleners et al., 2001; Vanagaite et al., 1997; Woodhouse & Drummond, 1993). The mechanism of this sensory dysmodulation of migraineurs during but also, at a lower degree, between attacks remains unknown. Only a few PET studies have been designed to investigate the hypothesis of a sensory hypersensitivity in migraineurs explaining photophobia and osmophobia.

OSMOPHOBIA

Osmophobia is an increased sensitivity to odors, which, during attacks, provokes an increase in discomfort (increase in headache and also in many patients increase in nausea and vomiting). A PET study has investigated migraineurs with interictal olfactory hypersensitivity in the hypothesis of different functional olfactory neural networks when compared to controls (Demarquay et al., 2008). Eleven migraineurs with olfactory hypersensitivity and 12 controls were studied by PET during olfactory stimulation and during exposure to only odorless air. Significant differences were found in cerebral activation patterns as well as in baseline rCBF between migraineurs and controls in both olfactory and nonolfactory brain regions. Higher rCBFs were observed in migraineurs compared to controls in the piriform cortex (which is a part of the primary olfactory cortex) during both olfactory and nonolfactory conditions. The authors suggest that hyperactivity of the piriform cortex could result in

facilitated triggering of the trigeminovascular system in response to odors during the interictal or preictal period. During olfactory stimulation, the neural network activated in migraineurs is different than in controls. This is consistent with the hypothesis of a hyperactive olfactory system in migraineurs with olfactory hypersensitivity.

PHOTOPHOBIA

The prevalence of photophobia is about 85% of patients during attacks (Aygul et al., 2005; Morillo et al., 2005). Some subjects even report bright lights as a trigger for their attacks, and others report photophobia as a signal symptom that announces their attacks (Giffin et al., 2003). In the International Classification of Headache Disorders (second edition), photophobia is defined as a hypersensitivity to light, usually causing avoidance (Headache Classification Subcommittee of the International Headache Society, 2004). But in clinical practice, and consistent with the definition by Lebensohn (1934), we can divide photophobia into two different symptoms in migraineurs: an increase of the headache when the patient is exposed to light during the migraine attack and an uncomfortable sense of glare reported between attacks.

Two PET studies deal with photophobia. The aim of the first $H_2{}^{15}O$ PET study was to explore the interaction between the visual cortex and trigeminal nociception (Boulloche et al., 2010). Seven migraineurs between attacks and seven matched controls were studied with three luminous intensities (obscurity, 600 Cd/m², and 1,800 Cd/m²) and with or without pain in the trigeminal territory. To facilitate habituation, the luminous stimulation was continuous, started 30 seconds before the beginning of each PET scan acquisition, and was performed through a white half-opaque mask covering the whole visual field to avoid any stimuli such as movement, shape, color, or contrast. When no concomitant pain stimulation was applied, luminous stimulations activated bilaterally the visual cortex in migraineurs (cuneus, lingual gyrus, posterior cingulate cortex), but not in controls. The absence of visual cortical activation was expected because of the stimuli characteristics that facilitate habituation. Concomitant pain stimulation allowed visual cortex activation in control subjects and potentiated its activation in migraineurs (see Fig. 21–2). These activations by luminous stimulations were luminance intensity dependent in both groups. Moreover, whatever the condition, the volume of the activations was larger in migraineurs than in control subjects. According to these results, migraineurs' visual cortex is hyperresponsive (or hyperexcitable) to light compared to controls, and there is an interaction between trigeminal pain and light in migraineurs and also in controls.

CONTROLS   MIGRAINEURS

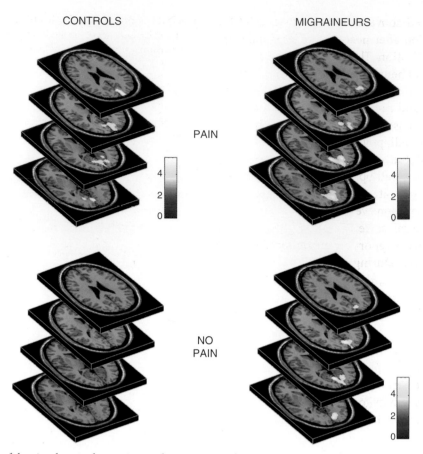

PAIN

NO
PAIN

FIGURE 21–2 *Activations of the visual cortex by continuous luminous stimulation in migraineurs during attack-free interval and in controls, with or without concomitant trigeminal pain. Axial cross-sections at z = 0, z = 8, z = 16, and z = 24. Activations by light at 1,800 Cd/m² were in the cuneus, lingual gyrus, posterior cingulate cortex, and precuneus. Note that the activation of the visual cortex is potentiated by pain and that the volume of activation is greater in migraineurs. From Boulloche, N., Denuelle, M., Payoux, P., Fabre, N., Trotter, Y., & Geraud. Photophobia in migraine: An interictal PET study of cortical hyperexcitability and its modulation by pain.* Journal of Neurology, Neurosurgery, and Psychiatry, 81, 978–984.

Interaction between visual and trigeminal pathways seems to play a key role in photophobia pathophysiology. Clinically, migraine headache increases photophobia, and light exposure can worsen acute migraine headache. Clinical studies have shown that pain stimulation in the V1 territory decreased tolerance to light (Drummond, 1997; Kowacs et al., 2001), while light stimulation lowered the trigeminal nociceptive threshold (Drummond & Woodhouse, 1993). The posterior thalamus could be an anatomical substrate for this interaction between visual cortex and trigeminal neurons (Maleki et al., 2011; Noseda et al., 2010). In a second H$_2$¹⁵O PET study, painful photophobia, defined as headache enhancement induced by continuous luminous stimulation covering the whole visual field (stimulation identical to the first PET study), was explored during spontaneous migraine attacks (Denuelle et al., 2011). Eight migraineurs were studied during migraine attacks, after headache relief by sumatriptan, and during the attack-free interval. Luminous stimulation with low intensity activated the visual cortex during migraine attacks and after headache relief but not during the attack-free interval. The visual cortex activation was statistically higher during migraine headache than after pain relief. Thus, migraine attacks seem to increase visual cortex excitability or responsiveness when compared to attack-free intervals. Moreover, independently of pain, the visual cortex remains hyperresponsive (or hyperexcitable) to light after headache relief by sumatriptan compared with the attack-free interval. The absence of cortical activation to light in migraineurs during the attack-free interval could be explained by the characteristics of the stimuli, which facilitate habituation, and by the low luminous intensity probably below the activation threshold, contrary to the first PET study using high luminous intensity in which the visual cortex of migraineurs was activated interictally. The visual cortex activation during migraine headache could be explained by the interaction between visual and trigeminal nerve pathways, as described above. But the persistence of the visual cortex activation after headache relief is independent of trigeminal activation. This hyperresponsiveness or hyperexcitability could be under brainstem nuclei modulation as brainstem activation persists after headache relief (Weiller et al., 1995) and can directly modulate neuronal excitability of the sensory cortex via the thalamus (Devilbiss et al., 2006; Filippov et al., 2004, 2008).

According to PET study results, a hypothesis could be proposed to explain the pathophysiology of photophobia in migraine. Between attacks, the visual cortex of migraineurs is hyperresponsive to light compared with controls, and this visual cortex hyperexcitability could explain why migraineurs report an uncomfortable sense of glare between attacks. During the ictal period (including the premonitory phase, the migraine headache, and after pain relief), the visual cortex excitability could possibly be enhanced by brainstem activation, explaining photophobia in migraineurs during the pre- and postictal phases (Giffin et al., 2003). And then the activation of the trigeminovascular system potentiates the visual cortex excitability via the posterior thalamus and could explain why headache and sensitivity to light increase in a vicious circle during migraine attack.

REFERENCES

Adams, R. W., Lambert, G. A., & Lance, J. W. (1989). Stimulation of brainstem nuclei in the cat: Effect on neuronal activity in the primary visual cortex of relevance to cerebral blood flow and migraine. *Cephalalgia, 9*, 107–118.

Afridi, S., Kaube, H., & Goadsby, P. J. (2005). Occipital activation in glyceryl trinitrate induced migraine with visual aura. *Journal of Neurology, Neurosurgery, and Psychiatry, 76*, 1158–1160.

Afridi, S. K., Giffin, N. J., Kaube, H., Friston, K. J., Ward, N. S., Frackowiak, R. S., et al. (2005). A positron emission tomographic study in spontaneous migraine. *Archives of Neurology, 62*, 1270–1275.

Afridi, S. K., Kaube, H., & Goadsby, P. J. (2004). Glyceryl trinitrate triggers premonitory symptoms in migraineurs. *Pain, 110*, 675–680.

Afridi, S. K., Matharu, M. S., Lee, L., Kaube, H., Friston, K. J., Frackowiak, R. S., et al. (2005). A PET study exploring the laterality of brainstem activation in migraine using glyceryl trinitrate. *Brain, 128*, 932–939.

Almeida, R., & Stetter, M. (2002). Modeling the link between functional imaging and neuronal activity: Synaptic metabolic demand and spike rates. *Neuroimage, 17*, 1065–1079.

Andersen, A. R., Friberg, L., Olsen, T. S., & Olesen, J. (1988). Delayed hyperemia following hypoperfusion in classic migraine. Single photon emission computed tomographic demonstration. *Archives of Neurology, 45*, 154–159.

Andersson, J. L., Muhr, C., Lilja, A., Valind, S., Lundberg, P. O., & Langstrom, B. (1997). Regional cerebral blood flow and oxygen metabolism during migraine with and without aura. *Cephalalgia, 17*, 570–579.

Aygul, R., Deniz, O., Kocak, N., Orhan, A., & Ulvi, H. (2005). The clinical properties of a migrainous population in eastern Turkey-Erzurum. *Southern Medical Journal, 98*, 23–27.

Bahra, A., Matharu, M. S., Buchel, C., Frackowiak, R. S., & Goadsby, P. J. (2001). Brainstem activation specific to migraine headache. *Lancet, 357*, 1016–1017.

Basarsky, T. A., Duffy, S. N., Andrew, R. D., & MacVicar, B. A. (1998). Imaging spreading depression and associated intracellular calcium waves in brain slices. *Journal of Neuroscience, 18*, 7189–7199.

Bednarczyk, E. M., Remler, B., Weikart, C., Nelson, A. D., & Reed, R. C. (1998). Global cerebral blood flow, blood volume, and oxygen metabolism in patients with migraine headache. *Neurology, 50*, 1736–1740.

Binder, J. R., Frost, J. A., Hammeke, T. A., Bellgowan, P. S., Rao, S. M., & Cox, R. W. (1999). Conceptual processing during the conscious resting state. A functional MRI study. *Journal of Cognitive Neuroscience, 11*, 80–95.

Bolay, H., Reuter, U., Dunn, A. K., Huang, Z., Boas, D. A., & Moskowitz, M. A. (2002). Intrinsic brain activity triggers trigeminal meningeal afferents in a migraine model. *Nature Medicine, 8*, 136–142.

Boulloche, N., Denuelle, M., Payoux, P., Fabre, N., Trotter, Y., & Geraud, G. (2010). Photophobia in migraine: An interictal PET study of cortical hyperexcitability and its modulation by pain. *Journal of Neurology, Neurosurgery, and Psychiatry, 81*, 978–984.

Brennan, K. C., Beltran-Parrazal, L., Lopez-Valdes, H. E., Theriot, J., Toga, A. W., & Charles, A. C. (2007). Distinct vascular conduction with cortical spreading depression. *Journal of Neurophysiology, 97*, 4143–4151.

Busija, D. W., Bari, F., Domoki, F., Horiguchi, T., & Shimizu, K. (2008). Mechanisms involved in the cerebrovascular dilator effects of cortical spreading depression. *Progress in Neurobiology, 86*, 379–395.

Cao, Y., Aurora, S. K., Nagesh, V., Patel, S. C., & Welch, K. M. (2002). Functional MRI-BOLD of brainstem structures during visually triggered migraine. *Neurology, 59*, 72–78.

Cao, Y., Welch, K. M., Aurora, S., & Vikingstad, E. M. (1999). Functional MRI-BOLD of visually triggered headache in patients with migraine. *Archives of Neurology, 56*, 548–554.

Charles, A., & Brennan, K. (2009). Cortical spreading depression-new insights and persistent questions. *Cephalalgia, 29*, 1115–1124.

Chuquet, J., Hollender, L., & Nimchinsky, E. A. (2007). High-resolution in vivo imaging of the neurovascular unit during spreading depression. *Journal of Neuroscience, 27*, 4036–4044.

Coghill, R. C., Sang, C. N., Maisog, J. M., & Iadarola, M. J. (1999) Pain intensity processing within the human brain: a bilateral, distributed mechanism. *Journal of Neurophysiology, 82*, 1934–1943.

De Luca, M., Beckmann, C. F., De Stefano, N., Matthews, P. M., & Smith, S. M. (2006). fMRI resting state networks define distinct modes of long-distance interactions in the human brain. *Neuroimage, 29*, 1359–1367.

Demarquay, G., Royet, J. P., Mick, G., & Ryvlin, P. (2008). Olfactory hypersensitivity in migraineurs: A H(2)(15)O-PET study. *Cephalalgia, 28*, 1069–1080.

Denuelle, M., Boulloche, N., Payoux, P., Fabre, N., Trotter, Y., & Geraud, G. (2011). A PET study of photophobia during spontaneous migraine attacks. *Neurology, 76*, 213–218.

Denuelle, M., Fabre, N., & Geraud, G. (2009). Posterior hypoperfusion in migraine without aura? *Cephalalgia, (Epub ahead of print)* doi:10.1111/j.1468-2982.2009.01949.x.

Denuelle, M., Fabre, N., Payoux, P., Chollet, F., & Geraud, G. (2007). Hypothalamic activation in spontaneous migraine attacks. *Headache, 47,* 1418–1426.

Denuelle, M., Fabre, N., Payoux, P., Chollet, F., & Geraud, G. (2008). Posterior cerebral hypoperfusion in migraine without aura. *Cephalalgia, 28,* 856–862.

Devilbiss, D. M., Page, M. E., & Waterhouse, B. D. (2006). Locus ceruleus regulates sensory encoding by neurons and networks in waking animals. *Journal of Neuroscience, 26,* 9860–9872.

Drummond, P. D. (1997). Photophobia and autonomic responses to facial pain in migraine. *Brain, 120*(Pt 10), 1857–1864.

Drummond, P. D., & Woodhouse, A. (1993). Painful stimulation of the forehead increases photophobia in migraine sufferers. *Cephalalgia, 13,* 321–324.

Filippov, I. V., Williams, W. C., & Frolov, V. A. (2004). Very slow potential oscillations in locus coeruleus and dorsal raphe nucleus under different illumination in freely moving rats. *Neuroscience Letters, 363,* 89–93.

Filippov, I. V., Williams, W. C., Krebs, A. A., & Pugachev, K. S. (2008). Dynamics of infraslow potentials in the primary auditory cortex: Component analysis and contribution of specific thalamic-cortical and non-specific brainstem-cortical influences. *Brain Research, 1219,* 66–77.

Fox, P. T., Mintun, M. A., Raichle, M. E., & Herscovitch, P. (1984). A noninvasive approach to quantitative functional brain mapping with H2 (15)O and positron emission tomography. *Journal of Cerebral Blood Flow and Metabolism, 4,* 329–333.

Frackowiak, R. S., Lenzi, G. L., Jones, T., & Heather, J. D. (1980). Quantitative measurement of regional cerebral blood flow and oxygen metabolism in man using 15O and positron emission tomography: Theory, procedure, and normal values. *Journal of Computer-Assisted Tomography, 4,* 727–736.

Giffin, N. J., Ruggiero, L., Lipton, R. B., Silberstein, S. D., Tvedskov, J. F., Olesen, J., et al. (2003). Premonitory symptoms in migraine: An electronic diary study. *Neurology, 60,* 935–940.

Goadsby, P. J., & Duckworth, J. W. (1989). Low frequency stimulation of the locus coeruleus reduces regional cerebral blood flow in the spinalized cat. *Brain Research, 476,* 71–77.

Goadsby, P. J., Lambert, G. A., & Lance, J. W. (1982). Differential effects on the internal and external carotid circulation of the monkey evoked by locus coeruleus stimulation. *Brain Research, 249,* 247–254.

Greicius, M. D., Krasnow, B., Reiss, A. L., & Menon, V. (2003). Functional connectivity in the resting brain: a network analysis of the default mode hypothesis. *Proceedings of the National Academy of Sciences of the United States of America, 100,* 253–258.

Greicius, M. D., & Menon, V. (2004). Default-mode activity during a passive sensory task: uncoupled from deactivation but impacting activation. *Journal of Cognitive Neuroscience, 16,* 1484–1492.

Grubb, R. L., Jr., Raichle, M. E., Higgins, C. S., & Eichling, J. O. (1978). Measurement of regional cerebral blood volume by emission tomography. *Annals of Neurology, 4,* 322–328.

Guthrie, P. B., Knappenberger, J., Segal, M., Bennett, M. V., Charles, A. C., & Kater, S. B. (1999). ATP released from astrocytes mediates glial calcium waves. *Journal of Neuroscience, 19,* 520–528.

Hadjikhani, N., Sanchez Del Rio, M., Wu, O., Schwartz, D., Bakker, D., Fischl, B., et al. (2001). Mechanisms of migraine aura revealed by functional MRI in human visual cortex. *Proceedings of the National Academy of Sciences of the United States of America, 98,* 4687–4692.

Hamilton, W. F., Riley, R. L., ., Attyah A M, Botvinick E, Sievers R, Higgins CB, et al. (1948). Comparison of the Fick and dye injection methods of measuring the cardiac output in man. *Am J Physiol, 153:* 309..

Headache Classification Subcommittee of the International Headache Society. (2004). The international classification of headache disorders: 2nd edition. *Cephalalgia, 24*(Suppl 1), 9–160.

Herscovitch, P., Markham, J., & Raichle, M. E. (1983). Brain blood flow measured with intravenous H2(15)O. I. Theory and error analysis. *Journal of Nuclear Medicine, 24,* 782–789.

Ibaraki, M., Shimosegawa, E., Miura, S., Takahashi, K., Ito, H., Kanno, I., et al. (2004). PET measurements of CBF, OEF, and CMRO2 without arterial sampling in hyperacute ischemic stroke: Method and error analysis. *Annals of Nuclear Medicine, 18,* 35–44.

Jones, T., Chesler, D. A., & Ter-Pogossian, M. M. (1976). The continuous inhalation of oxygen-15 for assessing regional oxygen extraction in the brain of man. *British Journal of Radiology, 49,* 339–343.

Jueptner, M., & Weiller, C. (1995). Review: Does measurement of regional cerebral blood flow reflect synaptic activity? Implications for PET and fMRI. *Neuroimage, 2,* 148–156.

Katayama, Y., Ueno, Y., Tsukiyama, T., & Tsubokawa, T. (1981). Long lasting suppression of firing of cortical neurons and decrease in cortical blood flow following train pulse stimulation of the locus coeruleus in the cat. *Brain Research, 216,* 173–179.

Kelman, L. (2004). The premonitory symptoms (prodrome): A tertiary care study of 893 migraineurs. *Headache, 44,* 865–872.

Kety, S. S., & Schmidt, C. F. (1948). The nitrous oxide method for the quantitative determination of cerebral blood flow in man: Theory, procedure and normal values. *Journal of Clinical Investigation, 27,* 476–483.

Kowacs, P. A., Piovesan, E. J., Werneck, L. C., Tatsui, C. E., Lange, M. C., Ribas, L. C., et al. (2001). Influence of intense light stimulation on trigeminal and cervical pain perception thresholds. *Cephalalgia, 21,* 184–188.

Kunkler, P. E., & Kraig, R. P. (2003). Hippocampal spreading depression bilaterally activates the caudal trigeminal nucleus in rodents. *Hippocampus, 13,* 835–844.

Lance, J. W., Lambert, G. A., Goadsby, P. J., & Duckworth, J. W. (1983). Brainstem influences on the cephalic circulation: Experimental data from cat and monkey of relevance to the mechanism of migraine. *Headache, 23,* 258–265.

Laufs, H., Krakow, K., Sterzer, P., Eger, E., Beyerle, A., Salek-Haddadi, A., & Kleinschmidt, A. (2003). Electroencephalographic signatures of attentional and cognitive default modes in spontaneous brain activity fluctuations at rest. *Proceedings of the National Academy of Sciences of the United States of America, 100:* 11053–11058.

Lauritzen, M., Skyhoj Olsen, T., Lassen, N. A., & Paulson, O. B. (1983). Changes in regional cerebral blood flow during the course of classic migraine attacks. *Annals of Neurology; 13:* 633–641.

Lauritzen, M., & Olesen, J. (1984). Regional cerebral blood flow during migraine attacks by Xenon-133 inhalation and emission tomography. *Brain, 107* (Pt 2), 447–461.

Lauritzen, M. (1985). On the possible relation of spreading cortical depression to classical migraine. *Cephalalgia, 5*(Suppl 2): 47–51.

Leao, A. A. (1944). Spreading depression of activity in the cerebral cortex. *Journal of Neurophysiology, 7,* 359–390.

Leao, A. A. P., & Morison, R. S. (1945). Propagation of spreading cortical depression. *Journal of Neurophysiology, 8,* 33–45.

Lebensohn, J. E. (1934). The nature of photophobia. *Archives of Ophthalmology, 12,* 380–390.

Lewellen, T. K. (2008). Recent developments in PET detector technology. *Physics in Medicine and Biology, 53,* R287–R317.

Maihofner, C., Handwerker, H. O., & Birklein, F. (2006). Functional imaging of allodynia in complex regional pain syndrome. *Neurology, 66,* 711–717.

Main, A., Dowson, A., & Gross, M. (1997). Photophobia and phonophobia in migraineurs between attacks. *Headache, 37,* 492–495

Maleki, N., Becerra, L., Upadhyay, J., Burstein, R., & Borsook, D. (2012). Direct optic nerve pulvinar connections defined by diffusion MR tractography in humans: Implications for photophobia. *Human Brain Mapping, 33*(1), 75–88.

Matharu, M. S., Bartsch, T., Ward, N., Frackowiak, R. S., & Weiner, R., & Goadsby, P. J. (2004). Central neuromodulation in chronic migraine patients with suboccipital stimulators: a PET study. *Brain, 127,* 220–230.

Mazoyer, B., Zago, L., Mellet, E., Bricogne, S., Etard, O., Houde, O., et al. (2001) Cortical networks for working memory and executive functions sustain the conscious resting state in man. *Brain Research Bulletin, 54,* 287–298.

Milner, P. M. (1958). Note on a possible correspondence between the scotomas of migraine and spreading depression of Leao. *Electroencephalography and Clinical Neurophysiology* Supplement, *10,* 705.

Morillo, L. E., Alarcon, F., Aranaga, N., Aulet, S., Chapman, E., Conterno, L., et al. (2005). Clinical characteristics and patterns of medication use of migraineurs in Latin America from 12 cities in 6 countries. *Headache, 45,* 118–126.

Moskowitz, M. A., Nozaki, K., Kraig, R. P. (1993). Neocortical spreading depression provokes the expression of c-fos protein-like immunoreactivity within trigeminal nucleus caudalis via trigeminovascular mechanisms. *Journal of Neuroscience, 13,* 1167–1177.

Mulleners, W. M., Aurora, S. K., Chronicle, E. P., Stewart, R., Gopal, S., & Koehler, P. J. (2001). Self-reported photophobic symptoms in migraineurs and controls are reliable and predict diagnostic category accurately. *Headache, 41,* 31–39.

Nariai, T., Senda, M., Ishii, K., Maehara, T., Wakabayashi, S., Toyama, H., et al. (1997). Three-dimensional imaging of cortical structure, function and glioma for tumor resection. *Journal of Nuclear Medicine, 38,* 1563–1568.

Noseda, R., Kainz, V., Jakubowski, M., Gooley, J. J., Saper, C. B., Digre, K., et al. (2010). A neural mechanism for exacerbation of headache by light. *Nature Neuroscience, 13,* 239–245.

Olesen, J., Friberg, L., Olsen, T. S., Iversen, H. K., Lassen, N. A., Andersen, A. R., et al. (1990). Timing and topography of cerebral blood flow, aura, and headache during migraine attacks. *Annals of Neurology, 28,* 791–798.

Olesen, J., Larsen, B., & Lauritzen, M. (1981). Focal hyperemia followed by spreading oligemia and impaired activation of rCBF in classic migraine. *Annals of Neurology, 9,* 344–352.

Peters, O., Schipke, C. G., Hashimoto, Y., & Kettenmann, H. (2003). Different mechanisms promote astrocyte Ca2+ waves and spreading depression in the mouse neocortex. *Journal of Neuroscience, 23,* 9888–9896.

Petrovic, P., Ingvar, M., Stone-Elander, S., Petersson, K. M., & Hansson, P. (1999). A PET activation study of dynamic mechanical allodynia in patients with mononeuropathy. *Pain, 83,* 459–470.

Peyron, R., Garcia-Larrea, L., Gregoire, M. C., Convers, P., Lavenne, F., Veyre, L., et al. (1998). Allodynia after lateral-medullary (Wallenberg) infarct. A PET study. *Brain, 121*(Pt 2), 345–356.

Phelps, M. E., Huang, S. C., Hoffman, E. J., Selin, C., Sokoloff, L., & Kuhl, D. E. (1979). Tomographic measurement of local cerebral glucose metabolic rate in humans with (F-18)2-fluoro-2-deoxy-D-glucose: Validation of method. *Annals of Neurology, 6,* 371–388.

Raichle, M. E. (1979). Quantitative in vivo autoradiography with positron emission tomography. *Brain Research, 180,* 47–68.

Raichle, M. E., Martin, W. R., Herscovitch, P., Mintun, M. A., & Markham, J. (1983). Brain blood flow measured with intravenous H2(15)O. II. Implementation and validation. *Journal of Nuclear Medicine, 24,* 790–798.

Raichle, M. E., & Snyder, A. Z. (2007). A default mode of brain function: A brief history of an evolving idea. *Neuroimage, 37,* 1083–1090; discussion 1097–1099.

Reivich, M., Kuhl, D., Wolf, A., Greenberg, J., Phelps, M., Ido, T., et al. (1979). The [18F]fluorodeoxyglucose method for the measurement of local cerebral glucose utilization in man. *Circulation Research, 44,* 127–137.

Sakai, F., & Meyer, J. S. (1978). Regional cerebral hemodynamics during migraine and cluster headaches measured by the 133Xe inhalation method. *Headache, 18,* 122–132.

Sanchez del Rio, M., Bakker, D., Wu, O., Agosti, R., Mitsikostas, D. D., Ostergaard, L., et al. (1999). Perfusion weighted imaging during migraine: Spontaneous visual aura and headache. *Cephalalgia, 19,* 701–707.

Shulman, G. L., Corbetta, M., Fiez, J. A., Buckner, R. L., Miezin, F. M., Raichle, M. E., & Petersen, S. E. (1997) Searching for activations that generalize over tasks. *Human Brain Mapping, 5,* 317–322.

Stewart, G. N. (1921). Researches on the circulation time and on the influences which affect it. V. The circulation time of the spleen, kidney, intestine, heart (coronary circulation) and retina, with some further observations on the time of the lesser circulation. *American Journal of Physiology, 58,* 278 –295.

Tagamets, M. A., & Horwitz, B. (2001). Interpreting PET and fMRI measures of functional neural activity: The effects of synaptic inhibition on cortical activation in human imaging studies. *Brain Research Bulletin, 54,* 267–273.

Vanagaite, J., Pareja, J. A., Storen, O., White, L. R., & Sand, T., & Stovner, L. J. (1997). Light-induced discomfort and pain in migraine. *Cephalalgia, 17,* 733–741.

Vingen, J. V., Sand, T., & Stovner, L. J. (1999). Sensitivity to various stimuli in primary headaches: a questionnaire study. *Headache, 39,* 552–558.

Warburton, E., Wise, R. J., Price, C. J., Weiller, C., Hadar, U., Ramsay, S., et al. (1996). Noun and verb retrieval by normal subjects. Studies with PET. *Brain, 119*(Pt 1), 159–179.

Weiller, C., May, A., Limmroth, V., Juptner, M., Kaube, H., Schayck, R. V., et al. (1995). Brain stem activation in spontaneous human migraine attacks. *Nature Medicine, 1,* 658–660.

Woodhouse, A., & Drummond, P. D. (1993). Mechanisms of increased sensitivity to noise and light in migraine headache. *Cephalalgia, 13,* 417–21.

Woods, R. P., Iacoboni, M., & Mazziotta, J. C. (1994). Brief report: Bilateral spreading cerebral hypoperfusion during spontaneous migraine headache. *New England Journal of Medicine, 331,* 1689–1692.

Zanchin, G., Dainese, F., Mainardi, F., Mampreso, E., Perin, C., & Maggioni, F. (2005). Osmophobia in primary headaches. *Journal of Headache and Pain, 6,* 213–215.

Zhang, X., Levy, D., Noseda, R., Kainz, V., Jakubowski, M., & Burstein, R. (2010). Activation of meningeal nociceptors by cortical spreading depression: implications for migraine with aura. *The Journal of Neuroscience, 30,* 8807–8814.

22 Imaging Activation in the Migraine State

TILL SPRENGER, CHRISTIAN SEIFERT, AND PETER J. GOADSBY

INTRODUCTION

Functional imaging of the human brain has tremendously improved our understanding of brain function as well as the activation pattern in the migraine state specifically. While basic science has much to offer and there are good animal models of components of migraine (Bergerot et al., 2006), no model comes close to mimicking the complexity of the disorder itself. We therefore need human studies to confirm results from animal research to make sure that research is moving in the right direction. Functional neuroimaging now provides the means to test hypotheses gained from clinical observations or animal research in awake humans suffering from migraine. As migraine is today regarded as a disorder of the brain (Goadsby et al., 2002), brain activation studies and related techniques offer much in terms of understanding the system's physiological dysfunction that characterizes the disorder (Afridi & Goadsby, 2006).

METHODS FOR IMAGING BRAIN ACTIVATION IN MIGRAINE

Most of the brain activation studies in migraine research have applied positron emission tomography (PET). Although this method contains some degree of invasiveness with injection of a radiopharmaceutical, it is extremely valuable as it is robust and allows the study of migraineurs during rest without experimental manipulation. Using the most widely applied radiotracer in headache research, $H_2{}^{15}O$, one can study cerebral blood flow as an indirect marker of neuronal activity. There is, however, an increasing number of studies applying other tracers also, such as 18-fluoro-deoxy-d-glucose (^{18}FDG) (Fumal et al., 2006; Sprenger, Henriksen, et al., 2007), or radioactively labeled ligands, which bind to specific receptors (Sprenger et al., 2006). Therefore, PET allows the investigation of brain activity and metabolism, as well as receptor neurochemistry (Sprenger et al., 2005; Sprenger, Henriksen, et al., 2007). In PET, the positron travels a few millimeters through tissue before colliding with an electron and generating the annihilation photons that are detected by the PET camera. This travel restricts the spatial resolution to about 5 mm; hence, investigations on the function of smaller brain areas are limited. PET is also limited in terms of temporal resolution, which is in the range of minutes.

Nowadays, functional magnetic resonance imaging (fMRI) is more and more employed with its noninvasive nature. It is based on the so-called blood oxygen level–dependent (BOLD) effect. Oxygenated hemoglobin (diamagnetic) differs in its magnetic characteristics from deoxygenated hemoglobin (paramagnetic). Because of neurovascular coupling in the brain, the blood flow and hence the oxyhemoglobin content increases with increasing neuronal activity (Jueptner & Weiller, 1995). Changes in neuronal activity can be visualized by changes in the BOLD contrast.

BRAIN ACTIVATION IN EXPERIMENTAL PAIN

By use of experimental pain models such as heat pain application with contact thermodes, a very consistent network of brain areas has been established, which is activated in response to painful stimulation (Peyron et al., 2000). This matrix consistently comprises the thalamus, insula, anterior cingulate cortex, prefrontal cortex, primary and secondary somatosensory cortex, and cerebellum (Peyron et al., 2000; Valet et al., 2004). Other than some differences related to the somatotopy of the activations and methodological aspects, basically the same network is also activated when stimulating in the area of the trigeminal nerve (May et al., 1998) instead of the extremities or trunk and when investigating migraine attacks (Afridi, Giffin, et al., 2005; Afridi, Matharu, et al., 2005; May et al., 1998; Weiller et al., 1995).

BRAIN ACTIVATION IN MIGRAINE ATTACKS

A key observation, perhaps the crucial observation of functional imaging in migraine to date, has been that brainstem areas are active during pain and that after successful treatment this activation persists, while it is not present between attacks (Afridi, Giffin, et al., 2005; Afridi, Matharu, et al., 2005; Bahra et al., 2001; Denuelle et al., 2007; Weiller et al., 1995). The areas active are in the dorsal midbrain and the dorsolateral pons, with most recently a suggestion of hypothalamic activation (Denuelle et al., 2007). This pattern of activation, specifically dorsolateral pontine activation, is also seen in chronic migraine (Matharu et al., 2004) and thus seems to provide a robust marker of the disorder. Because of the limited spatial resolution of PET, it is difficult to determine exactly which brainstem nuclei are corresponding to this activation. It has been suggested that the dorsal brainstem activation corresponds to the brain region that Raskin et al. (1987) initially reported, and Veloso et al. (1998) confirmed, to cause migrainelike headache when stimulated in patients with electrodes implanted for pain control in the periaqueductal gray matter. Other authors have suspected that the brainstem activation corresponds to locus coeruleus activity (Sprenger & Goadsby, 2009).

Interestingly, the same area was found not to be modulated in chronic migraine treated with suboccipital stimulation (Matharu et al., 2004), indicating that this potential therapy may not alter the underlying disorder, but rather act as a symptomatic treatment. Regarding laterality, the brainstem activations have been shown to occur ipsilaterally to the pain, which suggests that the lateralization of the pain is a matter of lateralized brainstem dysfunction (Afridi, Matharu, et al., 2005).

There are almost no data directly investigating the specificity of the above-cited neuroimaging results in migraine as compared to other headache or pain disorders, with the exception of a patient who had both migraine and cluster headache (Bahra et al., 2001). This patient had a typical migraine in the PET scanner and had findings of brainstem activation not of posterior hypothalamic activation, suggesting that the functional imaging data predicted the clinical phenotype. Differences in applied methodology make it difficult to compare results across studies. However, as noted above, some of the studies provided results on headache syndromes that are striking as compared to studies investigating other pain syndromes. Moreover, they are plausible as they fit to pathophysiological concepts derived from other research methods, such as electrophysiology and animal work. Future research will have to implement head-to-head comparisons to clarify whether findings such as brainstem involvement in migraine or hypothalamic activation in cluster headache are reliably specific to one or the other of the disorders.

Burstein and colleagues (2010) investigated the ictal role of the thalamus in response to painful experimental stimulation of extracephalic areas in patients who developed ictal allodynia and found increased thalamic responses as compared to the interictal phase, suggesting thalamic involvement in the extracephalic spread of allodynia observed in some patients.

Photophobia

Recent research has focused on specific aspects of migraine attacks such as photophobia. Denuelle and colleagues investigated visual cortex responses to continuous luminous stimulation in migraineurs with $H_2^{15}O$ PET and

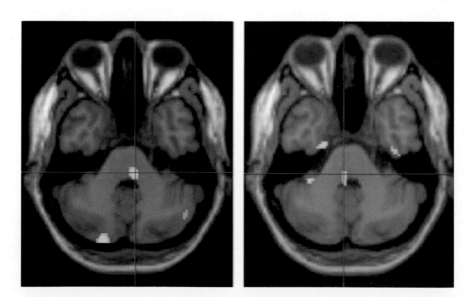

FIGURE 22–1 *Activation of the ipsilateral pons in patients with right-sided attacks* (n = 8, left image) *and left-sided attacks* (n = 8, right image).

found evidence for visual cortex hyperexcitability during the attack. Visual cortex activation in response to low luminous stimulation was stronger during the attack as compared to a period with headache relief after sumatriptan was applied. However, the activation during the headache relief phase just after the acute attack was still stronger than during an interictal scan, indicating that photophobia cannot be explained as a phenomenon exclusively produced by or secondary to trigeminal pain (Denuelle et al., 2011). The same group also studied visual cortex activation in migraineurs during the interictal state as compared to healthy subjects. They found increased cortical responses in migraineurs as compared to nonmigraineurs. In both groups, visual processing was modulated by concomitant trigeminal pain stimulation (Boulloche et al., 2010). The latter finding in the context of the above-mentioned study in acute migraine attacks indicates that, while light perception and processing can be augmented by trigeminal pain in both migraine and nonmigraine subjects, the existence of photophobia in migraineurs cannot be explained by the pain only, but could rather be driven by modulatory brainstem circuits.

The Interictal State

Few imaging studies such as the above-mentioned study on photophobia have investigated migraineurs interictally. One study indicated that cerebral glucose metabolism is increased in the pain network in migraineurs interictally (Kim et al., 2010). This could be a nonspecific finding in primary headache disorders as very similar findings were reported in cluster headache out of bout (Sprenger, Ruether, et al., 2007).

Interictal brain responses to experimental cephalic pain were shown to be increased in migraineurs in the area of the temporal pole and in the entorhinal cortex (Moulton et al., 2011), two areas that were previously not very much considered in migraine pathogenesis, although their activation had been occasionally reported in pain studies. Interestingly, though, the authors evidenced increased functional connectivity of the site of activation with several key areas of the pain network in migraineurs as compared to controls, arguing for a role of the temporal pole and entorhinal cortex in the pathophysiological process of migraine, although this role has yet to be defined.

A recent study investigated the role of the trigeminal nucleus caudalis in the interictal phase and a possible relation of its activity to the onset of migraine attacks (Stankewitz et al., 2011). Migraineurs were studied during painful trigeminal stimuli using a novel olfactory stimulation device. The authors found that the response in the trigeminal nucleus caudalis to the painful stimulation predicted the number of days to the next migraine attack

(Stankewitz et al., 2011). This study underlines that research has to be refocused to interictal and early attack stages instead of just investigating the ictal phase of migraine to better understand the mechanisms that are crucial for the generation of migraine attacks.

BRAIN ACTIVATION IN MIGRAINE AURA

Patients with migraine with aura experience both the typical migrainous head pain and often spectacular and sometimes frightening neurological phenomena, which usually precede the headache. Visual symptoms are the most common, such as scotoma with fortifications, and about 10% of all migraine patients have a characteristic march of symptoms starting with visual and evolving into sensory, speech, and rarely even motor symptoms within less than 60 minutes. Early clinical observations noted that the symptoms are consistent with a process transiently compromising cortical function at a speed of about 3 mm/min (Lashley, 1941), and Leao suggested that the so-called cortical spreading depression (CSD)—suppression of cortical activity advancing at about 3 mm/min over the cortex, which he observed in animals—was the electrophysiological correlate of fortification spectra in humans. It took more than 50 years until the existence of CSD in humans was proven electrophysiologically (Fabricius et al., 2006; Mayevsky et al., 1996; Strong et al., 2002) and human imaging studies using the [133]Xenon intra-arterial injection method in the pre-PET and fMRI era observed spreading oligemia in migraineurs (Olesen et al., 1991) as a surrogate of CSD. Regarding cerebral hypoperfusion, the latter results were confirmed by perfusion-weighted MRI in patients with visual migraine aura who showed decreased perfusion in the occipital cortex contralaterally to the aura symptoms (Sanchez del Rio et al., 1999). However, there have also been reports of occipital activation instead of hypoperfusion during migraine aura (Afridi, Kaube, et al., 2005). This apparent inconsistency between activation and deactivation of the occipital cortex in migraine aura is most likely related to the course and propagation of the aura with an early activation followed by prolonged deactivation (Cao et al., 1999). Hadjikhani and colleagues (2001) in an elegant study examined migraine aura in more detail taking advantage of the superior temporal and spatial resolution of fMRI. They observed decreases in stimulus-driven BOLD fluctuations in response to checkerboard stimulations, at a rate identical to CSD in the occipital cortex concurring with the onset of visual aura in the contralateral visual hemifield. Thereby, the retinotopic progression of the signal changes was consistent with the perceptual course and the changes

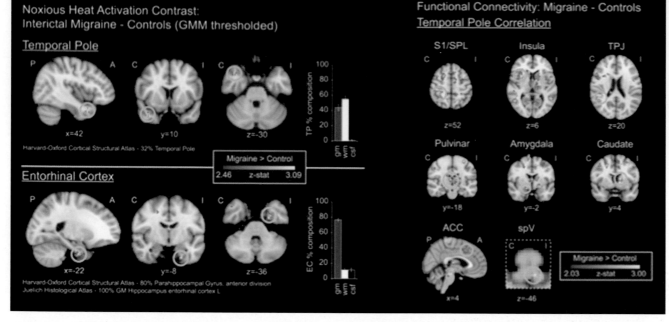

FIGURE 22–2 Left: *Contrast analysis of brain activation by noxious heat stimulation in interictal migraine patients versus healthy controls. Areas with a significant contrast (determined by Gaussian mixture modeling) are indicated by red-to-yellow voxels.* Right: *Functional connectivity contrast of the anterior temporal pole (TP) during intermittent painful heat stimulation in interictal migraine patients minus controls. The TP in interictal migraine patients has significantly enhanced functional connectivity within areas commonly activated by experimental pain, as well as in multimodal sensory processing areas. A, anterior; ACC, anterior cingulate cortex; C, contralateral; I, ipsilateral: P, posterior; S1, primary somatosensory cortex; SPL, superior parietal lobe; spV,; TPJ, temporoparietal junction. Reprinted from Moulton, E. A., Becerra, L., Maleki, N., et al. (2011). Painful heat reveals hyperexcitability of the temporal pole in interictal and ictal migraine states. Cerebral Cortex, 21, 435–448, with permission from Oxford University Press.*

crossed vascular territories. The authors located the source of the aura-related signal perturbations in the extrastriate cortex (V3A).

The role of CSD in migraine without aura, which involves the concept of clinically silent CSD, is an important question. The idea of silent aura was supported by an earlier imaging case of a patient developing an attack of migraine without aura during a PET scanning session and evidencing propagating cortical hypoperfusion, which started in the occipital cortex (Woods et al., 1994) and was believed by the authors to be the result of CSD. Although it has been questioned whether the patient studied using PET suffered from migraine with or without aura, which remains undetermined from the case description, a study on seven patients with migraine without aura from an independent group recently also reported a relative posterior cerebral hypoperfusion during migraine without aura

(Denuelle et al., 2008). Hypoperfusion—co-occurring with the headache—might also be the result of neuronal events in deeper brain structures, such as in the above-noted brainstem nuclei, and are certainly reported in pain studies (Coghill et al., 1998), while the marker of CSD is progression of the flow signal change, not anatomically static hypoperfusion. It has been shown in animals that stimulation of these brainstem nuclei can reduce the blood flow in the cortex, with maximal changes occurring in the occipital cortex (Goadsby & Duckworth; 1989; Lance et al., 1983). Moreover, activation changes in the brainstem have been shown to precede activation changes in posterior parts of the cortex (Cao et al., 2002). Thus, these results would fit an integrated concept of migraine with a primary brainstem dysfunction leading to secondary blood flow changes in the posterior circulation. Oligemia could then lead to CSD in susceptible patients (Denuelle et al., 2008).

SUMMARY AND FUTURE APPLICATION OF BRAIN ACTIVATION STUDIES IN MIGRAINE

One has to bear in mind that migraine is far more than isolated head pain. The key clinical features other than pain, such as photophobia, phonophobia, osmophobia, and nausea, argue for a severe episodic disturbance of sensory processing located in the central nervous system. The brain activation results agree with this view and demonstrate attack-related brain activation in brainstem areas coinciding with key areas for antinociception (Lothe et al., 2008). The results from functional imaging in migraine have helped not only to better understand the disorder but also to understand the mode of action of invasive treatment approaches (Matharu et al., 2004; May et al., 2006). Studies of the mechanisms underlying occipital nerve stimulation in migraine (Matharu et al., 2004) have supported the conduct of randomized controlled trials and clinical reports with that therapy in migraine (Saper et al., 2009). There are nowadays more and more new stimulation devices available, which can be used to investigate cranial somatic sensation in the setting of PET or fMRI studies and, even more important, to investigate cranial nociception in humans. This will help to better understand the course of abnormal nociceptive processing throughout migraine attacks, but also throughout the interictal phase, hopefully elucidating the episodic nature of migraine. New scanners combining PET and fMRI will allow the study of patients using different methodological approaches at the same time, for example, to better understand which neurotransmitter systems mediate brain activation changes in migraine. There is an increasing interest in developing radiotracers for PET targeting receptors thought to be implicated in pain and headache generation, such as serotonin, glutamate, and cannabinoid receptors (Li et al., 2005; Rstad et al., 2006). Studies using these tracers will again help to understand activation of specific neurochemical pathways, which were not accessible to research in humans in the past. Moreover, MRI techniques, which are suitable to study small-sized brain structures and detect subtle abnormalities, are rapidly evolving. Thus, there will be great opportunities to study brain activation and the contribution of well-defined anatomical areas to the development of the complex disorder and to furthermore elucidate causal neurochemical events.

REFERENCES

Afridi, S. K., Giffin, N. J., Kaube, H., et al. (2005). A positron emission tomographic study in spontaneous migraine. *Archives of Neurology, 62,* 1270–1275.

Afridi, S. K., & Goadsby, P. J. (2006). Neuroimaging of migraine. *Current Pain and Headache Reports, 10,* 221–224.

Afridi, S., Kaube, H., & Goadsby, P. J. (2005). Occipital activation in glyceryl trinitrate induced migraine with visual aura. *Journal of Neurology, Neurosurgery, and Psychiatry, 76,* 1158–1160.

Afridi, S. K., Matharu, M. S., Lee, L., et al. (2005). A PET study exploring the laterality of brainstem activation in migraine using glyceryl trinitrate. *Brain, 128,* 932–939.

Bahra, A., Matharu, M. S., Buchel, C., Frackowiak, R. S., & Goadsby, P. J. (2001). Brainstem activation specific to migraine headache. *Lancet, 357,* 1016–1017.

Bergerot, A., Holland, P. R., Akerman, S., et al. (2006). Animal models of migraine: Looking at the component parts of a complex disorder. *European Journal of Neuroscience, 24,* 1517–1534.

Boulloche, N., Denuelle, M., Payoux, P., Fabre, N., Trotter, Y., & Geraud, G. (2010). Photophobia in migraine: An interictal PET study of cortical hyperexcitability and its modulation by pain. *Journal of Neurology, Neurosurgery, and Psychiatry, 81,* 978–984.

Burstein, R., Jakubowski, M., Garcia-Nicas, E., et al. (2010). Thalamic sensitization transforms localized pain into widespread allodynia. *Annals of Neurology, 68,* 81–91.

Cao, Y., Aurora, S. K., Nagesh, V., Patel, S. C., & Welch, K. M. (2002). Functional MRI-BOLD of brainstem structures during visually triggered migraine. *Neurology, 59,* 72–78.

Cao, Y., Welch, K. M., Aurora, S., & Vikingstad, E. M. (1999). Functional MRI-BOLD of visually triggered headache in patients with migraine. *Archives of Neurology, 56,* 548–554.

Coghill, R. C., Sang, C. N., Berman, K. F., Bennett, G. J., & Iadarola, M. J. (1998). Global cerebral blood flow decreases during pain. *Journal of Cerebral Blood Flow and Metabolism, 18,* 141–147.

Denuelle, M., Boulloche, N., Payoux, P., Fabre, N., Trotter, Y., & Geraud, G. (2011). A PET study of photophobia during spontaneous migraine attacks. *Neurology, 76,* 213–218.

Denuelle, M., Fabre, N., Payoux, P., Chollet, F., & Geraud, G. (2007). Hypothalamic activation in spontaneous migraine attacks. *Headache, 47,* 1418–1426.

Denuelle, M., Fabre, N., Payoux, P., Chollet, F., & Geraud, G. (2008). Posterior cerebral hypoperfusion in migraine without aura. *Cephalalgia, 28,* 856–862.

Fabricius, M., Fuhr, S., Bhatia, R., et al. (2006). Cortical spreading depression and peri-infarct depolarization in acutely injured human cerebral cortex. *Brain, 129,* 778–790.

Fumal, A., Laureys, S., Di Clemente, L., et al. (2006). Orbitofrontal cortex involvement in chronic analgesic-overuse headache evolving from episodic migraine. *Brain, 129,* 543–550.

Goadsby, P. J., & Duckworth, J. W. (1989). Low frequency stimulation of the locus coeruleus reduces regional cerebral blood flow in the spinalized cat. *Brain Research, 476,* 71–77.

Goadsby, P. J., Lipton, R. B., & Ferrari, M. D. (2002). Migraine—current understanding and treatment. *New England Journal of Medicine, 346,* 257–270.

Hadjikhani, N., Sanchez Del Rio, M., Wu, O., et al. (2001). Mechanisms of migraine aura revealed by functional MRI in human visual cortex. *Proceedings of National Academy of Sciences of the United States of America, 98,* 4687–4692.

Jueptner, M., & Weiller, C. (1995). Review: Does measurement of regional cerebral blood flow reflect synaptic activity? Implications for PET and fMRI. *Neuroimage, 2,* 148–156.

Kim, J. H., Kim, S., Suh, S. I., Koh, S. B., Park, K. W., & Oh, K. (2010). Interictal metabolic changes in episodic migraine: A voxel-based FDG-PET study. *Cephalalgia, 30,* 53–61.

Lance, J. W., Lambert, G. A., Goadsby, P. J., & Duckworth, J. W. (1983). Brainstem influences on the cephalic circulation: Experimental data from cat and monkey of relevance to the mechanism of migraine. *Headache, 23,* 258–265.

Lashley, K. Patterns of cerebral integration indicated by the scotomas of migraine. *Archives of Neurology and Psychiatry, 46,* 331–339.

Li, Z., Gifford, A., Liu, Q., et al. (2005). Candidate PET radioligands for cannabinoid CB1 receptors: [18F]AM5144 and related pyrazole compounds. *Nuclear Medicine and Biology, 32,* 361–366.

Lothe, A., Merlet, I., Demarquay, G., Costes, N., Ryvlin, P., & Mauguiere, F. (2008). Interictal brain 5-HT1A receptors binding in migraine without aura: A 18F-MPPF-PET study. *Cephalalgia, 28,* 1282–1291.

Matharu, M. S., Bartsch, T., Ward, N., Frackowiak, R. S., Weiner, R., & Goadsby, P. J. (2004). Central neuromodulation in chronic migraine patients with suboccipital stimulators: A PET study. *Brain, 127,* 220–230.

May, A., Kaube, H., Buchel, C., et al. (1998). Experimental cranial pain elicited by capsaicin: A PET study. *Pain, 74,* 61–66.

May, A., Leone, M., Boecker, H., et al. (2006). Hypothalamic deep brain stimulation in positron emission tomography. *Journal of Neuroscience, 26,* 3589–3593.

Mayevsky, A., Doron, A., Manor, T., Meilin, S., Zarchin, N., & Ouaknine, G. E. (1996). Cortical spreading depression recorded from the human brain using a multiparametric monitoring system. *Brain Research, 740,* 268–274.

Moulton, E. A., Becerra, L., Maleki, N., et al. (2011). Painful heat reveals hyperexcitability of the temporal pole in interictal and ictal migraine states. *Cerebral Cortex, 21,* 435–448.

Olesen, J., Larsen, B., & Lauritzen, M. (1981). Focal hyperemia followed by spreading oligemia and impaired activation of rCBF in classic migraine. *Annals of Neurology, 9,* 344–352.

Peyron, R., Laurent, B., & Garcia-Larrea, L. (2000). Functional imaging of brain responses to pain. A review and meta-analysis. *Neurophysiology Clinics, 30,* 263–288.

Raskin, N. H., Hosobuchi, Y., & Lamb, S. (1987). Headache may arise from perturbation of brain. *Headache, 27,* 416–420.

Rstad, E., Platzer, S., Berthele, A., et al. (2006). Towards NR2B receptor selective imaging agents for PET-synthesis and evaluation of N-[11C]-(2-methoxy)benzyl (E)-styrene-, 2-naphthyl- and 4-trifluoromethoxyphenylamidine. *Bioorganic and Medicinal Chemistry, 14,* 6307–6313.

Sanchez del Rio, M., Bakker, D., Wu, O., et al. (1999). Perfusion weighted imaging during migraine: Spontaneous visual aura and headache. *Cephalalgia, 19,* 701–707.

Saper, J., Goadsby, P. J., Silberstein, S., & Dodick, D. W. (2009). Occipital nerve stimulation (ONS) for treatment of intractable chronic migraine (ICM): 3-Month results from the ONSTIM Feasibility Study. *Neurology, 72,* A252.

Sprenger, T., Berthele, A., Platzer, S., Boecker, H., & Tolle, T. R. (2005). What to learn from in vivo opioidergic brain imaging? *European Journal of Pain, 9,* 117–121.

Sprenger, T., & Goadsby, P. J. (2009). Migraine pathogenesis and state of pharmacological treatment options. *BMC Medicine, 7,* 71.

Sprenger, T., Henriksen, G., Valet, M., Platzer, S., Berthele, A., & Tolle, T. R. (2007). [Positron emission tomography in pain research. From the structure to the activity of the opiate receptor system]. *Schmerz, 21,* 503–513.

Sprenger, T., Ruether, K. V., Boecker, H., et al. (2007). Altered metabolism in frontal brain circuits in cluster headache. *Cephalalgia, 27,* 1033–1042.

Sprenger, T., Willoch, F., Miederer, M., et al. (2006). Opioidergic changes in the pineal gland and hypothalamus in cluster headache: A ligand PET study. *Neurology, 66,* 1108–1110.

Stankewitz, A., Aderjan, D., Eippert, F., & May, A. (2011). Trigeminal nociceptive transmission in migraineurs predicts migraine attacks. *Journal of Neuroscience, 31,* 1937–1943.

Strong, A. J., Fabricius, M., Boutelle, M. G., et al. (2002). Spreading and synchronous depressions of cortical activity in acutely injured human brain. *Stroke, 33,* 2738–2743.

Valet, M., Sprenger, T., Boecker, H., et al. (2004). Distraction modulates connectivity of the cingulo-frontal cortex and the midbrain during pain—an fMRI analysis. *Pain, 109,* 399–408.

Veloso, F., Kumar, K., & Toth, C. (1998). Headache secondary to deep brain implantation. *Headache, 38,* 507–515.

Weiller, C., May, A., Limmroth, V., et al. (1995). Brain stem activation in spontaneous human migraine attacks. *Nature Medicine, 1,* 658–660.

Woods, R. P., Iacoboni, M., & Mazziotta, J. C. (1994). Brief report: Bilateral spreading cerebral hypoperfusion during spontaneous migraine headache. *New England Journal of Medicine, 331,* 1689–1692.

23 Metabolites and Migraine

CATERINA TONON, GIULIA PIERANGELI, SABINA CEVOLI,

PIETRO CORTELLI, AND RAFFAELE LODI

INTRODUCTION

Magnetic resonance spectroscopy (MRS) has been utilized over the last three decades to characterize several metabolic pathways in living tissues by the direct assessment of biologically relevant metabolites. The noninvasive nature of this technique makes it an optimum tool for the investigation of the pathophysiological basis of human diseases as well as for enhancing routine clinical practice by improving differential diagnosis, prognosis, and the choice of treatment options.

Phosphorus and proton MRS techniques have been extensively applied to the study of brain and skeletal muscle metabolism in migraine patients and have revealed several pathophysiological aspects of this complex disorder mainly related to the tissue bioenergetic state.

MAGNETIC RESONANCE SPECTROSCOPY

Among advanced MR techniques, MRS has the ability to complement conventional magnetic resonance imaging (MRI) and enhance sensitivity to pathology by quantifying biologically significant molecules (Ross & Bluml, 2001). MRS is based on the same physical principles as MRI and uses the same hardware (Bloch et al., 1946; Purcell et al., 1946). Unlike conventional MRI, which gives structural information based on signals from water protons, the signals are collected, amplified, and then processed by Fourier transformation into a plot of frequency of nuclear rotation versus signal intensity. The variation in frequency of signal, defined as the chemical shift, is expressed in parts per million (ppm) of the field strength, thus normalizing frequency with respect to the intensity of the magnet field. The area of each peak is proportional to the concentration of the corresponding metabolite.

MRS techniques were introduced in the middle of the last century as analytical tools in chemistry and biochemistry (Jackmann & Sternhell, 1969). In vivo biomedical applications are mainly focused on proton (^{1}H) and phosphorus (^{31}P) nuclei. The first in vivo phosphorus (^{31}P) spectrum was obtained from excised rat skeletal muscle in high-resolution NMR instruments in the 1970s (Hoult et al., 1974), in 1980 the first ^{31}P magnetic resonance spectrum from intact rat brain was published (Ackerman et al., 1980), and in 1981 the first case of glycogenosis studied by muscle ^{31}P MRS was reported (Ross et al., 1981). The first in vivo ^{1}H magnetic resonance spectrum of the human brain was published in 1985 (Bottomley et al., 1985) and the first clinical applications soon followed.

Phosphorus Magnetic Resonance Spectroscopy

In both brain and skeletal muscle ^{31}PMRS can be used to noninvasively assay several metabolites that are present in millimolar concentrations in the tissue. Most of these metabolites are relevant to the tissue bioenergetic state: adenosine triphosphate (ATP) (γ–, α–, β–ATP), phosphocreatine (PCr), and inorganic phosphate (Pi) (Figs. 23–1 and 23–2). Other visible peaks include phosphomonoesters (PMEs) and phosphodiesters (PDEs). The PME peak in the skeletal muscle arises mainly from the hexose phosphate intermediates of glycolysis plus any inosine monophosphate from the net breakdown of ATP while in the brain it consists of various sugar monophosphates as well as phosphoethanolamine and phosphorylcholine. The PDE peak in both skeletal muscle and brain is constituted by the overlapping resonances of glycerophosphorylcholine and glycerophosphorylethanolamine, metabolites involved in cell membrane metabolism.

Intracellular pH (pH_i) and magnesium content can be calculated from the chemical shift of Pi and β-ATP from PCr, respectively. Through the creatine kinase reaction, it is possible to calculate the adenosine diphosphate (ADP) concentration (Arnold et al., 1985) that is too low to be measured directly. By knowing ATP, Pi, and ADP, it is possible to calculate the phosphorylation state ([ATP]/[Pi] × [ADP]) of a living tissue (Taylor et al., 2001).

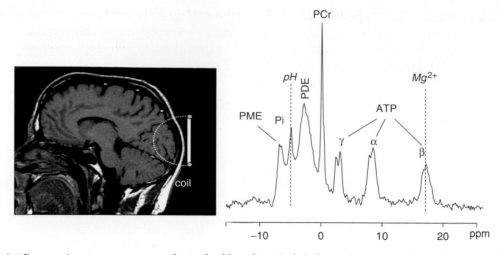

FIGURE 23–1 *Brain ³¹P magnetic resonance spectrum from a healthy subject (right) obtained using a surface coil placed, under the guide of magnetic resonance imaging, underneath the skull in the occipital region (left); the dashed line represents the approximate volume of signal acquisition of the coil. The spectrum was obtained by averaging 400 free induction decays (FIDs) acquired with a repetition time equal to 5 seconds. The abscissa reports the chemical shift in parts per million (ppm) and the ordinate the relative intensity. Cytosolic pH can be calculated from the chemical shift of Pi from PCr and free magnesium concentration [Mg²⁺] from the chemical shift of β–ATP from PCr. ATP, adenosine triphosphate (γ–, α–, β–ATP); PCr, phosphocreatine; Pi, inorganic phosphate; PME, phosphomonoesters; PDE, phosphodiesters.*

As the sensitivity of ³¹P is about one fifteenth of ¹H, it is necessary to study relatively large volumes of tissue using surface coils. Fat, fibrous tissue, blood, and extracellular fluid contribute no significant signal, and mitochondrial volume in cells is too small or mitochondrial metabolites are too tightly bound to interfere in measurements.

³¹P MRS of skeletal muscle has the capacity to evaluate tissue bioenergetics in a resting state as well as during dynamic processes resulting from skeletal muscle activity. Activity-related measurements are particularly valuable in detecting abnormalities of energy metabolism since these are often not apparent at rest, when demand for energy is low. A typical muscle ³¹P MR spectrum obtained from a healthy individual at rest is shown in Figure 23–2. In general, a surface coil is placed on/under the muscle of interest. Forearm finger flexors, calf muscle, and quadriceps

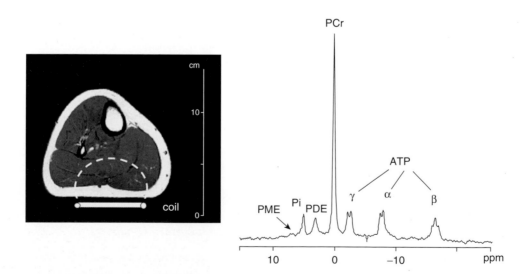

FIGURE 23–2 *Calf muscle ³¹P magnetic resonance spectrum at rest in a healthy subject (right) obtained using a surface coil placed, under the guide of magnetic resonance imaging, underneath the right calf muscle at the level of the maximum circumference. The spectrum was obtained by averaging 64 free induction decays (FIDs) acquired with a repetition time equal to 5 seconds. The dashed line indicates the approximate volume of signal acquisition of the coil. Abbreviations are as in Figure 23–1.*

muscle are the muscles most often studied (Taylor et al., 2001). The resulting spectrum represents an average of the energy state of all muscle fibers within the sensitive volume of the coil. The study of in vivo skeletal muscle bioenergetics, using ^{31}P-MRS–derived indices of metabolic recovery, requires an appropriate exercise ergometer to produce sufficient metabolic stress. ^{31}PMR spectra obtained during aerobic exercise show that the concentration of PCr falls, while that of Pi increases stoichiometrically. The magnitude of these changes corresponds to the extent of muscle work. Intracellular pH becomes acidic as lactate accumulates in the cell with increasing exercise intensity due to proportional increases in glycolytic flux. The calculated cytosolic free ADP rises with exercise and ATP remains constant. When muscle contraction stops, the rate of ATP turnover is immediately reduced, glycolysis stops, and ATP synthesis continues only through oxidative phosphorylation to restore high-energy phosphates to pre-exercise levels. There are several postexercise indices that can quantify mitochondrial ATP synthesis through oxidative phosphorylation (Kemp et al., 1993, 1994; Lodi, Kemp, et al., 1997): (a) *PCr recovery*: The rate of PCr repletion after exercise reflects the rate of mitochondrial ATP synthesis precisely. The resynthesis of PCr is directly visible in a recovery spectrum, and is the most commonly used index of mitochondrial oxidative phosphorylation rate. (b) *Maximum rate of mitochondrial ATP synthesis (V_{max})*: using the hyperbolic relationship between initial PCr resynthesis and end-exercise concentrations (ADP), Kemp et al. have estimated the apparent maximum rate of oxidative ATP synthesis (V_{max}) under the assumption that Michaelis constant (K_m) is normally equal to 30 μM. V_{max} provides a quantitative index of mitochondrial function that can be directly related to tissue respiratory rates and agrees reasonably well with enzyme analysis (Kemp et al., 1993, 1994).

There is a large body of evidence that primary mitochondrial disorders due to mitochondrial DNA (mtDNA) defects are characterized by a reduced rate of postexercise PCr resynthesis and V_{max} values (Argov et al., 1987; Taylor et al., 1994). These changes are also observed in mitochondrial disorders with no signs of myopathy and, in general, no ragged red fibers (RRFs) or cytochrome c oxidase (COX)–negative fibers in muscle biopsies, such as Leber hereditary optic neuropathy (LHON) or OPA1-related dominant optic atrophy (Lodi et al., 2000, 2004, 2011).

Proton Magnetic Resonance Spectroscopy

Proton MRS is based on the acquisition of signals from excitation of the nucleus of hydrogen or proton (^{1}H). It has two great advantages: The proton is the most sensitive stable nucleus and almost every compound in living tissue contains hydrogen atoms. However, whereas MRI generates images based on physical properties and distribution of water protons, MRS provides information on chemical compounds present at less than 1,000 times lower concentration than water. Thus, the signal to noise available and, consequently, the spatial resolution of ^{1}H MRS are much less than those available in conventional, water-based MRI. There are two ^{1}H MRS brain acquisition modalities: single voxel (SV) and multivoxel (chemical shift imaging [CSI]), resulting in single or multiple spectra, respectively. In both types of sequence the water signal is suppressed and the signal for metabolites is acquired either from a volume of interest (VOI) or from a two- or three-dimensional slice identified on the structural MRIs (Ross & Blum, 1999; Rudkin & Arnold, 1999).

The metabolites commonly observable with in vivo brain proton MRS (Fig. 23–3) are (a) *N*-acetyl-aspartate (NAA); (b) creatine plus phosphocreatine (Cr); (c) choline (Cho), constituted by a combination of choline-containing metabolites (phosphorylcholine, glyceryl-phosphoryl-choline); and (d) myoinositol (mI). Between 2.05 and 2.5 ppm, there is a pattern of resonances (Glx) that arise from the partially overlapping β- and γ-resonances of glutamine and glutamate (Rudkin & Arnold, 1999).

NAA represents the largest proton metabolic concentration in the human brain after H_2O (Ross & Blum, 1999; Rudkin & Arnold, 1999). NAA is contained primarily within neurons, axons, and their processes, and is used mainly as a marker of neuronal density or function. Reductions in NAA levels measured by ^{1}H MRS are a recognized index of neuronal loss or dysfunction in several neurological and psychiatric disorders including Alzheimer disease, HIV encephalopathy, multiple sclerosis, stroke, epilepsy, neoplasm, traumatic brain injury, drug abuse, and schizophrenia (Ross & Blum, 1999). Cho is a metabolic marker of membrane density and integrity, and its levels depend on the rates of phospholipid synthesis and degradation (Ross & Blum, 1999). An elevation in the Cho resonance within proliferative brain lesions is an accepted marker of malignancy (Rudkin & Arnold, 1999). Myoinositol, a cyclic sugar alcohol that is mainly located in astrocytes, can be used as a marker of cell osmolarity and glial cell proliferation (Ross & Blum, 1999). Lactate (Lac) is normally not resolved in the adult human brain under normal conditions (Boddaert et al., 2008; Ross & Blum, 1999) but can be detected as a doublet at 1.3 ppm (arising from methyl resonance) in disease states associated with an increased energy demand and/or impaired cellular capability for oxidative phosphorylation. A lactate peak can be readily observed by ^{1}H MRS in malignant tumors, ischemia, and other metabolic diseases, such as mitochondrial

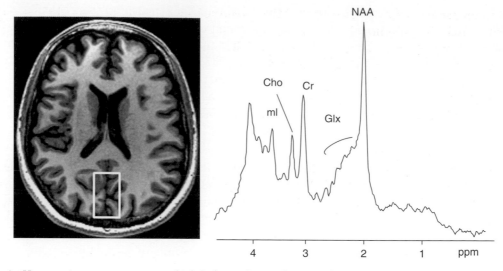

FIGURE 23–3 *Brain ¹H magnetic resonance spectrum (right) obtained using the PRESS localization technique (repetition time = 4 seconds, echo time = 35 milliseconds) from a volume of interest (VOI) localized in the midline occipital cortex (left). NAA, N-acetyl-aspartate; Glx, glutamate glutamine; Cr, creatine phosphocreatine; Cho, choline-containing compounds; mI, myoinositol; ppm, parts per million.*

disorders (Boddaert et al., 2008; José da Rocha et al., 2008; Ross & Blum, 1999; Rudkin & Arnold, 1999).

MITOCHONDRIAL DYSFUNCTION AND MIGRAINE

Migraine is a complex neurobiological disorder and its pathogenesis has yet to be completely defined. Migraine attacks seem to result from the intrinsic interaction of genetic background and environmental triggers in a susceptible brain (Montagna, 2000; Welch, 2003). Current evidence suggests that a generalized disorder of energy metabolism could be an important feature of the migraine brain since, in association with other susceptibility factors, it can lead to increased neuronal excitability that predisposes to migraine attacks (Aurora & Welch, 1998; Leao, 1944; Pietrobon & Striessnig, 2003; Schoenen, 1998).

Studies on energy metabolism dysfunction in migraine patients have addressed two main hypotheses: (a) that mitochondrial function is impaired and (b) that energy consumption is increased in migraine patients.

Biochemical and Pathological Studies

The frequent finding of migrainelike attacks in patients with mitochondrial encephalopathy, lactic acidosis, and strokelike episodes (MELAS), a mitochondrial encephalomyopathy due to the mtDNA 3243A>G mutation (Goto et al., 1990), prompted Montagna et al. (1988) to first look for mitochondrial dysfunction in migraine patients. Extraneural tissues such as skeletal muscle and platelets were investigated interictally in four patients with migraine with prolonged aura (defined as aura symptoms lasting more than 1 hour) and five patients with migraine stroke. Skeletal muscle was evaluated functionally, using a standardized effort test by means of a cycloergometer with determination of plasma lactate and subsequent histochemical and biochemical analyses of biopsy samples from triceps brachii or deltoid muscles. Venous lactate at rest was similar in migraine patients and healthy controls, but in patients it increased significantly with effort with no overlap to controls (Montagna et al., 1988). These findings were later reported in another patient with migraine stroke (Bresolin et al., 1991) and in two patients with familial hemiplegic migraine (FHM) and one with migraine without aura belonging to the same pedigree (Uncini et al., 1995), who showed increased levels of lactate after effort. Unfortunately, the exact genotype of patients in these preliminary studies was not determined. Okada et al. (1998) found increased plasma lactic acid and pyruvic acid at rest in 14 patients with migraine (11 with migraine without aura and 3 with migraine with aura) evaluated between attacks. Increased lactate production is indicative of defective oxidative metabolism and is a nonspecific hallmark of mitochondrial disorders. Lactic acidosis is secondary to an impaired utilization of pyruvate in the Krebs cycle that leads to an increased concentration of pyruvate, which, in turn, is reduced to lactate by lactate dehydrogenase (Finsterer et al., 1998). A compensatory increase in glycogenolytic/glycolytic activity may also contribute to the rise in lactate production in tissues with defective aerobic metabolism (Finsterer et al., 1998).

Among the 10 migraine patients studied by ^{31}P MRS who underwent muscle biopsy (Bresolin et al., 1991; Montagna et al., 1988; Uncini et al., 1995), two patients with migraine stroke (Bresolin et al., 1991; Montagna et al., 1988) and one patient with FHM (Uncini et al., 1995) showed histological evidence of mitochondrial impairment such as RRF and COX-negative fibers. Muscle biochemical analyses performed in seven out of nine patients by Montagna et al. (1988), revealed a mean activity of respiratory chain enzymes reduced from 16% for succinate dehydrogenase (complex II) to 30% for COX activity (complex IV) and 37% for NADH cytochrome c reductase (complex I–III) in migraine sufferers, while the activity of citrate synthetase, an enzyme of the Krebs cycle present in the mitochondrial matrix and used as an index of mitochondrial density, remained normal (Montagna et al., 1988). These findings were replicated in the muscle of the patient with migraine stroke reported by Bresolin et al. (1991), who found reduced COX activity (–30%) and NADH cytochrome c reductase (–39.4%), but not in the two FHM patients who showed normal muscle mitochondrial enzyme activity (Uncini et al., 1995).

Platelet spectrophotometric assays in the nine patients with migraine with prolonged aura or migraine stroke showed similar respiratory chain enzyme activities as in normal controls except for NADH cytochrome c reductase, which was reduced by 31% in migraine patients (Montagna et al., 1988). In a later study a more widespread interictal impairment of mitochondrial metabolism was demonstrated in the platelets of patients with migraine without aura ($n = 40$) and with aura ($n = 40$) (Sangiorgi et al., 1994). In both groups of patients there was a reduction in the activity of respiratory chain complex I and IV as well as of Krebs cycle enzyme citrate synthetase. The normal activity of other mitochondrial enzymes such as monoamine oxidase (MAO) and succinate dehydrogenase in migraine patients without and with aura (Sangiorgi et al., 1994) wasn't in agreement with a previous study that found reduced activity of both mitochondrial enzymes in the platelets of 48 patients with or without aura (Littlewood et al., 1984).

The relationship between mitochondrial impairment and migraine was further supported by the report of two female children suffering from migraine without aura, recurrent fatigue, muscle cramps, and multiple side effects from their migraine prophylactic treatment (Kabbouche et al., 2002). Both had low levels of carnitine, a major component of the mitochondrial fatty acid transportation system (Kabbouche et al., 2002). Muscle biopsy in one patient demonstrated a partial carnitine palmitoyltransferase II deficiency (Kabbouche et al., 2002). In a prior study, headache and carnitine deficiency had been reported in a subject on hemodialysis for renal failure (Wanic-Kossowska, 1997). Interestingly the headache in all three of these subjects responded to carnitine replacement therapy (Kabbouche et al., 2002; Wanic-Kossowska, 1997).

The molecular bases of mitochondrial dysfunction in migraine still remain to be fully understood. Only in the patient with migraine stroke reported by Bresolin et al. was a 5-kb mtDNA deletion, encompassing the genes for subunits of ATPase, COX, and complex I, detected (Bresolin et al., 1991). Conversely, the analysis of mtDNA variability suggested that haplogroup U represents a risk for migrainous stroke, being present in 83% of patients with it (Majamaa et al., 1998). However, the same study did not exclude the possible association with mtDNA mutations.

Systematic studies screening for mtDNA mutations in migraine-only subjects have, however, failed to recognize an association. An investigation of two maternal lineages with chronic progressive external ophthalmoplegia (CPEO) or MELAS subjects carrying the 3243 A>G tRNA^{leu} mutation compared to subjects with a high recurrence of migraine only led to the result that most of the latter did not carry the mutation. However, migraine subjects presented with mild mitochondrial abnormalities in skeletal muscle at biopsy, suggesting the possibility of an underlying mtDNA-associated genetic predisposition (Cevoli et al., 2010).

Magnesium Deficiency

Low magnesium content has been found interictally in serum, erythrocytes, saliva, and mononuclear cells of adult or pediatric patients with migraine without and with aura (Gallai et al., 1993, 1994; Sarchielli et al., 1992; Soriani et al., 1995; Thomas et al., 1992). No further reduction in magnesium content has been detected during attacks in both mononucleate and red cells (Gallai et al., 1992, 1993, 1994), while a significant further reduction was found during attacks in the serum of migraine patients (Gallai et al., 1992). Low cerebrospinal fluid magnesium levels have been detected inconsistently in migraine patients (Harrington et al., 2006; Jain et al., 1985). Although the link between brain energy metabolism deficit and reduced magnesium is not clear, low magnesium could contribute to increased neuronal instability and hyperexcitability by influencing neuronal glutamate NMDA receptor activity and calcium influx, thereby enhancing brain susceptibility to triggering an abnormal electric and metabolic event consistent with the cortical spreading depression (CSD) of Leao (Welch, 2005).

This is supported by a number of neurophysiological studies showing an association between increased cortical or neuromuscular hyperexcitability and low peripheral magnesium levels in migraineurs (Aloisi et al., 1997; Mazzotta et al., 1999).

MAGNETIC RESONANCE SPECTROSCOPY INVESTIGATION IN MIGRAINE

Phosphorus Magnetic Resonance Spectroscopy

Brain ^{31}P MRS has been employed since the late 1980s to investigate ischemia and deficits in energy homeostasis as two possible main determinants of aura and headache attacks in migraine (Table 23–1).

To test the hypothesis whether brain acidosis, secondary to vasospasm-induced ischemia, could lead subsequently to an increase in cerebral blood flow (CBF) and hence to throbbing headache (Skinhoj & Paulson, 1969), Welch et al. (1988, 1989) first used ^{31}P MRS to assess brain intracellular pH (pHi) and energy metabolism in migraine patients. Twelve patients with migraine without aura and eight patients with migraine with aura were studied. MR spectra were collected from up to four cortical regions (frontal, fronto-temporal, parieto-occipital, and occipital) during headache attacks (six patients with migraine without aura and five with migraine with aura) or interictally (six patients with migraine without aura and three with migraine with aura). In patients studied during attacks, cortical pHi was normal as it was in patients studied interictally. In migraine patients, scanned between 3 and 48 hours after the headache onset, normal pHi was associated with a 25% reduction in the PCr/Pi ratio (an index of tissue phosphorylation potential), whereas in patients studied interictally, the reduction in the PCr/Pi ratio was 15% but, due to the small size of the group, failed to reach statistical significance (Welch et al., 1989) (Fig. 23–4). In contrast, the same authors demonstrated, using the same technique, that patients with focal brain ischemia presented an early acidotic pH drop followed by subacute alkalosis. Acidosis was associated with reduced brain phosphorylation potential as shown by increased Pi and reduced ATP (Levine et al., 1992). Taken together, these findings lead to the conclusion that the defect of brain bioenergetics in migraine patients during headache attacks is unlikely to be secondary to brain ischemia, as normal brain pHi cannot support the presence of brain acidosis, and suggest therefore that the bioenergetic state of the brain could be impaired not only during attacks but also interictally.

The role of the interictal impairment of energy metabolism in migraine has been extensively investigated by the Bologna group of Lodi and colleagues (Barbiroli et al., 1990, 1992; Grimaldi et al., 2010; Lodi et al., 2001; Lodi, Kemp, Montagna et al., 1997; Lodi, Montagna et al., 1997;

Montagna et al., 1994). In studies spanning more than a decade, they used ^{31}P MRS to examine brain and skeletal muscle tissue bioenergetics in patients with different subtypes of migraine as well as other primary headaches.

In all studies brain bioenergetics were assessed in the occipital cortex using a surface coil positioned under the skull (Fig. 23–1). Eight patients with "complicated" migraine (four with prolonged aura and four with migraine strokes) were first investigated (Barbiroli et al., 1990). In the patient group the brain PCr/Pi was reduced by 35% and the PCr/ATP by 22%, indicating that a deficit of brain energy metabolism, at least in patients with severe forms of migraine, is present outside attack periods and may therefore be an intrinsic feature of the migraineurs' brain, predisposing it to headache attack triggers. This finding was confirmed only in part by a more recent study (Schulz et al., 2009) that used the one-dimensional CSI ^{31}P MRS technique. While patients with migraine with persistent aura showed reduced cortical PCr/Pi, patients with migraine stroke showed cortical PCr/Pi values similar to that found in healthy subjects. It is difficult to explain the different findings of these two studies, although some methodological differences were present. Barbiroli et al. (1990) obtained measurements from the occipital lobes, including the infarcted zone, while Schultz et al. (2009) included the noninfarcted cortex of the fronto-temporoparietal regions only. Interestingly, the assessment by Barbiroli et al. of the calf muscle mitochondrial ATP production rate, estimated from the rate of postexercise PCr resynthesis, revealed a particularly severe deficit of energy metabolism in the four patients with stroke who all presented with PCr $T_{1/2}$ (half-time constant of postexercise PCr resynthesis) above the 2 standard deviations (SD) of the normal mean (Barbiroli et al., 1990).

A deficit of brain and skeletal muscle energy metabolism was then detected interictally also in patients with milder forms of migraine such as migraine with aura (Barbiroli et al., 1992) and migraine without aura (Montagna et al., 1994). The reduction of PCr concentration in patients with migraine without aura was confirmed in a later two-dimensional CSI ^{31}P MRS study (Reyngoudt, et al., 2011) that used an external standard to calculate the absolute concentration of phosphorylated metabolites and did not use, as previous studies, ATP as internal standard. In migraine without aura, ATP concentrations were reduced by 16% compared to healthy controls, indicating that the studies (Barbiroli et al., 1990, 1992; Levine et al., 1992; Schulz et al., 2009) may have underestimated the reduction of PCr in migraine patients as ATP was assumed to be normal.

Similar findings to adults were obtained interictally in pediatric patients with migraine with aura who showed a deficit of both brain and muscle bioenergetics (Lodi,

TABLE 23–1 *Summary of Main Findings from Brain and Skeletal Muscle ^{31}P MRS Studies in Migraine Patients*

Reference	Type of Migraine (*n* patients)	Disease State	Magnet (Tesla, T)/^{31}P MRS Coil/Acquisition Technique	Metabolites' Quantification	Brain Region	Metabolites' Changes
Brain ^{31}P MRS studies						
Welch et al. (1988)	MwoA (12), MA (8)	Ictal: MA (5), MwoA (6) Interictal: MA (3), MwoA (6)	1.89 T/surface/volume	Relative	Bilateral: front, front-temp, par-occ, occ	Ictally and interictally pH = unchanged In at least two brain regions from those listed
Welch et al. (1989) [54]	MwoA (12), MA (8)	Ictal (11): MA (5), MwoA (6) Interictal (9): MA (5), MwoA (6)	1.89 T/surface/volume	Relative	Bilateral: front, front-temp, par-occ, occ	Ictal PCr/Pi= –25% Interictal PCr/Pi= –15% In at least two brain regions from those listed
Ramadan et al. (1989)	MwoA (11)	Ictal: MwoA (10) Interictal: MwoA (9)	1.89 T/surface/volume	Relative	Bilateral: front, front-temp, par-occ, occ	Ictal [Mg^{2+}] = –19% Ictal pH = unchanged In at least two brain regions from those listed
Barbiroli et al. (1990)	MwPA (4), MS (4)	Interictal	1.5 T/surface/volume	Relative	Bilateral occipital lobes	PCr/Pi= –35% PCr/ATP= –22%
Barbiroli et al. (1992)	MA (12)	Interictal	1.5 T/surface/volume	Relative[a]	Bilateral occipital lobes	[PCr]= –17% [Pi]= +24% pH= slightly reduced
Montagna et al. (1994)	MwoA (22)	Interictal	1.5 T/surface/volume	Relative[a]	Bilateral occipital lobes	[PCr]= –24% [Pi]= +5%
Lodi, Montagna et al. (1997)	Pediatric pts (15): MA (7 typical, 5 basilar), MwPA (3)	Interictal	1.5 T/surface/volume	Relative[a]	Bilateral occipital lobes	[PCr]= –21% [Pi]= +44% pH = slightly increased [Mg^{2+}] = –25%

(Continued)

TABLE 23–1 *Summary of Main Findings from Brain and Skeletal Muscle* ^{31}P *MRS Studies in Migraine Patients (Continued)*

Reference	Type of Migraine (n patients)	Disease State	Magnet (Tesla, T)/^{31}P MRS Coil/Acquisition Technique	Metabolites' Quantification	Brain Region	Metabolites' Changes
Lodi et al. (2001)	MwoA (21), MA (or basilar) (37), MwPA (13), MS (7)	Interictal	1.5 T/surface/volume	Relative[a]	Bilateral occipital lobes	ΔG ATP$_{hyd}$ (KJ/mol): MwoA = −0.94 MA = −1.06 MwPA = −1.15 MS = −1.47 [Mg^{2+}]: MwoA = −8% MA = −14% MwPA = −15% MS = −18%
Boska et al. (2002)	MwoA (19), MA (19), HM (8)	Interictal	3 T/birdcage ^{31}P (3D-CSI)	Relative[a]	Bilateral ant and post cortex (including occ)	[PCr]: MA= −14% (ant) HM= −11% (post) [Mg^{2+}]: MwoA= +7% (post) MA = −9% (ant) HM = −14% (post) [PDE]: MwoA= from +16% to +26% (ant-post)
Schulz et al. (2007)	MA (21): HM (11), MA nonmotor (10)	Interictal	2 T/surface coil 1D-CSI	Relative	Bilateral cortex and white matter: front-temp-pariet	Symptomatic hemisphere: gray matter HM PCr/Pi = −14% Pi/ATP= +20%
Schulz et al. (2009)	Mw persistent A (9), MS (5)	Interictal	2 T/surface coil 1D-CSI	Relative	Bilateral cortex and white matter: front-temp-pariet	Both hemispheres: gray matter MwPA PCr/Pi =−17%
Reyngoudt et al. (2011)	MwoA (19)	Interictal	3 T/Birdcage ^{31}P (2D-CSI)	Absolute external calibration using phantom replacement technique	Medial occipital lobes	[PCr] = −16% [ATP] = −16%

Skeletal Muscle ^{31}P MRS studies

Study	Subjects	Site	Quantification	Field/coil	Timing	Findings
Barbiroli et al. (1990) [56]	MwPA (4), MS (4)	Calf muscle	Relative	1.5 T/surface/volume	Interictal	*Rest* PCr/Pi = −11% *Postexercise* PCr $T_{1/2}$ = +53%
Barbiroli et al. (1992) [58]	MA (12)	Calf muscle	Relative	1.5 T/surface/volume	Interictal	*Postexercise* PCr TC = +41%
Montagna et al. (1994)	MwoA (22)	Calf muscle	Relative	1.5 T/surface/volume	Interictal	*Postexercise* PCr TC = delayed in 12 MwoA pts
Lodi, Montagna, et al. (1997)	Pediatric pts (15): MA (7 typical, 5 basilar), MwPA (3)	Calf muscle	Relative	1.5 T/surface/volume	Interictal	*Postexercise* PCr TC = delayed in 7 MA pts
Lodi, Kemp, Montagna, et al. (1997)	MwoA (23), MA (22), MS plus MwPA (18)	Calf muscle	Relative [ATP] assumed to be normal (8.2 mM)	1.5 T/surface/volume	MS Interictal	*Rest* [PCr]: MS-MwPA = +7% *End-exercise* pH: MS and MwPA, MA, MwoA (increased) [ADP]: MS-MwPA = +33%, MA = +18% *Postexercise* V_{max} MS plus MwPA = −38% MA = −18%
Grimaldi et al. (2010)	FHM2 (4)	Calf muscle	Relative	1.5 T/surface/volume	Interictal	*Rest* [Pi] = +22% *Exercise* Duration (min) = −39% *Postexercise* PCr $T_{1/2}$ = +68% V_{max} = −35%

Notes. ^{31}P MRS = ^{31} phosphorus magnetic resonance spectroscopy; MA = migraine with aura; front = frontal; temp = temporal; par = parietal; occ = occipital; MwoA = migraine without aura; MwPA = migraine with prolonged aura; MS = migraine stroke; [PCr], [Pi], [ATP], [Mg^{2+}], [PME], [PDE], [ADP] = concentration of phosphocreatine, inorganic phosphate, magnesium, adenosine triphosphate, phosphomonesters, phosphodiesters, adenosine diphosphate (mM); ΔG ATP_{hyd} = ∆ G of ATP hydrolysis (KJ/mol); HM = hemiplegic migraine; ant = anterior; post = posterior; PCr TC = time constant of postexercise PCr resynthesis (s); PCr $T_{1/2}$ = half-time constant of postexercise PCr resynthesis (s); FHM2 = familial hemiplegic migraine type 2; V_{max} = maximum rate of mitochondrial ATP synthesis (mM/min).

[a] [ATP] assumed to be normal (3 mM).

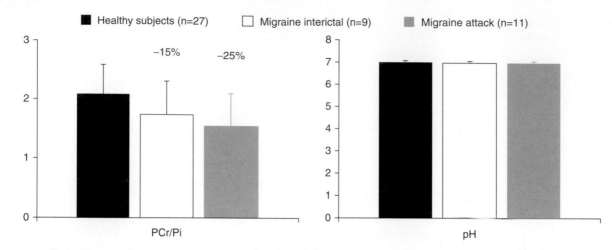

FIGURE 23-4 *Brain ^{31}P magnetic resonance spectroscopic data from the study of Welch et al. (1989). Phosphocreatine (PCr) to inorganic phosphate (Pi) ratio was evaluated in combined cortical regions (frontal, frontotemporal, parieto-occipital, or occipital) of migraine patients with and without aura during and in between attacks. In migraine patients PCr/Pi was more reduced during headache attacks while brain pH remained unchanged.*

Montagna, et al., 1997). These results strengthened the hypothesis that a defect in bioenergetics, unrelated to the age of migraine onset, number of attacks experienced, medications used, and age, (a) is an intrinsic feature of migraine and (b) has a pathogenic background that is able to enhance the susceptibility to develop headache when brain energy demand is increased and/or the supply of oxidizable substrates and oxygen is decreased.

When the bioenergetic state of the brain was compared in patients with different forms of migraine (7 with migraine stroke, 13 with migraine with prolonged aura, 37 with migraine with aura or basilar migraine, and 21 with migraine without aura) (Lodi, Montagna, et al., 1997), it was found that the free energy released by ATP hydrolysis (ΔG ATP$_{hyd}$, measured from ^{31}P MRS variables including Mg^{2+} concentration) in the occipital lobes presented a trend in keeping with the severity of headache attacks in migraine patients. The smallest mean amount of free energy released by ATP hydrolysis was found in patients with migraine stroke, and the highest in patients with migraine without aura (Figs. 23–5 and 23–6). This finding parallels ^{31}P MRS findings in the calf muscle of migraine patients (Lodi, Kemp, Montagna, et al. 1997), where the maximum rate of mitochondrial ATP production (V$_{max}$) was found to be the lowest in patients with migraine stroke and with prolonged aura and the highest in patients with migraine without aura (Fig. 23–7).

The availability of high field magnets (3 Tesla) and of chemical shift imaging sequences for ^{31}P allowed Welch's group to study multiple brain cortical regions in patients with migraine without aura (n = 19), migraine with aura

(n = 19) and hemiplegic migraine (HM) (n = 8), all in an interictal phase (Boska et al., 2002). Compared to their own (Welch et al., 1989) and the Bologna group's (Barbiroli et al., 1990, 1992; Montagna et al., 1994) previous findings, less persuasive changes in brain energetics were, however, found in these migraine patients. Reduced PCr content was detected only in the eight patients with HM (half of them familial) in the posterior cortical areas including the occipital cortex and in the anterior cortex of migraine with aura patients. The authors attributed the discrepancies between these observations and the results of previous ^{31}P MRS studies obtained using a surface coil to methodological differences. The results of Boska et al. (2002) were substantially confirmed by a later one-dimensional CSI ^{31}P MRS study (Schulz et al., 2007) that showed an association between interictal cortical reduction in the PCr/Pi ratio and severity and duration of aura in the symptomatic hemisphere. The PCr to Pi ratio (PCr/Pi) was significantly lower in patients with HM compared to those with nonmotor aura and in patients with aura duration greater than 7 days, while patients with nonmotor aura and aura duration from ≤1 hour to ≤7 days showed cortical PCr/Pi ratios similar to healthy controls (Schulz et al., 2007). In the study of Boska et al. (2002), the concentration of free Mg^{2+} was calculated and it was found to be reduced in the posterior cortex of HM patients and migraine with aura patients. In the posterior brain cortex, Mg^{2+} concentrations correlated with the severity of migraine, showing the highest values in migraine without aura and the lowest in HM patients. These findings were, however, in contrast to previous results reported by the

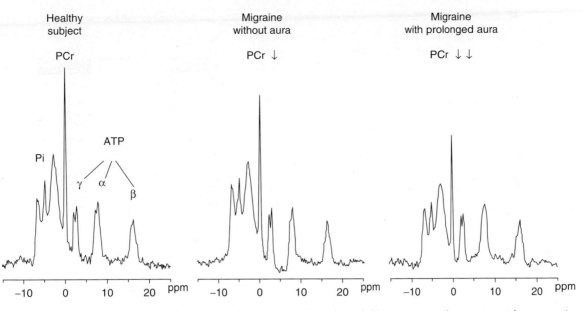

Healthy subject
PCr

Migraine without aura
PCr ↓

Migraine with prolonged aura
PCr ↓ ↓

Pi

ATP

γ α β

FIGURE 23–5 *^{31}P magnetic resonance spectra from occipital lobes of a healthy subject (left), a patient with migraine without aura (center), and a patient with migraine with prolonged aura (Right). PCr, Phosphocreatine; Pi, inorganic phosphate; ppm, parts per million. Modified from Lodi, R., Iotti, S., Cortelli, P., Pierangeli, G., Cevoli, S., Clementi, V., et al. (2001). Deficient energy metabolism is associated with low free magnesium in the brains of patients with migraine and cluster headache. Brain Research Bulletin, 54, 437–441.*

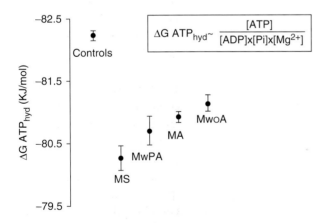

$$\Delta G\ ATP_{hyd} \sim \frac{[ATP]}{[ADP] \times [Pi] \times [Mg^{2+}]}$$

FIGURE 23–6 *Free energy released by the reaction of cytosolic adenosine triphosphate (ATP) hydrolysis (ΔG ATP$_{hyd}$) in the occipital lobes of patients with different types of migraine and healthy controls. ADP, adenosine diphosphate; Pi, inorganic phosphate; MS, migraine stroke; MwPA, migraine with prolonged aura; MA, migraine with typical aura or basilar migraine; MwoA, migraine without aura. Values are reported as means ± standard error (SE). Modified from Lodi, R., Iotti, S., Cortelli, P., Pierangeli, G., Cevoli, S., Clementi, V., et al. (2001). Deficient energy metabolism is associated with low free magnesium in the brains of patients with migraine and cluster headache. Brain Research Bulletin, 54, 437–441.*

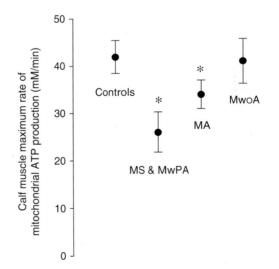

FIGURE 23–7 *Calf muscle maximum rate of mitochondrial adenosine triphosphate (ATP) production (V$_{max}$) in healthy controls and patients with migraine stroke (MS) and migraine with prolonged aura (MwpA), migraine with aura (MwA), and migraine without aura (MwoA). Values are reported as means ± standard error (SE). * p < .05 vs. healthy controls. Modified from Lodi, R., Kemp, G. J., Montagna, P., Pierangeli, G., Cortelli, P., Iotti, S., et al. (1997). Quantitative analysis of skeletal muscle bioenergetics and proton efflux in migraine and cluster headache. Journal of the Neurological Sciences, 146, 73–80.*

same group (Ramadan et al., 1989) that showed using a surface coil that free Mg^{2+} concentration was reduced by 19% in the cerebral cortex (average of frontal, frontotemporal, parieto-occipital, and occipital regions) during attacks but not in between attacks in a group of migraine patients with and without aura. Later studies by the Bologna group (Lodi et al., 2001) using a surface coil centered on the occipital cortex also found an interictal reduction in Mg^{2+} levels in all subtypes of migraine in comparison with healthy controls. Interestingly, migraine without aura patients had higher free Mg^{2+} concentrations than patients with migraine stroke and prolonged aura (Fig. 23–8). Similar findings were reported interictally in the occipital cortex of pediatric patients with migraine with aura who showed a 25% reduction in free $[Mg^{2+}]$ in the occipital cortex (Lodi, Montagna, et al., 1997).

The significant increase in PDE levels found by Boska et al. (2002) in the posterior and anterior cortical brain regions of patients with migraine without aura compared to healthy subjects, which was associated with lower, but not statistically significantly different, PDE levels in patients with migraine with aura and with hemiplegic migraine, led the authors to suggest that PDE levels could be related to the severity of migraine headache. However, neither migraine with aura nor hemiplegic migraine

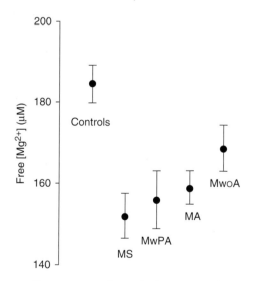

FIGURE 23–8 *Concentration of cytosolic free Mg^{2+} in the occipital lobes of patients with different types of migraine and healthy controls. MS, migraine stroke; MwPA, migraine with prolonged aura; MA, migraine with typical aura or basilar migraine; MwoA, migraine without aura. Values are reported as means ± standard error (SE). Modified from Lodi, R., Iotti, S., Cortelli, P., Pierangeli, G., Cevoli, S., Clementi, V., et al. (2001). Deficient energy metabolism is associated with low free magnesium in the brains of patients with migraine and cluster headache.* Brain Research Bulletin, 54, 437–441.

patients showed a significant reduction in PDE content compared to controls, in effect negating their own speculation concerning the role of altered metabolism of membrane phospholipids in the pathogenesis of headache attacks and aura.

Despite methodological differences and the heterogeneity of migraine patient populations that have been studied, impaired tissue bioenergetics and reduced Mg^{2+} have been demonstrated in both neural and extraneural tissues (see section Magnesium Deficiency) of patients affected by different types of migraine. In particular, brain ^{31}P MRS studies of migraine patients have overall shown an association between the bioenergetic deficit and reduced free magnesium concentration during attacks (Schulz et al., 2007) as well as interictally (Lodi et al., 2001; Lodi, Montagna, et al., 1997). However, the fundamental mechanisms leading to impaired oxidative phosphorylation and reduced brain Mg^{2+} concentration remain unknown. Low magnesium is known to lead to neuronal instability and hyperexcitability and so may be responsible for predisposing the brain to migraine attacks (Aurora et al., 1999; Welch & Ramadan, 1995).

The pathogenic role played by neuronal hyperexcitability is clear in the subgroup of FHM due to either mutations of the *CACNA1A* gene, encoding for a subunit of a neuronal calcium channel (FHM1); of the *ATP1A2* gene, encoding the α_2 subunit of the sodium/potassium ATPase (FHM2); or of the *SCN1A gene*, encoding for a neuronal sodium channel (FHM3). Interestingly, in patients with FHM2, the study of skeletal muscle by ^{31}P MRS revealed an impairment of mitochondrial oxidative metabolism (Grimaldi et al., 2010) as found in more common types of migraine.

The reduction of brain cytosolic free $[Mg^{2+}]$ is unlikely to be a direct consequence of hypomagnesemia. Magnesium ion, due to its large size, is thought not to cross the plasma membranes through channels or protein pores, and large quantities of Mg^{2+} are bound to intracellular phosphates and other anions, which would promptly release Mg^{2+} and re-equilibrate any systemic loss according to the specific affinity constant. Brain free $[Mg^{2+}]$ reduction is not specific for migraine, as it has been reported in patients with a deficit of oxidative phosphorylation due to mutations of mtDNA, suggesting that reduced cytosolic free $[Mg2+]$ may be secondary to a bioenergetic deficit (Barbiroli et al., 1999). From a bioenergetics point of view, the value of $\Delta G \ ATP_{hyd}$ varies as a function of free $[Mg^{2+}]$, as in most enzymatic reactions involving ATP the true substrate is $MgATP^{2-}$ and the actual amount of energy released by this highly exergonic reaction is that for $MgATP^{2-}$. The down-regulation of cytosolic free $[Mg^{2+}]$ re-equilibrates, at least in part, the rapidly available free energy in the cell, that is, increasing the absolute value of ΔG of ATP hydrolysis. As a consequence, in the presence of normal free cytosolic [Mg^{2+}], migraine as well as mitochondrial patients would display an even lower amount of energy released by ATP hydrolysis (Lodi et al., 2001).

In conclusion, there is a large body of evidence that deficits in brain bioenergetics and reduced Mg^{2+} concentration may play a pathogenic role in the genesis of migraine aura and headache attacks independently of any primary ischemia involving intracranial vessels. The extent of the deficit of in vivo neural and extraneural (skeletal muscle) bioenergetics and brain magnesium concentration has been shown by several studies to be somehow related to the severity of migraine. Overall, these findings point clearly to an unstable metabolic state of the migrainous brain and to a decreased ability to cope with further energy demand. It is noteworthy, however, that the mechanisms linking bioenergetics and Mg^{2+} to migraine may not be specific to the migraine condition and may be more a generalized phenomenon, since other forms of primary headache such as cluster headache have been shown to have similar neural and extraneural signatures in terms of tissue bioenergetics and Mg^{2+} levels (Lodi et al., 2001; Lodi, Kemp, Montagna, et al., 1997; Montagna et al., 1997).

Brain Proton Magnetic Resonance Spectroscopy

Proton MRS has been used to assess brain metabolites in migraine patients to evaluate bioenergetic homeostasis, cell membrane metabolism, and neuronal integrity in selected brain regions (Table 23–2).

As discussed in section "MR spectroscopy investigation in migraine", migraine pathophysiology possibly involves two functional brain changes: decreased mitochondrial energy reserve and abnormal central nervous system hyperexcitability. Several human neurophysiological and neuroimaging studies have provided evidence that these changes coexist and persist in the interictal period. In between attacks the cortex of migraineurs with and without aura, as a consequence of reduced phosphorylation potential and increased hyperexcitability due to impaired habituation (Schoenen et al., 2003), seems to be particularly vulnerable to cortical spreading depression and activation of the trigeminovascular system, the major human pain signaling system (Bolay et al., 2002; Moskowitz et al., 1993).

In addition to ^{31}P MRS, brain energy metabolism can be evaluated with high specificity using ^{1}H MRS to measure the regional brain content of lactate. Lactate is an intermediate of glucose metabolism that typically accumulates when ATP production switches to anaerobic glycolysis (Prichard, 1991). In healthy subjects brain lactate concentration is low at baseline conditions and increases when the energy demand increases. Early ^{1}H MRS data showed that photic stimulation, within the physiological range, raises the lactate concentration of human visual cortex. Such elevation is typically transient and tends to decline after the first few minutes of stimulation as the excess of glycolysis over mitochondrial respiration tends to normalize (Frahm et al., 1996; Prichard et al., 1991; Sappey-Marinier et al., 1992).

In patients with mitochondrial encephalomyopathies carrying either mtDNA point mutations (MELAS, Myoclonic Epilepsy with Ragged Red Fibers [MERFF]) (Frahm et al., 1996) or mtDNA deletions (Kearns-Sayre syndrome [KSS]) (Kuwabara et al., 1994; Mathews et al., 1993), brain lactate at rest has been reported to be higher than in healthy subjects. With photic stimulation, unlike in healthy subjects, who showed an increase in lactate content up to 200% of values at baseline, in KSS patients lactate did not rise significantly (Kuwabara et al., 1994), presumably because the brain of these individuals already had a greater reliance on glycolysis as an energy source.

Brain energy metabolism has been evaluated by ^{1}H MRS mainly in patients with migraine with aura. Since visual aura is the most common form of aura, most studies have investigated the occipital lobe both at rest and during photic stimulation.

Watanabe et al. (1996) first found increased lactate at rest in the occipital lobes of four out of five migraine patients with visual aura and in one patient with basilar migraine. The only patient without high lactate experienced his last attack 4 years before scanning, whereas the range was from 2 days to 2 months in the other patients. In the first functional ^{1}H MRS imaging study in migraine patients, performed using a one-dimensional CSI sequence, lactate levels were evaluated in the visual and nonvisual cortex (Sandor, Dydak, et al., 2005). At baseline, lactate, expressed relative to NAA, was increased in the visual cortex of patients with pure visual aura but not in patients with more complex aura (visual associated with paraesthesia, dysphasia, or paresis) (Fig. 23–9). In patients with pure visual aura, the lactate content was unchanged in the nonvisual cortex (Fig. 23–9). Photic stimulation resulted in a significant increase in lactate/NAA in the visual cortex of migraine patients with more complex aura, while it did not show a further increase in migraine patients with pure visual aura and was similar to baseline values in healthy volunteers (Sandor, Dydak, et al., 2005). Changes detected in the visual cortex in migraineurs with pure visual aura were exactly the same as those detected in mitochondrial patients, where the high lactate at baseline remained unchanged during visual

TABLE 23–2 *Summary of Main Findings from Brain 1H MRS Studies in Migraine Patients*

Reference	Type of Migraine (n patients)	Disease State	Magnet (Tesla, T)/¹H MRS coil/Acquisition Technique	Metabolites' Quantification	Brain Region	Metabolites' Changes
Watanabe et al. (1996)	MA (3), M with previous migrainous infarct (1), M basilar (1), M prolonged A/ migrainous infarct (1)	Interictal	1.5 T/surface/single voxel; Rest	Relative	Occipital	*Baseline* Lac/NAA increase (5/6 pts)
Sandor et al. (2005)	MA (10) Pure visual aura (5/10)	Interictal	1.5 T/quadrature head coil/CSI; Rest and visual stimulation (checkerboard)	Relative	Visual and nonvisual cortex	*Baseline* MA (pure visual) Lac/NAA (+31%) in visual cortex; *Stimulation* MA (complex) Lac/NAA (+43/+45%) in visual cortex
Sarchielli et al. (2005)	MA (22: 11 pure visual, 10 visual + sensory, 1 visual + sensory + dysphasic), MwoA (22)	Interictal	1.5 T/quadrature head coil/single-voxel PRESS; Rest and visual stimulation (flashing lights)	Relative	Occipital	*Baseline* MA NAA/Cho reduction ($p < .01$ vs. MwoA and healthy controls); *Stimulation* MA NAA (−14%) in visual cortex
Schulz et al. (2007)	MA (13): HM (7), MwA (nonmotor) (6)	Interictal	2 T/quadrature head coil/single-voxel PRESS	Relative	Bilateral basal ganglia	*Baseline* Normal metabolites' ratios; no lactate
Reyngoudt et al. (2010)	MwoA (22)	Interictal	3 T/quadrature head coil/PRESS	Absolute External calibration using phantom replacement technique	Medial occipital lobes	*Baseline* Normal metabolite concentrations; no lactate

Study	Group (n)	Condition	Technique	Quantification	Brain region	Findings
Reyngoudt, Paemeleire, Dierickx, et al. (2011)	MwoA (20)	Interictal	3 T/quadrature head coil/PRESS Rest and visual stimulation (checkerboard)	Absolute External calibration using phantom replacement technique	Medial occipital lobes	*Baseline* Normal metabolite concentrations; no lactate *Stimulation* Normal metabolite concentrations; no lactate
Gu et al. (2008)	MwoA (20)	Interictal	3 T/birdcage head coil/2D-CSI PRESS	Relative	Bilateral thalami	*Baseline* Left thalamus NAA/Cho (–14%)
Prescot et al. (2009)	Acute episodic MwoA (10)	Interictal	4 T/birdcage head coil/single-voxel modified PRESS 2D-J-resolved	Relative	Anterior cingulated cortex and insula	Glutamatergic changes on linear discriminant analysis
Sappey-Marinier et al. (1999)	EA2 (6)	Interictal	1.5 T/birdcage head coil/single-voxel PRESS	Relative	Cerebellum (including vermis) and occipital cortex	Increased cerebellar and occipital lactate in 50% of pts
Harno et al. (2005)	EA2 (9)	Interictal	1.5 T/birdcage head coil/single-voxel PRESS	Relative	Cerebellum, thalamus	Cerebellar hemispheres Cr (–12%) Vermis Cr (–16%)
Dichgans et al. (2005)	FHM1 (15)	Interictal	1.5 T/birdcage head coil/single-voxel PRESS	Absolute	Cerebellum (superior vermis), occipital and parietal cortex	Cerebellum NAA (–13%) mI (+20%) Glu (–15%)
Grimaldi et al. (2010)	FHM2 (4)	Interictal	1.5 T/birdcage head coil/single-voxel PRESS	Relative	Lateral ventricle CSF, parieto-occipital cortex and white matter	High lactate (1pt) Reduced NAA/Cr in the parieto-occipital cortex (1 pt)
Macri et al., (2003)	MA (8)	Interictal	1.5 T/birdcage head coil/single-voxel PRESS	Relative	Cerebellum	Cho/Cr (–12%)

Notes. ¹H MRS = proton magnetic resonance spectroscopy; MA = migraine with aura; Lac = lactate; NAA = *N*-acetyl-aspartate; CSI = chemical shift imaging; PRESS = Point RESolved Spectroscopy; MwoA = migraine without aura; HM = hemiplegic migraine; Cho = choline; EA2 = episodic ataxia type 2; FHM1 and FHM2 = familial hemiplegic migraine type 1 and type 2; Cr = creatine; mI = myoinositol; Glu = glutamate; CSF = cerebrospinal fluid.

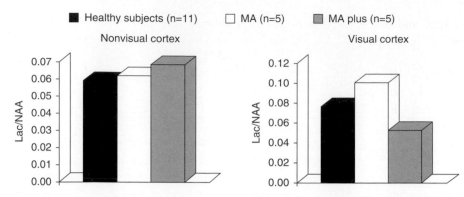

FIGURE 23-9 *Brain ¹H magnetic resonance spectroscopic data from the study of Sandor et al. (2005). Lactate–to–N-acetyl-aspartate (Lac/NAA) ratios before visual stimulation (mean values) in healthy controls, migraine patients with visual aura (MA), and migraine patients with visual symptoms and at least one of the following: paraesthesia, paresis, or dysphasia (MA plus).*

stimulation (Kuwabara et al., 1994). These findings (Sandor, Dydak, et al., 2005) were, however, not confirmed in a single-voxel ¹H MRS study of migraine patients with and without aura in which neither group showed a significant increase in occipital lobe lactate at baseline nor after visual stimulation (Sarchielli et al., 2005). The differences in the results of these studies (Sandor, Dydak, et al., 2005; Sarchielli et al., 2005) may be because migraine with aura patients with pure visual and more complex aura were not evaluated separately, the single-voxel technique (Sarchielli et al., 2005) may have also included some extra-visual cortex in the volume of interest (VOI) more easily than using multivoxel technique (Sandor, Dydak, et al., 2005), and finally, the visual stimulation was performed using flashing lights and not checkerboard (Sandor, Dydak, et al., 2005). Despite the lack of effect of photic stimulation on lactate content, in the same study Sarchielli et al. (2005) found that NAA content declined more markedly in migraine with aura patients than in migraine without aura patients or healthy subjects. They interpreted this as indirect evidence of mitochondrial dysfunction in migraine patients with aura. As NAA is synthesized in neuronal mitochondria, where it is thought to play a role in mitochondrial/cytosolic carbon transport, it can be considered as a marker of mitochondrial function (Clark, 1998). NAA (relative to Cho) was found to be reduced in migraine with aura patients at baseline in the occipital cortex (Sarchielli et al., 2005) but not in other brain regions such as the basal ganglia (Schulz et al., 2007), suggesting a region-specific occipital reduction in energy reserve and/or increased excitability in migraine with aura. This predisposing metabolic change found in migraine with aura patients was not detected in the occipital cortex of migraine without aura patients (Sarchielli et al., 2005) even when a careful absolute ¹H MRS quantification was performed (Reyngoudt et al., 2010) and a photic stimulation

was carried out (Reyngoudt, Paemeleire, Dierickx, et al., 2011).

Brain ¹H MRS has also been used in migraine patients to investigate the functional integrity of the brain structures involved in the sensory and emotional processing of pain stimuli. The study of the thalamus in patients with migraine without aura in the interictal state showed a significant decrease of NAA/Cho only in the left side compared to healthy controls (Gu et al., 2008). Patients with trigeminal neuralgia showed a similar reduction in NAA/Cho that was more severe than in migraine without aura patients and occurred bilaterally (Gu et al., 2008). The altered thalamic metabolism found in patients with migraine in between attacks (Gu et al., 2008) in association with positron emission tomography (PET) studies showing reduced thalamic activation during attacks (Weiller et al., 1995) points to an important pathophysiological role of the thalamus, which is the final gateway before nociceptive inputs reach the cortex, in the genesis of migraine headaches.

Other brain structures involved in pain processing have been investigated by ¹H MRS. The anterior cingulate cortex (ACC) has been suggested to play a role in antinociception and pain processing (Tracey & Dunckley, 2004) by exerting top–down influences on the brainstem sensory columns (Valet et al., 2004). Activation of the ACC has been consistently reported in functional MRI (fMRI) studies during a migraine attack (May, 2006).

¹H MRS studies of the ACC and insular cortex showed a normal metabolic profile in migraine without aura patients (Prescot et al., 2009). However, linear discriminant analysis (LDA) clearly separated migraine without aura patients and healthy subjects based on N-acetyl-aspartyl-glutamate (NAAG) and glutamine (Gln) concentration in both the ACC and insula. These findings are consistent with interictal glutamatergic

abnormalities in the ACC and insular cortex that may be a contributing factor for altered brain processing of pain stimuli in migraine.

Since the discovery that FHM1, episodic ataxia type 2 (EA2), and spinocerebellar ataxia type 6 (SCA6) are allelic channelopathies due to mutations within the *CACNA1A* gene (Ophoff et al., 1996), a great deal of interest was directed to the investigation of cerebellar functional, metabolic, and morphological aspects in FHM1 and later in FHM2.

In three of the six patients with EA2, most of them with interictal signs of cerebellar dysfunction, brain ^{1}H MRS demonstrated high lactate peaks and lower cerebellar total creatine in the occipital lobe and cerebellum. These findings were interpreted as indicating widespread altered energy metabolism (Sappey-Marinier et al., 1999) and early signs of calcium channel dysfunction, respectively (Harno et al., 2005). More pronounced ^{1}H MRS abnormalities were found in FHM1 patients. Fifteen patients from three FHM1 families, 11 of them with clinical signs of cerebellar involvement (Dichgans et al., 2005), showed decreased NAA and Glu concentrations and increased mI levels in the superior cerebellar vermis, compatible with neuronal damage and gliosis, in agreement with MRI measures of atrophy in the same volume studied by ^{1}H MRS. However, no changes in the energy metabolism markers were found in the parietal and occipital cortex, brain structures involved in the propagation of migraine aura (Dichgans et al., 2005).

Similar findings, though in a limited number of cases, have been reported in patients with FHM2 due to *ATP1A2* gene mutations (De Fusco et al., 2003). The study of four FHM2 patients by brain ^{1}H MRS and diffusion-weighted imaging (DWI) demonstrated in one patient an increase in cerebrospinal fluid (CSF) lactate and, in another, reduced NAA/Cr in the parieto-occipital cortex (Grimaldi et al., 2010). DWI revealed neurodegenerative changes in the vermis and cerebellar hemispheres of all patients, despite the fact that only two of them showed any interictal signs of cerebellar dysfunction (Grimaldi et al., 2010).

The clear cerebellar involvement in FHM1, later found also in FHM2, prompted additional investigations into the role of the cerebellum in the pathophysiology of more common forms of migraine. A subclinical cerebellar impairment, with hypermetria and other subtle cerebellar signs, was demonstrated in patients with migraine interictally (Sandor et al., 2001). These abnormalities were more pronounced in migraine patients with than without aura (Sandor et al., 2001). Patients with migraine, especially those affected by migraine with aura, have increased risk of cerebellar infarct and present with an increased prevalence of infratentorial hyperintense lesions predominantly in the cerebellum and pons (Kruit et al., 2004, 2005, 2006). These lesions correlate with the frequency of attacks. An ^{1}H MRS study of cerebellar hemispheres in eight patients with migraine with aura detected, as the only abnormality, a significant decrease in choline content (Macri et al., 2003). This finding was generically interpreted as indicative of altered membrane composition in migraine patients (Macri et al., 2003). A major flaw of the study was the absence of MRI scans, so it cannot be determined if choline changes were related to cerebellar signal intensity changes and/or atrophy.

Brain ^{1}H MRS and ^{31}P MRS studies have provided evidence that the more common types of migraine (without and with aura) can be characterized, interictally, by reduced energy reserve and/or increased excitability in brain regions commonly involved by aura symptoms, such as the occipital cortex, or part of the central pain processing pathway.

Some inconsistencies among different ^{1}H MRS studies might be due to small and inhomogeneous samples of patients, the possible presence of comorbidities, the coexistence in the same patients of different types of migraine attacks, differences in the temporal proximity to the last attack, attack frequency, disease duration, and the concurrent pharmacological treatment. Another confounding factor is the different criteria of migraine diagnosis used in these studies, due to the update of migraine classification over the years. In addition, different MR methodological approaches (intensity of the magnetic field, acquisition sequences, postprocessing analysis) enhance difficulties in comparing studies conducted at different clinical sites.

THERAPY BASED ON CORRECTING ENERGY METABOLISM DEFICIT IN MIGRAINE

Although no studies have yet used brain or skeletal muscle MRS to monitor in vivo the effect of drugs for the treatment or prevention of migraine, the results obtained by ^{31}P and ^{1}H MRS in migraine have provided strong rationales for specific pharmacological interventions. The evidence that brain-impaired energy metabolism and/or increased energy demand underlie different types of migraine has prompted the clinical evaluation of pharmacological treatments targeting oxidative metabolism. Several nutraceuticals have demonstrated some positive effects on migraine treatment, including in particular riboflavin and coenzyme Q10.

Riboflavin, vitamin B_2, is required for the activity of flavoenzymes in the mitochondrial electron transport chain. Some reports have demonstrated clinical and biochemical improvements with riboflavin administration in small groups of patients with mitochondrial disorders such as complex I deficiency (Bernsen et al., 1991, 1993; Gerards et al., 2011; Napolitano et al., 2000; Penn et al., 1992; Scholte et al., 1995) and complex II deficiency (Bugiani et al., 2006).

In the first randomized, double-blind, placebo-controlled trial riboflavin was administered (400 mg/day for 3 months) to 80 migraine patients with or without aura and resulted in reduced attack frequency and number of headache days (Schoenen et al., 1998) (Fig. 23–10). The efficacy of riboflavin on migraine was maximal at 3 months, when the study ended (Schoenen et al., 1998). A significant reduction of headache frequency was later confirmed in an open-label study (23 migraine patients with or without aura), where its use was associated with a reduction in the use of acute antimigraine drugs during attacks (Boehnke et al., 2004). In a pharmacogenetic study, Di Lorenzo et al. (2009) demonstrated that migraineurs belonging to the H haplogroup of mtDNA, which is mainly found in the European population, were less likely to respond to the riboflavin treatment in comparison to patients carrying other haplogroups, who responded significantly better. A potential explanation for this finding may be that haplogroup H is associated with higher complex I activity in the mitochondrial respiratory chain compared to other haplogroups, and thus that riboflavin might be unable to further increase oxidative phosphorylation (OXPHOS) metabolism. In contrast, riboflavin administration could show a beneficial effect in non-H haplogroups that are associated with lower complex I activity (Di Lorenzo et al., 2009). The encouraging

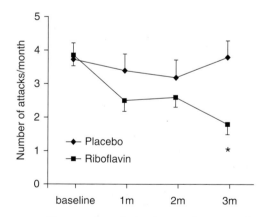

FIGURE 23–10 *Mean number of migraine attacks per month in the placebo (n = 26) and riboflavin (400 mg/day) groups (n = 28). The decrease of attack frequency is significant in the riboflavin group during the third month of the randomized phase. * p = .0001. From Schoenen, J., Jacquy, J., & Lenaerts, M. (1998). Effectiveness of high-dose riboflavin in migraine prophylaxis. A randomized controlled trial. Neurology, 50, 466–470.*

results obtained with riboflavin administration in adult migraineurs have not yet been confirmed in pediatric patients. A randomized, placebo-controlled, double-blind, cross-over trial, where riboflavin was administered at 50 mg daily for 4 months to 42 children (aged 6 to 13 years) with migraine, observed no reduction of mean frequency of migraine attacks in the last month of treatment compared to placebo (Bruijn et al., 2010).

Coenzyme Q10 is an electron transporter from complexes I and II to complex III in the mitochondrial respiratory chain. The effect of coenzyme Q10 administration in primary mitochondrial disease is controversial. Short-term administration of coenzyme Q10 plus riboflavin, vitamins K_3 and C, thiamine, and niacin was ineffective in 16 patients with different mitochondrial diseases (Matthews et al., 1993). However, in a separate randomized, double-blind, placebo-controlled, crossover study design in 16 patients with different mitochondrial diseases, coenzyme Q10, in combination with creatine and lipoic acid, lowered markers of oxidative damage and attenuated the decline in muscle strength (Rodriguez et al., 2007). A number of open-label studies and case reports of mitochondrial patients have suggested biochemical and clinical benefits with coenzyme Q10 administration (Abe et al., 1991; Bachmeyer et al., 2010; Goda et al., 1987; Ogasahara et al., 1985; Steele et al., 2004). The largest randomized, double-blind, crossover trial, with 30 patients with mitochondrial disease receiving 1,200 mg/day of coenzyme Q10 for 60 days, demonstrated only minor effects on cycle exercise aerobic capacity and postexercise lactate and did not show any coenzyme Q10 effect on clinically relevant variables such as strength or resting lactate levels (Glover et al., 2010).

In contrast to mitochondrial disease, as for riboflavin, the administration of coenzyme Q10 to migraine patients seems to have some beneficial effects. The treatment, in an open-label study, with coenzyme Q10 (150 mg/day) of 31 patients with migraine with or without aura resulted in reduced attack frequency and headache days per month (Rozen et al., 2002). This finding was confirmed in a later double-blind, randomized, placebo-controlled trial in 42 migraine patients (only 2 with migraine with aura), where coenzyme Q10 administration (300 mg/day) reduced attack frequency, headache days, and days with nausea in the third treatment month (Sandor, Di Clemente, et al., 2005). More recently, coenzyme Q10 supplementation was also suggested to be effective in the prevention of migraine attacks in children and adolescents. About one third of 1,550 young migraine patients, with low blood levels of coenzyme Q10, were treated with 1 to 3 mg/kg per day of coenzyme Q10, and showed reduced headache frequency (Hershey et al., 2007). However, when confirmation was sought in a more rigorous placebo-controlled, double-blinded, cross-over, add-on trial, children and adolescents with migraine improved over time regardless of supplementation with coenzyme Q10 or placebo (Slater et al., 2011).

Thioctic acid enhances mitochondrial oxygen metabolism and ATP production. Its administration produced a clinical and biochemical improvement in various mitochondriopathies such as Leigh encephalomyopathy (Byrd et al., 1989), pyruvate dehydrogenase deficiency (Yoshida et al., 1990), and pyruvate carboxylase deficiency (Maesaka et al., 1976). However, in a double-blind trial (600 mg/day), thioctic acid was administrated to 26 patients with migraine (21 without aura and 5 with aura) and only a nonsignificant trend to reduced frequency of migraine attacks was found (Magis et al., 2007).

Creatine is a precursor of phosphocreatine, and it is used to increase mass and aerobic fitness of muscles. A pilot double-blind, placebo-controlled, crossover trial did not show efficacy of creatine (5 g by mouth four times a day for 1 week followed by 5 g once a day for 3 months) in the prevention of migraine without aura in a small sample of patients (Pierangeli et al., 2001).

Overall, the administration of drugs enhancing mitochondrial function in migraine patients was safe and well tolerated, and some studies have found that they are effective in reducing headache attacks, supporting their use in the prophylaxis of migraine attacks.

The evidence of low ictal (Ramadan et al., 1989) and interictal (Boska et al., 2002; Lodi et al., 2001; Lodi, Montagna, et al., 1997) free $[Mg^{2+}]$ in the brain and low interictal $[Mg^{2+}]$ in serum and erythrocytes of patients with different forms of migraine (Gallai et al., 1992, 1993, 1994; Sarchielli et al., 1992; Soriani et al., 1995; Thomas et al., 1992) has suggested that hypomagnesemia may be a predisposing factor in migraine attacks. Magnesium administration has been evaluated for acute and prophylactic treatment of different forms of migraine and cluster headache. The efficacy of acute magnesium administration was reported in different anecdotal studies (Mauskop et al., 1995, 1996) and in a single-blind (Demirkaya et al., 2001) and double-blind randomized controlled study (Bigal et al., 2002). In contrast, two randomized control studies performed in emergency room settings didn't find any difference between magnesium and placebo in acute use (Cete et al., 2005; Corbo et al., 2001). The prophylactic efficacy of magnesium administration (from 300 to 600 mg/day) was evaluated in a randomized controlled trial in 20 women with menstrual migraine and showed a reduction in the number of headache days (Facchinetti et al., 1991); and, in larger studies, magnesium was shown to reduce migraine attack frequency and severity in patients with and without

aura (Köseoglu et al., 2008; Peikert et al., 1996). Unfortunately, while there is evidence that oral magnesium administration may have a beneficial prophylactic effect in migraine patients, the high frequency of diarrhea, the most common adverse effect recorded in almost all studies, which in one study was so frequent and severe that the trial was discontinued (Pfaffenrath et al., 1996), is a substantial limitation to the clinical use of oral magnesium.

In conclusion, MRS studies of migraine have given a mechanistic rationale for pharmacotherapy with agents that enhance oxidative metabolism and magnesium content in the brain, and subsequent clinical efficacy studies have shown that these agents can benefit patients. Future MRS investigations may provide the basis for further improvements in the prognosis, diagnosis, and treatment of migraineurs.

REFERENCES

Abe, K., Fujimura, H., Nishikawa, Y., Yorifuji, S., Mezaki, T., Hirono, N., et al. (1991). Marked reduction in CSF lactate and pyruvate levels after CoQ therapy in a patient with mitochondrial myopathy, encephalopathy, lactic acidosis and stroke-like episodes (MELAS). *Acta Neurologica Scandinavica*, *83*, 356–359.

Ackerman, J. J., Grove, T. H., Wong, G. G., Gadian, D. G., & Radda, G. K. (1980). Mapping of metabolites in whole animals by 31P NMR using surface coils. *Nature*, *283*, 167–170.

Aloisi, P., Marrelli, A., Porto, C., Tozzi, E., & Cerone, G. (1997). Visual evoked potentials and serum magnesium levels in juvenile migraine patients. *Headache*, *37*(6), 383–385.

Argov, Z., Bank, W. J., Maris, J., Peterson, P., & Chance, B. (1987). Bioenergetic heterogeneity of human mitochondrial myopathies: Phosphorus magnetic resonance spectroscopy study. *Neurology, 37*, 257–262.

Arnold, D. L., Taylor, D. J., & Radda, G. K. (1985). Investigation of human mitochondrial myopathies by phosphorus magnetic resonance spectroscopy. *Annals of Neurology, 18*, 189–196.

Aurora, S. K., Cao, Y., Bowyer, S. M., & Welch, K. M. (1999). The occipital cortex is hyperexcitable in migraine: Experimental evidence. *Headache, 39*(7), 469–476.

Aurora, S. K., & Welch, K. M. A. (1998). Brain excitability in migraine: Evidence from transcranial magnetic stimulation studies. *Current Opinion in Neurology, 11*, 205–209.

Bachmeyer, C., Ferroir, J. P., Eymard, B., Maïer-Redelsperger, M., Lebre, A. S., & Girot, R. (2010). Coenzyme Q is effective on anemia in a patient with sideroblastic anemia and mitochondrial myopathy. *Blood, 116*(18), 3681–3682.

Barbiroli, B., Iotti, S., Cortelli, P., Martinelli, P., Lodi, R., Carelli, V., et al. (1999). Low brain intracellular free magnesium in mitochondrial cytopathies. *Journal of Cerebral Blood Flow and Metabolism, 19*, 528–532.

Barbiroli, B., Montagna, P., Cortelli, P., Funicello, R., Iotti, S., Monari, L., et al. (1992). Abnormal brain and muscle energy metabolism shown by 31P magnetic resonance spectroscopy in patients affected by migraine with aura. *Neurology, 42*, 1209–114.

Barbiroli, B., Montagna, P., Cortelli, P., Martinelli, P., Sacquegna, T., Zaniol, P., et al. (1990). Complicated migraine studied by phosphorus magnetic resonance spectroscopy. *Cephalalgia, 10,* 263–72.

Bernsen, P. L., Gabreels, F. J., Ruitenbeek, W., & Hamburger, H. L. (1993). Treatment of complex I deficiency with riboflavin. *Journal of the Neurological Sciences, 118,* 181–187.

Bernsen, P. L., Gabreëls, F. J., Ruitenbeek, W., Sengers, R. C., Stadhouders, A. M., & Renier, W. O. (1991). Successful treatment of pure myopathy, associated with complex I deficiency, with riboflavin and carnitine. *Archives of Neurology, 48*(3), 334–338.

Bigal, M. E., Bordini, C., Tepper, S. J., & Speciali, J. G. (2002). Intravenous magnesium sulphate in the acute treatment of migraine without aura and migraine with aura. A randomized, double-blind, placebocontrolled study. *Cephalalgia, 22,* 345–353.

Bloch, F., Hansen, W. W., & Packard, M. E. (1946). Nuclear induction. *Physical Review, 69,* 127.

Boddaert, N., Romano, S., Funalot, B., Rio, M., Sarzi, E., Lebre, A. S., et al. (2008). 1H MRS spectroscopy evidence of cerebellar high lactate in mitochondrial respiratory chain deficiency. *Molecular Genetics and Metabolism, 93*(1), 85–88.

Boehnke, C., Reuter, U., Flach, U., Schuh-Hofer, S., Einhaupl, K. M., & Arnold, G. (2004). High-dose riboflavin treatment is efficacious in migraine prophylaxis: An open study in a tertiary care centre. *European Journal of Neurology, 11,* 475–477.

Bolay, H., Reuter, U., Dunn, A. K., Huang, Z., Boas, D. A., & Moskowitz, M. A. (2002). Intrinsic brain activity triggers trigeminal meningeal afferents in a migraine model. *Nature Medicine, 8*(2), 136–142.

Boska, M. D., Welch, K. M., Barker, P. B., Nelson, J. A., & Schultz, L. (2002). Contrasts in cortical magnesium, phospholipid and energy metabolism between migraine syndromes. *Neurology, 58*(8), 1227–1233.

Bottomley, P. A., Edelstein, W. A., Foster, T. H., & Adams, W. A. (1985). In vivo solvent suppressed localized hydrogen nuclear magnetic resonance spectroscopy: A window to metabolism? *Proceedings of the National Academy of Sciences of the United States of America, 82*(7), 2148–2252.

Bresolin, N., Martinelli, P., Barbiroli, B., Zaniol, P., Ausenda, C., Montagna, P., et al. (1991). Muscle mitochondrial DNA deletion and 31P-NMR spectroscopy alterations in a migraine patient. *Journal of the Neurological Sciences, 104*(2), 182–189.

Bruijn, J., Duivenvoorden, H., Passchier, J., Locher, H., Dijkstra, N., & Arts, W. F. (2010). Medium-dose riboflavin as a prophylactic agent in children with migraine: A preliminary placebo-controlled, randomised, double-blind, cross-over trial. *Cephalalgia, 30*(12), 1426–1434.

Bugiani, M., Lamantea, E., Invernizzi, F., Moroni, I., Bizzi, A., Zeviani, M., et al. (2006). Effects of riboflavin in children with complex II deficiency. *Brain Development, 28*(9), 576–581.

Byrd, D. J., Krohn, H. P., Winkler, L., Steinborn, C., Hadam, M., Brodehl, J., et al. (1989). Neonatal pyruvate dehydrogenase deficiency with lipoate responsive lactic acidaemia and hyperammonaemia. *European Journal of Pediatrics, 148*(6), 543–547.

Cete, Y., Dora, B., Ertan, C., Ozdemir, C., & Oktay, C. (2005). A randomized prospective placebo-controlled study of intravenous magnesium sulphate vs. metoclopramide in the management of acute migraine attacks in the emergency department. *Cephalalgia, 25,* 199–204.

Cevoli, S., Pallotti, F., La Morgia, C., Valentino, M. L., Pierangeli, G., Cortelli, P., et al. (2010). High frequency of migraine-only patients negative for the 3243 A>G tRNA^leu mtDNA mutation in two MELAS families. *Cephalalgia, 30,* 919–927.

Clark, J. B. (1998). N-acetyl aspartate: a marker for neuronal loss or mitochondrial dysfunction. *Developmental Neuroscience, 20,* 271–276.

Corbo, J., Esses, D., Bijur, P. E., Iannaccone, R., & Gallagher, E. J. (2001). Randomized clinical trial of intravenous magnesium sulfate as an adjunctive medication for emergency department treatment of migraine headache. *Annals of Emergency Medicine, 38,* 621–627.

De Fusco, M., Marconi, R., Silvestri, L., Atorino, L., Rampoldi, L., Morgante, L., et al. (2003). Haploinsufficiency of ATP1A2 encoding the Na+/K+ pump alpha2 subunit associated with familial hemiplegic migraine type 2. *Nature Genetics, 33*(2), 192–196.

Demirkaya, S., Vural, O., Dora, B., & Topcuoglu, M. A. (2001). Efficacy of intravenous magnesium sulfate in the treatment of acute migraine attacks. *Headache, 41,* 171–177.

Di Lorenzo, C., Pierelli, F., Coppola, G., Grieco, G. S., Rengo, C., Ciccolella, M., et al. (2009). Mitochondrial DNA haplogroups influence the therapeutic response to riboflavin in migraineurs. *Neurology, 72*(18), 1588–1594.

Dichgans, M., Freilinger, T., Eckstein, G., Babini, E., Lorenz-Depiereux, B., Biskup, S., et al. (2005). Mutation in the neuronal voltage-gated sodium channel SCN1A causes familial hemiplegic migraine. *Lancet, 366,* 371–377.

Facchinetti, F., Sances, G., Borella, P., Genazzani, A. R., & Nappi, G. (1991). Magnesium prophylaxis of menstrual migraine: effects on intracellular magnesium. *Headache, 31*(5), 298–301.

Finsterer, J., Shorny, S., Capek, J., Cerny-Zacharias, C., Pelzl, B., Messner, R., et al. (1998). Lactate stress test in the diagnosis of mitochondrial myopathy. *Journal of the Neurological Sciences, 159*(2), 176–180

Frahm, J., Krüger, G., Merboldt, K. D., Hänicke, W., & Kleinschmidt, A. (1996). Dynamic uncoupling and recoupling of perfusion and oxidative metabolism during focal brain activation. *Magnetic Resonance Medicine, 35,* 143–148.

Gallai, V., Sarchielli, P., Coata, G., Firenze, C., Morucci, P., & Abbritti, G. (1992). Serum and salivary magnesium levels in migraine. Results in a group of juvenile patients. *Headache, 32*(3), 132–135.

Gallai, V., Sarchielli, P., Morucci, P., & Abbritti, G. (1993). Red blood cell magnesium levels in migraine patients. *Cephalalgia, 13*(2), 94–81; discussion 73.

Gallai, V., Sarchielli, P., Morucci, P., & Abbritti, G. (1994). Magnesium content of mononuclear cells in migraine patients. *Headache, 34,* 160–165.

Gerards, M., van den Bosch, B. J., Danhauser, K., Serre, V., van Weeghel, M., Wanders, R. J., et al. (2011). Riboflavin-responsive oxidative phosphorylation complex I deficiency caused by defective ACAD9: New function for an old gene. *Brain, 134*(Pt 1), 210–219.

Glover, E. I., Martin, J., Maher, A., Thornhill, R. E., Moran, G. R., & Tarnopolsky, M. A. (2010). A randomized trial of coenzyme Q10 in mitochondrial disorders. *Muscle and Nerve, 42*(5), 739–748.

Goda, S., Hamada, T., Ishimoto, S., Kobayashi, T., Goto, I., & Kuroiwa, Y. (1987). Clinical improvement after administration of coenzyme Q10 in a patient with mitochondrial encephalomyopathy. *Journal of Neurology, 234,* 62–63.

Goto, Y., Nonaka, I., & Horai, S. (1990). A mutation in the tRNA(Leu) (UUR) gene associated with the MELAS subgroup of mitochondrial encephalomyopathies. *Nature, 348*(6302), 651–653.

Grimaldi, D., Tonon, C., Cevoli, S., Pierangeli, P., Malucelli, E., Rizzo, G., et al. (2010). Clinical and neuroimaging evidence of interictal cerebellar dysfunction in FHM2. *Cephalalgia, 30,* 552–559.

Gu, T., Ma, X. X., Xu, Y. H., Xiu, J. J., & Li, C. F. (2008). Metabolite concentration ratios in thalami of patients with migraine and trigeminal neuralgia measured with 1H-MRS. *Neurological Research, 30,* 229–233.

Harno, H., Heikkinen, S., Kaunisto, M. A., Kallela, M., Häkkinen, A. M., Wessman, M., et al. (2005). Decreased cerebellar total creatine in episodic ataxia type 2: A 1H MRS study. *Neurology, 64*(3), 542–544.

Harrington, M. G., Fonteh, A. N., Cowan, R. P., Perrine, K., Pogoda, J. M., Biringer, R. G., et al. (2006). Cerebrospinal fluid sodium increases in migraine. *Headache, 46*(7), 1128–1135.

Hershey, A. D., Powers, S. W., Vockell, A. L., Lecates, S. L., Ellinor, P. L., Segers, A., et al. (2007). Coenzyme Q10 deficiency and response to supplementation in pediatric and adolescent migraine. *Headache, 47*(1), 73–80.

Hoult, D. I., Busby, S. J., Gadian, D. G., Radda, G. K., Richards, R. E., & Seeley, P. J. (1974). Observation of tissue metabolites using 31P nuclear magnetic resonance. *Nature, 252*(5481), 285–287.

Jackmann, L. M., & Sternhell, S. (1969). *Application of nuclear magnetic resonance spectroscopy in organic chemistry.* New York: Academic Press.

Jain, A. C., Sethi, N. C., & Balbar, P. K. (1985). A clinical electroencephalographic and trace element study with special reference to zinc, copper and magnesium in serum and cerebrospinal fluid (CSF) in cases of migraine. *Journal of Neurology Supplement, 232,* 161.

José da Rocha, A., Túlio Braga, F., Carlos Martins Maia, A., Jr., Jorge da Silva, C., Toyama, C., Pereira Pinto Gama, H., et al. (2008). Lactate detection by MRS in mitochondrial encephalopathy: Optimization of technical parameters. *Journal of Neuroimaging, 18*(1), 1–8.

Kabbouche, M. A., Powers, S. W., Vockell, A-L. B., LeCates, S. L., & Hershey, A. D. (2002). Carnitine palmityltransferase II (CPT2) deficiency and migraine headache: Two case reports. *Headache, 43,* 490–495.

Kemp, G. J., Taylor, D. J., Thompson, C. H., Hands, L. J., Rajagopalan, B., Styles, P., et al. (1993). Quantitative analysis by 31P magnetic resonance spectroscopy of abnormal mitochondrial oxidation in skeletal muscle during recovery from exercise. *NMR in Biomedicine, 6,* 302–310.

Kemp, G. J., Thompson, C. H., Barnes, P. R., & Radda, G. K. (1994). Comparisons of ATP turnover in human muscle during ischemic and aerobic exercise using 31P magnetic resonance spectroscopy. *Magnetic Resonance Medicine, 31,* 248–258.

Köseoglu, E., Talaslioglu, A., Gönül, A. S., & Kula, M. (2008). The effects of magnesium prophylaxis in migraine without aura. *Magnesium Research, 21*(2), 101–108.

Kruit, M. C., Launer, L. J., Ferrari, M. D., & van Buchem, M. A. (2005). Infarcts in the posterior circulation territory in migraine. The population-based MRI CAMERA study. *Brain, 128,* 2068–2077.

Kruit, M. C., Launer, L. J., Ferrari, M. D., & van Buchem, M. A. (2006). Brain stem and cerebellar hyperintense lesions in migraine. *Stroke, 37,* 1109–1112.

Kruit, M. C., van Buchem, M. A., Hofman, P. A., Bakkers, J. T., Terwindt, G. M., Ferrari, M. D., et al. (2004). Migraine as a risk factor for subclinical brain lesions. *Journal of the American Medical Association, 291,* 427–434

Kuwabara, T., Wanatabe, H., Tanaka, K., Tsuji, S., Ohkubo, M., Ito, T., et al. (1994). Mitochondrial encephalopathy: Elevated visual cortex lactate unresponsive to photic stimulation—a localized 1H MRS study. *Neurology, 44,* 557–559.

Leao, A. A. P. (1944). Pial circulation and spreading depression of activity in the cerebral cortex. *Journal of Neurophysiology, 7,* 391–396.

Levine, S. R., Helpern, J. A., Welch, K. M., Vande Linde, A. M., Sawaya, K. L., Brown, E. E., et al. (1992). Human focal cerebral ischemia: Evaluation of brain pH and energy metabolism with P-31 NMR spectroscopy. *Radiology, 185*(2), 537–544.

Littlewood, J., Glover, V., Sandler, M., Peatfield, R., Petty, R., & Rose, F. C. (1984). Low platelet monoamine oxidase activity in headache: No correlation with phenolsulphotransferase, succinate dehydrogenase, platelet preparation method or smoking. *Journal of Neurology, Neurosurgery, and Psychiatry, 47,* 338–343.

Lodi, R., Iotti, S., Cortelli, P., Pierangeli, G., Cevoli, S., Clementi, V., et al. (2001). Deficient energy metabolism is associated with low free magnesium in the brains of patients with migraine and cluster headache. *Brain Research Bulletin, 54,* 437–441.

Lodi, R., Kemp, G. J., Iotti, S., Radda, G. K., & Barbiroli, B. (1997). Influence of cytosolic pH on in vivo assessment of human muscle mitochondrial respiration by phosphorus magnetic resonance spectroscopy. *MAGMA, 5,* 165–171.

Lodi, R., Kemp, G. J., Montagna, P., Pierangeli, G., Cortelli, P., Iotti, S., et al. (1997). Quantitative analysis of skeletal muscle bioenergetics and proton efflux in migraine and cluster headache. *Journal of the Neurological Sciences, 146,* 73–80.

Lodi, R., Montagna, P., Cortelli, P., Iotti, S., Cevoli, S., Carelli, V., et al. (2000). "Secondary" 4216/ND1 and 13708/ND5 Leber's hereditary optic neuropathy mtDNA mutations do not further impair mitochondrial oxidative metabolism deficit due to 11778/ND4 mtDNA mutation. An in vivo brain and skeletal muscle phosphorus MR spectroscopy study. *Brain, 123,* 1896–1902.

Lodi, R., Montagna, P., Soriani, S., Iotti, S., Arnaldi, C., Cortelli, P., et al. (1997). Deficit of brain and skeletal muscle bioenergetics and low brain magnesium in juvenile migraine: An in vivo 31P magnetic resonance spectroscopy interictal study. *Pediatric Research, 42,* 866–871.

Lodi, R., Tonon, C., Valentino, M. L., Iotti, S., Clementi, V., Malucelli, E., et al. (2004). Deficit of *in vivo* mitochondrial ATP production in OPA1-related dominant optic atrophy. *Annals of Neurology, 56*(5), 719–723.

Lodi, R., Tonon, C., Valentino, M. L., Manners, D., Testa, C., Malucelli, E., et al. (2011). Defective mitochondrial ATP production in skeletal muscle from patients with dominant optic atrophy due to *OPA1* mutations. *Archives of Neurology, 68*(1), 67–73.

Macri, M. A., Garreffa, G., Giove, F., Ambrosini, A., Guardati, M., Pierelli, F., et al. (2003). Cerebellar metabolite alterations detected in vivo by proton MR spectroscopy. *Magnetic Resonance Imaging, 21,* 1201–1206.

Maesaka, H., Komiya, K., Misugi, K., & Tada, K. (1976). Hyperalaninemia, hyperpyruvicemia and lactic acidosis due to pyruvate carboxylase deficiency of the liver; treatment with thiamine and lipoic acid. *European Journal of Pediatrics, 122,* 159–168.

Magis, D., Ambrosini, A., Sandor, P., Jacquy, J., Laloux, P., & Schoenen, J. (2007). A randomized double blind placebo controlled trial of thioctic acid in migraine prophylaxis. *Headache, 47,* 52–77.

Majamaa, K., Finnilä, S., Turkka, J., & Hassinen, I. E. (1998). Mitochondrial DNA haplogroup U as a risk factor for occipital stroke in migraine. *Lancet, 352*(9126), 455–456.

Mathews, P. M., Andermann, F., Silver, K., Karpati, G., & Arnold, D. L. (1993). Proton MR spectroscopic characterization of differences in regional brain metabolic abnormalities in mitochondrial encephalomyopathies. *Neurology, 43*(12), 2484–2490.

Matthews, P. M., Ford, B., Dandurand, R. J., Eidelman, D. H., O'Connor, D., Sherwin, A., et al. (1993). Coenzyme Q10 with multiple vitamins is generally ineffective in treatment of mitochondrial disease. *Neurology, 43*(5), 884–890.

Mauskop, A., Altura, B. T., Cracco, R. Q., & Altura, B. M. (1995). Intravenous magnesium sulfate relieves cluster headaches in patients with low serum ionized magnesium levels. *Headache, 35*, 597–600.

Mauskop, A., Altura, B. T., Cracco, R. Q., & Altura, B. M. (1996). Intravenous magnesium sulfate rapidly alleviates headaches of various types. *Headache, 36*, 154–160.

May, A. (2006). A review of diagnostic and functional imaging in headache. *Journal of Headache and Pain, 7*, 174–184.

Mazzotta, G., Sarchielli, P., Alberti, A., & Gallai, V. (1999). Intracellular Mg++ concentration and electromyographical ischemic test in juvenile headache. *Cephalalgia, 19*(9), 802–809.

Montagna, P. (2000). Molecular genetics of migraine headache: A review. *Cephalalgia, 20*, 3–14.

Montagna, P., Cortelli, P., Monari, L., Pierangeli, G., Parchi, P., Lodi, R., et al. (1994). 31P-magnetic resonance spectroscopy in migraine without aura. *Neurology, 44*, 666–669.

Montagna, P., Lodi, R., Cortelli, P., Pierangeli, G., Iotti, S., Cevoli, S., et al. (1997). Phosphorus magnetic resonance spectroscopy in cluster headache. *Neurology, 48*, 113–118.

Montagna, P., Sacquegna, T., Martinelli, P., Cortelli, P., Bresolin, N., Moggio, M., et al. (1988). Mitochondrial abnormalities in migraine. Preliminary findings. *Headache, 28*, 477–480.

Moskowitz, M. A., Nozaki, K., & Kraig, R. P. (1993). Neocortical spreading depression provokes the expression of c-fos protein-like immunoreactivity within trigeminal nucleus caudalis via trigeminovascular mechanisms. *Journal of Neuroscience, 13*(3), 1167–1177.

Napolitano, A., Salvetti, S., Vista, M., Lombardi, V., Siciliano, G., & Giraldi, C. (2000). Long-term treatment with idebenone and riboflavin in a patient with MELAS. *Neurological Sciences, 21*(5 Suppl), S981–S982.

Ogasahara, S., Yorifuji, S., Nishikawa, Y., Takahashi, M., Wada, K., Hazama, T., et al. (1985). Improvement of abnormal pyruvate metabolism and cardiac conduction defect with coenzyme Q10 in Kearns–Sayre syndrome. *Neurology, 35*, 372–377.

Okada, H., Araga, S., Takeshima, T., & Nakashima, K. (1998). Plasma lactic acid and pyruvic levels in migraine and tension-type headache. *Headache, 38*, 39–42.

Ophoff, R. A., Terwindt, G. M., Vergouwe, M. N., van Eijk, R., Oefner, P. J., Hoffman, S. M., et al. (1996). Familial hemiplegic migraine and episodic ataxia type-2 are caused by mutations in the Ca2+ channel gene CACNL1A4. *Cell, 87*(3), 543–552.

Peikert, A., Wilimzig, C., & Kohne-Volland, R. (1996). Prophylaxis of migraine with oral magnesium: Results from a prospective, multi-center, placebo-controlled and double-blind randomized study. *Cephalalgia, 16*, 257–263.

Penn, A. M. W., Lee, J. W. K., Thuillier, P., Wagner, M., Maclure, K. M., Menard, M. R., et al. (1992). MELAS syndrome with mitochondrial tRNALeu(UUR) mutation: Correlation of clinical state, nerve conduction, and muscle 31P magnetic resonance spectroscopy during treatment with nicotinamide and riboflavin. *Neurology, 42*, 2147–2152.

Pfaffenrath, V., Wessely, P., Meyer, C., Isler, H R., Evers, S., Grotemeyer, K. H., et al. (1996). Magnesium in the prophylaxis of migraine—a double-blind placebo-controlled study. *Cephalalgia, 16*, 436–440.

Pierangeli, G., Cortelli, P., Cevoli, S., Albani, F., & Montagna, P. (2001). Creatine phosphate as a prophylactic agent in migraine. A pilot study. *Cephalalgia, 21*, 381.

Pietrobon, D., & Striessnig, J. (2003). Neurobiology of migraine. *Nature Reviews, 4*, 386–398.

Prescot, A., Becerra, L., Pendse, G., Tully, S., Jensen, E., Hargreaves, R., et al. (2009). Excitatory neurotransmitters in brain regions in interictal migraine patients. *Molecular Pain, 5*, 34.

Prichard, J. W. (1991). What the clinician can learn from MRS lactate measurements. *NMR in Biomedicine, 4*(2), 99–102.

Prichard, J., Rothman, D., Novotny, E., Petroff, O., Kuwabara, T., Avison, M., et al. (1991). Lactate rise detected by 1H NMR in human visual cortex during physiologic stimulation. *Proceedings of the National Academy of Sciences of the United States of America, 88*, 5829–5831.

Purcell, E. M., Torrey, H. C., & Pound, R. V. (1946). Resonance absorption by nuclear magnetic moments in a solid. *Physical Review, 69*, 37–38.

Ramadan, N. M., Halvorson, H., Vande-Linde, A., Levine, S. R., Helpern, J. A., & Welch, K. M. (1989). Low brain magnesium in migraine. *Headache, 29*, 416–419.

Reyngoudt, H., De Deene, Y., Descamps, B., Paemeleire, K., & Achten, E. (2010). (1)H-MRS of brain metabolites in migraine without aura: Absolute quantification using the phantom replacement technique. *MAGMA, 23*(4), 227–241.

Reyngoudt, H., Paemeleire, K., Descamps, B., De Deene, Y., & Achten, E. (2011). 31P-MRS demonstrates a reduction in high-energy phosphates in the occipital lobe of migraine without aura patients. *Cephalalgia, 31*(12),1243–1253.

Reyngoudt, H., Paemeleire, K., Dierickx, A., Descamps, B., Vandemaele, P., De Deene, Y., et al. (2011). Does visual cortex lactate increase following photic stimulation in migraine without aura patients? A functional (1)H-MRS study. *Journal of Headache and Pain, 12*(3), 295–302.

Rodriguez, M. C., MacDonald, J. R., Mahoney, D. J., Parise, G., Beal, M. F., & Tarnopolsky, M. A. (2007). Beneficial effects of creatine, CoQ10, and lipoic acid in mitochondrial disorders. *Muscle and Nerve, 35*, 235–242.

Ross, B. D., & Blum, S. (1999). Neurospectroscopy. In: J. O. Greenberg (Ed.), *Neuroimaging: A Companion to Adam's and Victor's Principles of Neurology* (2nd edition, pp. 727–774). New York:McGraw-Hill.

Ross, B., & Bluml, S. (2001). Magnetic resonance spectroscopy of the human brain. *Anatomical Record, 265*(2), 54–84.

Ross, B. D., Radda, G. K., Gadian, D. G., Rocker, G., Esiri, M., & Falconer-Smith, J. (1981). Examination of a case of suspected McArdle's syndrome by 31P nuclear magnetic resonance. *New England Journal of Medicine, 304*, 1338–1342.

Rozen, T. D., Oshinsky, M. L., Gebeline, C. A., Bradley, K. C., Young, W. B., Shechter, A. L., & Silberstein, S. D. (2002). Open label trial of coenzyme Q10 as a migraine preventive. *Cephalalgia, 22*, 137–141.

Rudkin, T. M., & Arnold, D. L. (1999). Proton magnetic resonance spectroscopy for the diagnosis and management of cerebral disorders. *Archives of Neurology, 56*, 919–926.

Sandor, P. S., Di Clemente, L., Coppola, G., Saenger, U., Fumal, A., Magis, D., et al. (2005). Efficacy of coenzyme Q10 in migraine prophylaxis: A randomized controlled trial. *Neurology, 64*, 713–715.

Sandor, P. S., Dydak, U., Schoenen, J., Kollias, S. S., Hess, K., Boesiger, P., et al. (2005). MR-spectroscopic imaging during visual stimulation in subgroups of migraine with aura. *Cephalalgia, 25,* 507–518.

Sandor, P. S., Mascia, A., Seidel, L., de Pasqua, V., & Schoenen, J. (2001). Subclinical cerebellar impairment in the common types of migraine: A three-dimensional analysis of reaching movements. *Annals of Neurology, 49,* 668–672.

Sangiorgi, S., Mochi, M., Riva, R., Cortelli, P., Monari, L., Pierangeli, G., et al. (1994). Abnormal platelet mitochondrial function in patients affected by migraine with and without aura. *Cephalalgia, 14,* 21–23.

Sappey-Marinier, D., Calabrese, G., Fein, G., Hugg, J. W., Biggins, C., & Weiner, M. W. (1992). Effect of photic stimulation on human visual cortex lactate and phosphates using 1H and 31P magnetic resonance spectroscopy. *Journal of Cerebral Blood Flow and Metabolism, 12,* 584–592.

Sappey-Marinier, D., Vighetto, A., Peyron, R., Broussolle, E., & Bonmartin, A. (1999). Phosphorus and proton magnetic resonance spectroscopy in episodic ataxia type 2. *Annals of Neurology, 46*(2), 256–259.

Sarchielli, P., Costa, G., Firerize, C., Morucci, P., Abritti, G., & Galla, V. (1992). Serum and salivary magnesium levels in migraine and tension-type headaches. Results in a group of adult patients. *Cephalalgia, 12,* 21.

Sarchielli, P., Tarducci, R., Presciutti, O., Gobbi, G., Pelliccioli, G. P., Stipa, G., et al. (2005). Functional 1H-MRS findings in migraine patients with and without aura assessed interictally. *Neuroimage, 24,* 1025–1031.

Schoenen, J. (1998). Cortical electrophysiology in migraine and possible pathogenetic implications. *Clinical Neuroscience, 5,* 10–17.

Schoenen, J., Ambrosini, A., Sándor, P. S., & Maertens de Noordhout, A. (2003). Evoked potentials and transcranial magnetic stimulation in migraine: Published data and viewpoint on their pathophysiologic significance. *Clinical Neurophysiology, 114*(6), 955–972.

Schoenen, J., Jacquy, J., & Lenaerts, M. (1998). Effectiveness of high-dose riboflavin in migraine prophylaxis. A randomized controlled trial. *Neurology, 50,* 466–470.

Scholte, H. R., Busch, H. F., Bakker, H. D., Bogaard, J. M., Luyt-Houwen, I. E., & Kuyt, L. P. (1995). Riboflavin-responsive complex I deficiency. *Biochimica Biophysica Acta, 1271,* 75–83.

Schulz, U. G., Blamire, A. M., Corkill, R. G., Davies, P., Styles, P., & Rothwell, P. M. (2007). Association between cortical metabolite levels and clinical manifestations of migrainous aura: An MR-spectroscopy study. *Brain, 130*(Pt 12), 3102–3110.

Schulz, U. G., Blamire, A. M., Davies, P., Styles, P., & Rothwell, P. M. (2009). Normal cortical energy metabolism in migrainous stroke: A 31P-MR spectroscopy study. *Stroke, 40*(12), 3740–3744.

Skinhoj, E., & Paulson, O. B. (1969). Regional blood flow in internal carotid distribution during migraine attack. *BMJ, 3,* 569–70.

Slater, S. K., Nelson, T. D., Kabbouche, M., Lecates, S. L., Horn, P., Segers, A., et al. (2011). A randomized, double-blinded, placebo-controlled, crossover, add-on study of CoEnzyme Q10 in the prevention of pediatric and adolescent migraine. *Cephalalgia. 31*(8), 897–905.

Soriani, S., Arnaldi, C., DeCarlo, L., Arcudi, D., Mazzotta, D., Battistella, P. A., et al. (1995). Serum and red blood cell magnesium levels in juvenile migraine patients. *Headache, 35,* 14–16.

Steele, P. E., Tang, P. H., DeGrauw, A. J., & Miles, M. V. (2004). Clinical laboratory monitoring of coenzyme Q10 use in neurologic and muscular diseases. *American Journal of Clinical Pathology, 121*(suppl), S113–S120.

Taylor, D. J., Fleckenstein, J. L., & Lodi, R. (2001). Magnetic resonance imaging and spectroscopy of muscle. In: G. Karpati, D. Hilton-Jones, & R. C. Griggs (Eds.), *Disorders of voluntary muscle* (7th ed., pp. 319–346). Cambridge: Cambridge University Press.

Taylor, D. J., Kemp, G. J., & Radda, G. K. (1994). Bioenergetics of skeletal muscle in mitochondrial myopathy. *Journal of the Neurological Sciences, 127,* 198–206.

Thomas, J., Thomas, E., & Tomb, E. (1992). Serum and erythrocyte magnesium concentrations and migraine. *Magnesium Research, 5,* 127–130.

Tracey, I., & Dunckley, P. (2004). Importance of anti- and pro-nociceptive mechanisms in human disease. *Gut, 53,* 1553–1555.

Uncini, A., Lodi, R., Di Muzio, A., Silvestri, G., Servidei, S., Lugaresi, A., et al. (1995). Abnormal brain and muscle energy metabolism shown by 31P-MRS in familial hemiplegic migraine. *Journal of the Neurological Sciences, 129*(2), 214–222.

Valet, M., Sprenger, T., Boecker, H., Willoch, F., Rummeny, E., Conrad, B., et al (2004). Distraction modulates connectivity of the cingulo-frontal cortex and the midbrain during pain—an fMRI analysis. *Pain, 109,* 399–408.

Wanic-Kossowska, M. (1997). Protective role of carnitine in acetate metabolism of patients with uremia treated by hemodialysis. *Polskie archiwum medycyny wewnetrznej, 97,* 534–540.

Watanabe, H., Kuwabara, T., Ohkubo, M., Tsuji, S., & Yuasa, T. (1996). Elevation of cerebral lactate detected by localized 1H-magnetic resonance spectroscopy in migraine during the interictal period. *Neurology, 47,* 1093–1095.

Weiller, C., May, A., Limmoroth, V., Limmroth, V., Jüptner, M., Kaube, H., Schayck, R.V., et al. (1995). Brain stem activation in spontaneous human migraine attacks. *Nature Medicine, 1,* 658–660.

Welch, K. M. (2005). Brain hyperexcitability: The basis for antiepileptic drugs in migraine prevention. *Headache, 45*(Suppl 1), S25–S32.

Welch, K. M. A. (2003). Contemporary concepts of migraine pathogenesis. *Neurology, 61*(Suppl 4), S2–S8.

Welch, K. M., Levine, S. R., D'Andrea, G., & Helpern, J. A. (1988). Brain pH in migraine: an in vivo phosphorus-31 magnetic resonance spectroscopy study. *Cephalalgia, 8,* 273–227.

Welch, K. M., Levine, S. R., D'Andrea, G., Schultz, L. R., & Helpern, J. A. (1989). Preliminary observations on brain energy metabolism in migraine studied by in vivo phosphorus 31 NMR spectroscopy. *Neurology, 39,* 538–541.

Welch, K. M., & Ramadan, N. M. (1995). Mitochondria, magnesium and migraine. *Journal of the Neurological Sciences, 134*(12), 9–14.

Yoshida, I., Sweetman, L., Kulovich, S., Nyhan, W. L., & Robinson, B. H. (1990). Effect of lipoic acid in a patient with defective activity of pyruvate dehydrogenase, 2-oxoglutarate dehydrogenase, and branched-chain keto acid dehydrogenase. *Pediatric Research, 27*(1), 75–79.

24 Visual Aura

NOUCHINE HADJIKHANI AND MAURICE B. VINCENT

"The process which precedes the headache of migraine is very mysterious, whether it is referred to the eye or the arm; there is a process of intense activity which seems to spread, like the ripples in a pond into which a stone is thrown. But the activity is slow, deliberate, occupying twenty minutes or so in passing through the centre affected." —Sir William Richard Gowers. (1906). *Clinical lectures on the borderland of epilepsy III – migraine. The British Medical Journal, Dec 8, 1617–1622.*

INTRODUCTION

Migraine is a complex neurological disorder. Although headache stands out as its most obvious manifestation, several aura symptoms, usually preceding the typical headache phase, may occur. The most frequent aura type is visual, characterized mostly by flashes of light or typically bright zigzag, horseshoe-shaped expanding visual perceptions (Cologno et al., 1998). Patients may experience diverse visual (Golden, 1979; Lendvai et al., 1999; Lewis et al., 1989; Lippman, 1952; Mattsson & Lundberg, 1999; Queiroz, et al., 1997) as well as sensory (Jensen et al., 1986), motor (Estevez & Gardner, 2004; Ophoff et al., 1997; Thomsen & Olesen, 2004), or language disturbances (Vincent & Hadjikhani, 2007), isolated or in various combinations. The way the multitude of neurological dysfunctions manifests during aura indicates that the cerebral cortex is most likely the center of such manifestations. When multiple symptoms are present, their progressive and building-up nature demonstrates that the cerebral cortex is pivotal in aura pathophysiology. The spreading nature of visual and sensory symptoms, which respects functional somatotopy, fits with a cortical origin. Clinical and experimental evidence (Lauritzen, 2001; Leão & Morison, 1945; Milner, 1958) suggests that aura is the symptomatic counterpart of cortical spreading depression (CSD) (Leão, 1944b). Since the majority of migraine auras are visual, the occipital cortex appears as the area where most of them would start, and therefore consists of a natural target for functional neuroimaging approaches.

THE VISUAL AURA

The typical teichopsia (τειχος, town wall; ooΨις vision) starts as a grayish spot somewhere in the visual field and expands during the following 5 to 20 minutes or so, edged by a bright horseshoe-shaped zigzag group of lines, and disappearing usually within 60 minutes (Richards, 1971). The disturbance starts at the center or, more frequently, paracentrally to the focus of vision, and shortly after, the perception starts to shine and expands to the periphery, becoming brighter as it proceeds. The front of this spreading abnormality consists of positive visual phenomena, such as bright, glowing lines constituting the so-called fortification spectrum, as named by John Fothergill. Sometimes a complex interlacement of lines may occur, resembling a "chevaux de frises" in the opinion of Gowers (Plant, 1986). The angles between these zigzag lines are not serendipitous and seem to follow a particular trend based on visual physiology. Richards, observing patterns obtained from sketches drawn by his migrainous wife, estimated the inner angle of the zigzag serrations as 45 degrees close to the center, increasing up to 70 degrees at the periphery. He suggested that this pattern is caused by the spatial layout of a specific type of neuron in the visual cortex specialized in detecting edges with a particular orientation (Richards, 1971). This expanding visual abnormality may be followed by a bean-shaped loss of visual acuity, a scotoma that blocks vision and impedes activities such as driving or reading. In contrast to the spreading front of bright teichopsias, this hemianoptic homonymous scotoma is a negative phenomenon.

Apart from the more typical and frequent visual aura, a large number of variations have been described, including visual noise (or TV noise), the frequently reported visual illusions similar to looking through heat rising from the asphalt, bright-colored spots, and distortions of perception. Complex illusions, such as lilliputian (objects being smaller) and Brobdingnagian (objects in colossal sizes) vision, zoom misperception independently of size, and misinterpretations of distances and mosaic vision, among other changes, may occur in the so-called Alice in

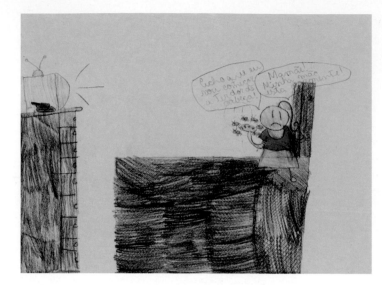

FIGURE 24–1 *Drawing of an aura by a 9-year-old girl with migraine. Her sad face indicates sufferance; the relative proportion of her size as compared to the furniture denotes her perception of being too small (microsomatognosia); and the insects around her right hand indicate paraesthesia. The texts say, "I think a headache will start" and "Mom, my hand is numb."*

Wonderland syndrome (Evans & Rolak, 2004; Golden, 1979; Lippman, 1953; Sacks, 1999). Body image misperceptions, such as having the sensation of being too tall or too small, or as if a vertical line separates the body in two halves, or the false impression of movements going too fast or too slowly, are further examples of migraine visual auras (Evans & Rolak, 2004; Golden, 1979; Lippman, 1952; Sacks, 1999). Figure 24–1 illustrates the perception of complex aura symptoms by a young girl.

Visual agnosias, characterized by difficulty in recognizing faces or objects (Vincent & Hadjikhani, 2007), have also been described. Sensations such as anxiety and strange feelings such as being separated from one's own body can also be considered under the category of migraine aura. A recent survey of 143 patients with migraine, which specifically targeted rare or strange symptoms, revealed that close to 50% of patients considered as migraineurs without aura were in fact experiencing abnormalities associated with higher tier areas related to migraine attack (face and color recognition difficulties, language and memory abnormalities, irritability, sleep disturbance) (Vincent & Hadjikhani, 2007). The complexity of these descriptions indicate that aura resides in a dysfunctional visual cortex, which produces both positive and negative symptoms in functionally distinct areas.

The visual cortex occupies a large part of the brain, and this may be one of the reasons why so many auras seem to be of a visual nature. The relatively greater density of neurons at the visual cortex may also justify a lower threshold for CSD in this part of the cortex, as suggested by Leão himself:

It seems well established that an essential part of the mechanism of SD is transmission of a disturbance of cell membrane function, from one cell to its neighbours, by diffusion of substances in the extracellular fluid. Therefore, close proximity of the cells certainly facilitates SD. The density of packing of the cells varies with the region of cortex, and is by far highest in visual area. Thus, one would expect this area to be the most liable to suffer from SD, and in fact visual symptoms are the most frequent in the migraine aura. They may be the only symptoms (SD restricted to the visual area), and if they are not the only ones, they most often precede the other symptoms (SD originated in the visual area and propagated to other areas). (Leao, 1987)

A number of other types of auras are described by patients, including somatosensory or aphasic auras. However, other parts of the brain may be less prone as compared to the occipital cortex to revert into symptoms of the pathophysiological processes typical of migraine aura. In such places, symptoms may be much more subtle, or even go unnoticed. For example, some patients may describe auditory (buzzes, modulation of sounds) and olfactory misperceptions (strange smells), as well as changes in reasoning or thoughts.

Many migraineurs describe similar behavior of their visual aura, with a progression reminiscent of the cortical representation of the visual field. This is the reason why a closer look at the retinotopic organization in participants with migraine aura and visual brain activation during the subjective experience of aura may reveal more about the pathophysiology of aura.

VISUAL CORTEX: RETINOTOPIC ORGANIZATION

Neurons in the visual cortex are organized spatially to reflect the visual space, in an orderly arrangement. The visual system is composed of the primary visual cortex (also known as striate cortex, V1, area 17, Brodmann area 17) and several so-called extrastriate areas (including V2, V3, V3A, V4v, V6, V7, V8, LOC, and MT), every one with specific functions in visual processing, such as motion, color, etc. Each visual area contains a map of the visual field, with a specific topographic organization. Retinotopic boundaries define areas of the early-tier areas of the visual cortex (e.g., the vertical meridian defines the border between V1 and V2). Maps of the visual field can be defined in terms of eccentricity (distance from the center of the visual field) and polar angle (representation of the lower or higher visual quarter-field).

Foveal regions of the visual field are represented at the occipital pole, while peripheral regions are represented more anteriorly, along the calcarine sulcus. This anatomo-functional structure is particularly important for the understanding of visual aura from the neuroimaging perspective, as the aura description echoes precisely the anatomical evolvement. More cortex is devoted to the central 1.3 degrees (fovea)—a phenomenon known as the cortical magnification factor. There is a continuous representation of the visual field from central to peripheral location, and the representation of eccentricity (distance from the center of gaze) is typically investigated with the use of a constantly expanding, phase-encoded wave traveling from the center to the periphery of the visual field. This type of stimulus elicits periodic excitation at the dilation frequency at each point of the cortical retinotopic map (Sereno et al., 1995). It is important to note that while all the lower tier visual areas have a continuous foveal representation at the occipital pole, a number of other areas (V3A, V7, V8, and MT) have their own foveal representation situated elsewhere in the cortex.

CORTICAL SPREADING DEPRESSION AND ITS ROLE IN MIGRAINE AURA IMAGING

CSD is a neurophysiological phenomenon characterized by a self-propagating wave of neuronal hyperexcitability followed by a temporary hypoexcitability, firstly identified in the rabbit cerebral cortex by Leão (1944a). CSD propagates at a rate of 2 to 3 mm/min in all directions through the gray matter. This phenomenon is widespread in nature, being present in many areas of the nervous system of several vertebrates, including humans (Gorji et al., 2001; Strong et al., 2002). The most characteristic electrophysiological feature of CSD is a direct current (DC) triphasic potential transient shift, which begins by a relatively small positive component, followed first by a 30- to 50-second negative wave of 5 to 20 mV, and finally by a

positive wave of smaller amplitude and longer duration. A depression of normal neuronal activity appears with the onset of the negative slow-voltage shift and persists for several minutes. This phenomenon reflects a dramatic ion distribution change and an intense tissue activity. K^+ and H^+ are released from the cells, exchanged by Na^+, Ca^{2+}, Cl^-, and water. As a consequence, cells swell and the extracellular compartment volume decreases, with consumption of O_2 and glucose (Martins-Ferreira et al., 2000).

One of the first and most relevant developments about visual aura (VA) and its relationship with CSD came by the American neuropsychologist Karl Spencer Lashley[1] (Lashley, 1941). Recording his own VAs, Lashley showed that a small initial scotoma would start close to the macular area, within 1 degree adjacent to the foveal field, rapidly increasing in size and spreading toward the temporal field, although the opposite might well occur. The symmetrical nature of the scotoma led him to the conclusion of a cortical origin. From his several scotoma maps, observing the shape, rate, distribution, and pace of scintillations in contrast with the retinotopic distribution of vision in the human cortex, Lashley concluded that "a wave of intense excitation is propagated at a rate of about 3 mm per min. across the visual cortex. This wave is followed by complete inhibition of activity, with recovery progressing at the same rate." This is in total accordance with the physiology of spreading depression, described 3 years later.[2]

One migraineur, P.V.V., has provided a rich series of these drawings that have been used to model aura progression in the cortex (Dahlem & Hadjikhani, 2009, and Fig. 24–2).

Interestingly, a computerized model of possible visual experiences secondary to a cortical spreading depression wave, assuming that a continuous excitation front would propagate across the V1 area at the occipital cortex, has shown a pattern rather similar to real VA drawings (Fig. 24–3) (Dahlem et al., 2000). The authors came to this finding based on the physiology of neurons in V1,

---

1. *It is remarkable that Lashley himself did not suffer from headache, as he said in his original paper: "the scotomas characteristic of ophthalmic migraine have been described by a number of investigators". Further down, it reads: "Over a period of years I have had opportunity to observe and map a large number of such scotomas, uncomplicated by any other symptoms of migraine", and finally "Except for a very slight torticollis associated with complete hemianopia, I have been unable to detect any additional symptoms during or after the scotoma."*

2. *Leão was not aware of Lashley's work when he described CSD and, with Morrison in 1945, first suggested a possible link between CSD and migraine (personal communication to Professor Péricles Maranhão-Filho, Universidade Federal do Rio de Janeiro).*

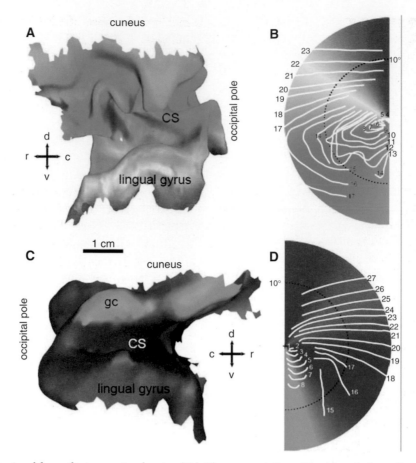

FIGURE 24–2 *Three-dimensional form of primary visual cortex (V1). The representation of the azimuthal coordinate of the two visual hemifields is given by the hue, value, saturation color model: (A) right V1, (B) left visual hemifield, (C) left V1, and (D) right visual hemifield. The current position of the visual field defect, occurring during two different migraine aura attacks and each exclusively in one visual hemifield, are indicated by white lines, with numbers denoting the time in minutes after onset. CS: calcarine Sulcus gc: gyral crown. From Dahlem, M. A., & Hadjikhani, N. (2009). Migraine aura: Retracting particle-like waves in weakly susceptible cortex. PLoS One, 4(4), e5007.*

considering their precise response to visual orientation and their organized retinotopy.

NEUROIMAGING OF THE AURA

Until recently, no imaging technology able to detect cortical abnormalities putatively related to visual aura was available. The development of positron emission tomography (PET), magnetic resonance with functional imaging, and new anatomic imaging approaches led to the possibility of looking upon migraine aura pathophysiology from new perspectives, although these new techniques added yet few if any subsidies to headache diagnosis for the practicing physician.

To understand the mechanisms behind VA and comprehend the meaning of the neuroimaging data, its clinical picture must be carefully considered (Schott, 2007). Descriptions of aura vary in many ways. The nature, duration, intensity, type, and frequency of visual auras are far from being uniform, even in the same subject. Some patients experience visual disturbances of such a small magnitude that they do not even bother mentioning them to the physician. On the other extreme, some may demand specifically for aura treatment, as the extremely unpleasant visual disturbances may impact them comparatively much more than the headache itself. Thus, this phenomenon must involve underlying mechanisms that do not lead to constant, stereotyped symptoms. Neuroimaging may therefore display changes not necessarily proportional to the clinical picture. Likewise, abnormalities may even be expected to occur in both migraine with aura and migraine without aura.

Neuroimaging of VA must be considered from three distinct viewpoints: permanent anatomical changes specific for migraine with aura, functional studies performed interictally, and functional studies aimed to image aura while it occurs. The first two approaches are covered elsewhere and will not be focused on in this section.

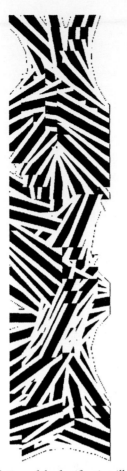

FIGURE 24–3 *Simulation of the fortification illusion. Multiple bars with white margins were plotted in the order of their dominance. The pattern resembles a snapshot of a fraction of the moving zigzag front. From Dahlem, M. A., Engelmann, R., Lowel, S., & Muller, S. C. (2000). Does the migraine aura reflect cortical organization?* European Journal Neuroscience, 12(2), 767–770. Copyright Wiley. *Reproduced with permission.*

CSD is coupled with metabolic and vascular changes. Leão firstly called attention to pial vascular changes in connection with CSD. He observed that a wave of marked arterial dilation in pial vessels parallels CSD over the affected hemisphere (Leão, 1944a). The so-called "spreading oligoemia," as described 40 years later by Olesen's group in migraineurs, also fits with the possible association between vascular changes and CDS (Olesen et al., 1981). These authors used regional cerebral blood flow measurement techniques in 254 areas of the cerebral hemisphere using ^{133}Xe during migraine aura induced by carotid catheterization. They found that changes in cerebral blood flow (CBF) start 5 to 15 minutes prior to aura symptoms, consisting of reduction in flow (hypoperfusion), starting at the posterior area of the brain. The oligemia, as named by the authors, spreads into the parietal and temporal lobes at a rate of 2 to 3 mm/min, reaching

a maximal decrease of CBF by 30% to 40% (Lauritzen et al., 1983).

Imaging VA therefore implies a series of provisos. Since recording and reproducing the actual personal visual experience of migraine aura is not yet possible, imaging would necessarily rather catch putative CSD waves as measured by its consequences in blood flow and/or metabolism. Whatever technology used, a spread with a pace similar to what has been recorded for CSD is necessarily required.

In migraine with aura (MWA), several studies have reported the presence of changes that can be related to CSD (Cao et al., 1999; Hadjikhani, et al., 2001) and supported the neurogenic theory of migraine, holding that a phenomenon similar to CSD underlies occipital lobe dysfunction during visual aura (Barkley et al, 1990; Cao et al., 1999; Hadjikhani et al., 2001; Kraig & Nicholson, 1978; Lauritzen, 1987, 1994; Lauritzen et al., 1982; Okada et al., 1988; Olesen et al., 1981; Welch et al., 1992). Accumulating data are converging to support increased susceptibility to CSD in migraineurs (for review, see Pietrobon, 2005; Pietrobon & Striessnig, 2003).

BLOOD FLOW

Concerning ictal blood flow studies, one of the most important contributions was performed in 1994 by Woods et al. (1994). In this case report, a 21-year-old woman, recruited as a normal volunteer for a PET study of cerebral blood flow, happened to be a migraine sufferer with an attack every 1 to 2 weeks, some of which were unilateral and associated with nausea, vomiting, or photophobia. Noteworthy is the fact that she had never had migraine with aura or neurological deficits. While undergoing 12 serial blood flow measurements with intervals of 15 minutes apart, a few minutes after the sixth measurement, she presented with a throbbing headache in the center of the back of her head, accompanied by nausea and photophobia. She denied aura symptoms, although during one measurement believed to the ninth, she was unable to focus her vision clearly. The headache, together with nausea, mild vertigo, and anorexia, persisted for the entire next day and gradually subsided. Bilateral decreases in blood flow became evident at the occipital regions in the first measurement after the headache onset. This decrease was shown in subsequent measurements to progress forward with time across the cortical surface at a relatively constant rate, sparing the cerebellum, the basal ganglia, and the thalamus, ultimately spanning the vascular distributions of four major cerebral arteries. The authors considered CSD as the most plausible explanation for their findings. The fact that this subject had no aura suggests that CSD may occur in migraine even without overt aura symptoms. It remains to be clarified, therefore, which mechanisms drive the conversion of CSD into symptoms.

Perfusion-weighted imaging (PWI) and diffusion-weighted imaging (DWI) have been used as techniques to approach circulatory changes associated with aura during migraine attacks. Four migraine with aura patients were examined ictally by Cutrer et al. (1998). The time span between aura onset and the data acquisition varied from 25 to 45 minutes. Scans showed mainly a decrease (16% to 53%) in cerebral blood flow (rCBF), a decrease (6% to 33%) in relative cerebral blood volume (rCBV), and an increase (10% to 36%) in the mean transit time (MTT). The apparent diffusion coefficient (ADC) increased in two, decreased in two, and was not available in the other two attacks. As the authors concluded, if ischemia is present, it is less severe or not persistent enough to cause whatever changes ADC abnormalities represent. The findings with such a new technology supported the circulatory abnormities detected previously.

Sanchez del Rio et al. (1999) also used PWI to study 19 migraine patients, 7 with aura, 6 of them scanned during 7 spontaneous visual auras within 31 ± 6 minutes of the attack onset. Perfusion deficits were noticed at the occipital cortex in all subjects contralateral to the visual field defect. The regional cerebral blood flow (rCBF) and rCBV decreased by 27% and 15%, respectively, whereas the MTT increased by 32%. After 150 minutes, however, there were increases in rCBF (+20%) and rCBV (+2%) and a reduction in MTT (−21%), suggesting a late hyperperfusion phase, contrary to the initial changes (Fig. 24–4). In one particular case, repeated measurements during four attacks suggested that the perfusion deficit evolves over time, reaching its peak during aura. Since the circulatory changes were not observed in any of the migraine without aura subjects, data suggest that the circulatory changes in these two forms of migraine do not reach the same order or magnitude.

Long-lasting VAs were also studied with the PWI and DWI techniques. Jager et al. (2005) studied two patients with persistent VA without infarction as defined by the International Headache Society under the code 1.3.5. The DWI and the ADC maps were not abnormal. The MTT maps and rCBVs did not vary and were symmetrical. These findings suggest that persistent visual changes in migraine, putatively related to prolonged auralike phenomena, do not lead to the same circulatory changes in the brain as detected by similar studies. It is also possible that the abnormalities were too small to be detected with the technology used.

FUNCTIONAL MAGNETIC RESONANCE IMAGING

The blood oxygenation level–dependent functional magnetic resonance imaging (fMRI-BOLD) technique was first used to address migraine and VA in 1999. Cao et al. (1999) visually stimulated 12 migraineurs (10 with aura) and 6 controls using a red-green checkerboard in an MRI scanner. In case of migrainous symptoms, subjects were instructed to inform the researchers immediately. Six of the 12 patients with migraine with aura developed headache, and 2 of those experienced visual changes together or right after the headache onset they described as atypical of their usual aura. In the beginning of the stimulation, fMRI activation over primary and association visual areas at the visual cortex were equal between controls and migraineurs, with the exception of one patient, who presented with headache immediately. The migraineurs who did not develop attacks kept an activation indistinguishable to controls, contrasting with suppression observed in previously activated pixels in six out of eight patients who developed headache, visual change, or both, occurring 4.6 $\pm$ 4.2 minutes after the stimulation onset. Interestingly, in five of these six patients, suppression was detected before headache. Both the movement of the suppression as it progressed along the gyri and the recovery of activation (or at least loss of suppression) at the end of the experiment were registered. The latter occurred in a timed and ordered way along the track of the original suppression wave. The suppression and recovery spreads differentiated patients with migraine who experienced headache and visual change from those who did not. The speed at which the suppression spread ranged from 2.9 to 6.0 mm/min, with a mean $\pm$ standard deviation (SD) of 4.1 $\pm$ 1.3.

Although in the majority of the cases the suppression was present on the same side of the headache, this proved not always to be the case. In fact, a common clinical situation is a disagreement between the side of the headache and the visual field affected by VA, suggesting that there is no obligatory correlation between the side CSD is detected and the occurrence of pain. In conformity with the study by Woods et al., the spreading suppression seemed to be associated with an initial activation of a migraine attack, regardless of the presence of aura symptoms. These data suggest that a CDS-like phenomenon does occur in migraine, that it is not necessarily related to the presence of aura, that it precedes symptoms in many cases, and that metabolic suppression is probably associated with its presence.

While an aura can be a good predictor that a headache may follow, it is very difficult to predict when an aura will start. Many migraineurs know of food or behaviors that may trigger an attack, but it is usually not possible to know

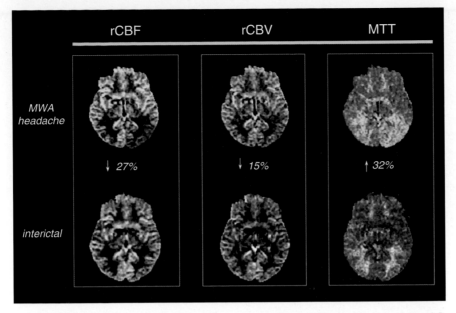

FIGURE 24-4 *Perfusion-weighted imaging during migraine, showing transient reduction of regional cerebral blood flow (rCBF) and regional cerebral blood volume (rCBV), accompanied by transient increase of meant transit time (MTT) (see also Sanchez del Rio et al., 1999). MWA, migraine with aura.*

exactly when it will start. The same goes for the premonitory symptoms, frequently detected by patients as a reliable sign of a coming migraine attack.

Hadjikhani et al. (2001) had the opportunity to collaborate with migraineurs who could reliably and quite precisely predict the occurrence of an aura. Anecdotally, in two cases aura triggering was associated with intense basketball playing. Although a link to basketball playing is not obvious, it may be related to the concomitant loss of electrolytes because of transpiration and very abrupt changes of visual information, in the context of a predisposition to migraine. One patient, P.R., agreed to try to induce a series of attacks. The scanning room was prepared to receive him and start acquiring imaging as soon as he would arrive—but before that the team went to the next-door gym with him, where P.R. played intense basketball for about 80 minutes. When he felt that this would be sufficient to induce an attack, the team went back to the scanner and started to acquire functional images. Alternate periods of radial checkerboard stimulation, known to activate the entire visual cortex, were presented in alternation with periods of black screen during which only a central small red fixation cross was present. P.R. was instructed to look at the stimuli and indicate by pressing the scanner squeeze-ball if/when he felt that an aura was starting, as well as when he felt that the aura had disappeared, and when the headache began. For safety reasons, a code was also defined to convey whether he was not feeling well and wanted to interrupt the scanning to get out. P.R. was able to induce two attacks in the scanner.

Two other patients, who were working in the building where the scanner was located, also were caught at the very beginning of an aura, but only in P.R. were the very first seconds of a visual aura propagating in the brain observable.

A number of other measurements had to be done prior to data interpretation. First, at the time, there was no report of visual response to an alternating checkerboard for a stimulation going for as long as 34 minutes, and responses needed to be proved to be stable interictally (Fig. 24-5).

Second, participants were asked to draw the progression of one or several of their auras. To make sure that angles could be calculated, they had to sit and remain at the same distance from the paper, and keep their eyes on a fixation cross at the center, while sketching the progression of the front of scintillations, indicating the time on each line of the sketch

Third, to study the relationship between subjective aura propagation and visual cortex organization, interictal data of the retinotopy of all participants were acquired.

The following observations were made (see Fig. 24-6):

1. Interictally, it was possible to stimulate the visual cortex for prolonged periods of time and not having either a drop in signal or the induction of an aura.
2. The retinotopic maps of all migraineurs were normal, comparable to other participants without migraine.

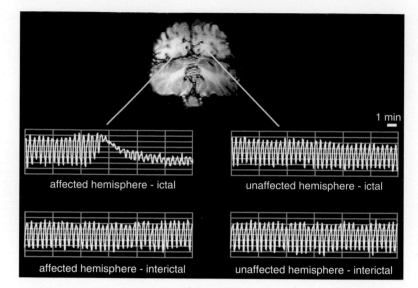

FIGURE 24–5 *Blood oxygenation level–dependent (BOLD) responses to a flickering checkerboard, ictally and interictally, in the affected and unaffected hemisphere. Adapted from Hadjikhani, N., Sanchez del Rio, M., Wu, O., Schwartz, D., Bakker, D., Fischl, B., et al. (2001). Mechanisms of migraine aura revealed by functional MRI in human visual cortex. Proceedings of the* National Academy of Sciences of the United States of America, 98(8), 4687–4692. *Copyright (2001) National Academy of Sciences, USA.*

3. During a migraine attack, at the beginning of the aura, profound changes were observed in the visual cortex on the side contralateral to the perceived aura. Those consisted of
   a. increased MR signal (5% ± 0.7%),
   b. accompanied by decreased amplitude, lasting 3.3 ± 1.9 minutes,
   c. followed by decreased baseline (5% ± 0.7%) and
   d. recovery of the decreased amplitude to 80% after 15 ± 3 minutes.
4. Those changes did not happen at the same time in the entire cortex: rather, they started at the occipital pole and spread anteriorly along the calcarine sulcus.
5. The procession of the changes mirrored the subjective progression of the aura and the retinotopic organization of the visual cortex.
6. The source of this signal change was not as expected in area V_1, but rather in area V3A, an area involved in the processing of coherent motion, in two attacks in participant P.R. An early activation of this area could explain the description of his aura given by P.R., who described it as "moving TV noise."

This value, the nature of the signal change with time, and its topography as contrasted with the patient visual perception make CSD the sole possible underlying mechanism. Furthermore, comparing the CSD-induced CBF changes over time obtained in rats with the MR signal

changes detected here showed remarkable correspondence between these two phenomena.

The same group searched for anatomical changes at different cerebral structures in migraine using MRI high-resolution cortical thickness measurement and diffusion tensor imaging (DTI) technology. They found that two cortical areas related with visual perception of motion—namely, areas V3A and MT+ located, respectively, in the transverse occipital sulcus and at the occipitotemporal region, between the lateral and the inferior occipital sulcus—are relatively thicker in migraineurs as compared to controls (Granziera et al., 2006, and Fig. 24–7). When the location of these cortical thickened areas was compared with the cortical areas where the BOLD signal started to change in their previous study (Hadjikhani et al., 2001), it became clear that area V3A was functionally related with the aura (namely, CSD) start from the functional point of view, and was anatomically thicker from the structural perspective.

IMAGING OTHER AURAS

As indicated above, visual auras are not the only type of auras, and when asked specifically a lot of patients report symptoms in other modalities.

Vincent and Hadjikhani reported two patients with complex auras that seemed to indicate continuous involvement

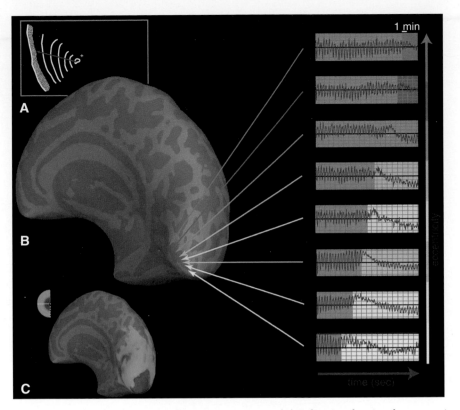

FIGURE 24-6 *Spreading suppression of cortical activation during migraine aura. (A) A drawing showing the progression over 20 minutes of the scintillations and the visual field defect affecting the left hemifield, as described by the patient (P.R.). The fixation point appears as a small white cross. The red line shows the overall direction of progression of the visual percept. The front of the scintillation at different times within the aura is indicated by a white line. (B) A reconstruction of the same patient's brain (P.R.), based on anatomical magnetic resonance (MR) data. The posterior medial aspect of the occipital lobe is shown in an inflated cortex format. In this format, the cortical sulci and gyri appear in darker and lighter gray, respectively, on a computationally inflated surface. MR signal changes over time are shown to the right. Each time course was recorded from one in a sequence of voxels that were sampled along the calcarine sulcus, in the primary visual cortex (V1), from the posterior pole to more anterior location, as indicated by arrowheads. A similar blood oxygenation level–dependent (BOLD) response was found within all of the extrastriate areas, differing only in the time of onset of the MR perturbation. The MR perturbations developed earlier in the foveal representation, compared with more eccentric representations of retinotopic visual cortex. This finding was consistent with the progression of the aura from central to peripheral eccentricities in the corresponding visual field (A and C). (C) The MR maps of retinotopic eccentricity from this same subject, acquired during interictal scans. As shown in the logo in the upper left, voxels that show retinotopically specific activation in the fovea are coded in red (centered at 1.5° eccentricity). Parafoveal eccentricities are shown in blue, and more peripheral eccentricities are shown in green (centered at 3.8° and 10.3°, respectively). From Hadjikhani, N., Sanchez del Rio, M., Wu, O., Schwartz, D., Bakker, D., Fischl, B., et al. (2001). Mechanisms of migraine aura revealed by functional MRI in human visual cortex.* Proceedings of the National Academy of Sciences of the United States of America, 98(8), 4687–4692. Copyright (2001) National Academy of Sciences, USA.

of different brain areas. Unfortunately, no data are available about brain signals during these episodes. However, the comparison of the progression of these auras with what is known of the functional organization of the human cortex is revealing of a probable continuous cortical involvement.

In one of the patients, a 31-year-old male migraineur since the age of 14, the complex aura would always begin with scintillations in the center of the visual field, expanding toward the periphery. The scintillations would then be followed by distorted vision, with dysmorphopsia and dyschromatopsia, followed by a difficulty to recognize specifically human faces. Twenty minutes later, paresthesia would appear in the middle of the forearm and expand toward both the face and the hand, followed by the leg, until a total hemianesthesia (with no paresia) would be present and persist for 2 to 3 hours. This would then be followed by aphasia, which could last up to 3 days, as well as ideational apraxia (Fig. 24–8). Interestingly, this patient reported that in spite of the fact that paraesthesia and visual disturbances could occur in either side from one attack to another, aphasia was present only when the paraesthesia would affect the right arm.

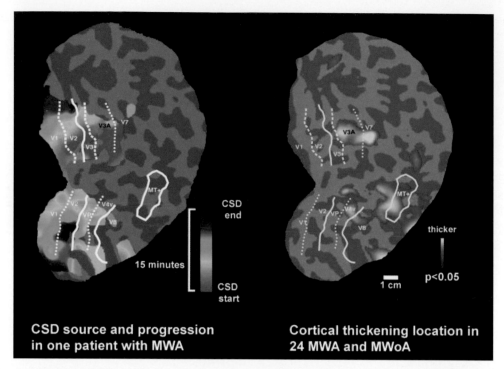

FIGURE 24-7 *Two representations of flattened maps of the right occipital cortex are shown, the gyri and sulci indicated as light and dark gray, respectively. The borders of retinotopic areas are indicated in white (horizontal meridians, solid lines; upper vertical meridians, dotted lines; lower vertical meridians, dashed lines). The image on the left is taken from a previous study that shows the progression of cortical spreading depression (CSD) during a visual aura. According to the color code, in that patient, aura started in area V3A. As an attempt to correlate structure and dysfunction, the image on the right is placed for comparison, showing the average map of the mean cortical thickness difference between 24 migraineurs and 15 matched controls, projected on the same brain, with the superimposed retinotopy for one participant. A clear correspondence can be seen between the area of CSD origin in V3A in the left image and cortical thickness difference in the right image. In addition, areas of thickening can be observed in visual area MT+. MWA, migraine with aura; MWoA, migraine without aura. From Granziera, C., DaSilva, A. F., Snyder, J., Tuch, D. S., & Hadjikhani, N. (2006). Anatomical alterations of the visual motion processing network in migraine with and without aura. PLoS Medicine, 3(10), e402.*

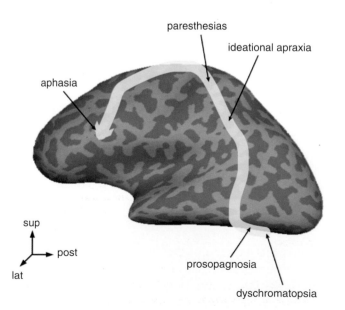

FIGURE 24-8 *The symptoms presented by a patient with complex aura are related to the successive effect on contiguous cortical areas (yellow arrow). Adapted from Vincent, M. B., & Hadjikhani, N. (2007). Migraine aura and related phenomena: Beyond scotomata and scintillations. Cephalalgia, 27(12), 1368–1377.*

CONCLUSIONS

Taken together, data obtained from different studies using diverse approaches seem to indicate that the human brain shows functional and structural abnormalities during aura that may be objectively measured. The changes detected so far indicate that CSD is the most probable phenomenon underlying the neuroimaging abnormalities related to VA. Several aspects, however, remain to be clarified. Even in the absence of overt clinical aura, spreading circulatory changes sometimes have been detected in migraine. Besides, similar changes at the "wrong hemisphere" have also been documented. This may indicate that CSD-like waves are probably more frequent in migraine than hitherto supposed, and that they do not imply necessarily the presence of aura symptoms. On the other hand, aura symptoms are frequently related to circulatory and metabolic changes compatible with CSD, as detected by many modern neuroimaging studies. Whether such changes are a consequence of an anatomically predisposed cerebral cortex or the structural changes observed in the brain are a consequence of a constant dysfunction of the cortex with frequent CSD waves remains as an unanswered question.

REFERENCES

Barkley, G. L., Tepley, N., Simkins, R., Moran, J., & Welch, K. M. (1990). Neuromagnetic fields in migraine: Preliminary findings. *Cephalalgia, 10*(4), 171–176.

Cao, Y., Welch, K. M., Aurora, S., & Vikingstad, E. M. (1999). Functional MRI-BOLD of visually triggered headache in patients with migraine. *Archives of Neurology, 56*(5), 548–554.

Cologno, D., Torelli, P., & Manzoni, G. C. (1998). Migraine with aura: A review of 81 patients at 10–20 years' follow-up. *Cephalalgia, 18*(10), 690–696.

Cutrer, F. M., Sorensen, A. G., Weisskoff, R. M., Ostergaard, L., Sanchez del Rio, M., Lee, E. J., et al. (1998). Perfusion-weighted imaging defects during spontaneous migrainous aura. *Annals of Neurology, 43*(1), 25–31.

Dahlem, M. A., & Hadjikhani, N. (2009). Migraine aura: Retracting particle-like waves in weakly susceptible cortex. *PLoS One, 4*(4), e5007.

Dahlem, M. A., Engelmann, R., Lowel, S., & Muller, S. C. (2000). Does the migraine aura reflect cortical organization? *European Journal Neuroscience, 12*(2), 767–770.

Estevez, M., & Gardner, K. L. (2004). Update on the genetics of migraine. *Human Genetics, 114*(3), 225–235.

Evans, R. W., & Rolak, L. A. (2004). The Alice in Wonderland syndrome. *Headache, 44*(6), 624–625.

Golden, G. S. (1979). The Alice in Wonderland syndrome in juvenile migraine. *Pediatrics, 63*, 517–519.

Gorji, A., Scheller, D., Straub, H., Tegtmeier, F., Köhling, R., Höhling, J. M., et al. (2001). Spreading depression in human neocortical slices. *Brain Research, 906*(1–2), 74–83.

Granziera, C., Dasilva, A. F., Snyder, J., Tuch, D. S., & Hadjikhani, N. (2006). Anatomical alterations of the visual motion processing network in migraine with and without aura. *PLoS Medicine, 3*(10), e402.

Hadjikhani, N., Sanchez del Rio, M., Wu, O., Schwartz, D., Bakker, D., Fischl, B., et al. (2001). Mechanisms of migraine aura revealed by functional MRI in human visual cortex. *Proceedings of the National Academy of Sciences of the United States of America, 98*(8), 4687–4692.

Jager, H. R., Giffin, N. J., & Goadsby, P. J. (2005). Diffusion- and perfusion-weighted MR imaging in persistent migrainous visual disturbances. *Cephalalgia, 25*(5), 323–332.

Jensen, K., Tfelt-Hansen, P., Lauritzen, M., & Olesen, J. (1986). Classic migraine. A prospective recording of symptoms. *Acta Neurologica Scandinavica, 73*(4), 359–362.

Kraig, R. P., & Nicholson, C. (1978). Extracellular ionic variations during spreading depression. *Neuroscience, 3*(11), 1045–1059.

Lashley, K. S. (1941). Patterns of cerebral integration indicated by the scotomas of migraine. *Archives of Neurology and Psychiatry, 46*, 259–264.

Lauritzen, M. (1987). Cerebral blood flow in migraine and cortical spreading depression. *Acta Neurologica Scandinavica Supplementum, 113*, 1–40.

Lauritzen, M. (1994). Pathophysiology of the migraine aura. The spreading depression theory [see comments]. *Brain, 117*(Pt 1), 199–210.

Lauritzen, M. (2001). Cortical spreading depression in migraine. *Cephalalgia, 21*(7), 757–760.

Lauritzen, M., Jorgensen, M. B., Diemer, N. H., Gjedde, A., & Hansen, A. J. (1982). Persistent oligemia of rat cerebral cortex in the wake of spreading depression. *Annals of Neurology, 12*(5), 469–474.

Lauritzen, M., Skyhøj Olsen, T., Larsen, N. A., & Paulson, O. B. (1983). Changes in regional cerebral blood flow during the course of classic migraine attacks. *Annals of Neurology, 13*, 633–641.

Leao, A. A. (1987). On the inferred relationship of migraine and spreading depression. In: Rose, F. C., *Advances in headache research* (pp. 19–24). London: John Libbey & Co.

Leão, A. A. P. (1944a). Pial circulation and spreading depression of activity in the cerebral cortex. *Journal of Neurophysiology, 7*, 391–396.

Leão, A. A. P. (1944b). Spreading depression of activity in cerebral cortex. *Journal of Neurophysiology, 7*, 359–390.

Leão, A. A. P., & Morison, R. S. (1945). Propagation of spreading cortical depression. *Journal of Neurophysiology, 8*, 33–45.

Lendvai, D., Crenca, R., Verdecchia, P., Redondi, A., Turri, E., Pittella, S., et al. (1999). Migraine with visual aura in developing age: visual disorders. *European Review for Medical and Pharmacological Sciences, 3*(2), 71–74.

Lewis, R. A., Vijayan, N., & Watson, C. (1989). Visual field loss in migraine. *Ophthalmology, 96*, 321–326.

Lippman, C. W. (1952). Certain hallucinations peculiar to migraine. *Journal of Nervous and Mental Disease, 116*(4), 346–351.

Lippman, C. W. (1953). Hallucinations of physical duality in migraine. *Journal of Nervous and Mental Disease, 117*(4), 345–350.

Martins-Ferreira, H., Nedergaard, M., & Nicholson, C. (2000). Perspectives on spreading depression. *Brain Research: Brain Research Reviews, 32*(1), 215–234.

Mattsson, P., & Lundberg, P. O. (1999). Characteristics and prevalence of transient visual disturbances indicative of migraine visual aura. *Cephalalgia, 19*(5), 479–484.

Milner, P. M. (1958). Note on a possible correspondence between the scotomas of migraine and spreading depression of Leão. *Electroencephalography and Clinical Neurophysiology*, *10*, 705.

Okada, Y. C., Lauritzen, M., & Nicholson, C. (1988). Magnetic field associated with spreading depression: A model for the detection of migraine. *Brain Research*, *442*(1), 185–190.

Olesen, J., Larsen, B., & Lauritzen, M. (1981). Focal hyperemia followed by spreading oligemia and impaired activation of rCBF in classic migraine. *Annals of Neurology*, *9*(4), 344–352.

Ophoff, R. A., Terwindt, G. M., Vergouwe, M. N., Frants, R. R., & Ferrari, M. D. (1997). Familial hemiplegic migraine: Involvement of a calcium neuronal channel. *Neurologia*, *12*(Suppl 5), 31–37.

Pietrobon, D. (2005). Migraine: New molecular mechanisms. *Neuroscientist*, *11*(4), 373–386.

Pietrobon, D., & Striessnig, J. (2003). Neurobiology of migraine. *Nature Reviews Neuroscience*, *4*(5), 386–398.

Plant, G. T. (1986). The fortification spectra of migraine. *BMJ*, *293*(20–27), 1613–1617.

Queiroz, L. P., Rapoport, A. M., Weeks, R. E., Sheftell, F. D., Siegel, S. E., & Baskin, S. M. (1997). Characteristics of migraine visual aura. *Headache*, *37*(3), 137–141.

Richards, W. (1971). The fortification illusions of migraines. *Scientific American*, *224*, 89–96.

Sacks, O. (1970). Migraine. London: Faber and Faber.

Sanchez del Rio, M., Bakker, D., Wu, O., Agosti, R., Mitsikostas, D. D., Ostergaard, L., et al. (1999). Perfusion weighted imaging during migraine: Spontaneous visual aura and headache. *Cephalalgia*, *19*(8), 701–707.

Schott, G. D. (2007). Exploring the visual hallucinations of migraine aura: The tacit contribution of illustration. *Brain (England)*, *130*(Pt 6), 1690–1703.

Sereno, M. I., Dale, A. M., Reppas, J. B., Kwong, K. K., Belliveau, J. W., Brady, T. J., et al. (1995). Borders of multiple visual areas in humans revealed by functional magnetic resonance imaging [see comments]. *Science*, *268*(5212), 889–893.

Strong, A. J., Fabricius, M., Boutelle, M. G., Hibbins, S. J., Hopwood, S. E., Jones, R., et al. (2002). Spreading and synchronous depressions of cortical activity in acutely injured human brain. *Stroke*, *33*(12), 2738–2743.

Thomsen, L. L., & Olesen, J. (2004). Sporadic hemiplegic migraine. *Cephalalgia*, *24*(12), 1016–1023.

Vincent, M. B., & Hadjikhani, N. (2007). Migraine aura and related phenomena: Beyond scotomata and scintillations. *Cephalalgia*, *27*(12), 1368–1377.

Welch, K. M., Barkley, G. L., Ramadan, N. M., & D'Andrea, G. (1992). NMR spectroscopic and magnetoencephalographic studies in migraine with aura: Support for the spreading depression hypothesis. *Pathologie-Biologie (Paris)*, *40*(4), 349–354.

Woods, R. P., Iacoboni, M., & Mazziotta, J. C. (1994). Bilateral spreading cerebral hypoperfusion during spontaneous migraine headache. *New England Journal of Medicine*, *331*, 1689–1692.

25 Functional Imaging of the Migraine Brain
New Insights into Brain Dysfunction

ERIC A. MOULTON

INTRODUCTION

Though neuroimaging in migraine research has largely focused on the symptomatic attack phase, the interictal phase poses distinct challenges and opportunities in developing treatments for migraine headache. Defined as the time period between migraine attacks, the interictal phase can present a significant burden to patients, including a state of heightened anxiety and impairment in performing ordinary daily tasks. Such symptoms are perhaps related to experimental findings of altered sensory, autonomic, and emotional processing in patients during the interictal phase. Note that the discussion of the interictal phase of migraine as presented in this chapter is separate from the phenomenon of auras that can precede migraine attacks.

Understanding of the migraine brain has advanced through imaging techniques such as positron emission tomography (PET), and more recently through the use of functional magnetic resonance imaging (fMRI). fMRI is a noninvasive method that has helped provide insight into the physiological mechanisms potentially behind these perceptual and systemic changes. Fundamentally, MRI measures the magnetic properties of the tissue being scanned. Since hemoglobin has different magnetic properties depending on its state of oxygenation, fMRI can measure regional changes in the ratio of oxygenated to deoxygenated hemoglobin. This hemoglobin-dependent signal is also known as the blood oxygen level–dependent (BOLD) signal. Fluctuations in the BOLD signal represent changes in the oxygen demand of neural tissues and provide an indirect measure of neural activation. Though functional imaging of the interictal phase of migraine is still in its infancy, current fMRI research offers exciting insights that bolster the existing foundation of data generated by clinical migraine research and animal studies.

INTERICTAL ALTERATIONS IN PERCEPTUAL, PHYSIOLOGICAL, AND PSYCHOLOGICAL STATES

Findings from a variety of studies suggest that the interictal migraine brain is changed relative to healthy subjects. Migraine patients have been shown to have altered brain morphology (DaSilva, Granziera, Snyder, et al., 2007; Granziera et al., 2006; Rocca et al., 2006; Valfre et al., 2008; Welch et al., 2001), brain vasculature (de Hoon et al., 2003), neurotransmitter levels (Prescot et al., 2009), and 5-HT$_{1A}$ receptor occupancy (Lothe et al., 2008). Gastrointestinal (Aurora et al., 2006; Boyle et al., 1990), autonomic (Melek et al., 2007; Peroutka, 2004), and psychological changes (Hamelsky & Lipton, 2006; Lanteri-Minet et al., 2005; Radat et al., 2009) have been found during the interictal phase.

Electroencephalography (EEG) studies also suggest that brain function is altered in the interictal migraine brain when considering evoked responses from visual (Afra et al., 2000; Backer et al., 2001; Chen et al., 2011; Coppola, Ambrosini, et al., 2007), auditory (Afra et al., 2000; Ambrosini et al., 2003; Wang et al., 1996), somatosensory (Lang et al., 2004), and nociceptive (noxious) stimuli (de Tommaso et al., 2005, 2007; Di Clemente et al., 2007; Katsarava et al., 2003; Valeriani et al., 2003). The latter EEG studies indicate that cortical habituation to noxious laser stimuli is reduced in interictal migraine patients, and that these patients have a reduced capacity for modulating pain through diffuse noxious inhibitory control (DNIC). Note that behavioral findings indicate that interictal migraine patients are not significantly different from healthy subjects in regards to heat pain thresholds (Burstein et al., 2000; Moulton et al., 2008) and suprathreshold pain ratings to noxious heat (Moulton et al., 2008) and to intranasal ammonia (Aderjan et al., 2010; Stankewitz et al., 2011).

THE NEUROLOGICAL BASIS OF INTERICTAL ALTERATIONS IN MIGRAINE

The predominant theories regarding migraine headache are also applicable to the mechanisms underlying the expression of interictal changes in migraine. Major mechanisms involve descending modulatory circuitry in the brainstem and changes in cortical excitability.

Brainstem Descending Modulatory Circuitry

The brainstem contains modulatory circuitry that can reduce the experience of pain in healthy subjects (Fields et al., 2006). These descending circuits consist of a variety of brainstem structures, including the periaqueductal gray, nucleus raphe magnus in the rostroventral medulla, and nucleus cuneiformis. In migraine, these structures are thought to inadequately inhibit pain-related signals conducted by trigeminovascular primary afferents to the trigeminal nucleus (Fig. 25–1). By failing to fully inhibit nociceptive processing at the first relay station in the trigeminal nociceptive pathway, nociceptive processing proceeds uninhibited into the thalamus and cortical processing areas related to pain.

These same modulatory brainstem structures can also facilitate nociceptive processing in healthy subjects. This suggests the possibility that migraine patients have dysfunctional brainstem circuits that may not just fail to inhibit pain, but may actually enhance the facilitation of pain. A dysfunction of descending modulation, whether it features a lack of inhibition or increased facilitation of pain, may cause downstream changes in cortical sensory processing that result in multisensory interictal changes. Ultimately, this disruption may lead to hyperexcitability along the trigeminovascular pathway (Burstein & Jakubowski, 2005; Lambert & Zagami, 2009) and has been hypothesized to be an underlying cause for migraine pathology (Bahra et al., 2001; Burstein & Jakubowski, 2005; Knight & Goadsby, 2001; Welch, 2003).

Structural changes in the brainstem support the notion that descending modulatory circuits are dysfunctional in migraineurs. The periaqueductal gray (PAG) in patients with episodic migraine contains high levels of nonheme iron accumulation, an indirect measure of neural dysfunction or damage (Welch et al., 2001). In migraine patients, increased gray matter density, an indication of neuronal loss and secondary reactive gliosis, was also found in the PAG as well as the dorsolateral pons (Rocca et al., 2006). Furthermore, the ventrolateral PAG in migraine patients without aura has been reported to exhibit decreased fractional anisotropy of diffusion, an indication of change in cellular consistency (DaSilva, Granziera, Tuch, et al., 2007).

Altered Brainstem Processing: New Insights into Nucleus Cuneiformis

Functional magnetic resonance imaging has identified physiological changes in descending brainstem circuitry in migraine patients during the interictal phase (Fig. 25–1). The nucleus cuneiformis (NCF), a brainstem structure that directly modulates nociceptive transmission neurons in the spinal cord, may be dysfunctional in interictal migraine patients. An fMRI study that compared brainstem responses to thermal stimuli found decreased NCF activation in interictal migraine patients relative to healthy controls (Moulton et al., 2008). NCF hypofunction was interpreted as a characteristic of migraine sufferers that could reflect a dysfunction of descending modulation. Note that this study did not directly test the hypothesis of impaired descending modulation, but the findings are suggestive. The NCF shares extensive connections with the PAG (Bernard et al., 1989; Zemlan & Behbehani, 1984), and the structures are cytoarchitecturally similar (Fields et al., 2006), suggesting that the structural changes detected in the PAG and surrounding brainstem regions may be related to the functional changes observed in the NCF. Functional brainstem abnormalities in these regions have also been observed during migraine attacks (Afridi, Giffin, et al., 2005; Bahra et al., 2001; Stankewitz et al., 2011; Weiller et al., 1995).

The etiology of these structural and functional changes in the brainstem is unknown, though it has been suggested to be a result of damage arising from a history of repeated migraine attacks (Kurth et al., 2005; Olsen et al., 1987; Rocca et al., 2000) but may be a result of a predisposed condition (i.e., genetic).

The Cerebral Cortex

Though sensitized trigeminovascular afferents and hypofunctional descending modulatory circuits represent the early stages of neural processing that participate in migraine, one cannot overlook the cerebral cortex, where the highest levels of sensory processing occur and where neural activity most closely parallels conscious perception. All the stages of nociceptive processing, including the fine-tuning of ascending trigeminovascular information, culminates into the final result of cortical activity. Interictal alterations in a variety of sensory processing modalities suggest the possibility of a "dys-excitable" brain (Coppola, Pierelli, & Schoenen, 2007; Stankewitz & May, 2009), in which a number of functional abnormalities may be preconditioned and show fulminate manifestation in the migraine state.

Structural changes relating to gray matter composition have been reported in the interictal migraine brain. In migraine patients with and without aura, cortical thickness

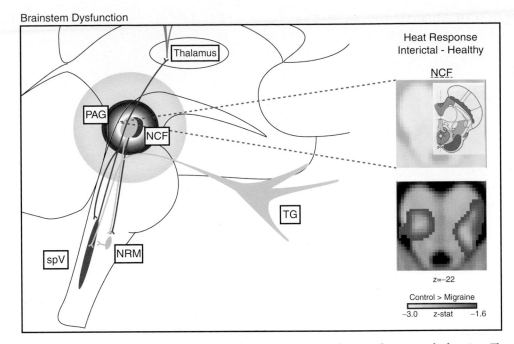

Brainstem Dysfunction

Heat Response
Interictal - Healthy

FIGURE 25–1 *Proposed neural mechanisms underlying interictal changes in migraine relating to brainstem dysfunction. The schematic highlights the hypothesized area of brainstem dysfunction (magenta halo), based on reported structural and functional abnormalities (DaSilva, Granziera, Tuch, et al., 2007b; Moulton et al., 2008; Rocca et al., 2006; Welch et al., 2001). Dysfunctional descending modulatory circuits result in enhanced nociceptive processing in the trigeminal nucleus as it receives trigeminovascular inputs from the trigeminal ganglion. Ascending and descending pathways are depicted in warm and cool colors, respectively. The anatomical cross-section of the brainstem on the right highlights the nucleus cuneiformis in green. The corresponding statistical parametric map indicates that interictal migraine patients have significantly decreased NCF responses to heat relative to age- and gender-matched controls. NCF, nucleus cuneiformis; NRM, nucleus raphe magnus; PAG, periaqueductal gray; TG, trigeminal ganglion; spV, trigeminal nucleus. Statistical map adapted from Moulton, E. A., Burstein, R., Tully, S., Hargreaves, R., Becerra, L., & Borsook, D. (2008). Interictal dysfunction of a brainstem descending modulatory center in migraine patients. PLoS One, 3, e3799. doi:10.1371/journal.pone.0003799.*

is increased in the primary somatosensory cortex (DaSilva, Granziera, Snyder, et al., 2007), as well as in visual areas in the occipital lobe related to motion processing (Granziera et al., 2006). Note that fMRI studies using visual stimuli indicate that the visual cortex in interictal migraineurs has enhanced reactivity that has been related to aura and motion processing (Antal et al., 2005; Vincent et al., 2003). Reductions in gray matter density that correlate with migraine frequency and disease duration have also been found in the frontal and temporal lobes (Rocca et al., 2006; Valfre et al., 2008).

Altered Cortical Processing: New Insights into Temporal Lobe

Functional neuroimaging has identified several cortical areas that show differential neural activity in interictal migraine patients and healthy controls (Fig. 25–2). Converging lines of evidence suggest that structures in the temporal lobe, in particular the temporal pole (TP) and the entorhinal cortex (EC), are sensitized in migraineurs even outside of a migraine attack (Moulton et al., 2011). Both of these areas show increased BOLD responses to noxious heat in migraineurs relative to gender- and age-matched healthy controls. TP dysfunction could perhaps relate to previous reports of impaired memory in interictal migraine patients (Calandre et al., 2002; Vincent & Hadjikhani, 2007), as the TP has been linked to the assignment of affective tone to short-term memories relating to pain (Godinho et al., 2006). In migraineurs in their interictal phase, the evidence of enhanced TP and EC sensitivity to noxious heat extends to their heightened functional connectivity with brain areas related to the processing of orofacial pain (Fig. 25–3), such as the trigeminal nucleus, insula, anterior cingulate gyrus, and primary somatosensory cortex. These temporal lobe structures with hypersensitivity to noxious heat in the interictal period also show increased activation during migraine attacks. Together, this evidence suggests that temporal lobe dysfunction in migraine patients may contribute to some of their perceptual changes.

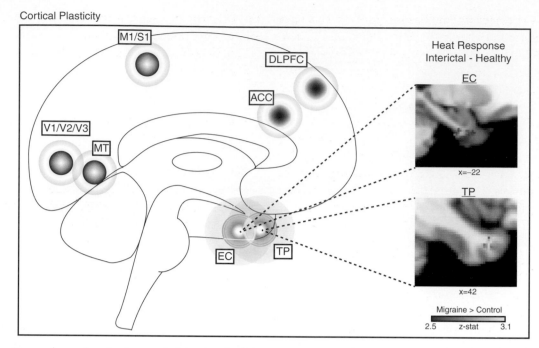

Cortical Plasticity

Heat Response
Interictal - Healthy

EC

x=−22

TP

x=42

Migraine > Control
2.5   z-stat   3.1

FIGURE 25–2 *Proposed neural mechanisms underlying interictal changes in migraine relating to cortical plasticity. The schematic highlights cortical structures in interictal migraine patients that have structural (white circles = cortical thickening; black circles = thinning) and functional abnormalities to painful stimuli (orange halos = hypersensitivity) (DaSilva et al., 2007a; Granziera et al., 2006; Moulton et al., 2011; Rocca et al., 2006; Valfre et al., 2007). Statistical parametric maps on the right indicate heightened responses to noxious heat in the temporal pole and entorhinal cortex (EC) of interictal migraine patients (Moulton et al., 2011). ACC, anterior cingulate cortex; DLPFC, dorsolateral prefrontal cortex; EC, entorhinal cortex; M1/S1, sensorimotor cortex; MT, middle temporal cortex; TP, temporal pole; V1/V2/V3, primary visual cortex, prestriate cortex, and third visual complex. Statistical maps were adapted from Moulton, E. A., Becerra, L., Maleki, N., Pendse, G., Tully, S., Hargreaves, R., et al. (2011). Painful heat reveals hyperexcitability of the temporal pole in interictal and ictal migraine states. Cerebral Cortex, 21, 435–448, by permission of Oxford University Press.*

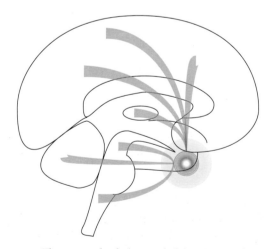

FIGURE 25–3 *The temporal pole (orange halo) in interictal migraine patients has enhanced functional connectivity with cortical areas related to experimental pain and multimodal sensory processing (Moulton et al., 2011). Functional connectivity refers to neural activation correlated with a seed region, in this case the temporal pole.*

Though a specific role for the TP in migraine is not clear, other studies support the hypothesis of hyperexcitable temporal regions in migraine: (a) in interictal migraine, higher order sensory processing related to the temporal lobe, including vision (Antal et al., 2005; Granziera et al., 2006; Harle et al., 2006) and odor (Demarquay et al., 2008), is disrupted; (b) increased temporal lobe activation during migraine attacks and aura has been observed in functional neuroimaging studies (Afridi, Giffin, et al., 2005; Afridi, Matharu, et al., 2005; Hall et al., 2004; Weiller et al., 1995); and (c) headache and epilepsy are comorbid, particularly in regards to temporal lobe epilepsy and migraine (Bigal et al., 2003; Castro et al., 2009; De Simone et al., 2007; Ito et al., 2003; Kors et al., 2004; Kwan et al., 2008; Lipton et al., 1994; Vanmolkot et al., 2003; Yankovsky et al., 2005), and resection of the anterior temporal lobe in epileptic patients with migraine headaches resolves their migraines in addition to their epilepsy (Yankovsky et al., 2005).

The TP is an associative multisensory area that encodes visual, auditory, and odor information (Asari et al., 2008; Bougeard & Fischer, 2002; Clarke et al., 2002; Moran et al., 1987; Olson et al., 2007). Odor hypersensitivity during the interictal period in migraineurs has been correlated with greater attack frequency, a greater incidence of odor-induced migraines, and visual hypersensitivity (Demarquay et al., 2006). In interictal migraine patients, a PET study found that olfactory stimuli produced significantly greater activation in the TP and the cuneus relative to healthy controls (Demarquay et al., 2008). This finding corresponds intriguingly with disrupted odor perception in temporal lobe epilepsy (Grant, 2005).

Both migraine attacks and aura have previously been reported to activate the temporal lobe (Afridi, Giffin, et al., 2005; Afridi, Matharu, et al., 2005; Hall et al., 2004; Weiller et al., 1995). These previous imaging reports have suggested that temporal lobe activations may relate to migraine patient reports of visual and auditory irregularities. Combined with recent neuroimaging findings regarding the TP and EC, hyperexcitability of the temporal lobe during both the interictal and ictal state may contribute to symptoms of migraine.

Patients with temporal lobe epilepsy often also suffer from migraine headaches (De Simone et al., 2007; Deprez et al., 2007). Also, these patients recover from their migraine symptoms following resection of the anterior temporal lobe or hippocampus to reduce epileptic seizures (Yankovsky et al., 2005). Both epilepsy and migraine have been associated with abnormal functioning within the pulvinar nucleus (Burstein et al., 2010; Moulton et al., 2011; Rosenberg et al., 2006), which has extensive functional connectivity with the temporal lobe in patients with epilepsy (Rosenberg et al., 2009) and migraine (Moulton et al., 2011). Such data suggest that the association between epilepsy and migraine may be due to abnormal temporal pole function.

The entorhinal cortex in migraineurs showed hypersensitivity to noxious heat as well. Part of the medial temporal lobe member system, the EC is connected structurally and functionally to the hippocampus (Eichenbaum & Lipton, 2008). In addition to memory processing, the hippocampus has also been related to the exacerbation of pain by anxiety (Ploghaus et al., 2001) and spatial navigation (Jeffery, 2007). Little is known about how the EC may play a role in migraine. However, electrical stimulation to areas proximal to the EC produces emotional, dysautonomic states known as "dreamy state syndromes" (Bartolomei et al., 2004). This suggests that the EC may be related to the storage and retrieval of multisensory information to and from parietal association areas (Sakai, 2003). Repeated migraine attacks may sensitize the EC.

The EC may also serve a role in the elaboration of the painful migraine state based on the experience of previous attacks (Casey & Tran, 2006), which may be related to Hebbian conditioning (Hebb, 2002).

CAVEATS IN THE NEUROIMAGING OF INTERICTAL MIGRAINE

Several considerations should be acknowledged and addressed in the neuroimaging of the interictal phase of migraine patients. The interictal phase should be clearly delineated beyond simply migraine attacks and "between attacks." Most clearly with migraine accompanied by aura, the period of time that precedes a migraine attack is different from a state of rest or reprieve, as implied by the interictal phase. With or without aura, premonitory symptoms can appear hours or days before a migraine attack, a phase known as prodrome. Similarly, the time following an acute attack (postdrome) may feature a gradual degradation of symptoms over the course of several days before returning to a migraine-free state. The variation in migraine attack frequency from subject to subject should be taken into consideration when determining an interictal phase clearly separate from the other phases with their associated symptoms. For example, pain thresholds are significantly lower 24 hours before an attack relative to the interictal phase (Sand et al., 2008). Indeed, recent neuroimaging evidence indicates that the spinal trigeminal nucleus may exhibit cyclic sensitivity to painful stimuli that can predict the timing of migraine attacks (Stankewitz et al., 2011).

Another important caveat is that brain physiology may be altered by the influence of migraine medications. Chronic medication usage could reduce cortical responsiveness to painful stimuli in migraine patients. Also, another uncertainty is the possibility that acute abortive migraine medications could have potential unknown long-term effects on nociceptive processing. Central processing of noxious stimuli in migraine patients could be altered by medications, such as triptans (De Felice et al., 2010), but the effects of such medications on fMRI activation remain unclear.

Implications for Future Studies

Findings of physiological changes in interictal migraine patients indicate that therapies and treatments for migraines can be evaluated between migraine attacks as well as during them. The above evidence suggests that the interictal phase is a state that is not directly comparable with migraine-free healthy subjects. As noted above, the migraine brain may differ from the normal brain for a variety of reasons. Some of the behavioral symptoms reported in migraine patients in the interictal phase may originate from neuroplastic changes driven by repeated migraine attacks. Genetic factors likely also play a role. Prospective and/or twin studies may help determine the extent of how these interictal changes may preexist or are acquired with migraine.

While the studies summarized above help us better understand the underlying dysfunctions of migraine during the interictal phase, much remains to be discovered. A relatively unexplored area of migraine research that is of vital therapeutic importance is the transformation of episodic migraine into chronic migraine. Using neuroimaging to track this transformation with regard to the development of interictal abnormalities in episodic migraine is in need of further study. The impact of dysfunctional brainstem descending circuits on pain modulation in migraine also remains to be determined. Also, the basis for the greater occurrence of migraine in females relative to males remains unknown.

Perhaps the biggest opportunity lies in the measurement of specific features of the interictal brain that can form the basis for the development of preventive migraine therapies. The study of migraine during the interictal phase has many logistical advantages over research geared toward migraine attacks. By considering the interictal phase rather than the attack, migraine patients will not have to be suffering from an attack when participating in a migraine study. Likewise, patients are more likely to volunteer for such studies, and their physicians are also more likely to encourage them to do so. As the focus of migraine research is to reduce the burden of the illness, the interictal phase of migraine is a window of opportunity to predict and retard impending attacks before they happen. A migraine headache is best prevented before it starts, and the interictal phase preceding an attack may hold the underlying precipitating mechanisms that lead to migraine. Such insights have significant and important applications in the ability to inhibit migraine progression or transformation (Lipton, 2009). These and other investigations regarding the interictal phase hold promise toward developing our understanding of the etiology of migraine and, in turn, the development of more effective ways to treat it.

REFERENCES

Aderjan, D., Stankewitz, A., & May, A. (2010). Neuronal mechanisms during repetitive trigemino-nociceptive stimulation in migraine patients. *Pain, 151*, 97–103.

Afra, J., Proietti Cecchini, A., Sandor, P. S., & Schoenen, J. (2000). Comparison of visual and auditory evoked cortical potentials in migraine patients between attacks. *Clinical Neurophysiology, 111*, 1124–1129.

Afridi, S. K., Giffin, N. J., Kaube, H., Friston, K. J., Ward, N. S., Frackowiak, R. S., et al. (2005). A positron emission tomographic study in spontaneous migraine. *Archives of Neurology, 62*, 1270–1275.

Afridi, S. K., Matharu, M. S., Lee, L., Kaube, H., Friston, K. J., Frackowiak, R. S., et al. (2005). A PET study exploring the laterality of brainstem activation in migraine using glyceryl trinitrate. *Brain, 128*, 932–939.

Ambrosini, A., Rossi, P., De Pasqua, V., Pierelli, F., & Schoenen, J. (2003). Lack of habituation causes high intensity dependence of auditory evoked cortical potentials in migraine. *Brain, 126*, 2009–2015.

Antal, A., Temme, J., Nitsche, M. A., Varga, E. T., Lang, N., & Paulus, W. (2005). Altered motion perception in migraineurs: evidence for interictal cortical hyperexcitability. *Cephalalgia, 25*, 788–794.

Asari, T., Konishi, S., Jimura, K., Chikazoe, J., Nakamura, N., & Miyashita, Y. (2008). Right temporopolar activation associated with unique perception. *NeuroImage, 41*, 145–152.

Aurora, S. K., Kori, S. H., Barrodale, P., McDonald, S. A., & Haseley, D. (2006). Gastric stasis in migraine: More than just a paroxysmal abnormality during a migraine attack. *Headache, 46*, 57–63.

Backer, M., Sander, D., Hammes, M. G., Funke, D., Deppe, M., Conrad, B., et al. (2001). Altered cerebrovascular response pattern in interictal migraine during visual stimulation. *Cephalalgia, 21*, 611–616.

Bahra, A., Matharu, M. S., Buchel, C., Frackowiak, R. S., & Goadsby, P. J. (2001). Brainstem activation specific to migraine headache. *Lancet, 357*, 1016–1017.

Bartolomei, F., Barbeau, E., Gavaret, M., Guye, M., McGonigal, A., Regis, J., et al. (2004). Cortical stimulation study of the role of rhinal cortex in deja vu and reminiscence of memories. *Neurology, 63*, 858–864.

Bernard, J. F., Peschanski, M., & Besson, J. M. (1989). Afferents and efferents of the rat cuneiformis nucleus: An anatomical study with reference to pain transmission. *Brain Research, 490*, 181–185.

Bigal, M. E., Lipton, R. B., Cohen, J., & Silberstein, S. D. (2003). Epilepsy and migraine. *Epilepsy Behavior, 4*(Suppl 2), S13–S24.

Bougeard, R., & Fischer, C. (2002). The role of the temporal pole in auditory processing. *Epileptic Disorders, 4*(Suppl 1), S29–S32.

Boyle, R., Behan, P. O., & Sutton, J. A. (1990). A correlation between severity of migraine and delayed gastric emptying measured by an epigastric impedance method. *British Journal of Clinical Pharmacology, 30*, 405–409.

Burstein, R., & Jakubowski, M. (2005). Unitary hypothesis for multiple triggers of the pain and strain of migraine. *Journal of Comparative Neurology, 493*, 9–14.

Burstein, R., Jakubowski, M., Garcia-Nicas, E., Kainz, V., Bajwa, Z., Hargreaves, R., et al. (2010). Thalamic sensitization transforms localized pain into widespread allodynia. *Annals of Neurology, 68*, 81–91.

Burstein, R., Yarnitsky, D., Goor-Aryeh, I., Ransil, B. J., & Bajwa, Z. H. (2000). An association between migraine and cutaneous allodynia. *Annals of Neurology, 47*, 614–624.

Calandre, E. P., Bembibre, J., Arnedo, M. L., & Becerra, D. (2002). Cognitive disturbances and regional cerebral blood flow abnormalities in migraine patients: Their relationship with the clinical manifestations of the illness. *Cephalalgia, 22*, 291–302.

Casey, K. L., & Tran, T. D. (2006). Cortical mechanisms mediating acute and chronic pain in humans. In: F. Cervero & T. S. Jensen (Eds.), *Handbook of clinical neurology* (pp. 159–177). Edinburgh, New York: Elsevier.

Castro, M. J., Stam, A. H., Lemos, C., de Vries, B., Vanmolkot, K. R., Barros, J., et al. (2009). First mutation in the voltage-gated Nav1.1 subunit gene SCN1A with co-occurring familial hemiplegic migraine and epilepsy. *Cephalalgia, 29,* 308–313.

Chen, W. T., Wang, S. J., Fuh, J. L., Lin, C. P., Ko, Y. C., & Lin, Y. Y. (2011). Persistent ictal-like visual cortical excitability in chronic migraine. *Pain, 152,* 254–258.

Clarke, S., Bellmann Thiran, A., Maeder, P., Adriani, M., Vernet, O., Regli, L., et al. (2002). What and where in human audition: selective deficits following focal hemispheric lesions. *Experimental Brain Research, 147,* 8–15.

Coppola, G., Ambrosini, A., Di Clemente, L., Magis, D., Fumal, A., Gerard, P., et al. (2007). Interictal abnormalities of gamma band activity in visual evoked responses in migraine: An indication of thalamocortical dysrhythmia? *Cephalalgia, 27,* 1360–1367.

Coppola, G., Pierelli, F., & Schoenen, J. (2007). Is the cerebral cortex hyperexcitable or hyperresponsive in migraine? *Cephalalgia, 27,* 1427–1439.

DaSilva, A. F., Granziera, C., Snyder, J., & Hadjikhani, N. (2007). Thickening in the somatosensory cortex of patients with migraine. *Neurology, 69,* 1990–1995.

DaSilva, A. F., Granziera, C., Tuch, D. S., Snyder, J., Vincent, M., & Hadjikhani, N. (2007). Interictal alterations of the trigeminal somatosensory pathway and periaqueductal gray matter in migraine. *Neuroreport, 18,* 301–305.

De Felice, M., Ossipov, M. H., Wang, R., Lai, J., Chichorro, J., Meng, I., et al. (2010). Triptan-induced latent sensitization: A possible basis for medication overuse headache. *Annals of Neurology, 67,* 325–337.

de Hoon, J. N., Willigers, J. M., Troost, J., Struijker-Boudier, H. A., & van Bortel, L. M. (2003). Cranial and peripheral interictal vascular changes in migraine patients. *Cephalalgia, 23,* 96–104.

De Simone, R., Ranieri, A., Marano, E., Beneduce, L., Ripa, P., Bilo, L., et al. (2007). Migraine and epilepsy: Clinical and pathophysiological relations. *Neurological Sciences, 28*(Suppl 2), S150–S155.

de Tommaso, M., Difruscolo, O., Sardaro, M., Libro, G., Pecoraro, C., Serpino, C., et al. (2007). Effects of remote cutaneous pain on trigeminal laser-evoked potentials in migraine patients. *Journal of Headache and Pain, 8,* 167–174.

de Tommaso, M., Libro, G., Guido, M., Losito, L., Lamberti, P., & Livrea, P. (2005). Habituation of single CO_2 laser-evoked responses during interictal phase of migraine. *Journal of Headache and Pain, 6,* 195–198.

Demarquay, G., Royet, J. P., Giraud, P., Chazot, G., Valade, D., & Ryvlin, P. (2006). Rating of olfactory judgements in migraine patients. *Cephalalgia, 26,* 1123–1130.

Demarquay, G., Royet, J. P., Mick, G., & Ryvlin, P. (2008). Olfactory hypersensitivity in migraineurs: A H(2)(15)O-PET study. *Cephalalgia, 28,* 1069–1080.

Deprez, L., Peeters, K., Van Paesschen, W., Claeys, K. G., Claes, L. R., Suls, A., et al. (2007). Familial occipitotemporal lobe epilepsy and migraine with visual aura: Linkage to chromosome 9q. *Neurology, 68,* 1995–2002.

Di Clemente, L., Coppola, G., Magis, D., Fumal, A., De Pasqua, V., Di Piero, V., et al. (2007). Interictal habituation deficit of the nociceptive blink reflex: An endophenotypic marker for presymptomatic migraine? *Brain, 130,* 765–770.

Eichenbaum, H., & Lipton, P. A. (2008). Towards a functional organization of the medial temporal lobe memory system: Role of the parahippocampal and medial entorhinal cortical areas. *Hippocampus, 18,* 1314–1324.

Fields, H. L., Basbaum, A. I., & Heinricher, M. M. (2006). Central nervous system mechanisms of pain modulation. In: *Wall and Melzack's textbook of pain.* New York: Elsevier, Churchill Livingstone.

Godinho, F., Magnin, M., Frot, M., Perchet, C., & Garcia-Larrea, L. (2006). Emotional modulation of pain: Is it the sensation or what we recall? *Journal of Neuroscience, 26,* 11454–11461.

Grant, A. C. (2005). Interictal perceptual function in epilepsy. *Epilepsy Behavior, 6,* 511–519.

Granziera, C., DaSilva, A. F., Snyder, J., Tuch, D. S., & Hadjikhani, N. (2006). Anatomical alterations of the visual motion processing network in migraine with and without aura. *PLoS Medicine, 3,* e402.

Hall, S. D., Barnes, G. R., Hillebrand, A., Furlong, P. L., Singh, K. D., & Holliday, I. E. (2004). Spatio-temporal imaging of cortical desynchronization in migraine visual aura: a magnetoencephalography case study. *Headache, 44,* 204–208.

Hamelsky, S. W., & Lipton, R. B. (2006). Psychiatric comorbidity of migraine. *Headache, 46,* 1327–1333.

Harle, D. E., Shepherd, A. J., & Evans, B. J. (2006). Visual stimuli are common triggers of migraine and are associated with pattern glare. *Headache, 46,* 1431–1440.

Hebb, D. O. (2002). *The organization of behavior: A neuropsychological theory.* Mahwah, NJ: Lawrence Erlbaum Associates.

Ito, M., Adachi, N., Nakamura, F., Koyama, T., Okamura, T., Kato, M., et al. (2003). Multi-center study on post-ictal headache in patients with localization-related epilepsy. *Psychiatry and Clinical Neuroscience, 57,* 385–389.

Jeffery, K. J. (2007). Self-localization and the entorhinal-hippocampal system. *Current Opinion in Neurobiology, 17,* 684–691.

Katsarava, Z., Giffin, N., Diener, H. C., & Kaube, H. (2003). Abnormal habituation of "nociceptive" blink reflex in migraine—evidence for increased excitability of trigeminal nociception. *Cephalalgia, 23,* 814–819.

Knight, Y. E., & Goadsby, P. J. (2001). The periaqueductal grey matter modulates trigeminovascular input: A role in migraine? *Neuroscience, 106,* 793–800.

Kors, E. E., Melberg, A., Vanmolkot, K. R., Kumlien, E., Haan, J., Raininko, R., et al. (2004). Childhood epilepsy, familial hemiplegic migraine, cerebellar ataxia, and a new CACNA1A mutation. *Neurology, 63,* 1136–1137.

Kurth, T., Slomke, M. A., Kase, C. S., Cook, N. R., Lee, I. M., Gaziano, J. M., et al. (2005). Migraine, headache, and the risk of stroke in women: A prospective study. *Neurology, 64,* 1020–1026.

Kwan, P., Man, C. B., Leung, H., Yu, E., & Wong, K. S. (2008). Headache in patients with epilepsy: A prospective incidence study. *Epilepsia, 49,* 1099–1102.

Lambert, G. A., & Zagami, A. S. (2009). The mode of action of migraine triggers: A hypothesis. *Headache, 49,* 253–275.

Lang, E., Kaltenhauser, M., Neundorfer, B., & Seidler, S. (2004). Hyperexcitability of the primary somatosensory cortex in migraine—a magnetoencephalographic study. *Brain, 127,* 2459–2469.

Lanteri-Minet, M., Radat, F., Chautard, M. H., & Lucas, C. (2005). Anxiety and depression associated with migraine: Influence on migraine subjects' disability and quality of life, and acute migraine management. *Pain, 118,* 319–326.

Lipton, R. B. (2009). Tracing transformation: Chronic migraine classification, progression, and epidemiology. *Neurology, 72,* S3–S7.

Lipton, R. B., Ottman, R., Ehrenberg, B. L., & Hauser, W. A. (1994). Comorbidity of migraine: The connection between migraine and epilepsy. *Neurology, 44*, S28–S32.

Lothe, A., Merlet, I., Demarquay, G., Costes, N., Ryvlin, P., & Mauguiere, F. (2008). Interictal brain 5-HT1A receptors binding in migraine without aura: A 18F-MPPF-PET study. *Cephalalgia, 28*, 1282–1291.

Melek, I. M., Seyfeli, E., Duru, M., Duman, T., Akgul, F., & Yalcin, F. (2007). Autonomic dysfunction and cardiac repolarization abnormalities in patients with migraine attacks. *Medical Science Monitor, 13*, RA47–RA49.

Moran, M. A., Mufson, E. J., & Mesulam, M. M. (1987). Neural inputs into the temporopolar cortex of the rhesus monkey. *Journal of Comparative Neurology, 256*, 88–103.

Moulton, E. A., Becerra, L., Maleki, N., Pendse, G., Tully, S., Hargreaves, R., et al. (2011). Painful heat reveals hyperexcitability of the temporal pole in interictal and ictal migraine states. *Cerebral Cortex, 21*, 435–448.

Moulton, E. A., Burstein, R., Tully, S., Hargreaves, R., Becerra, L., & Borsook, D. (2008). Interictal dysfunction of a brainstem descending modulatory center in migraine patients. *PLoS One, 3*, e3799.

Olsen, T. S., Friberg, L., & Lassen, N. A. (1987). Ischemia may be the primary cause of the neurologic deficits in classic migraine. *Archives of Neurology, 44*, 156–161.

Olson, I. R., Plotzker, A., & Ezzyat, Y. (2007). The enigmatic temporal pole: A review of findings on social and emotional processing. *Brain, 130*, 1718–1731.

Peroutka, S. J. (2004). Migraine: A chronic sympathetic nervous system disorder. *Headache, 44*, 53–64.

Ploghaus, A., Narain, C., Beckmann, C. F., Clare, S., Bantick, S., Wise, R., et al. (2001). Exacerbation of pain by anxiety is associated with activity in a hippocampal network. *Journal of Neuroscience, 21*, 9896–9903.

Prescot, A., Becerra, L., Pendse, G., Tully, S., Jensen, E., Hargreaves, R., et al. (2009). Excitatory neurotransmitters in brain regions in interictal migraine patients. *Molecular Pain, 5*, 34.

Radat, F., Lanteri-Minet, M., Nachit-Ouinekh, F., Massiou, H., Lucas, C., Pradalier, A., et al. (2009). The GRIM2005 study of migraine consultation in France. III: Psychological features of subjects with migraine. *Cephalalgia, 29*, 338–350.

Rocca, M. A., Ceccarelli, A., Falini, A., Colombo, B., Tortorella, P., Bernasconi, L., et al. (2006). Brain gray matter changes in migraine patients with T2-visible lesions: A 3-T MRI study. *Stroke, 37*, 1765–1770.

Rocca, M. A., Colombo, B., Pratesi, A., Comi, G., & Filippi, M. (2000). A magnetization transfer imaging study of the brain in patients with migraine. *Neurology, 54*, 507–509.

Rosenberg, D. S., Mauguiere, F., Catenoix, H., Faillenot, I., & Magnin, M. (2009). Reciprocal thalamocortical connectivity of the medial pulvinar: A depth stimulation and evoked potential study in human brain. *Cerebral Cortex, 19*, 1462–1473.

Rosenberg, D. S., Mauguiere, F., Demarquay, G., Ryvlin, P., Isnard, J., Fischer, C., et al. (2006). Involvement of medial pulvinar thalamic nucleus in human temporal lobe seizures. *Epilepsia, 47*, 98–107.

Sakai, K. (2003). Reactivation of memory: Role of medial temporal lobe and prefrontal cortex. *Reviews in the Neurosciences, 14*, 241–252.

Sand, T., Zhitniy, N., Nilsen, K. B., Helde, G., Hagen, K., & Stovner, L. J. (2008). Thermal pain thresholds are decreased in the migraine preattack phase. *European Journal of Neurology, 15*, 1199–1205.

Stankewitz, A., Aderjan, D., Eippert, F., & May, A. (2011). Trigeminal nociceptive transmission in migraineurs predicts migraine attacks. *Journal of Neuroscience, 31*, 1937–1943.

Stankewitz, A., & May, A. (2009). The phenomenon of changes in cortical excitability in migraine is not migraine-specific—A unifying thesis. *Pain, 145*, 14–17.

Valeriani, M., de Tommaso, M., Restuccia, D., Le Pera, D., Guido, M., Iannetti, G. D., et al. (2003). Reduced habituation to experimental pain in migraine patients: A CO(2) laser evoked potential study. *Pain, 105*, 57–64.

Valfre, W., Rainero, I., Bergui, M., & Pinessi, L. (2008). Voxel-based morphometry reveals gray matter abnormalities in migraine. *Headache, 48*, 109–117.

Vanmolkot, K. R., Kors, E. E., Hottenga, J. J., Terwindt, G. M., Haan, J., Hoefnagels, W. A., et al. (2003). Novel mutations in the Na +, K + -ATPase pump gene ATP1A2 associated with familial hemiplegic migraine and benign familial infantile convulsions. *Annals of Neurology, 54*, 360–366.

Vincent, M., Pedra, E., Mourao-Miranda, J., Bramati, I. E., Henrique, A. R., & Moll, J. (2003). Enhanced interictal responsiveness of the migraineous visual cortex to incongruent bar stimulation: A functional MRI visual activation study. *Cephalalgia, 23*, 860–868.

Vincent, M. B., & Hadjikhani, N. (2007). Migraine aura and related phenomena: Beyond scotomata and scintillations. *Cephalalgia, 27*, 1368–1377.

Wang, W., Timsit-Berthier, M., & Schoenen, J. (1996). Intensity dependence of auditory evoked potentials is pronounced in migraine: An indication of cortical potentiation and low serotonergic neurotransmission? *Neurology, 46*, 1404–1409.

Weiller, C., May, A., Limmroth, V., Juptner, M., Kaube, H., Schayck, R. V., et al. (1995). Brain stem activation in spontaneous human migraine attacks. *Nature Medicine, 1*, 658–660.

Welch, K. M. (2003). Contemporary concepts of migraine pathogenesis. *Neurology, 61*, S2–S8.

Welch, K. M., Nagesh, V., Aurora, S. K., & Gelman, N. (2001). Periaqueductal gray matter dysfunction in migraine: Cause or the burden of illness? *Headache, 41*, 629–637.

Yankovsky, A. E., Andermann, F., Mercho, S., Dubeau, F., & Bernasconi, A. (2005). Preictal headache in partial epilepsy. *Neurology, 65*, 1979–1981.

Zemlan, F. P., & Behbehani, M. M. (1984). Afferent projections to the nucleus cuneiformis in the rat. *Neuroscience Letters, 52*, 103–109.

26 Transcranial Magnetic Stimulation and Magnetoencephalographic Studies in Migraine

SHEENA K. AURORA, SIDRA SAEED, AND SUSAN M. BOWYER

INTRODUCTION

Migraine is a very common disorder, occurring in 20% of women and 6% of men. Central neuronal hyperexcitability is proposed to be the putative basis for the physiological disturbances in migraine. Since there are no consistent structural disturbances in migraine, physiological studies have provided insight into the underlying mechanisms. The exact pathogenesis of migraine remains to be determined. Migraine is an episodic disorder involving head pain and cortical phenomena without consistent structural abnormalities. Therefore, only investigations aimed at studying the function of the brain provide insight into migraine pathophysiology. Some studies that have been reviewed in the literature support the concept of central neuronal hyperexcitability as a pivotal physiological disturbance predisposing to migraine (Welch et al., 1980). The reasons for increased neuronal excitability may be multifactorial. Through genetic studies, the abnormality of calcium channels has been introduced as a potential mechanism of interictal neuronal excitability (Ophoff et al., 1996). Mutant voltage-gated P/Q-type calcium channel genes likely influence presynaptic neurotransmitter release, possibly via the excitatory amino acid systems or the inhibitory system. Other genetic studies have demonstrated dysfunction in the ATP1A2 gene, which encodes an ion pump (Ophoff et al., 1996). Data in episodic ataxia and hemiplegic migraine patients with no mutation in either CACNA1A or ATP1A2 demonstrated that a heterozygous mutation in EAAT1 can lead to decreased glutamate uptake, which can contribute to neuronal hyperexcitability leading to seizures, hemiplegia, and episodic ataxia (Jenet al., 2005). It could therefore be hypothesized that genetic abnormalities result in a lowered threshold of response to trigger factors (Haan et al., 2005). A genetic mouse model with the FHM1 mutation has recently been developed (van den Maagdenberg et al., 2004). Experimental models carried out on these genetically modified mice have demonstrated a reduced threshold for cortical spreading depression (CSD) (Eikermann-Haerter et al., 2011), which

may be the result of enhanced glutamate release at pyramidal cell synapses (Tottene et al., 2009). In addition, DC MEG waveforms arising during migraine aura were also used to determine the effectiveness of prophylactic medication therapy with valproate on neuronal hyperexcitability. Using visual stimulation, widespread regions of hyperexcitability were detected throughout the occipital cortex in migraine patients, explaining the susceptibility for triggering CSD and migraine aura. After 30 days of prophylactic treatment (valproate), reduced DC MEG shifts in the occipital cortex and reduced incidence of migraine attacks were observed. This study confirmed that MEG can noninvasively determine the status of neuronal excitability before and after therapy (Bowyer et al., 2005). Similar findings have been found with topiramate (unpublished HFH MEG lab).

This chapter is a review of the transcranial magnetic stimulation (TMS) and magnetoencephalographic (MEG) studies that have provided insight into migraine pathogenesis supporting the theory of hyperexcitability.

TRANSCRANIAL MAGNETIC STIMULATION

TMS has been developed to non-invasively study cortical physiology (Barker et al., 1985, 1987). Motor and occipital cortices have been extensively investigated with magnetic stimulation in migraineurs.

Transcranial Magnetic Stimulation of Motor Cortex in Migraine

Several studies have investigated the motor cortex of migraineurs using TMS; these studies are summarized in Table 26–1. Three studies have been performed on the motor cortex, two of which reported an increase in excitability threshold in migraineurs and suggested that this neurophysiological correlate may be useful in the study of migraine mechanisms (Bettucci et al., 1992; Maertens de Noordhout et al., 1992). The first study compared subjects with migraine with aura (MwA) and migraine without

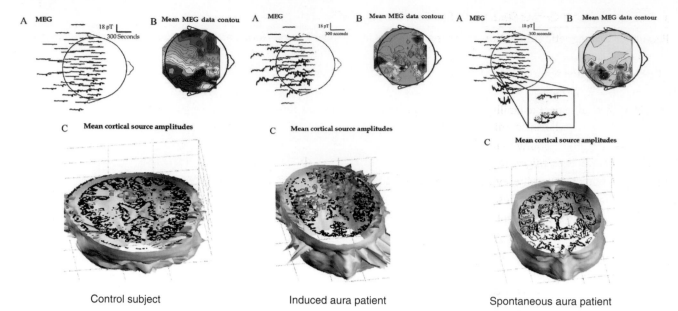

FIGURE 26–1 Left: *Control subject.* **(A)** *Direct current magnetoencephalographic (DC MEG) data from control subject during visual stimulation. Total time interval is 300 seconds. The channels at the back of the head have been laid out flat for ease of viewing. Small spikes (2- to 5-second shifts from baseline) in the recording are an artifact of patient movement.* **(B)** *Data contour average over the first 200 seconds is shown. Red corresponds to points where the magnetic field exits the subject's head and blue corresponds to points where the magnetic field enters.* **(C)** *Two-dimensional inverse imaging (2DII) localization of neuronal activity from analysis of the MEG signals during visual stimulation coregistered with control subject's magnetic resonance image (MRI). The 2DII analysis of an averaged 200 seconds of cortical source amplitudes localized focally in the striate cortex. This is representative of the entire 18 minutes of data. Red indicates region of most intense cortical activity.* Middle: *Induced aura patient.* **(A)** *DC MEG data collected during visually induced migraine aura, 150 seconds after onset of stimulus. Total time interval is 300 seconds.* **(B)** *Data contour average over the first 200 seconds is shown.* **(C)** *The 2DII analysis of the average cortical source amplitude locations for 200 seconds is displayed on the patient's MRI. Significant areas of neuronal activation are seen in the primary visual cortex, right temporal area, and left occipital cortex during visually evoked stimulation. External distortion of the patient skull is caused by artifacts in the MRI data used to generate the three-dimensional surface.* Right: *Spontaneous aura patient.* **(A)** *DC MEG data collected during spontaneous visual aura. Data collection started 3 minutes after onset of visual symptoms. Total time interval is 300 seconds. Inset of selected channels depicting large DC MEG shifts.* **(B)** *Data contour average over the first 200 seconds is shown.* **(C)** *2DII analysis of the location of DC MEG shifts during spontaneous visual aura mapped onto patient's MRI. An average of the first 200 seconds of data is displayed showing minimal neuronal activity in the primary visual cortex as well as in the left occipitoparietal cortex; most activation occurred in the right occipitoparietal/temporal region. From Bowyer, S. M., Aurora, K. S., Moran, J. E., Tepley, N., & Welch, K. M. (2001). Magnetoencephalographic fields from patients with spontaneous and induced migraine aura.* Annals of Neurology, 50(5), 582–587. *Reprinted with permission from John Wiley & Sons.*

aura (MwoA) to controls and demonstrated an increased motor threshold in classic migraine (Maertens de Noordhout et al., 1992). The motor threshold was increased on the side corresponding to the aura. The threshold difference could not be attributed to attack frequency. The second study was performed on menstrual migraineurs during their cycle compared to controls (Bettucci et al., 1992). An increased threshold was demonstrated similar to the first study but in this study all patients had migraine without aura. There were no differences found between the ictal and interictal phases. The last two studies were done by the same investigators. In the first study a difference was found in amplitude of motor evoked potentials in MwA

compared to controls, but no differences were found in the motor threshold (van der Kamp et al., 1996). The differences in this study compared to previous reports of increased threshold were explained on the basis of attack frequency, which was higher in their group of patients.

In a second study performed on familial hemiplegic migraine, the threshold of the motor cortex was higher on the side corresponding to the aura (van der Kamp et al., 1997). The amplitudes were also lower with prolonged central motor conduction time. Although the differences in the above studies pertaining to motor threshold in migraine were attributed to attack frequency, there were also some important technical differences (Aurora & Welch, 1998).

TABLE 26-1 *Motor Cortex Studies of Migraineurs Using TMS*

Percutaneous magnetic stimulation of the motor cortex in migraine.	Maertens de Noordhout, A. L., Pepin, J. L., Schoenen, J., & Delwaide, P. J. (1992)
Menstrual migraine without aura: Cortical excitability to magnetic stimulation.	Bettucci, D., Cantello, R., Gianelli, M., Naldi, P., & Mutani, R. (1992)
Interictal cortical hyperexcitability in migraine patients demonstrated with transcranial magnetic stimulation.	van der Kamp, W., Maassenvandenbrink, A., Ferrari, M. D., & vanDijk, J. G. (1996)
Interictal cortical excitability to magnetic stimulation in familial hemiplegic migraine	van der Kamp, W., Maassenvandenbrink, A., Ferrari, M. D., & vanDijk, J. G. (1997)
Brain excitability in migraine; evidence from transcranial magnetic stimulation studies.	Aurora, S. K., & Welch, K. M. A. (1998)
Effects of serotonin 1B/1D receptor agonist zolmitriptan on motor cortical excitability in humans.	Werhahn, K. J., Förderreuther, S., & Straube, A., (1998).
Reduced cerebellar inhibition in migraine with aura: A TMS study.	Brighina, F., Palermo, A., Panetta, M. L., Daniele, O., Aloisio, A., Cosentino, G., et al. (2009)
The dynamic regulation of cortical excitability is altered in episodic ataxia type 2.	Helmich, R. C., Siebner, H. R., Giffin, N., Bestmann, S., Rothwell, J. C., & Bloem, B. R. (2010)
Impaired glutamatergic neurotransmission in migraine with aura? Evidence by an input-output curves transcranial magnetic stimulation study.	Cosentino, G., Fierro, B., Vigneri, S., Talamanca, S., Palermo, A., Puma, A., et al. (2011)

Paired stimulation of the motor cortex has been studied in episodic ataxia type 2. Compared to normal controls, patients with episodic ataxia type 2 showed an excessive increase in motor cortex excitability following a brief facilitatory input consisting of a test stimulus (Helmich et al., 2010). Of late, physiological studies of the cerebellum using TMS have also been conducted (Minks et al., 2010). Using a conditioning pulse prior to a test stimulus to the motor cortex, the inhibitory function of the cerebellum was studied. There was a significant deficit of cerebellar inhibition in migraine compared to controls (Brighina et al., 2009).

Using paired pulses, a recent study demonstrated reduced motor cortical excitability after administration of zolmitriptan, a centrally acting 5-$HT_{1B/D}$ agonist used in the treatment of migraine (Werhahn et al., 1998). A more recent study measured input–output curves with paired stimuli of resting motor thresholds before and after treatment with levetiracetam. At baseline the findings were increased facilitation in migraine with aura compared to controls, which normalized after treatment. These studies demonstrate a new window of opportunity to study cortical physiology and the effects of drugs in migraine (Cosentino et al., 2011).

Cortical Silent Period in Migraine

Two studies have examined the cortical silent period (CSP). Both studies reported no differences in CSP at high levels of stimulation. One study found a shorter CSP in MwA compared to controls at low stimulus intensity (Aurora, Al Sayed, et al., 1998). Since the CSP, in part, is a measure of central inhibition of motor pathways, the shortened CSP that was measured in MwA patients may suggest reduced central inhibition, thus inferring increased excitability. Recently another study has confirmed the findings of a shortened CSP in a blinded study (Curra et al., 2007).

Transcranial Magnetic Stimulation of Occipital Cortex in Migraine

Perhaps more relevant to migraine is to study TMS of the occipital cortex, since enhanced excitability of the occipital cortex is possibly the basis for either spontaneous or triggered migraine aura (Welch et al., 1980). Occipital cortex excitability in migraine has been evaluated by the generation of phosphenes by TMS of the occipital cortex. The very first study using this technique reported a low threshold for generation of phosphenes in MwA, inferring hyperexcitability of the occipital cortex in migraine (Aurora, Ahmad, et al., 1998). Since this early study there have been several other studies performed on the occipital cortex using TMS to measure phosphenes, both confirming the initial reports of hyperexcitability (Aggugia et al., 1999; Aurora et al., 1999, 2005; Battelli et al., 2002; Young et al., 2004). In one of the studies the threshold of phosphenes correlated with studies investigating visually triggered headache (Aurora et al., 1999). In the study by Young et al. (2004), phosphenes were measured repeatedly in the same subjects and no relationship was found in threshold and timing of migraine attack or menstrual period. Battelli and colleagues (2002) investigated the extrastriate visual area V5, which is important for the perception of motion. Both migraine with aura and migraine without aura groups required significantly lower magnetic field strength for the induction of moving phosphenes, compared to the control group; this difference was significant for V5 in both the left and right hemispheres. In addition, the phosphenes were better defined and had clearer presentation in migraine groups, whereas in controls they tended to be more transient and ill-defined. Recently longitudinal studies have showed variability in the phosphene threshold in children (Siniatchkin et al., 2009), during menstrual periods (Boros et al., 2009), and with severity of headache (Lo et al., 2008), and in general greater variability in patients with migraine (Antal et al., 2006). Compared to single-pulse TMS, double pulse produced phosphenes more reliably in migraine and demonstrated lower phosphene thresholds in migraineurs compared to controls (Gerwig et al., 2005).

Repetitive Transcranial Magnetic Stimulation

Hyperexcitability of the visual cortex was also demonstrated using repetitive (rTMS) (Brighina et al., 2002). In a study using 1-IIz rTMS, the phosphene threshold was assessed before and after 15 minutes of rTMS. In normal controls there was an increased phosphene threshold after rTMS; conversely, in migraine there was a reduction in phosphene threshold, suggesting visual cortex excitability. The physiological basis for rTMS in normal cortex demonstrates facilitation after low-frequency and inhibition after high-frequency stimulation. In an effort to explore normalizing excitability, Brighina and colleagues used 10-Hz high-frequency priming stimulation of the motor cortex. This resulted in normalized excitability following a short interstimulus interval compared to previous facilitation. Valproate was also studied with a similar paradigm of 1-Hz stimulation; patients who were treated with valproate had a normalization of intracortical facilitation (Palermo et al., 2009). Therapeutic effects of TMS have been studied in a sham-controlled, small double-blind study in migraine with aura. The primary endpoint of the study was to treat patients with single-pulse TMS during aura. They found pain-free responses were higher in the active versus sham-treated patients (Lipton et al., 2010).

Magnetic Suppression of Perceptual Accuracy

Most studies with TMS utilized the subjective sensation of phosphenes as a measure of excitability. Although these studies have shown important differences in migraine, the lack of objectivity makes data interpretation difficult. We have therefore developed objective physiological measures to assess differences in cortical excitability (Chronicle et al., 2006). To assess inhibitory function of the occipital cortex, a visual suppression method, magnetic suppression of perceptual accuracy (MSPA), was utilized. Timed TMS impulses, usually 10% above phosphene threshold or where suppression was noted, were delivered to the visual cortex. Subjects were asked to report letters projected at a fixed luminance on a screen in front of them. Visual suppression was calculated based on the number of errors the subjects made. Using an automated analysis, we confirmed that migraineurs had reduced errors, demonstrating a reduction in visual suppression (Palmer et al., 2000). We completed a study demonstrating a spectrum of illness in chronic migraine (Aurora et al., 2005). A cohort of these subjects demonstrated decreased metabolism in cerebral metabolism, thus correlating with the MSPA studies. Using this objective model, we have collected data on medication treatment (topiramate) demonstrating dynamic changes in episodic and chronic migraine in two subjects. Topiramate seemed to balance the dysfunction in cortical inhibition seen in chronic migraine (Aurora et al., 2010; Lauritzen et al., 1982).

Functional Imaging in Migraine Demonstrating Hyperexcitability

A link between CSD and migraine pathogenesis has been hypothesized for more than 40 years (Lauritzen et al., 1982), and recent evidence has strengthened the concept that the neurological symptoms that can precede or accompany an attack (e.g., aura) arise from CSD, whereas migraine headache results, in part, from the ensuing trigeminal-induced meningeal inflammation and central activation (Bolay et al., 2002). Using functional magnetic resonance imaging (fMRI) during spontaneous migraine auras, Hadjikhani et al. (2001) discovered at least eight neurovascular events in the human occipital cortex that resembled CSD observed in experimental animals, expanding a previous fMRI study of visually triggered migraine, which showed a suppression of blood oxygenation level–dependent (BOLD) response propagating into contiguous occipital cortical areas at a rate of 3 to 6 mm/min (Cao et al., 1999). These studies demonstrated indirect evidence for CSD in migraine. In animals, the CSD's band of hyperexcited neurons travels into sulci or fissures, eliciting signals that can be detected on MEG (Bowyer, Okada, et al., 1999; Bowyer, Tepley, et al., 1999). Using seven-channel MEG, Barkley et al. reported DC shifts in spontaneous migraine (Barkley et al., 1980). A further study of a larger number of patients has not been possible because of the unpredictable nature of migraine and time of capture of these spontaneous events. Using the visual trigger modeled by Cao et al (Cao, Welch, et al., 1999), Bowyer et al. (2001) was able to detect DC shifts when headache or aura was precipitated. These studies were performed using a whole-head MEG (148 channels), which permits a precise localization of signals. In this study headache was triggered in five of eight migraine patients and none of six controls. DC MEG shifts were observed in migraine subjects during visually triggered aura and in a patient studied during the first few minutes of spontaneous aura. No DC MEG shifts were seen in control subjects. This is additional evidence supporting the primary neural basis of migraine and confirms MEG-recorded DC shifts typical of those found during CSD reported previously in migraine attacks. MEG has been used to detect the underlying cortical activity in a case study of migraine aura without headache (Hall et al., 2004). MEG detected alpha desynchronization in the generation of phosphenes, indicating an increase in the neuronal oscillations. MEG also detected gamma desynchronization for approximately 10 minutes after aura; this may underlie the sustained inhibition of visual function. Increased cellular excitability results in a low-amplitude desynchronized electroencephalogram (Steriade & Llinás, 1988).

DC MEG waveforms arising during migraine aura were used to determine the effectiveness of prophylactic medication therapy valproate on neuronal hyperexcitability. Using visual stimulation, widespread regions of hyperexcitability were detected throughout the occipital cortex in migraine patients, explaining the susceptibility for triggering CSD and migraine aura. After 30 days of prophylactic treatment, reduced DC MEG shifts in the occipital cortex and reduced incidence of migraine attacks were observed. This study confirmed that MEG can noninvasively determine the status of neuronal excitability before and after therapy (Bowyer et al., 2005). Similar findings have been found with topiramate by this group.

The somatosensory cortex was also tested in migraineurs, using magnetoencephalography (Lang et al., 2004). The study concluded that the population of neurons in the primary somatosensory cortex underlying the N20m was hyperexcitable and that this hyperexcitability was linked to the frequency of migraine attacks. A recent MEG study on the motor cortex excitability in children with migraine found high-amplitude cortical activity in the motor cortex and longer latencies, indicating neurophysiological changes in the motor cortices of children with migraine (Wang et al., 2010). The auditory cortex in migraine has also been investigated with MEG (Korostenskaja et al., 2011). Acute migraine could be associated with neurophysiological and cognitive changes. A mismatch negativity (MMN) paradigm was used to detect cortical differences between migraineurs and healthy controls. Results indicated that the function of neural substrates, responsible for different stages of auditory information processing, is impaired during the acute migraine.

A recent study evaluated structural abnormalities in the motion-processing network in migraineurs and compared it to age-matched controls (Granziera et al., 2006). High-resolution cortical thickness was measured by diffusion tensor imaging. The authors concluded that a structural abnormality in the network of motion-processing areas could account for, or be the result of, the cortical hyperexcitability observed in migraineurs. The authors also proposed that the finding in patients with both MwA and MwoA of thickness abnormalities in area V3A, previously described as a source in spreading changes involved in visual aura, raised the question as to whether a "silent" cortical spreading depression develops as well in MwoA.

CONCLUSION

To summarize, no one single neurophysiological technique can be ascribed to best define differences in migraineurs versus nonmigraineurs. Further, even when the same technique is used, uniform results have not been demonstrated in migraine. These differences may be due to not only technical factors but also the important fact that migraine has shifts of physiology and therefore is difficult to ascertain. However, some physiological studies, where an increased excitability was inferred in migraine, are in keeping with the genetic studies in familial hemiplegic migraine, which also lend support to the theory of central neuronal excitability. Other studies that support this hypothesis are a disorder of mitochondrial energy metabolism (Barbiroli et al., 1990; Welch et al., 1989), deficiency of systemic and brain Mg^{2+} (Ramadan et al., 1989), and abnormalities of glutamate metabolism (D'Andrea et al., 1989). As well as contributing to excitability of neurons, these same factors may be involved in sustaining the propagation of spreading depression (Van Harreveld et al., 1984). It should now be possible to investigate how closely these abnormalities correlate with direct measurements of brain excitability using TMS and MEG techniques. Independent of mechanism, these results add to the increasingly substantial body of evidence that enhanced excitability of brain cortex may be important in the overall pathogenesis of migraine. The future of MEG and TMS will be to help identify underlying cortical dysfunction and provide neurophysiological biomarkers for diagnosing and evaluating response to treatment for this disorder.

REFERENCES

Aggugia, M., Zibetti, M., Febbraro, A., & Mutani, R. (1999). Transcranial magnetic stimulation in migraine with aura: Further evidence of occipital cortex hyperexcitability. *Cephalalgia, 19*, 465.

Antal, A., Arlt, S., Nitsche, M. A., Chadaide, Z., & Paulus, W. (2006). Higher variability of phosphene thresholds in migraineurs than in controls: A consecutive transcranial magnetic stimulation study. *Cephalalgia, 26*(7), 865–870.

Aurora, S. K., Ahmad, B. K., Welch, K. M. A., Bhardhwaj, P., & Ramadan, N. M. (1998). Transcranial magnetic stimulation confirms hyperexcitability of occipital cortex in migraine. *Neurology, 50*, 1111–1114.

Aurora, S. K., Al Sayed, F., Norris, L., & Welch, K. M. A. (1998). Cortical stimulation silent period is shortened in migraine with aura. *Cephalalgia, 18*, 397.

Aurora, S. K., Barrodale, P., Chronicle, E. P., & Mulleners, W. M. (2005). Cortical inhibition is reduced in chronic and episodic migraine and demonstrates a spectrum of illness. *Headache, 45*, 546–552.

Aurora, S. K., Barrodale, P. M., Vermaas, A. R., & Rudra, C. B. (2010). Topiramate modulates excitability of the occipital cortex when measured by transcranial magnetic stimulation. *Cephalalgia, 30*(6), 648–654.

Aurora, S. K., Cao, Y., Bowyer, S. M., & Welch, K. M. (1999). The occipital cortex is hyperexcitable in migraine: Experimental evidence. *Headache, 39*(7), 469–476.

Aurora, S. K., & Welch, K. M. A. (1998). Brain excitability in migraine; evidence from transcranial magnetic stimulation studies. *Current Opinion in Neurology, 11*, 205–209.

Barbiroli, B., Montagna, P., Cortelli, P., Martinelli, P., Sacquegna, T., Zaniol, P., et al. (1990). Complicated migraine studied by phosphorous magnetic resonance spectroscopy. *Cephalalgia, 10*, 263–272.

Barker, A. T., Freeston, I. L., Jalinous, R., & Jarratt, J. A. (1987). Magnetic stimulation of the human brain and peripheral nervous system: An introduction and the results of an initial clinical evaluation. *Neurosurgery, 20*, 100–109.

Barker, A. T., Jalinous, R., & Freeston, I. L. (1985). Non-invasive magnetic stimulation of human motor cortex. *Lancet, 1*, 1106–1107.

Barkley, G. L., Tepley, N., Nagel-Leiby, S., Moran, J. E., Simkins, R. T., & Welch, K. M. A. (1990). Magnetoencephalographic studies of migraine. *Headache, 30*, 428–434.

Battelli, L., Black, K. R., & Wray, S. H. (2002). Transcranial magnetic stimulation of visual area V5 in migraine. *Neurology, 58*(7), 1066–1069.

Bettucci, D., Cantello, R., Gianelli, M., Naldi, P., & Mutani, R. (1992). Menstrual migraine without aura: Cortical excitability to magnetic stimulation. *Headache, 32*, 345–347.

Bolay, H., Reuter, U., Dunn, A. K., Huang, Z., Boas, D. A., & Moskowitz, M. A. (2002). Intrinsic brain activity triggers trigeminal meningeal afferents in a migraine model. *Nature Medicine, 8*, 136–142.

Boros, K., Poreisz, C., Paulus, W., & Antal, A. (2009). Does the menstrual cycle influence the motor and phosphene thresholds in migraine? *European Journal of Neurology, 16*(3), 367–374.

Bowyer, S. M., Aurora, K. S., Moran, J. E., Tepley, N., & Welch, K. M. (2001). Magnetoencephalographic fields from patients with spontaneous and induced migraine aura. *Annals of Neurology, 50*(5), 582–587.

Bowyer, S. M., Okada, Y. C., Papuashvili, N., Moran, J. E., Barkley, G. L., Welch, K. M., et al. (1999). Analysis of MEG signals of spreading cortical depression with propagation constrained to a rectangular cortical strip. I. Lissencephalic Rabbit Model. *Brain Research, 843*, 79–86.

Bowyer, S. M., Tepley, N., & Mitsias, P. D. Cortical hyperexcitability in a migraine patient before and after sodium valproate treatment. *Journal of Clinical Neurophysiology, 22*, 65–67.

Bowyer, S. M., Tepley, N., Papuashvili, N., Kato, S., Barkley, G. L., Welch, K. M. A., et al. (1999). Analysis of MEG signals of spreading cortical depression with propagation constrained to a rectangular cortical strip: II. Gyrencephalic swine model. *Brain Research, 843*, 71–78.

Brighina, F., Palermo, A., Panetta, M. L., Daniele, O., Aloisio, A., Cosentino, G., et al. (2009). Reduced cerebellar inhibition in migraine with aura: A TMS study. *Cerebellum, 3*, 260–266.

Brighina, F., Piazza, A., Daniele, O., & Fierro, B. (2002). Modulation of visual cortical excitability in migraine with aura: Effects of 1 Hz repetitive transcranial magnetic stimulation. *Experimental Brain Research, 145*(2), 177–181.

Cao, Y., Welch, K. M. A., Aurora, S., & Vikingstad, E. M. (1999). Functional MRI-Bold of visually triggered headache in patients with migraine. *Archives of Neurology, 56*(5), 548–554.

Chronicle, E. P., Pearson, A. J., & Mulleners, W. M. (2006). Objective assessment of cortical excitability in migraine with and without aura. *Cephalalgia, 26*, 801–808.

Cosentino, G., Fierro, B., Vigneri, S., Talamanca, S., Palermo, A., Puma, A., et al. (2011). Impaired glutamatergic neurotransmission in migraine with aura? Evidence by an input-output curves transcranial magnetic stimulation study. *Headache, 51*(5), 726–733.

Curra, A., Pierelli, F., Coppola, G., Barbanti, P., Buzzi, M. G., Galeotti, F., et al. (2007). Shortened cortical silent period in facial muscles of patients with migraine. *Pain, 132*(1–2), 124–131.

D'Andrea, G., Cananzi, A. R., Joseph, R., Morra, M., Zamberlan, F., Ferro Milone, F., et al. (1989). Platelet glycine, glutamate and aspartate in primary headache. *Cephalalgia, 9*, 105–106.

Eikermann-Haerter, K., Yuzawa, I., Qin, T., Wang, Y., Baek, K., Kim, Y. R., et al. (2011). Enhanced subcortical spreading depression in familial hemiplegic migraine type 1 mutant mice. *Journal of Neuroscience, 31*(15), 5755–5763.

Gerwig, M., Niehaus, L., Kastrup, O., Stude, P., & Diener, H. C. (2005). Visual cortex excitability in migraine evaluated by single and paired magnetic stimuli. *Headache, 45*(10), 1394–1399.

Granziera, C., DaSilva, A. F. M., Snyder, J., Tuch, D. S., & Hadjikhani, N. (2006). Anatomical alterations of the visual motion processing network in migraine with and without aura. *PLoS Medicine, 3*(10), e402.

Haan, J., Kors, E. E., Vanmolkot, K. R., van den Maagdenberg, A. M., Frants, R. R., & Ferrari, M. D. (2005). Migraine genetics: An update. *Current Pain and Headache Reports, 9*(3), 213–220.

Hadjikhani, N., Sanchez Del Rio, M., Wu, O., Schwartz, D., Bakker, D., Fischl, B., et al. (2001). Mechanisms of migraine aura revealed by functional MRI in human visual cortex. *Proceedings of the National Academy of Science of the United States of America, 98*(8), 4687–4692.

Hall, S. D., Barnes, G. R., Hillebrand, A., Furlong, P. L., Singh, K. D., & Holliday, I. E. (2004). Spatio-temporal imaging of cortical desynchronization in migraine visual aura: A magnetoencephalography case study. *Headache, 44*(3), 204–208.

Helmich, R. C., Siebner, H. R., Giffin, N., Bestmann, S., Rothwell, J. C., & Bloem, B. R. (2010). The dynamic regulation of cortical excitability is altered in episodic ataxia type 2. *Brain, 133,* 3519–3529.

Jen, J. C., Wan, J., Palos, T. P., Howard, B. D., & Baloh, R. W. (2005). Mutation in the glutamate transporter EAAT1 causes episodic ataxia, hemiplegia, and seizures. *Neurology, 65*(4), 529–534.

Korostenskaja, M., Pardos, M., Kujala, T., Rose, D. F., Brown, D., Horn, P., et al. (2011). Impaired auditory information processing during acute migraine: A magnetoencephalography study. *International Journal of Neuroscience, 121*(7), 355–365.

Lang, E., Kaltenhauser, M., Neundorfer, B., & Seidler, S. (2004). Hyperexcitability of the primary somatosensory cortex in migraine-a magnetoencephalographic study. *Brain, 127,* 2459–2469.

Lauritzen, M., Jorgensen, M. B., Diemer, N. H., Gjedde, A., & Hansen, A. J. (1982). Persistent oligemia of rat cerebral cortex in the wake of spreading depression. *Annals of Neurology, 12,* 469–474.

Lipton, R. B., Dodick, D. W., Silberstein, S. D., Saper, J. R., Aurora, S. K., Pearlman, S. H., et al. (2010). Single-pulse transcranial magnetic stimulation for acute treatment of migraine with aura: A randomised, double-blind, parallel-group, sham-controlled trial. *Lancet Neurology, 9*(4), 373–380.

Lo, Y. L., Lum, S. Y., Fook-Chong, S., Cui, S. L., & Siow, H. C. (2008). Clinical correlates of phosphene perception in migraine without aura: An Asian study. *Journal of Neurological Sciences, 264*(1–2), 93–96.

Maertens de Noordhout, A. L., Pepin, J. L., Schoenen, J., & Delwaide, P. J. (1992). Percutaneous magnetic stimulation of the motor cortex in migraine. *Electroencephalography and Clinical Neurophysiology, 85,* 110–115.

Minks, E., Kopickova, M., Marecek, R., Streitova, H., & Bares, M. (2010). Transcranial magnetic stimulation of the cerebellum. *Biomedical Papers of the Medical Faculty of the University Palacky, Olomouc, Czechoslovakia, 154*(2), 133–139.

Okada, Y. C., Lauritzen, M., & Nicholson, C. (1988). Magnetic field associated with spreading depression: A model for the detection of migraine. *Brain, 442,* 185–190.

Ophoff, R. A., Terwindt, G. M., Vergouwe, M. N., van Eijk, R. V., Oefner, P. J., Hoffman, S. M. G., et al. (1996). Familial hemiplegic migraine and episodic ataxia type-2 are caused by mutations in the Ca+2 channel gene CACNL1A4. *Cell, 87,* 543–552.

Palermo, A., Fierro, B., Giglia, G., Cosentino, G., Puma, A. R., & Brighina, F. (2009). Modulation of visual cortex excitability in migraine with aura: Effects of valproate therapy. *Neuroscience Letters, 467*(1), 26–29.

Palmer, J. E., Chronicle, E. P., Rolan, P., & Mulleners, W. M. (2000). Cortical hyperexcitability is cortical under-inhibition: Evidence from a novel functional test of migraine patients. *Cephalalgia, 20,* 525–532.

Ramadan, N. M., Halvorson, H., Vande-Linde, A. M., Levine, S. R., Helpern, J. A., et al. (1989). Low brain magnesium in migraine. *Headache, 29,* 590–593.

Siniatchkin, M., Reich, A. L., Shepherd, A. J., van Baalen, A., Siebner, H. R., & Stephani, U. (2009). Peri-ictal changes of cortical excitability in children suffering from migraine without aura. *Pain, 147*(1–3), 132–140.

Steriade, M., & Llinás, R. R. (1988). The functional states of the thalamus and the associated neuronal interplay. *Physiological Reviews, 68*(3), 649–742.

Tottene, A., Conti, R., Fabbro, A., Vecchia, D., Shapovalova, M., Santello, M., et al. (2009). Enhanced excitatory transmission at cortical synapses as the basis for facilitated spreading depression in Ca(v)2.1 knockin migraine mice. *Neuron, 61*(5), 762–773.

van den Maagdenberg, A. M., Pietrobon, D., Pizzorusso, T., Kaja, S., Broos, L. A., Cesetti, T., et al. (2004). A Cacna1a knockin migraine mouse model with increased susceptibility to cortical spreading depression. *Neuron, 41*(5), 701–710.

van der Kamp, W., Maassenvandenbrink, A., Ferrari, M. D., & vanDijk, J. G. (1996). Interictal cortical hyperexcitability in migraine patients demonstrated with transcranial magnetic stimulation. *Journal of Neurological Sciences, 139,* 106–110.

van der Kamp, W., Maassenvandenbrink, A., Ferrari, M. D., & vanDijk, J. G. (1997). Interictal cortical excitability to magnetic stimulation in familial hemiplegic migraine. *Neurology, 48,* 1462–1464.

Van Harreveld, A. (1984). The nature of the chick's magnesium sensitive retinal spreading depression. *Journal of Neurobiology, 15,* 333–344.

Wang, X., Xiang, J., Wang, Y., Pardos, M., Meng, L., Huo, X., et al. (2010). Identification of abnormal neuromagnetic signatures in the motor cortex of adolescent migraine. *Headache, 50*(6), 1005–1016.

Welch, K. M. A., D'Andrea, G., Tepley, N., Barkley, G., & Ramadan, N. M. (1990). The concept of migraine as a state of central neuronal hyperexcitability. *Neurological Clinics, 8,* 817–882.

Welch, K. M. A., Levine, S. R., D'Andrea, G., Schultz, L. R., & Helpern, J. A. (1989). Preliminary observations on brain energy metabolism in migraine studied by in-vivo phosphorous 31 NMR spectroscopy. *Neurology, 39,* 538–541.

Werhahn, K. J., Förderreuther, S., & Straube, A. (1998). Effects of serotonin 1B/1D receptor agonist zolmitriptan on motor cortical excitability in humans. *Neurology, 51,* 896–898.

Young, W. B., Oshinsky, M. L., Shechter, A. L., Gebeline-Myers, C., Bradley, K. C., & Wassermann, E. M. (2004). Consecutive transcranial magnetic stimulation: Phosphene thresholds in migraineurs and controls. *Headache, 44*(2), 131–135.

27 Magnetic Resonance Angiography and Migraine

M. SOHAIL ASGHAR AND MESSOUD ASHINA

VASCULAR HYPOTHESIS OF MIGRAINE

Vasodilatation as causative for migraine pain has been a subject of intense debate for centuries. In the second century, Galen suggested that the throbbing pain during headache originated from blood vessels (Olesen et al., 2005). In the Middle Ages, Avicenna (Ibn Sina) suggested in his famous Canon of Medicine that the head pain may elicit from the bone of the skull, from the membrane underneath, or because of substances reaching the side of the headache via the blood vessels (Abokrysha, 2009). In 1672, Thomas Wills proposed the first vascular theory of migraine and suggested that "megrim" was due to dilatation of blood vessels within the head (Olesen et al., 2005). More than 70 years ago, Graham and Wolff provided the first observations in humans demonstrating that focal head pain may be elicited from both extra- and intracranial vessels (Graham & Wolff, 1938). In 1940, Ray and Wolff reported that stimulation or distention of the large cranial arteries and dural arteries evoked head pain associated with the feeling of nausea or sickness (Ray & Wolff, 1940). The similarity between referred pain locations following stimulation of large cerebral arteries and headache patterns in migraine provides the strongest support yet for the involvement of perivascular nociceptors in migraine pain. More recently it was reported that focal headache may be induced by balloon dilatation of cerebral arteries (Nichols et al., 1990, 1993). The advent of new techniques such as ultrasonography and magnetic resonance angiography (MRA) has provided new insights into the role of cerebral vessels in migraine pathophysiology. In this chapter, we present a concise review of previous transcranial Doppler (TCD) data and the most recent MRA data, recorded during spontaneous and provoked migraine attacks.

Imaging Techniques: Transcranial Doppler and Magnetic Resonance Angiography

Previous human studies have primarily focused on the intracerebral arteries. Possible diameter changes in the middle cerebral artery (MCA) have been estimated indirectly by Transcranial Doppler (TCD) (Iversen, 1995).

Given that cerebral blood flow is constant, changes in blood velocity in the MCA can indirectly indicate relative diameter changes (i.e., MCA contraction or dilatation). To ensure a constant cerebral blood flow, TCD measurements are usually supplemented with single-photon emission computed tomography (SPECT) recordings (Iversen et al., 2008). Limitations of this method are (a) the recordings are only indirect and therefore one has to be cautious with interpretation of data; (b) it is not possible to examine the extracerebral compartment, such as measuring changes in the meningeal arteries by the TCD; and (c) the radiation exposure does not permit multiple scans.

Magnetic resonance angiography is a powerful tool to examine arteries in the brain in vivo without contrast material. Recent advances in image analysis software allow direct, noninvasive, and repetitive investigation of diameter changes of cerebral arteries (de Koning et al., 2003). To detect these changes, however, it is important to use a voxel size with a high image resolution. If instead a large voxel size is used, it would be impossible to detect a subthreshold dilatation and thereby lead to false-negative results. Therefore, high-resolution MRA is recommended, and to avoid prolonged scan duration, high-field MR scanners (3 Tesla or more) are preferred.

Spontaneous Migraine Attacks

Friberg et al. (1991) examined migraine patients with half-sided headache during spontaneous attacks by TCD and reported MCA dilatation of 20% on the headache side compared to the nonheadache side. Moreover, the MCA dilatation was reversible by treatment with sumatriptan. Thomsen et al. (1995) reported decreased velocity (9%) in the MCA on the pain side in half-sided migraine attacks, but these findings have been challenged by Zwetsloot et al. (1993). However, the results are not directly comparable because Zwetsloot et al. (1993) examined patients on average 6 hours (range 1 to 35 hours) after onset of attack. In contrast, the previous studies recorded diameter changes close to onset of attack (Friberg et al., 1991; Thomsen et al., 1995). One study (Iversen et al., 1990) employed Dermascan C (Cortex Technology, Hadsund, Denmark) to record diameter changes in the superficial temporal artery (STA) and found 9.4% dilatation of the STA on the headache side.

To our knowledge, there have been two previously published cases employing MRA during spontaneous migraine attack. Yanagawa et al. (2004) reported one patient with half-sided headache and found a relative decrease in the diameter of the arteries on the nonheadache side compared to the headache side during migraine attack. After treatment with eletriptan, the authors found no difference between sides. Using a 3-Tesla MRA, Nagata et al. (2009) examined diameter changes of the middle meningeal artery (MMA) in one female patient 2 hours after onset of migraine attack. The authors reported a slight dilatation on the headache side (~5%) and bilateral contraction of the MMA after sumatriptan administration. This study did not report time of postsumatriptan MR scans. Moreover, a rather large voxel size (0.36 mm × 0.36 mm × 0.50 mm) was used and the authors reported partial volume–related problems with detecting the rims of the arteries. In our opinion, with a voxel size close to double the size of the dilatation, it is quite remarkable that the authors were able to detect a dilatation at all.

Provoked Migraine Attacks

Human models of migraine offer a unique opportunity to study migraine attacks in a controlled setup. Intravenous infusion of the nitric oxide (NO) donor glyceryl trinitrate (GTN) (Afridi et al., 2005; Olesen et al., 1993; Thomsen et al., 1994) and calcitonin gene–related peptide (CGRP) provokes migraine attacks in patients with (Hansen et al., 2010) and without aura (Lassen et al., 2002). Moreover, the provoked attacks are reported as indistinguishable from spontaneous migraine attacks and effectively treated with triptans.

Using the GTN model of migraine, Schoonmann et al. (2008) examined migraine patients during delayed migraine attacks using 3-Tesla MRA. Schoonmann el al. included 32 migraine patients (5 with aura and 27 without aura). Twenty-seven received 0.5 mg/kg/min of GTN and five received placebo. Twenty patients reported delayed migraine attacks, and the attacks occurred on average 3.75 hours postinfusion (range 1.5 to 5.5 hours), where MRA and flow measurements were performed. The major outcome of this study was that provoked migraine attacks were *not* associated with dilatation of the MMA or MCA. Asghar et al. (2011) used the CGRP model of migraine to investigate possible diameter changes in the MMA and MCA during delayed migraine attacks. Migraine patients were examined before and during delayed migraine attacks. In addition, diameter changes were recorded 20 minutes after subcutaneous sumatriptan administration. The study reported that migraine attacks were associated

with dilatation of both the MMA (9.22%) and MCA (11.24%). Explorative analyses showed that in half-sided headache there was dilatation on the headache side and in double-sided headache there was bilateral dilatation. Sumatriptan administration resulted in bilateral MMA contraction and amelioration of the headache while the MCA was left unchanged (Fig. 27–1).

The two studies of Schoonman et al. (2008) and Asghar et al. (2011) are similar in many aspects (Table 27–1). Thus, both studies used the same type of MR scanner (Philips Achiva) and the same radiofrequency head coil (eight-channel SENSE). Both employed the same software (QMRA, Leiden, The Netherlands) to measure the same part of the MMA and MCA. The main differences between the two studies are that Schoonmann et al. used GTN to induce migraine attacks, whereas Asghar et al. used CGRP. But this can hardly explain the discrepancy, because patients in both studies reported migraine attacks indistinguishable from spontaneous attacks. The discrepancy is probably due to the practical execution of the study combined with the scan setup (Table 27–1). Asghar et al. (2011) (a) applied predefined pain intensity criteria (Verbal Rating Scale ≥4) before a migraine attack qualified for MRA scans; (b) used artery circumference measurements instead of diameter measurements for the calculation because circumference more precisely represents the irregular shape of arteries in situ; and (c) used a high-resolution MRA with a very small voxel size, resulting in images with sufficient voxels across the vessels to avoid possible partial volume problems while fulfilling the software requirements of at least three voxels across the artery. In contrast, Schoonmann et al. (2008) did not report predefined pain criteria. The majority of the patients were scanned when they reported headache equal to VRS = 2 (0, no headache; 1, a very mild headache or prepain [including a feeling of pressing or throbbing]; 2, very mild headache; 10, worst imaginable headache; Iversen et al., 1989). Furthermore, the authors used an image resolution with the approximately double voxel, allowing less than the required three voxels across the arteries to perform reliable measurements. In conclusion, Schoonmann et al. performed probably less detailed recordings with approximately double voxel size compared to Asghar et al. Thus, the method applied allows detecting large dilatation and but makes it impossible to detect subvoxel size dilatation because reliable vessel wall analysis requires at least three voxels across the measured area.

The question arises whether the modest dilatation by 9% to 12% (Asghar et al., 2011) is sufficient to activate normal sensory afferents in the perivascular space or whether it has an effect only on sensitized nociceptors. We suggest the latter since arterial diameters may dilate

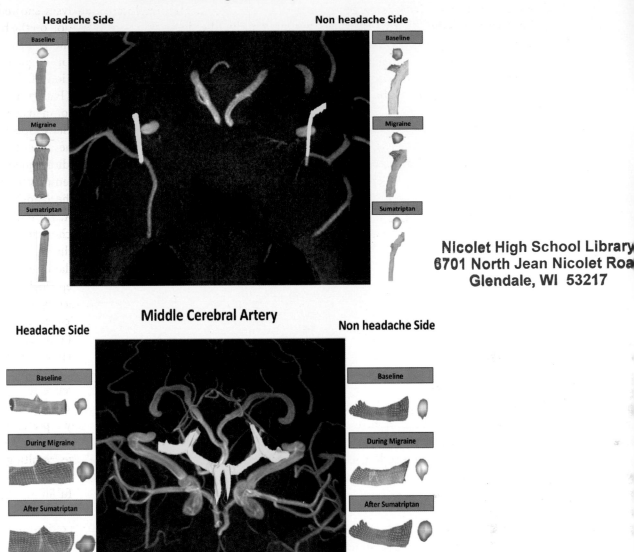

Middle Meningeal Artery

Headache Side · Non headache Side

Middle Cerebral Artery

Headache Side · Non headache Side

FIGURE 27–1 *Three-dimensional data from one subject with half-sided headache during migraine attack.* Top: *Middle meningeal artery (MMA) dilates on the headache side during migraine attack, whereas no dilatation is observed on the nonheadache side. After injection of sumatriptan MMA contracts on both sides.* Bottom: *Middle cerebral artery (MCA) dilates on the headache side during migraine attack, whereas no dilatation is observed on the nonheadache aside. After injection of sumatriptan no contraction of MCA is observed.* Source: *Asghar, M. S., et al. (2011). Evidence for a vascular factor in migraine.* Annals of Neurology. *2011 Apr;69(4):635-45. Reproduced with the permission from* Annals of Neurology.

markedly (e.g., during blood pressure decreases and during pulsation, which may increase during physical exercise without accompanying head pain). But what are the possible mechanisms of sensitization and excitation of the nerve terminals? If migraine attacks start in the brain (Goadsby et al., 2009) and cause nociception, this can only be caused by efferent activity in perivascular nerves (Olesen et al., 2009). Release of vasoactive substances from the perivascular nerve terminals is the only plausible way to explain why arteries in the intracerebral vascular compartment (i.e., the MCA) are dilated when exogenous CGRP cannot pass the blood-brain barrier and therefore cannot cause MCA dilatation per se when given intravenously. In addition, this also explains why the dilatation is limited to the headache side. Furthermore, the studies suggest that dilatation of the MMA and probably also other arteries supplying the dura plays an important role in provoking migraine attacks, while reversal is associated with amelioration of the headache. Sensitization could be caused by leakage of vasoactive/sensitizing substances

TABLE 27–1 *Comparison Between the Studies of Asghar et al. and Schoonman et al.*[a]

	Asghar et al.[a]	Schoonmann et al.[b]
Patients	Migraine without aura (*n* = 24)	Migraine without aura (*n* = 27)
		Migraine with aura (*n* = 5)
Migraine attacks	18 out 24 (75%)	20 out of 27 (74%)
Drugs	CGRP	GTN
	Intervention with sumatriptan	
Migraine criteria during MRA	Migraine attack and pain score ≥4 on VRS	Migraine attack
MRI scanner	3-Tesla Philips Achiva	3-Tesla Philips Achiva
Software	QMRA, Leiden, The Netherlands	QMRA, Leiden, The Netherlands
Resolution	High-resolution MRA	Low-resolution MRA
Voxel size	MMA: 0.2 mm × 0.2 mm × 0.35 mm (*2.8 × 5 voxels across*)	MMA: 0.39 mm × 0.39 mm × 0.25 mm (*2 × 2 voxels across*)
	MCA: 0.2 mm × 0.2 mm × 0.5 mm (*2 × 5 voxels across*)	MCA: 0.42 mm × 0.432 mm × 0.65 mm (*1.5 × 2.3 voxels across*)

Notes: CGRP = calcitonin gene–related peptide; GTN = glyceryl trinitrate; MRA = magnetic resonance angiography; VRS =; MRI = magnetic resonance imaging; MMA = middle meningeal artery; MCA = middle cerebral artery.

[a] Asghar, M. S., et al. (2011). Evidence for a vascular factor in migraine. *Annals of Neurology.* 2011 Apr;69(4):635–45.

[b] Schoonman, G., et al. (2008). Migraine headache is not associated with cerebral or meningeal vasodilatation—a 3T magnetic resonance angiography study. *Brain, 131*(Pt 8), 2192–2200.

from trigeminal nerve terminals (Mayberg et al., 1981; Strassman et al., 1996) or by efferent activity in parasympathetic nerves (Burstein & Jakubowski, 2005) and consequent release of substances that may sensitize sensory afferents.

We conclude that migraine attacks may be evoked in deep brain structures but these initiating mechanisms trigger perivascular release of vasoactive substances, causing sensitization of trigeminal afferents, vasodilatation, and migraine pain.

CONCLUSION

To date, two MRA studies during pharmacologically triggered attacks provided conflicting results probably due to methodological differences. The most recent study (Asghar et al., 2011) found that migraine attacks were associated with extra- and intracerebral arterial dilatation, in particular on the headache side. Furthermore, contraction of dural arteries by sumatriptan was associated with headache relief, suggesting primarily an extracerebral vascular site of action of sumatriptan. More studies are needed, in particular during spontaneous attacks, to confirm these data.

REFERENCES

Abokrysha, N. (2009). Ibn Sina (Avicenna) on pathogenesis of migraine compared with the recent theories. *Headache, 49*(6), 923–927.

Afridi, S. K., Matharu, M. S., Lee, L., Kaube, H., Friston, K. J., Frackowiak, R. S., & Goadsby, P. J. (2005). A PET study exploring the laterality of brainstem activation in migraine using glyceryl trinitrate. *Brain: A Journal of Neurology, 128*(Pt 4), 932–939.

Asghar, M. S., Hansen, A. E., Amin, F. M., van der Geest, R. J., Koning, P., Larsson, H. B., et al. (2011). Evidence for a vascular factor in migraine. *Annals of Neurology, 69*(4), 635–645.

Burstein, R., & Jakubowski, M. (2005). Unitary hypothesis for multiple triggers of the pain and strain of migraine. *Journal of Comparative Neurology, 493*(1), 9–14.

de Koning, P. J., Schaap, J. A., Janssen, J. P., Westenberg, J. J., van der Geest, R. J., & Reiber, J. H.(2003). Automated segmentation and analysis of vascular structures in magnetic resonance angiographic images. *Magnetic Resonance Medicine, 50*(6), 1189–1198.

Friberg, L., Friberg, L., Olesen, J., Iversen, H. K., & Sperling, B. (1991). Migraine pain associated with middle cerebral artery dilatation: Reversal by sumatriptan. *Lancet, 338*(8758), 13–17.

Goadsby, P. J., Charbit, A. R., Andreou, A. P., Akerman, S., & Holland, P. R. . (2009). Neurobiology of migraine. *Neuroscience, 161*(2), 327–341.

Graham, J. R., & Wolff, H. G. (1938). Mechanism of migraine headache and action of ergotamine tartrate. *Archives of Neurology and Psychiatry, 39*(4), 737–763.

Hansen, J. M., Hauge A. W., Olesen J., & Ashina M. (2010). Calcitonin gene-related peptide triggers migraine-like attacks in patients with migraine with aura. *Cephalalgia*, 30(10), 1179–1186.

Iversen, H. (1995). Experimental headache in humans. *Cephalalgia*, 15(4), 281–287.

Iversen, H. K., Olesen, J., & Tfelt-Hansen, P. (1989). Intravenous nitroglycerin as an experimental model of vascular headache. Basic characteristics. *Pain, 38*, 17–24.

Iversen, H. K.,Nielsen, T. H., Olesen, J., & Tfelt-Hansen, P. (1990). Arterial responses during migraine headache. *Lancet*, 336(8719), 837–839.

Iversen, H., Holm, S., Friberg, L., & Tfelt-Hansen, P. (2008). Intracranial hemodynamics during intravenous infusion of glyceryl trinitrate. *Journal of Headache and Pain*, 9(3), 177–180.

Lassen, L., Haderslev P. A., Jacobsen V.B., Iversen H.K., Sperling B., & Olesen J. (2002). CGRP may play a causative role in migraine. *Cephalalgia*, 22(1), 54–61.

Mayberg, M., Langer, R. S., Zervas, N. T., & Moskowitz, M. A. (1981). Perivascular meningeal projections from cat trigeminal ganglia: Possible pathway for vascular headaches in man. *Science (New York, NY)*, 213(4504), 228–230.

Nagata, E., Moriguchi, H., Takizawa, S., Horie, T., Yanagimachi, N., & Takagi, S. (2009). The middle meningeal artery during a migraine attack: 3T magnetic resonance angiography study. *Internal Medicine (Tokyo, Japan)*, 48(24), 2133–2135.

Nichols, F. T. 3rd, Mawad, M., Mohr, J. P., Stein, B., Hilal, S., & Michelsen, W. J. (1990). Focal headache during balloon inflation in the internal carotid and middle cerebral arteries. *Stroke*, 21(4), 555–559.

Olesen, J., Iversen, H. K., & Thomsen, L. L., (1993). Nitric oxide supersensitivity: A possible molecular mechanism of migraine pain. *Neuroreport*, 4(8), 1027–1030.

Olesen, J., Tfelt-Hansen, P., & Welch, K. (2005). History of headache. In: *The headaches*. Philadelphia, PA: Lippincott Williams & Wilkins.

Olesen, J., Burstein, R., Ashina, M., & Tfelt-Hansen, P. (2009). Origin of pain in migraine: Evidence for peripheral sensitisation. *Lancet Neurology*, 8(7), 679–690.

Ray, B. S., & Wolff, H. G. (1940). Experimental studies on headache: Pain-sensitive structures of the head and their significance in headache. *Archives of Surgery*, 41(4), 813–856.

Schoonman, G., van der Grond, J., Kortmann, C., van der Geest, R. J., Terwindt G. M., & Ferrari M. D. . (2008). Migraine headache is not associated with cerebral or meningeal vasodilatation—a 3T magnetic resonance angiography study. *Brain*, 131(Pt 8), 2192–2200.

Strassman, A. M., Raymond, S. A., & Burstein, R. (1996). Sensitization of meningeal sensory neurons and the origin of headaches. *Nature*, 384(6609), 560–564.

Thomsen, L. L., Iversen, H. K., & Olesen, J. (1995). Cerebral blood flow velocities are reduced during attacks of unilateral migraine without aura. *Cephalalgia*, 15(2), 109–116.

1994#Thomsen, L. L., Kruuse, C., Iversen, H. K., & Olesen, J. (1994). A nitric oxide donor (nitroglycerin) triggers genuine migraine attacks. *European Journal of Neurology, 1*, 73–80.

Yanagawa, Y., Katoh, H., Yoshikawa, T., Sakamoto, T., & Okada, Y. (2004). [A case of the usefulness of MR angiography and diffusion weighted image to evaluate migraine]. *No Shinkei Geka. Neurological Surgery*, 32(10), 1059–1062.

Zwetsloot, C. P., Caekebeke, J. F., & Ferrari, M. D. (1993). Lack of asymmetry of middle cerebral artery blood velocity in unilateral migraine. *Stroke: A Journal of Cerebral Circulation*, 24(9), 1335–1338.

28 Transcranial Magnetic Stimulation/Repetitive Transcranial Magnetic Stimulation

MAGDALENA SARAH VOLZ AND FELIPE FREGNI

INTRODUCTION

Transcranial magnetic stimulation (TMS) was first introduced in 1985 (Barker et al., 1985). In the last decades, the relevance and significance of TMS has been growing continuously. TMS is a method of non-invasive brain stimulation using a pulsed magnetic field. This technique involves the utilization of a rapidly changing and powerful magnetic field (0 to 2 Tesla) applied to the brain in a non-invasive manner. A TMS pulse induces an electromagnetic current in a focal area of the brain cortex (approximately 1 to 4 cm^3). There are a variety of different applications of TMS. It can be applied as only one stimulus at a time, called single-pulse TMS, or in pairs of stimuli with different inter-stimulus intervals, called paired-pulse TMS. Often, single- and paired-pulse TMS are used as an assessment and diagnostic tool, for instance, to measure motor and visual cortex global excitability, study central motor conduction time, measure intracortical facilitation and inhibition, and study other cortico-cortical interactions. Repetitive transcranial magnetic stimulation (rTMS) is a technique where multiple stimuli of TMS are delivered in trains. rTMS and its induced after-effects offer the opportunity to reveal a better understanding about human brain plasticity (Thickbroom, 2007), and it is utilized as a therapeutic treatment in clinical application. Thus, a very broad range of usage led to an enormous number of studies investigating TMS and rTMS and exploring their effects as a clinical intervention.

The effects of rTMS have widely been investigated in clinical applications, for instance, in psychiatric and neurological diseases such as depression, stroke, tinnitus, schizophrenia, and Parkinson disease (Elahi & Chen, 2009; Fregni & Pascual-Leone, 2005; Lopez-Ibor et al., 2008; Ridding & Rothwell, 2007). A major and very important effort in rTMS research is dedicated to the development of a therapeutic tool for chronic pain treatment, including for different forms of neuralgia, fibromyalgia, and peripheral and central nerve lesions (Avery et al., 2007; Borckardt et al., 2008; Fregni et al., 2007;

Lefaucheur, 2008; Sampson et al., 2006). In fact, there is evidence suggesting that rTMS can alleviate pain, and furthermore, modify neurophysiological correlates of the perception of pain. These results led researchers to become interested in the testing of rTMS as a therapeutic tool in migraine (Brighina et al., 2004).

BASIC PRINCIPLES OF TRANSCRANIAL MAGNETIC STIMULATION

TMS uses the basic principle of electromagnetic induction, as it was discovered two centuries ago by Faraday. A pulse of a stimulator needs to have a fast changing current, which has powerful strength and appropriate duration to create a magnetic field (Kobayashi & Pascual-Leone, 2003). When applied over a human's head, the magnetic pulse passes through the scalp and skull non-invasively to target the brain in a relatively painlessly manner and with insignificant attenuation (Fig. 28–1). The time frame of the pulse is approximately 50 μs. These magnetic pulses secondary produce an ionic current in the brain, and this in turn penetrates the nerve cells' membranes, which eventually results in modified postsynaptic potential or direct action potentials (Kobayashi & Pascual-Leone, 2003; Terao & Ugawa, 2002). Stimulation usually takes place at a location along a nerve fiber, where the largest amount of current flows through the membrane. This induces a depolarization of the neuron's membrane. Because the current will progress in a straight line, when a nerve fiber bends, a potential location of stimulation and depolarization is the bended site of the fiber (Kobayashi & Pascual-Leone, 2003). TMS preferentially activates interneurons, which will activate pyramidal cells indirectly through a synaptic connection, generating an indirect wave. In contrast, a direct wave can be evoked directly through activating the axon hillock of a pyramidal cell. TMS preferentially excites neurons at the surface of the brain also when stimulation intensity is increased. This is, because the magnetic field attenuates immediately with increased distance from the coil. Given the current TMS equipment, TMS is considered to be capable of activating neurons that are within approximately 2.0 cm below the scalp surface. Thus, this technique is desirable to investigate the cortical excitability and its changes within the brain cortex (Kobayashi & Pascual-Leone, 2003).

TMS can also be used to modify intracortical excitability and activate distant cortical and subcortical structures along specific connections and networks. Currently available TMS stimulators usually generate a magnetic field of 2 to 3 Tesla. The precise mechanism and specific cellular effects underlying TMS still remain unclear (Kobayashi & Pascual-Leone, 2003). There are a variety of different coil types, which usually differ in the extent of their induced focus. A circular coil (Fig. 28–2) produces current in the opposite direction just underneath its winding, and therefore is capable of exciting brain regions more widely. A circular coil mostly is approximately 14 cm in diameter (Terao & Ugawa, 2002). This makes it suitable for bihemispheric stimulation (e.g., for the study of central motor conduction times). A figure-of-eight coil is consisted of two circular coils placed beside each other (Fig. 28–2). Both coils are usually approximately 9 cm in diameter. This coil allows increased focality of the induced magnetic field (Kobayashi & Pascual-Leone, 2003; Terao & Ugawa, 2002). During TMS, the focality and stimulation site can also be determined by controlling the intensity of stimulation. Therefore,

the operator can change the intensity of current applied through the coil by changing the magnitude of the delivered magnetic field and thus, secondarily, the induced electrical field (Kobayashi & Pascual-Leone, 2003). In addition, one can control the frequency of the applied stimuli. If TMS is delivered in trains of stimuli, it is so-called repetitive TMS (see paragraph "Repetitive Transcranial Magnetic Stimulation"). Furthermore, the location of the stimulated site can be varied and thus, according to the brain region, different behavioral effects can be obtained (Kobayashi & Pascual-Leone, 2003; Terao & Ugawa, 2002). In migraine the mainly cortical targets for TMS are the primary motor cortex (M1), the occipital cortex (V1), and the dorsolateral prefrontal cortex (DLPFC).

TECHNIQUE OF TRANSCRANIAL MAGNETIC STIMULATION AND REPETITIVE TRANSCRANIAL MAGNETIC STIMULATION

TMS is most commonly used as single- and paired-pulse TMS or rTMS.

Single-Pulse Transcranial Magnetic Stimulation

If TMS is applied in one single pulse at a time (with an interval of at least 8 seconds between pulses), it is called single-pulse TMS. Single-pulse TMS can be used, for instance, for mapping motor cortical outputs, inducing phosphenes, and studying central motor conduction time. Overall, it is an assessment tool for studying and measuring cortical excitability.

When a single pulse of TMS is applied to the motor cortex at suprathreshold intensity, it generates electrical currents in the motor cortex that indirectly induce motor evoked potentials (MEPs) via the activation of interneurons.

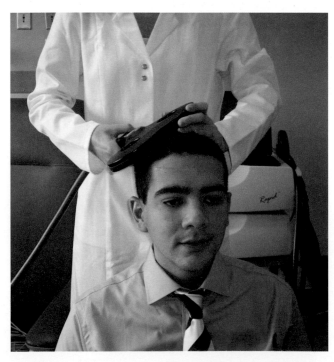

FIGURE 28–1 *Picture of transcranial magnetic stimulation (TMS) application.*

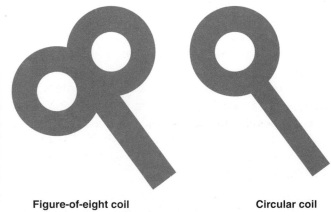

Figure-of-eight coil　　　　　　　　**Circular coil**

FIGURE 28–2 *Drawing of different transcranial magnetic stimulation (TMS) coils.*

By measuring electromyographic (EMG) signal recordings from muscles corresponding to the topographic area of the motor cortex stimulated, it is possible to measure the latency and amplitude of MEPs, which can be interpreted as a general measure of corticospinal excitability (Petersen et al., 2003). Since MEPs measure cortical excitability at any given moment in time, valuable information about the electrophysiology of the corticospinal tract can be acquired using this technique (Ilmoniemi et al., 1997; Petersen et al., 2003).

Motor threshold (MT), another parameter that can be obtained with single-pulse TMS, is defined as the lowest stimulator output intensity capable of producing a recordable MEP with a peak-to-peak amplitude of at least 50 μV (or 100 μV) in 3 out of 5 trials (or 6 out of 10 trials). Measurement of MT is also useful to determine the intensity of stimulation.

The cortical silent period is another useful parameter of cortical excitability that can be investigated with TMS. It can be assessed by applying a single pulse to the cortical representation area of a specific muscle during a slight contraction (usually about 10% of maximal contraction) of this muscle. The muscle contraction as indexed by EMG is followed by a silent period. The silent period is believed to be due to inhibitory mechanisms at the motor cortex. It is believed to be mediated by γ-aminobutyric acid B ($GABA_B$) receptors (Werhahn et al., 1999).

Relating to above-mentioned parameters of stimulation of the motor cortex, single-pulse TMS can be applied over the occipital lobe to elicit phosphenes. A phosphene is a phenomenon defined by the experience of seeing light or flashes of light without the stimulation of the peripheral visual system. Similar to the MT, a phosphene threshold (PT) can be determined and used to study the occipital cortex, visual pathways, and state of excitability. PT is defined as the minimal stimulus intensity at which the subject reports phosphenes in at least 5 out of 10 stimulations while maintaining the same coil positioning (Marg & Rudiak, 1994). Although TMS-elicited phosphenes might be useful to study the visual excitability of the visual cortex, phosphenes are not easily perceived by subjects and there is a learning curve that the investigator needs to consider when using this neurophysiological parameter.

Additionally, when a TMS pulse is administered to the occipital cortex during the presentation of a visual stimulus, it is possible to record changes in the waveform and topography of visual evoked potentials (VEPs) via electroencephalography (EEG) recordings and, therefore, to investigate modulation of VEPs by TMS.

Paired-Pulse Transcranial Magnetic Stimulation

TMS can also be applied in pairs of stimuli separated by a short inter-stimulus interval. This method is called paired-pulse TMS. During paired-pulse technique, TMS can be applied over only one cortical area utilizing the same coil, which is generating two pulses, or to two different brain regions using two separated coils (Rossi et al., 2009).

This technique of administering two consecutive stimuli using one coil can provide measures of intracortical facilitation and inhibition, and reveals insights into local intracortical excitability (Rossi et al., 2009; Terao & Ugawa, 2002).

For the measurement of short intracortical inhibition (SICI) (Wagle-Shukla et al., 2009), two stimuli are applied over the motor cortex with an interstimulus interval of 1 to 5 ms for short ICI and 50 to 100 ms for long LICI. The intensity of the first stimulus is set at subthreshold, usually 60% to 80% of the individual MT value. The second stimulus has a suprathreshold intensity, most commonly set as the value to obtain an MEP of 1 mV (most commonly 130% of MT). The amplitude of the evoked MEP is usually smaller compared to stimulation with a single pulse.

Intracortical facilitation (ICF) is assessed by delivering two stimuli with an interstimulus interval of 7 to 20 ms. Similarly to ICI, the intensity of the first stimulus is at subthreshold and the second is at suprathreshold intensity. In contrast, short-interval intracortical facilitation can be explored by two stimuli both at threshold intensity or the first at suprathreshold and the second at subthreshold intensity (Wagle-Shukla et al., 2009).

Paired-pulse stimulation can also be applied as two single pulses with two different coils. This application technique allows the examination of interhemispheric interactions. The most common one is the method to investigate transcallosal inhibition in which both motor cortices are stimulated with suprathreshold TMS with an interval of 7 to 15 ms. This interhemispheric interaction is influenced by the intensity of the first TMS stimulus: The stronger the stimulus, the greater and longer the induced interhemispheric inhibition (Kobayashi & Pascual-Leone, 2003). Overall, these techniques can be used to measure neurophysiological correlates of the motor cortex associated with migraine pain.

Repetitive Transcranial Magnetic Stimulation

A train of multiple TMS stimuli of the same intensity delivered to a single brain area at a given frequency is known as rTMS. Currently, repetitive stimulators of as much as 100 Hz are available commercially. Figure 28–3 shows a variety of different application methods. Patterned rTMS comprises the repetitive application of short rTMS bursts with a high frequency separated by phases without stimulation. Theta burst stimulation (TBS) is a specific type of patterned TMS in which short bursts of 50-Hz rTMS are applied using a theta range rate of 5 Hz (Rossi et al., 2009). The main difference of this technique as compared to regular TMS is that theta burst stimulation has been shown to induce longer lasting after-effects on cortical excitability; however, to date, it has not been shown to induce larger behavioral effects.

During conventional rTMS the frequency can range from 1 stimulus per second to 20 or more. The higher the stimulation frequency, the greater is the disruption of cortical function during the train of stimulation. Fast or high-frequency rTMS is defined by stimulus rates of more than 3 Hz. Slow or low-frequency rTMS refers to stimulus rates of 1 Hz or less (Terao & Ugawa, 2002).

The effects of a TMS train can be described as induction of a modulation of cortical excitability. These effects range from inhibition to facilitation. Lower frequencies of rTMS can suppress excitability of the motor cortex, while higher stimulation trains lead to a transient enhancement in cortical excitability (Kobayashi & Pascual-Leone, 2003). However, there is an important variability in the effects of rTMS: For example, in some subjects low-frequency TMS induces an increase in cortical excitability, whereas high-frequency TMS induces a decrease in cortical excitability—the opposite of what is expected. Lasting inhibitory

after-effects have also been shown for continuous TBS and facilitatory after-effects following intermittent TBS. The underlying mechanisms include synaptic changes, long-term depression-like (LTD) and long-term potentiation-like (LTP) mechanisms, shifts in network excitability, activation of feedback loops, and activity-dependent metaplasticity (Rossi et al., 2009).

Studies in animals indicate that modulation of neurotransmitters and gene induction also contributes to these modulatory effects of rTMS. Furthermore, combined rTMS and functional neuroimaging techniques have confirmed the neurophysiological changes induced by rTMS by demonstrating that there is suppressed or increased cerebral blood flow and metabolism in the stimulated area after slow-frequency or fast-frequency rTMS of the motor cortex and dorsolateral prefrontal cortex (Kobayashi & Pascual-Leone, 2003; Terao & Ugawa, 2002).

Transcranial Direct Current Stimulation

Transcranial direct current stimulation (tDCS) is another non-invasive brain stimulation technique based on the application of low-intensity (up to 2 mA) constant direct current to the scalp through electrodes to modulate excitability of cortical areas. Its effects depend on stimula-

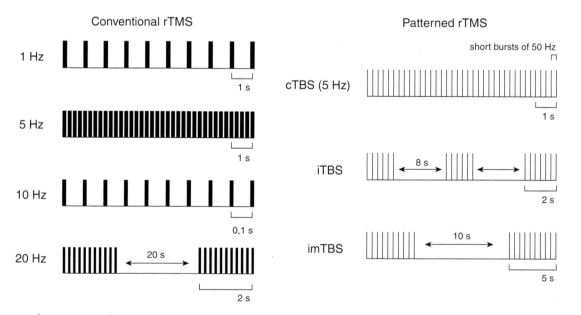

FIGURE 28–3 Left: *Conventional repetitive transcranial magnetic stimulation (rTMS). From the top: Examples of rTMS at 1 Hz (first trace), at 5 Hz (second trace), and at 10 Hz, and an example of 20-Hz application with trains of 2 seconds and a pause interval of 20 seconds (third trace).* Right: *Patterned rTMS. From the top: Continuous theta burst (first trace), intermittent theta burst (second trace), and intermediate theta burst (third trace). CTBS, continuous theta burst stimulation; iTBS, intermittent theta burst stimulation; imTBS, intermediate theta burst stimulation. Modified from Rossi, S., Hallett, M., Rossini, P. M., & Pascual-Leone, A. (2009). Safety, ethical considerations, and application guidelines for the use of transcranial magnetic stimulation in clinical practice and research.* Clinical Neurophysiology, 120(12), 2008–2039.

tion polarity, location, duration, and intensity. Anodal stimulation leads to an increase in cortical excitability, whereas cathodal stimulation decreases cortical excitability. In clinical and experimental approaches, tDCS is usually applied over the primary motor cortex.

USE OF TRANSCRANIAL MAGNETIC STIMULATION ASSESSMENT IN MIGRAINE

Central neuronal hyperexcitability associated with changes in a distributed cortico-subcortical network is proposed to play a key role for the manifestation of a migraine (Aurora & Welch, 1998) and seems to be a predisposing factor (Welch et al., 1990). Due to the fact that rTMS is a non-invasive technique of brain stimulation that can modulate excitability in specific regions of the brain cortex, it is reasonable to assume that rTMS can alleviate pain in migraine. Indeed, there is evidence that rTMS serves as abortive (Lipton et al., 2010) and prophylactic intervention (Brighina et al., 2004) for migraine patients. Application of rTMS for prevention of migraine is based on long-term modifications of cortical excitability, whereas, in the acute phase, it is proposed that rTMS can block neurophysiological processes associated with a migraine attack such as cortical spreading depression (CSD) (May & Jurgens, 2011). There is compelling evidence that cortical excitability is modified in migraine patients between attacks, which supports use of TMS as a preventive intervention. In the setting of experience with potential targets of TMS, the motor cortex and visual cortex have emerged as effective sites for investigating the migraine brain. In addition, targeting one of these cortices has an important advantage as they are easily accessible.

For this chapter we reviewed data available from the current literature in order to summarize and present the results of TMS for the treatment of migraine and the findings of TMS used as an assessment tool in migraine patients. We selected articles published from 1985 to December 2010 from PUBMED (http://www.ncbi.nlm.nih.gov/sites/entrez?db=pubmed). Reference lists in systematic reviews were examined and clinical experts on the field were contacted in an attempt to find more references (published or unpublished). Key search terms were "transcranial magnetic stimulation" and "migraine," and "transcranial direct current stimulation" and "migraine." Also, we searched using following terms specifically: "transcranial magnetic stimulation migraine prophylaxis," "transcranial magnetic stimulation migraine prevention," "transcranial magnetic stimulation migraine acute," "transcranial magnetic stimulation migraine abort,"

"transcranial magnetic stimulation migraine assessment," and "transcranial magnetic stimulation migraine intervention." We reviewed all studies that met our search criteria, excluding those not written in English or German.

Numerous studies investigated migraine with aura (MwA) and migraine without aura (MwoA) using TMS as an assessment tool (Aurora & Welch, 1998). The results of these previous studies using TMS have produced equivocal findings concerning changes in cortical excitability in migraine. Contrary findings include either a hyperexcitability or hypoexcitability in different cortical areas. Results of previous studies suggest an increase of cortical excitability rather than a decrease (Boulloche et al., 2010).

Transcranial Magnetic Stimulation/Repetitive Transcranial Magnetic Stimulation in Migraine

TMS has been used to test the hypotheses that there is a change in cortical excitability in the motor cortex and visual cortex. Measurement of MT or PT is a non-invasive method to reveal the excitability state of the motor cortex or the visual cortex.

Some studies do not support the concept of a general change of cortical excitability in migraineurs; for instance, Werhahn et al. (2000) investigated the state of excitability of the motor cortex in patients with MwA ($n = 12$). They could not find any significant differences between the patient group compared to controls ($n = 17$) with measurement of MT and intracortical inhibition and facilitation (Werhahn et al., 2000). In contrast, Conte et al. (2010) found opposite results when studying inhibitory cortical interneuron excitability assessed by 5-Hz rTMS delivered over the primary motor cortex. The study, including patients with MwA ($n = 19$), patients with MwoA ($n = 18$), and control subjects ($n = 19$), showed that 5-Hz rTMS induced MEP facilitation, being significantly highest in MwA patients. This suggests an abnormal motor cortex susceptibility to 5-Hz rTMS and that cortical potentiation patterns differ in MwA and MwoA (Conte et al., 2010). A subsequent study confirms this finding by evaluating the effects of rTMS (1-Hz frequency, 900 stimuli, 90% MT intensity) on the excitability of inhibitory and facilitatory circuits of the motor cortex. Investigators explored whether an abnormal pattern of excitability is measurable at motor cortex areas in MwA ($n = 9$). Results showed that migraineurs present significantly reduced levels of intracortical inhibition compared to controls ($n = 8$). Moreover, after 1-Hz rTMS was applied, opposite findings were obtained in migraineurs compared to controls. Specifically, intracortical facilitation significantly decreased in controls, whereas it significantly increased in migraineurs (Brighina et al., 2005). These results show that the motor cortex of migraine patients presents an abnormal modulation of cortical excitability, suggesting that inefficiency of inhibitory circuits may play a relevant role.

Aurora et al. (Aurora, al-Sayeed, et al., 1999) also studied the silent period elicited by TMS in MwA patients (n = 9). The mean MT was higher in MwA patients compared with controls (n = 9), but the difference was not significant. They found that applying a stimulus at MT intensity, result in a shortening of the cortical silent period in MwA patients compared to controls. Furthermore, there was an inverse correlation between the duration of the cortical silent period and an increase in the frequency of headache (Aurora, al-Sayeed, et al. 1999). These findings suggest reduced central inhibition resulting in increased excitability of cortical neurons in migraineurs. The association of cortical silent period reduction with an increased frequency of migraine is further suggestive that brain excitability is the basis of susceptibility to migraine attacks. Another study (Gunaydin et al., 2006) proposed that there is no hyperexcitable dysfunction in the motor cortex, but in the occipital cortex of migraine patients. In this study, MTs, MEPs, the central motor conduction time, and the cortical silent period were measured over the motor cortex in patients with MwA (n = 15), patients with MwoA (n = 15), and normal controls (n = 31). Additionally, phosphenes and the PT were determined by stimulation of the visual cortex. No significant differences were observed between the groups with respect to all measurements of the motor cortex. Although not statistically significant, the proportion of the migraineurs with phosphene generation (90%) was found to be higher than that of normal controls (71%). PT levels in migraine patients were significantly lower than those of the controls. Patients with MwA had the lowest levels of PT (Gunaydin et al., 2006).

Contrary to these results, a study investigating patients with MwA (n = 10) and MwoA (n = 10) through measurement of MT, cortical silent period, MEP, and PT suggests that both motor and visual cortices are hyperexcitable (Khedr et al., 2006). Patients in this study had lower MT, shorter cortical silent periods, and increased MEP. Moreover, there was an increased prevalence of phosphene in migraineurs compared with the control group (n = 20) (85% versus 75%) as well as lower PT (63% versus 72%). Additionally, there was a significant negative correlation between duration of attacks and PT and no significant differences between patients with aura and without aura in different parameters of cortical excitability measurements (Khedr et al., 2006).

In contrast, a study evoking VEPs after low- and high-frequency rTMS (900 pulses, 1 or 10 Hz) showed opposite results. In 30 migraine patients (n = 20 for MwoA, n = 10 for MwA), 10-Hz rTMS was followed by a significant increase of VEP amplitude. In controls (n = 24), VEP amplitude was significantly decreased after 1-Hz rTMS. There were no significant changes of VEP amplitudes after 1-Hz rTMS in migraineurs and after 10-Hz rTMS in healthy volunteers, nor after sham stimulation (Bohotin et al., 2002). The authors of the study suggest that this would lead one to conclude that the deficient VEP habituation in migraine could be due to dysfunctional visual cortex excitability. Interestingly, most studies of the visual cortex investigating PTs indicate a central neuronal hyperexcitability. Aurora et al. (1998) evaluated the differences in the threshold of occipital cortex excitation in MwA patients (n = 11) and controls (n = 11). The difference in the proportion of subjects with phosphene generation between MwA patients and controls was significant. Furthermore, all threshold levels for MwA patients were lower than the lowest threshold for the control group, and the threshold for excitability of the occipital cortex was lower in MwA patients compared with normal subjects (Aurora et al., 1998). This could indicate a direct neurophysiological correlate that migraineurs have a hyperexcitability of the occipital cortex. The same finding of a difference in the threshold for excitability of the occipital cortex in migraineurs revealed a study comparing the threshold for eliciting phosphenes and the ability to visually trigger headache in individuals with MwA and MwoA (n = 15). A significant proportion of the migraineurs (86.7%) developed phosphenes compared to controls (25%) (n = 8). Additionally, a significant correlation was found between the threshold for phosphenes on TMS and visually triggered headache (Aurora, Cao, et al., 1999). The hyperexcitable visual cortex in migraine seems to predispose to visually triggered headache. Moreover, Mulleners et al. (2001b) found that the occipital cortex is hyperexcitable interictally in both MwA and MwoA. The research group studied magnetophosphene thresholds in MwA (n = 16) and MwoA (n = 12). There were no significant differences across patient groups in the proportion of subjects seeing phosphenes (47% and 46%), but the mean threshold at which phosphenes were reported was significantly lower in both migraine groups than in controls (66%). Furthermore, there was no significant correlation between individual PT and the time interval to the closest migraine attack (Mulleners et al. 2001b).

Other results confirm that patients with migraine in the interictal state have an increased excitability of visual cortical areas. In this study, they determined the excitability of the visual cortex by PTs in patients with MwA (n = 19) and MwoA (n = 19) within 3 days before or after an acute migraine attack. In both single-pulse and paired-pulse TMS, mean PTs were reduced in MwoA patients and in MwA patients compared with control subjects (Gerwig et al., 2005).

Further experimental evidence trying to explain the underlying mechanism speaks in favor of impairment of inhibitory circuits. Chronicle et al. (2006) demonstrated functional changes in the visual cortex of migraine patients using an objective TMS technique—magnetic suppression of perceptual accuracy (MSPA). In their study they investigated MwA ($n = 8$) and MwoA ($n = 14$), expressing MSPA performance as a marker for response accuracy across target-pulse delay intervals. The profiles of migraine-free controls and MwoA patients exhibited a normal U-shape. MwA patients had significantly shallower profiles, showing little or no suppression at intermediate-delay intervals. They indicate that the U-shape of the normal MSPA function is caused by preferential activation of inhibitory neurons. Shallower MPSA profiles in MwA patients are therefore likely to indicate a functional hyperexcitability caused by impaired inhibition (Chronicle et al., 2006). Moreover, Mulleners et al. (2001a) tested patients with MwA ($n = 7$) using a test where letter combinations had to be recognized, which were followed by a magnetic pulse. In the MwA group, the mean proportion of correctly identified letters was significantly higher. These findings can be interpreted that inhibitory systems are activated to a lesser extent by TMS pulses in patients (Mulleners et al., 2001a).

Overall, although mixed, these previous studies point to the hypothesis that there is a deficiency of intracortical inhibition of the visual cortex and also possibly of the primary motor cortex.

Rationale for Transcranial Magnetic Stimulation in Migraine

Migraine is a disease that has a high prevalence in the human population (about 10%). Migraine leads to extensive suffering and work loss in the most productive years of life since the manifestation of migraine is typically at younger ages. Usually, acute migraine attacks can be treated with drugs, such as triptans, and a growing number of patients have to take preventive medication. However, not all attacks respond to acute treatment, some patients with migraine have contraindications to migraine medication (e.g., pregnancy or cardiovascular co-morbidity), and sometimes the drugs are not effective or approved during the aura phase of a migraine attack. This is also true for prophylactic medications. Therefore, nonmedical treatments of migraine are needed. TMS can be a relatively safe, non-invasive alternative to treat migraine in both phases: during the acute phase and also in between attacks as a prophylactic treatment.

The rationale for the use of TMS for migraine treatment is based on known changes in cortical excitability in the migraine brain. The visual cortex especially seems to be in a hyperexcitable state. These alterations are found in the interictal (Gerwig et al., 2005) as well as the ictal state (Conte et al., 2010). The reduction of PT levels in migraineurs supports the notion of excitability changes in the migraine cortex. Studies of PT using TMS and other electrophysiological techniques have suggested that effective prophylactic migraine medications reduce cortical hyperexcitability (Young et al., 2008).

Transcranial Magnetic Stimulation in Migraine

Several studies have investigated the effects of TMS in migraine. There is evidence that rTMS has a positive effect on alleviation of pain in migraine, especially when rTMS is applied for several sessions and a longer period. Thus, rTMS is a potential prophylactic intervention for migraine attacks. Furthermore, several clinical studies have shown that TMS, when applied as a single pulse, can be an effective and well-tolerated prospective alternative for abortive medication in the acute therapy of migraine with or without aura. Thus, TMS is suggested to offer a nonpharmacologic, nonbehavioral therapeutic approach to the currently prescribed drugs for patients who suffer from migraine. Mulleners and co-workers (2002) have even gone as far as suggesting that the PTs may prove useful in the monitoring of antimigraine medication efficacy (Mullners et al., 2002). Since Young et al. (2008) found that headache frequency and PT are negatively correlated, one can suggest that PT might be a predictor of migraine severity.

Transcranial Magnetic Stimulation as an Acute Therapy and Abortive Intervention in Migraine

In a recent study the application of single-pulse TMS over the occipital cortex was investigated in the early onset of a migraine attack during the aura phase. The verum group had a significantly higher rate of pain relief after 2 hours (39%) as compared to the sham stimulation group (22%). These effects were explained by the hypothesis that TMS interrupted the related neurophysiological marker of migraine—CSD; thus, effects might be valid only for migraine patients with aura (May & Jurgens, 2011). Also, Clarke et al. (2006) investigated migraineurs during their acute onset of headache or their aura phase. They found that high-frequency and low-frequency TMS often offered immediate pain relief and the frequency of headache recurrence decreased by 48%. They also reported improvement after more than one trial, and this may be due to cumulative effects of TMS (Clarke et al., 2006). In another very elegant study, Lipton et al. (2010) investigated the effects of single-pulse TMS for acute treatment of MwA in a randomized, double-blind, parallel-group, sham-controlled trial. The early treatment of MwA ($n = 82$)

resulted in pain-free response rates (39%) after 2 hours of the first attack and were significantly higher with single-pulse TMS compared with sham stimulation (22%, $n = 82$). Sustained pain-free response rates were enhanced with TMS at 24 hours and 48 hours post treatment. In addition, adverse effects such as nausea, photophobia, and phonophobia were not different between the two groups of treatment (Lipton et al., 2010). These findings suggest that single-pulse TMS may be effective for acute treatment of migraine with aura. Overall, initial results suggest that TMS might be an effective adjunct treatment to block migraine attacks.

Repetitive Transcranial Magnetic Stimulation for Prophylaxis and Prevention of Migraine Attacks

Brighina et al. (2010) proposed that high-frequency rTMS is a potential prophylactic treatment for migraine. They based this on the idea that there is reduced interictal intracortical inhibition in migraineurs and the notion of rTMS's homeostatic effects, such as that low-frequency inhibitory rTMS actually leads to *facilitation* of cortical excitability when the baseline activity is decreased, such as in migraine, and the opposite results after facilitatory high-frequency rTMS. In their study, therefore, they showed that high-frequency rTMS normalized excitability in migraine, increasing short intracortical inhibition and so confirming the notion of homeostatic-related rTMS effects (Brighina et al., 2010). These findings could open perspectives for new treatment strategies in migraine prevention to normalize cortical excitability and consequently to avoid abnormal responsiveness to external and internal stimuli.

On the other hand, Teepker et al. (2010) did not find a significant effect. They conducted a placebo-controlled blinded study to evaluate the therapeutic effects of low-frequency (1 Hz, two trains of 500 pulses) rTMS in migraine. rTMS was applied over the vertex in 27 migraineurs. A significant decrease of migraine attacks could be observed in the verum group, but when compared with placebo, no significance was evident. The same was true concerning days with migraine and total hours with migraine. No effects were evident for pain intensity and use of analgesics. Thus, rTMS stimulation over the vertex with 1 Hz was not effective in migraine prophylaxis when compared with placebo (Teepker et al., 2010). However, the positive effects regarding migraine attacks and days and total hours with migraine in the verum group deserve further investigation.

Another study investigated 12 sessions of high-frequency rTMS over the left DLPFC. Six patients received real rTMS, whereas sham stimulation was delivered to five patients. The results of the study showed that high-frequency rTMS trains delivered over the left DLPFC are able to ameliorate migraine. rTMS treatment significantly reduced headache attacks, headache index, and number of abortive medications as compared to sham treatment. These effects were still stable 1 month after the end of the treatment (Brighina et al., 2004).

Furthermore, a case report of a 51-year-old woman with a history of major depressive disorder and a migraine diagnosis, which was made by a neurologist and predated her first depressive episode, showed an alleviation of migraine suffering after rTMS treatment. In the study, the patient initially received 10-Hz-frequency rTMS with 120% of her MT, including 3,000 pulses per session over the left DLPFC with five sessions per week. After a 4-week period, her headache diary showed a reduction in migraine frequency, along with a subjective impression of their severity being reduced. Prior to treatment, 50% of her migraine attacks were characterized as severe, compared with 10% afterwards. The patient did not change her migraine prophylactic medications. Her improvement in migraine frequency and severity was sustained for 1 month following termination of rTMS treatment. In an additional maintenance phase of the study over 1 year, where rTMS was provided prophylactically as a maintenance antidepressant treatment, the patient reported a sustained benefit in migraine reduction, which she classified as "much improved." This suggests an improvement during repeated episodes of migraine, as well as a benefit in prophylactic treatment of migraine (O'Reardon et al., 2007). Overall, these results suggest that rTMS may have a potential in migraine prevention therapy; however, optimal parameters of stimulation, such as stimulation site, frequency, and intensity, still need to be defined.

Interestingly, a study investigating whether repeated rTMS sessions on 5 consecutive days can modify VEPs for longer periods showed that in eight control subjects the 1-Hz rTMS-induced dishabituation increased in duration over consecutive sessions. It persisted between several hours and several weeks. In six out of eight migraineurs, the normalization of VEP habituation by 10-Hz rTMS lasted longer after each stimulation, but did not exceed several hours after the last session. Exceptions were recorded in two patients, where it persisted for 2 days and 1 week. Thus, rTMS can induce long-lasting changes in cortical excitability and VEP habituation (Fumal et al., 2006). It remains to be investigated whether this effect may be useful in preventative migraine therapy.

Transcranial Direct Current Stimulation and Migraine

Although tDCS has not been investigated extensively in migraine, it is reasonable to hypothesize, based on previous studies showing that tDCS alleviates pain in a variety of different chronic pain syndromes (Fregni et al., 2007; Lefaucheur et al., 2008), that this method of brain stimulation would also lead to positive effects. Although it is easy to use, is a relatively cheap device, and has a robust paradigm for sham stimulation, it is necessary to investigate it in controlled trials before any conclusions are made.

Nevertheless, the use of these techniques—tDCS and TMS—may contribute to the understanding of mechanisms associated with migraine. For instance, Antal et al. (2008) preconditioned the primary motor cortex with tDCS to shape the magnitude and direction of excitability changes. It was found out that short-term homeostatic plasticity is altered in patients with visual aura between the attacks. Thus, such trials reveal novel insights of metaplasticity in the migraine brain (Antal et al., 2008). Chadaide et al. (2007) observed the dynamics of this basic interictal state by further modulating the excitability level of the visual cortex using tDCS in MwA and MwoA. Compared with healthy controls, migraine patients tend to show lower baseline PT values. Anodal stimulation decreases PT in migraineurs similarly to controls, having a larger effect in MwA. This result strengthens the notion of deficient inhibitory processes in the cortex of migraineurs, which is selectively revealed by activity-modulating cortical input (Chadaide et al., 2007).

There is also evidence that abnormal cortical excitability influences susceptibility to CSD in migraine. A study investigated the after-effects of tDCS on the propagation velocity of CSD in rats and found that anodal tDCS induced a significant increase in propagation velocity. Because anodal tDCS is known to induce a lasting enhancement of cortical excitability, this supports the notion that CSD propagation velocity reflects cortical excitability. Since cortical excitability and susceptibility to CSD is elevated in migraine patients, anodal tDCS—by increasing cortical excitability—might increase the probability of migraine attack in these patients, even beyond the end of its application (Liebetanz et al., 2006), or, in contrast, might have similar homeostatic effects as high-frequency rTMS as demonstrated by Brighina et al. (2010).

RELATED ISSUES

Safety in Transcranial Magnetic Stimulation

Although TMS is a non-invasive and relatively safe brain stimulation technique, it should be noted that there is the possibility to induce adverse effects. The most common side effects are local pain, discomfort, headache, syncope, and defective hearing. The most severe, though not common, adverse effect associated with rTMS is seizures induction. To avoid this serious incident, subjects should be carefully screened for conditions that may increase cortical excitability. Therefore, migraine patients might have increased risk of seizures especially if receiving high-frequency rTMS. In addition, researchers should follow the safety guidelines (Rossi et al., 2009) before applying TMS and refer to its recommended stimulation parameters and application guidelines before establishing a new protocol.

Transcranial Magnetic Stimulation as a Clinical Tool and Intervention

TMS has a broad range of demands as a clinical tool, and recently there has been intensive testing of its various abilities. The most widespread clinical use of TMS is for the treatment of mood disorders—particularly major depression. Many such conditions are comorbid in migraine patients.

FUTURE DIRECTIONS

Results from studies to date show that TMS and tDCS seem to be useful tools for the study of the pathophysiology of the migraine brain and the migraine aura. Further studies are needed to explore the therapeutic potential of rTMS in migraine, especially for prophylactic treatment. Additionally, more studies investigating the effects of single-pulse TMS as an abortive intervention for migraine attacks are needed. An important next step is to explore optimal stimulation parameters and the duration of the long-term effects. Furthermore, further work is needed to assess whether TMS would have any long-lasting effects.

REFERENCES

Antal, A., Lang, N., Boros, K., Nitsche, M., Siebner, H. R., & Paulus, W. (2008). Homeostatic metaplasticity of the motor cortex is altered during headache-free intervals in migraine with aura. *Cerebral Cortex, 18*(11), 2701–2705.

Aurora, S. K., Ahmad, B. K., Welch, K. M., Bhardhwaj, P., & Ramadan, N. M. (1998). Transcranial magnetic stimulation confirms hyperexcitability of occipital cortex in migraine. *Neurology, 50*(4), 1111–1114.

Aurora, S. K., al-Sayeed, F., & Welch, K. M. (1999). The cortical silent period is shortened in migraine with aura. *Cephalalgia, 19*(8), 708–712.

Aurora, S. K., Cao, Y., Bowyer, S. M., & Welch, K. M. (1999). The occipital cortex is hyperexcitable in migraine: Experimental evidence. *Headache, 39*(7), 469–476.

Aurora, S. K., & Welch, K. M. (1998). Brain excitability in migraine: Evidence from transcranial magnetic stimulation studies. *Current Opinion in Neurology, 11*(3), 205–209.

Avery, D. H., Holtzheimer, P. E., 3rd, Fawaz, W., Russo, J., Neumaier, J., Dunner, D. L., et al. (2007). Transcranial magnetic stimulation reduces pain in patients with major depression: A sham-controlled study. *Journal of Nervous and Mental Disorders, 195*(5), 378–381.

Barker, A. T., Jalinous, R., & Freeston, I. L. (1985). Non-invasive magnetic stimulation of human motor cortex. *Lancet, 1*(8437), 1106–1107.

Bohotin, V., Fumal, A., Vandenheede, M., Gerard, P., Bohotin, C., Maertens de Noordhout, A., et al. (2002). Effects of repetitive transcranial magnetic stimulation on visual evoked potentials in migraine. *Brain, 125*(Pt 4), 912–922.

Borckardt, J. J., Reeves, S. T., Weinstein, M., Smith, A. R., Shelley, N., Kozel, F. A., et al. (2008). Significant analgesic effects of one session of postoperative left prefrontal cortex repetitive transcranial magnetic stimulation: A replication study. *Brain Stimulation, 1*(2), 122–127.

Boulloche, N., Denuelle, M., Payoux, P., Fabre, N., Trotter, Y., & Geraud, G. (2010). Photophobia in migraine: An interictal PET study of cortical hyperexcitability and its modulation by pain. *Journal of Neurology, Neurosurgery, and Psychiatry, 81*(9), 978–984.

Brighina, F., Giglia, G., Scalia, S., Francolini, M., Palermo, A., & Fierro, B. (2005). Facilitatory effects of 1 Hz rTMS in motor cortex of patients affected by migraine with aura. *Experimental Brain Research, 161*(1), 34–38.

Brighina, F., Palermo, A., Daniele, O., Aloisio, A., & Fierro, B. (2010). High-frequency transcranial magnetic stimulation on motor cortex of patients affected by migraine with aura: A way to restore normal cortical excitability? *Cephalalgia, 30*(1), 46–52.

Brighina, F., Piazza, A., Vitello, G., Aloisio, A., Palermo, A., Daniele, O., et al. (2004). rTMS of the prefrontal cortex in the treatment of chronic migraine: A pilot study. *Journal of Neurological Sciences, 227*(1), 67–71.

Chadaide, Z., Arlt, S., Antal, A., Nitsche, M. A., Lang, N., & Paulus, W. (2007). Transcranial direct current stimulation reveals inhibitory deficiency in migraine. *Cephalalgia, 27*(7), 833–839.

Chronicle, E. P., Pearson, A. J., & Mulleners, W. M. (2006). Objective assessment of cortical excitability in migraine with and without aura. *Cephalalgia, 26*(7), 801–808.

Clarke, B. M., Upton, A. R., Kamath, M. V., Al-Harbi, T., & Castellanos, C. M. (2006). Transcranial magnetic stimulation for migraine: Clinical effects. *Journal of Headache and Pain, 7*(5), 341–346.

Conte, A., Barbanti, P., Frasca, V., Iacovelli, E., Gabriele, M., Giacomelli, E., et al. (2010). Differences in short-term primary motor cortex synaptic potentiation as assessed by repetitive transcranial magnetic stimulation in migraine patients with and without aura. *Pain, 148*(1), 43–48.

Elahi, B., & Chen, R. (2009). Effect of transcranial magnetic stimulation on Parkinson motor function—systematic review of controlled clinical trials. *Movement Disorders, 24*(3), 357–363.

Fregni, F., Freedman, S., & Pascual-Leone, A. (2007). Recent advances in the treatment of chronic pain with non-invasive brain stimulation techniques. *Lancet Neurology, 6*(2), 188–191.

Fregni, F., & Pascual-Leone, A. (2005). Repetitive transcranial magnetic stimulation for the treatment of depression. *Journal of Psychiatry and Neuroscience, 30*(6), 434; author reply 434–435.

Fumal, A., Coppola, G., Bohotin, V., Gerardy, P. Y., Seidel, L., Donneau, A. F., et al. (2006). Induction of long-lasting changes of visual cortex excitability by five daily sessions of repetitive transcranial magnetic stimulation (rTMS) in healthy volunteers and migraine patients. *Cephalalgia, 26*(2), 143–149.

Gerwig, M., Niehaus, L., Kastrup, O., Stude, P., & Diener, H. C. (2005). Visual cortex excitability in migraine evaluated by single and paired magnetic stimuli. *Headache, 45*(10), 1394–1399.

Gunaydin, S., Soysal, A., Atay, T., & Arpaci, B. (2006). Motor and occipital cortex excitability in migraine patients. *Canadian Journal of Neurological Sciences, 33*(1), 63–67.

Ilmoniemi, R. J., Virtanen, J., Ruohonen, J., Karhu, J., Aronen, H. J., Naatanen, R., et al. (1997). Neuronal responses to magnetic stimulation reveal cortical reactivity and connectivity. *Neuroreport, 8*(16), 3537–3540.

Khedr, E. M., Ahmed, M. A., & Mohamed, K. A. (2006). Motor and visual cortical excitability in migraineurs patients with or without aura: Transcranial magnetic stimulation. *Neurophysiology Clinics, 36*(1), 13–18.

Kobayashi, M., & Pascual-Leone, A. (2003). Transcranial magnetic stimulation in neurology. *Lancet Neurology, 2*(3), 145–156.

Lefaucheur, J. P. (2008). Use of repetitive transcranial magnetic stimulation in pain relief. *Expert Reviews in Neurotherapy, 8*(5), 799–808.

Lefaucheur, J. P., Antal, A., Ahdab, R., Ciampi de Andrade, D., Fregni, F., Khedr, E. M., et al. (2008). The use of repetitive transcranial magnetic stimulation (rTMS) and transcranial direct current stimulation (tDCS) to relieve pain. *Brain Stimulation, 1*(4), 337–344.

Liebetanz, D., Fregni, F., Monte-Silva, K. K., Oliveira, M. B., Amancio-dos-Santos, A., Nitsche, M. A., et al. (2006). After-effects of transcranial direct current stimulation (tDCS) on cortical spreading depression. *Neuroscience Letters, 398*(1–2), 85–90.

Lipton, R. B., Dodick, D. W., Silberstein, S. D., Saper, J. R., Aurora, S. K., Pearlman, S. H., et al. (2010). Single-pulse transcranial magnetic stimulation for acute treatment of migraine with aura: A randomised, double-blind, parallel-group, sham-controlled trial. *Lancet Neurology, 9*(4), 373–380.

Lopez-Ibor, J. J., Lopez-Ibor, M. I., & Pastrana, J. I. (2008). Transcranial magnetic stimulation. *Current Opinion in Psychiatry, 21*(6), 640–644.

Marg, E., & Rudiak, D. (1994). Phosphenes induced by magnetic stimulation over the occipital brain: Description and probable site of stimulation. *Optometry and Vision Science, 71*(5), 301–311.

May, A., & Jurgens, T. P. (2011). [Therapeutic neuromodulation in primary headaches.] *Nervenarzt, 82*(6), 743–752.

Mulleners, W. M., Chronicle, E. P., Palmer, J. E., Koehler, P. J., & Vredeveld, J. W. (2001a). Suppression of perception in migraine: Evidence for reduced inhibition in the visual cortex. *Neurology, 56*(2), 178–183.

Mulleners, W. M., Chronicle, E. P., Palmer, J. E., Koehler, P. J., & Vredeveld, J. W. (2001b). Visual cortex excitability in migraine with and without aura. *Headache, 41*(6), 565–572.

Mulleners, W. M., Chronicle, E. P., Vredeveld, J. W., & Koehler, P. J. (2002). Visual cortex excitability in migraine before and after valproate prophylaxis: A pilot study using TMS. *European Journal of Neurology, 9*(1), 35–40.

O'Reardon, J. P., Fontecha, J. F., Cristancho, M. A., & Newman, S. (2007). Unexpected reduction in migraine and psychogenic headaches following rTMS treatment for major depression: A report of two cases. *CNS Spectrum, 12*(12), 921–925.

Petersen, N. T., Pyndt, H. S., & Nielsen, J. B. (2003). Investigating human motor control by transcranial magnetic stimulation. *Experimental Brain Research, 152*(1), 1–16.

Ridding, M. C., & Rothwell, J. C. (2007). Is there a future for therapeutic use of transcranial magnetic stimulation? *Nature Reviews Neuroscience, 8*(7), 559–567.

Rossi, S., Hallett, M., Rossini, P. M., & Pascual-Leone, A. (2009). Safety, ethical considerations, and application guidelines for the use of transcranial magnetic stimulation in clinical practice and research. *Clinical Neurophysiology, 120*(12), 2008–2039.

Sampson, S. M., Rome, J. D., & Rummans, T. A. (2006). Slow-frequency rTMS reduces fibromyalgia pain. *Pain Medicine, 7*(2), 115–118.

Teepker, M., Hotzel, J., Timmesfeld, N., Reis, J., Mylius, V., Haag, A., et al. (2010). Low-frequency rTMS of the vertex in the prophylactic treatment of migraine. *Cephalalgia, 30*(2), 137–144.

Terao, Y., & Ugawa, Y. (2002). Basic mechanisms of TMS. *Journal of Clinical Neurophysiology, 19*(4), 322–343.

Thickbroom, G. W. (2007). Transcranial magnetic stimulation and synaptic plasticity: Experimental framework and human models. *Experimental Brain Research, 180*(4), 583–593.

Wagle-Shukla, A., Ni, Z., Gunraj, C. A., Bahl, N., & Chen, R. (2009). Effects of short interval intracortical inhibition and intracortical facilitation on short interval intracortical facilitation in human primary motor cortex. *Journal of Physiology, 587*(Pt 23), 5665–5678.

Welch, K. M., D'Andrea, G., Tepley, N., Barkley, G., & Ramadan, N. M. (1990). The concept of migraine as a state of central neuronal hyperexcitability. *Neurological Clinics, 8*(4), 817–828.

Werhahn, K. J., Kunesch, E., Noachtar, S., Benecke, R., & Classen, J. (1999). Differential effects on motorcortical inhibition induced by blockade of GABA uptake in humans. *Journal of Physiology, 517*(Pt 2), 591–597.

Werhahn, K. J., Wiseman, K., Herzog, J., Forderreuther, S., Dichgans, M., & Straube, A. (2000). Motor cortex excitability in patients with migraine with aura and hemiplegic migraine. *Cephalalgia, 20*(1), 45–50.

Young, W., Shaw, J., Bloom, M., & Gebeline-Myers, C. (2008). Correlation of increase in phosphene threshold with reduction of migraine frequency: Observation of levetiracetam-treated subjects. *Headache, 48*(10), 1490–1498.

29 Measures of Cortical Excitability

GIANLUCA COPPOLA AND JEAN SCHOENEN

INTRODUCTION

Among the various neuronal structures that appear to be involved in migraine pathophysiology, the cerebral cortex has raised interest for a long time, because the aura of the migraine attack clearly seems to have a cortical origin pointing toward an abnormal cortical excitability. However, neither the pathophysiology of the aura nor that of the attack itself is likely to fully explain why the attacks recur and the disorder perpetuates itself (i.e., the so-called migraine diathesis or predisposition). Hints for such an explanation may be better looked for in the interictal period.

Several studies have searched for interictal neural abnormalities that may predispose to migraine attacks. During the last decades the methods of clinical neurophysiology have allowed the in vivo measurement of the migraineur's electrocortical responses to various sensory stimuli. In particular, the visual, auditory, somatosensory, and cognitive evoked potentials have undoubtedly demonstrated that lack of habituation during stimulus repetition is a reproducible central nervous system (CNS) dysfunction in the commonest forms of migraine. Lack of habituation has a familial character and undergoes periodic fluctuations in strict relationship with the development of the migraine cycle as well as modifications after certain pharmacological or non-pharmacological treatments. In addition, recent more selective and sophisticated electrophysiological techniques, such as quantitative electroencephalography and the analysis of the high-frequency bands embedded in the common evoked response signals, have been valuable contributions for the understanding of migraine pathophysiology.

We will review here the available neurophysiological data providing information about the response properties of the cerebral cortex in migraineurs, with emphasis on the more recent data. We will limit ourselves to the electrophysiological methods and not comment in detail on the functional neuroimaging studies of cortical responsivity in migraine, as they are discussed in other chapters of this book.

AVAILABLE DATA

Electroencephalography

Electroencephalography (EEG) was the first electrophysiological method allowing the detection of an abnormal cortical responsivity in migraine patients. Although the EEG is not as useful for diagnosis of nonacute primary headache disorders (Sandrini et al., 2011), it may provide some useful information in a research setting.

A so-called *H-response* (i.e., enhanced brain waves produced by repetitive light stimulation at high frequency and synchronized with this frequency or enhanced "photic driving") was consistently reported in migraineurs during the last 50 years (Chorlton & Kane, 2000; de Tommaso et al., 1998; Genco et al., 1994; Golla & Winter, 1959; Péchadre & Gibert, 1987; Puca et al., 1992, 1996; Schoenen et al., 1987; Simon et al., 1982, 1983; Smyth & Winter, 1964; Tsounis & Varfis, 1992). All these studies, however, were conducted during different phases of the migraine cycle. Recently, Bjørk et al. addressed this issue, recording visual evoked EEG responses in 41 migraineurs and 32 healthy subjects and comparing recordings between attacks with those performed before, during, and after an attack, as well as with the EEGs of healthy subjects (Bjørk et al., 2010). They found actually depressed photic driving both during and between attacks in migraineurs without aura, while photic driving was increased immediately before an attack.

EEG power mapping using quantitative topographical EEG (qEEG) showed two parameters to be particularly significant in migraine: alpha activity abnormalities and the presence of slowing. The alpha abnormalities consisted mostly of alpha rhythm asymmetries and alpha total power abnormalities (Facchetti et al., 1990; Jonkman & Lelieveld 1981). Alpha power was decreased in migraine with aura patients contralateral to the visual hemifield affected by the aura during (Seri et al., 1993) and within 3 days of an attack (Schoenen et al., 1987). Alpha power was also reduced in migraine without aura on the headache side and in patients with menstrual migraine up to 24 hours before the attack (Schoenen, et al. 1987). In some studies an increase in alpha power was observed (Facchetti et al., 1990; Hughes & Robbins 1990; Sauer et al., 1997).

In a source localization qEEG study using low-resolution electromagnetic tomography (LORETA) in migraine without aura patients, alpha power was found to be increased in parts of the precuneus and the posterior part of the middle temporal gyrus of the right hemisphere, and decreased bilaterally in medial parts of the frontal cortex including the anterior cingulate and the superior and medial frontal gyri (Clemens et al., 2008). In a blinded paired qEEG study, Bjørk and Sand suggested that migraineurs are most susceptible to have an attack when anterior qEEG delta power and posterior alpha and theta asymmetry values are high (Bjørk & Sand, 2008). The changes in alpha rhythm seem to be related to increased migraine load and clinical photophobia (Bjørk, Stovner, Nilsen et al., 2009). In one study, nonspecific EEG abnormalities were modified by treatment with flunarizine in parallel with clinical improvement (Formisano et al., 1988). Multichannel EEG in migraine without aura patients between attacks during repetitive flash stimulation identified hypersynchronization of the alpha rhythm in all regions of the scalp (de Tommaso, Marinazzo, et al., 2005), a phenomenon that was reverted by preventive treatment with levetiracetam (de Tommaso, Marinazzo, et al., 2007), but not by low-frequency repetitive transcranial magnetic stimulation (rTMS) over the occipital cortex (de Tommaso et al., 2011).

Migraine patients also may have widespread increase in slow activities (theta and/or delta) mostly over temporo-occipital areas (Facchetti et al., 1990; Hughes & Robbins, 1990; Sauer et al., 1997; Seri et al., 1993; Valdizán et al., 1994). A global increase in theta and delta activity was found interictally in a blinded controlled study (Bjørk, Stovner, Engstrøm et al., 2009). With the method of nonlinear multielectrode sleep EEG analysis, a pronounced focus of maximum change in dimensional complexity was observed in the preictal period over the scalp area where subsequently the migraine headache would be perceived (Fritzer et al., 2004).

Because of the clinical report by patients of a possible relationship between sleep and migraine attacks, several studies have monitored the EEG during sleep. A relation seems to emerge between rapid eye movement (REM) sleep and the appearance of nighttime headache (Dexter & Weitzman, 1970), and between morning arousals with migraine and larger amounts of stage III to IV and REM sleep during the preceding night (Dexter, 1979). During the latter, a significant decrease in the number of arousals, a decrease in REM sleep density, a significant decrease in beta power in the slow-wave sleep, and a decrease of alpha power during the first REM period were also reported (Göder et al., 2001) and interpreted as a decrease in cortical activation during sleep preceding migraine attacks.

Moreover, loss of dimensional complexity in the second sleep cycle was observed examining nonlinear EEG measures during the development of a spontaneous migraine attack (Strenge et al., 2001). The study by Della Marca et al. is the only full-night polysomnographic study in a group of adult migraine without aura patients during pain-free nights compared with healthy subjects (Della Marca et al., 2006). It reported a reduction in the cyclic alternating pattern and a lower index of high-frequency EEG arousals during REM sleep, which was interpreted by the authors as reflecting a general hypoactivity of the arousal systems in migraineurs during sleep. Taken together, these studies tend to indicate a reduction of cortical activation during sleep, especially during the night preceding an attack.

Magnetoencephalography

Since magnetoencephalography (MEG) records activity from tangentially oriented cortical dipoles, it was thought to be the most suitable atraumatic method to detect cortical equivalents of cortical spreading depression (CSD) in migraine. In the first published study, various combinations of large-amplitude waves, suppression of spontaneous cortical activity, and slow potential shifts were indeed recorded during attacks of migraine with aura (Barkley et al., 1990). In a subsequent study (Bowyer et al., 2001), the same group confirmed during spontaneous and visual stimulation-induced migraine aura the occurrence of slow potential shifts very similar to those found during CSD in animals and abnormal spread of visual evoked activity, but the large-amplitude waves were found to be ocular artifacts (Bowyer et al., 1999). After effective prophylactic therapy with valproate, direct current (DC) MEG shifts were reduced (Bowyer et al., 2005). In a patient having a migrainous scintillating scotoma in the right hemifield, an MEG study found alpha band desynchronization in the opposite extrastriate and temporal cortices for the duration of the visual disturbance, and gamma band desynchronization peaking 10 minutes following the aura (Hall et al., 2004).

Taken together, the MEG findings favor of the occurrence of a cortical phenomenon similar to CSD during the migraine aura. They provide no evidence, however, in favor of cortical dysexcitability between attacks.

Evoked Potentials

During the last 40 years, evoked cortical responses with various paradigms were extensively studied in migraine. Almost every sensory stimulus modality has been explored, but particularly visual and auditory stimulations. Various interictal abnormalities have been reported by analyzing the evoked responses in a classical way of averaging a large number of single responses. However, when amplitude change is calculated in successive blocks of 50/100 averaged evoked responses without stimulus interruption, deficient lack of habituation, that is, of the normal response decrement, was the most reproducible functional abnormality.

VISUAL EVOKED RESPONSES

An abnormal steady-state visual evoked response (SS-VEP) by a sine-wave visual stimulus was seen in migraineurs (Nyrke & Lang, 1982; Nyrke et al., 1989, 1990; Shibata et al., 2008) and improved after administration of propranolol or femoxetine (Nyrke et al., 1984).

Amplitude of flash or pattern reversal visual evoked response (PR-VEP) was found normal in the majority of studies (Áfra et al., 1998, 2000; Drake et al., 1990; Lai et al., 1989; Mariani et al., 1988; Sand & Vingen 2000; Schoenen et al., 1995; Sener et al., 1997; Wang et al., 1999), but in some studies it was increased (Connolly et al., 1982; Kennard et al., 1978; Khalil et al., 2000; Lehtonen, 1974; Mariani et al., 1988; Sand et al., 2009; Shibata et al., 1997a, 2005) and in others decreased (Khalil et al., 2000; Polich et al., 1986; Tagliati et al., 1995) compared to controls. Interhemispheric asymmetry of VEP amplitude was reported in several studies (Benna et al., 1985; Coppola, Parisi, et al., 2007; Coutin-Churchman & Padrón de Freytez, 2003; Khalil et al., 2011; Logi et al., 2001; Shibata et al., 1997b, 1998; Tagliati et al., 1995; Tsounis et al., 1993).

When *habituation* of the evoked potential is assessed by averaging successive blocks of responses, a deficit of habituation seems to be the hallmark of migraineurs between attacks (Fig. 29–1)

After the first description of a deficient habituation to a stereotyped presentation of a checkerboard pattern in 1995 (Schoenen et al., 1995), it was confirmed in several other studies (Áfra et al., 1998; Bohotin et al., 2002; Coppola, Ambrosini, et al., 2007; Coppola, Currà, Serrao, et al., 2010; Coppola, Currà, Sava, et al., 2010; Di Clemente et al., 2005; Fumal et al., 2006; Ozkul & Bozlar, 2002; Wang et al., 1999). Interestingly, selective serotonin reuptake inhibitors, which are not consistently effective in migraine preventive treatment, may be able to increase amplitude of the first VEP block and to normalize habituation (Ozkul & Bozlar, 2002).

Short-term habituation or adaptation is defined as a response decrement as a result of repeated stimulation and usually exhibits an exponential course (Rankin et al., 2009). It is a common feature of any cortical response that helps limit the response range of neurons to encode sensory signals with much larger dynamic ranges. The mechanism of habituation protects the cortex against the overflow of inward information and, at the same time,

prepares the stimulated neuronal networks for the appearance of subsequent stimuli. Habituation is also a seminal phenomenon in learning processes (Thompson & Spencer, 1966).

In theory, the habituation deficit in migraine could be due to hyperexcitability (secondary to hyperexcitable excitatory neurons) (Aurora et al., 1998) or hypoexcitable inhibitory interneurons (Mulleners et al., 2001). The data showing that evoked potentials in response to all non-painful sensory modalities are characterized in migraine by a normal or slightly lower amplitude in the first block of averaged responses (i.e., after a low number of stimuli) (Ambrosini et al., 2003; Ozkul & Uckardes, 2002; Schoenen et al., 1995; Wang et al., 1995), and that this initial amplitude is inversely related to the degree of habituation (Áfra et al., 2000), suggest that in migraine the cortical habituation deficit may be a consequence of an initial hypoactivation of sensory cortices (Fig. 29–1). Further support in favor of this hypothesis comes from studies of cortical activity modulation by transcranial magnetic stimulation (TMS), of high-frequency oscillations embedded in standard evoked cortical potentials, and of paired-pulse suppression of VEPs.

In migraine patients, high-frequency (10-Hz) rTMS that facilitates the underlying visual cortex increased moderately the amplitude in the first VEP block and normalized habituation over successive blocks, while low-frequency (1-Hz) rTMS, which has an inhibitory effect, had no effect. By contrast, in healthy subjects, low-frequency rTMS reduced first-block amplitude as well as habituation, whereas rapid rTMS had no effect (Bohotin et al., 2002; Fumal et al., 2006). These rTMS data suggest that deactivating the visual cortex produces deficient habituation and that the habituation deficit of migraineurs can be reversed by activating the visual cortex.

Tonic pain induced by using the cold pressor test was able to significantly decrease first VEP block amplitude and abolish normal habituation in healthy subjects, probably by acting on brainstem structures that modulate thalamocortical activation. By contrast, tonic pain left the deficient VEP habituation unchanged in migraineurs, suggesting an abnormality of the subcortical structures subserving tonic pain (Coppola, Serrao, Currà, et al., 2010; Coppola, Currà, Serrao, et al., 2010).

Three minutes of forced *hyperventilation* also decreased VEP amplitude in block 1 and abolished the normal VEP habituation in healthy subjects. In migraine patients, hyperventilation further decreased the already low first-block amplitude and worsened the interictal habituation deficit (Coppola, Currà, Sava, et al., 2010). The effects of hyperventilation can be attributed to the modulation of thalamocortical activity leading to reduced preactivation

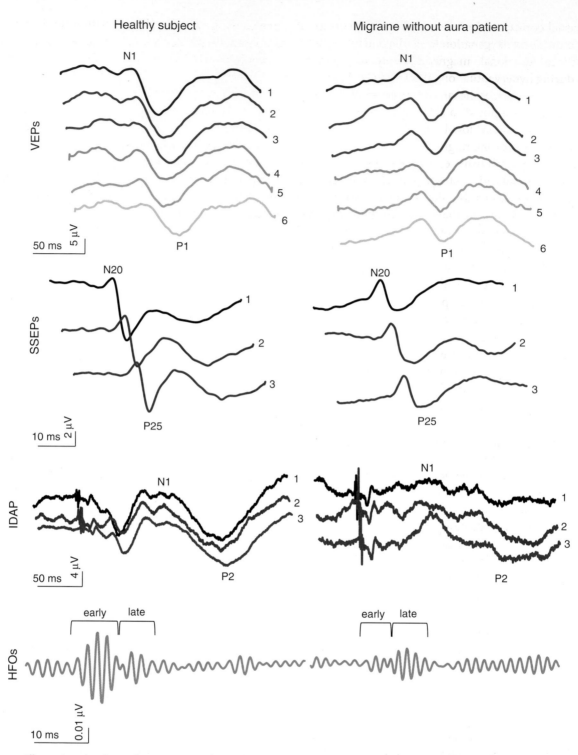

FIGURE 29–1 *Illustrative recordings of pattern reversal visual evoked potentials (VEPs), somatosensory evoked potentials (SSEPs), cortical auditory evoked potentials (intensity dependence of auditory evoked cortical potentials [IDAP]), and SSEP high-frequency oscillations (HFOs) in a healthy subject and a migraine without aura patient between attacks. VEPs and SSEPs are successive blocks of averaged responses during continuous stimulation; IDAP shows responses for stimulations at 40, 60, and 90 dB; HFOs show early and late components. Compared to the healthy subject, the migraineur is characterized by a lower amplitude of the first block of averaged responses (VEPs and SSEPs), lack of habituation over successive blocks of responses (VEPs and SSEPs), amplitude increase with increasing intensity of auditory stimuli (IDAP), and decreased amplitude of the early burst of HFOs. For explanations, see text.*

of the visual cortex, as also evidenced by the decrease of the occipital blood oxygenation level–dependent (BOLD) contrast on functional magnetic resonance imaging (fMRI) during hyperventilation (Weckesser et al., 1999).

Lack of habituation of the late visual *gamma band oscillations* (>20 Hz), supposed to be of postsynaptic cortical origin, parallels standard low-band VEP habituation loss in both migraine with and migraine without aura between attacks (Coppola, Ambrosini, et al., 2007). We interpreted these results as indicative of a dysfunction in cortical oscillatory networks possibly due to an abnormal thalamic control. A change in thalamocortical activity due, for instance, to an anatomical or functional disconnection of the thalamus from its controlling inputs (e.g., aminergic brainstem nuclei) can favor low-frequency activity, which at the cortical level will reduce lateral inhibition and enhance high-frequency phase-locked discharges in cortical networks of inhibitory interneurons. This is postulated to underlie the so-called thalamocortical dysrhythmia syndromes (Llinás et al., 1999; Walton et al., 2010), which, when applied to migraine, would imply that a serotonergic disconnection of the thalamus can enhance low-frequency and gamma frequency activity, leading, respectively, to a deficit in habituation of low-band VEP and visual-evoked gamma band oscillations (Coppola, Ambrosini, et al., 2007).

Further evidence for reduced cortical preactivation came recently from a study of *paired-pulse suppression* using short-stimulus-onset asynchronies. Höffken et al. found at baseline lower VEP amplitudes with subsequently reduced paired-pulse inhibition in migraine without aura patients compared to healthy subjects (Höffken et al., 2009). The authors conclude that in migraine the cortical preactivation via thalamocortical transmission is reduced as a part of a compensatory mechanism to protect the cortex against overstimulation. Interestingly, similar results were recently obtained with another visual-stimulus-onset asynchrony psychophysical paradigm, the metacontrast masking test (Shepherd et al., 2011).

AUDITORY EVOKED POTENTIALS

The short-latency *brainstem auditory evoked responses* (BAERs), assessing the function of auditory pathways in the brainstem, are normal interictally in the majority of studies (Benna et al., 1985; Bussone et al., 1985; Drake et al., 1990; Podoshin et al., 1987; Sand & Vingen, 2000). However, prolonged absolute latencies and interpeak differences, when present, seem not to be related to the presence of vertigo (Dash et al., 2008). In agreement with VEP studies, a significant increase of side asymmetries of BAER has been reported (Bussone et al., 1985; Schlake et al., 1990). Lack of habituation of wave IV to V was found in one study, in which a direct relationship between BAER amplitudes and blood 5-HT levels was also reported in controls but not in migraineurs (Sand et al., 2008a).

Sensory gating—a filtering of external stimuli by central sensory pathways—can be assessed by the suppression of the cortical response to a test stimulus delivered after an identical conditioning stimulus. In a paired-stimulus auditory P50 event-related potential paradigm, sensory gating was markedly reduced in migraine patients compared to control subjects (Ambrosini et al., 2001; Siniatchkin et al., 2003), which was considered to reflect reduced short-term habituation.

Another interictal electrophysiological abnormality in migraine is marked stimulus *intensity dependence of auditory evoked cortical potentials* (IDAP) (Wang et al., 1996), a phenomenon attributed to deficient habituation, especially for higher stimulus intensities (Ambrosini et al., 2003), and to reduced serotoninergic activity (Fig. 29–1). This phenomenon was, however, not confirmed in two works from another group, possibly because of methodological differences (Sand & Vingen, 2000; Sand, Zhitniy, et al., 2008a).

Recently, we studied the interference of light stimulation with IDAP and found that migraineurs can have larger modifications of their cortical reactivity during sensory overload than controls, possibly because of an altered EEG response (alpha rhythm hypersynchronization) (de Tommaso, Marinazzo, et al., 2005) and/or a reduced cross-modal sensory gating (Ambrosini et al., 2011).

SOMATOSENSORY EVOKED POTENTIALS

Somatosensory evoked potentials (SSEPs) are generated in afferent pathways, subcortical structures, and various regions of the cerebral cortex after electrical stimulation of a peripheral nerve. Amplitude and latency of the standard SSEPs after median nerve stimulation recorded between attacks were normal in the majority of studies (Coppola et al., 2005; Coppola, Currà, Di Lorenzo, et al., 2010; Firenze et al., 1988; Marlowe, 1995; Sakuma et al., 2004), although in some studies delayed latencies (Montagna et al., 1985) and decreased (de Tommaso et al., 1997) or increased (Lang et al., 2004) amplitudes were reported respective to controls. In one subject, the parietal N20 SSPE component was significantly prolonged and reduced in amplitude during the hemiparesthetic migraine aura, and these abnormalities gradually returned to normal during the headache phase (Chayasirisobhon, 1995). In agreement both with VEP and BAER studies, a significant increase of interhemispheric asymmetries in amplitude of the N30 SSEP component has been observed (de Tommaso et al., 1997). Deficient habituation has been confirmed interictally also for the SSEP components. In fact, both cervical N13 (Ozkul & Uckardes, 2002) and sensorimotor N20 (Coppola, Currà, Di Lorenzo, et al., 2010; Lang et al., 2004; Ozkul & Uckardes, 2002) and P35 (Lang et al., 2004) components showed an augmenting, instead of a reducing, response during stimulus repetition.

Appropriate band-pass filtering allows the detection of high-frequency oscillations (HFOs) that are embedded within the classical N20 broadband components of standard SSEPs. They are thought to reflect spike activity in thalamocortical cholinergic fibers (early HFOs) and in cortical inhibitory/excitatory fast-spiking neurons (late HFOs). Two independent groups found that early HFOs were decreased in migraine between attacks (Coppola et al., 2005; Sakuma et al., 2004), which suggests that activity in thalamocortical afferents is reduced, while late HFOs were normal (Coppola et al., 2005) or decreased (Sakuma et al., 2004). This again supports the hypothesis that the habituation deficit in migraine is likely due to a reduced preactivation level of sensory cortices (Fig. 29–1).

CONTINGENT NEGATIVE VARIATION AND P300

Contingent negative variation (CNV) is a slow cortical potential related to higher mental functions, which consists of a negative wave generated in a reaction-time paradigm, which is supposed to reflect expectancy, attention, preparation, and motivation. Its early component (related to the warning stimulus) may represent the level of expectation and it is supposed to be modulated by the noradrenergic system, while its late component is thought to be related to motor readiness and to be under dopaminergic control (Birbaumer et al., 1990).

Increased CNV amplitude, more pronounced for the early component (iCNV), has been consistently found interictally in migraine by several independent groups (Böcker et al., 1990; Kropp & Gerber, 1993a; Maertens de Noordhout et al., 1986). The iCNV augmentation is supposed to reflect an excess of excitatory versus inhibitory processes, and seems to be enhanced by stress and the premenstrual phase of the ovarian cycle (Siniatchkin, Averkina, Andrasik, et al., 2006; Siniatchkin, Averkina, & Gerber, 2006), but not by pregnancy (Darabaneanu et al., 2008). iCNV abnormalities correlate inversely with disease duration (Kropp et al., 2000).

CNV habituation is reported to be markedly decreased or even abolished in patients affected by migraine without aura between attacks (Kropp & Gerber, 1993a, 1995; Schoenen & Timsit-Berthier, 1993; Schoenen et al., 1985). This abnormality was observed especially for the early and not for the late CNV component (Kropp & Gerber 1993a, 1993b; Siniatchkin, Gerber, et al., 2000; Siniatchkin et al., 2001; Siniatchkin, Averkina, Andrasik, et al., 2006;

Siniatchkin, Averkina, & Gerber, 2006; Siniatchkin et al., 2007). Prophylactic treatment with β-blockers (Ahmed, 1999; Schoenen, 1986; Schoenen et al., 1986; Siniatchkin et al., 2007) and anticonvulsants such as topiramate and levetiracetam (Tommaso et al., 2008) decrease CNV amplitude and increase habituation. A loss of habituation in migraine was also described for the cognitive functions, as measured by event-related P300 potential. This can only be seen during the migraine interval with a visual (Evers et al., 1997, 1999) or auditory (Siniatchkin et al., 2003; Wang & Schoenen, 1998; Wang et al., 1995) oddball paradigm, and is inversely correlated with platelet 5-HT content (Evers et al., 1999).

During the event-related potential paradigms, the subject is often asked to respond to a stimulus, which allows measures of *reaction times* in parallel to the electrophysiological recording. Reaction times have also been assessed in dedicated psychophysical studies. Reaction times (RTs) and error data (omissions to respond or false responses) recorded during a cognitive paradigm were found either normal (Buodo et al., 2004; Evers et al., 1997, 1998, 1999; Mulder et al., 2002), prolonged (Annovazzi et al., 2004; Wang et al., 1995), or shortened (Woestenburg et al., 1993). In several studies, migraineurs were found to make more errors than controls (Wang et al., 1995). Neurophysiological tests also found either normal (Antal et al., 2005; Conlon & Hine, 2000; Fierro et al., 2003; Mazzucchi et al., 1988; Palmer & Chronicle, 1998), slower (Mulder et al., 1999), or faster RTs (Wray et al., 1995). Interestingly, RTs increase just before (Siniatchkin, Averkina, et al., 2006), during (Evers et al., 1999; Mazzucchi et al., 1988), and for some time after the migraine attack (Siniatchkin, Averkina, et al., 2006), which might explain in part the variability of results reported in the literature. Another possible explanation for this variability could be the inverted U-shape relation between performance and level of arousal (reviewed in Hebb, 1955).

PAIN-RELATED EVOKED POTENTIALS

Brief radiant heat pulses, generated by CO_2 laser stimulation able to excite Aδ and C thermal nociceptors in the superficial skin, have been used frequently to study nociceptive evoked brain responses in the trigeminal or extracranial systems. The laser-evoked potential (LEP) comprises two main complexes, N1–P1 and N2–P2, of which the latter originates in the anterior cingulate cortex, an area that is primarily devoted to the attentive and emotional aspects of pain (Treede et al., 2003).

In migraine, during the interictal phase, the N2–P2 LEP complex is normal in basal conditions after both cephalic and extracephalic stimulation. Remote heterotopic capsaicin application (de Tommaso, Difruscolo, et al., 2007) as well as a distraction task (de Tommaso et al., 2008) reduces LEP amplitude in healthy subjects but not in migraineurs, probably because of a defective brainstem inhibitory control. In women suffering from migraine and healthy controls, there was a significant increase in amplitude of the N2–P2 complex in parallel with increased pain perception in the premenstrual phase (de Tommaso et al., 2009).

LEPs have confirmed that the reduced habituation during repetitive stimulation between migraine attacks also exists for the noxious stimulus modality during short (de Tommaso, Libro, et al., 2005) as well as long periods of stimulation (de Tommaso, Losito, Di Fuscolo, Sardaro et al., 2005; Valeriani et al., 2003). Moreover, patients had a lack of LEP habituation both after cephalic (supraorbital zone) and extracephalic (hand dorsum) stimulation (de Tommaso, Lo Sito, Di Fruscolo, Sardaro, et al., 2005; Valeriani et al., 2003). Interestingly, during the premenstrual phase, the N2–P2 LEP complex failed to habituate both in migrainous and healthy women (de Tommaso et al., 2009).

PERI-ICTAL CHANGES IN CORTICAL RESPONSIVITY

The cortical neurophysiological abnormalities summarized above for the interictal phase undergo marked changes across the migraine cycle. These changes occur immediately before (preictally) and during (ictally) the migraine attack.

Consecutive recordings over several days have shown that during the days preceding the attack, CNV amplitude and habituation deficit (Kropp & Gerber, 1998; Siniatchkin, Kropp, et al., 2000) as well as P300 habituation deficit (Evers et al., 1999) become maximal. During this time period migraineurs also have an exaggerated CNV amplitude increase and habituation decrease to stressful events (Siniatchkin, Averkina, et al., 2006). In a longitudinal study, increased VEP P1–N2 amplitude was observed within a few days before the attack compared with interictal recordings (Sand et al., 2008b), especially for large checks (Sand et al., 2009).

Within the 12 to 24 hours that immediately precede the attack (i.e., at a time point when so-called premonitory symptoms may occur), the habituation pattern of evoked potentials surprisingly normalizes. This has been shown for intensity dependence of auditory evoked potentials (Judit et al., 2000); CNV (Kropp & Gerber, 1998; Siniatchkin, Kropp, Gerber, Stephani, 2000), VEP (Chen et al., 2009; Judit et al., 2000), and SSEP (Coppola, Currà, Di Lorenzo, et al., 2010) amplitude; and visual P300

latency (Evers et al., 1999). The normalization of habituation may be due to activation of the rostral brainstem aminergic nuclei projecting to the thalamus and cortex (Bahra et al., 2001; Weiller et al., 1995), since early somatosensory high-frequency oscillation bursts, which reflect activity in thalamocortical projections and are reduced in migraine interictally, also normalize during an attack (Coppola et al., 2005) (Fig. 29–2). By contrast, pain evoked potentials tend to increase during the attack (de Tommaso et al., 2002) in parallel with a lowering of cutaneous pain thresholds (de Tommaso et al., 2002) and a reorganization of cortical areas devoted to pain processing (Buchgreitz et al., 2010; de Tommaso et al., 2004). Moreover, contrary to nonnoxious cortical responses, nociceptive evoked potentials show a persistent lack of habituation during the attack (de Tommaso, Lo Sito, Di Fruscolo, Sardaro, et al., 2005). The changes in pain evoked potentials have been attributed to central sensitization.

MEASURES OF CORTICAL EXCITABILITY IN CHRONIC MIGRAINE

Although most migraineurs suffer on average one or two attacks per month, about 4% of adults in the general population have evolved to chronic headache; that is, they have 15 or more headache days per month (Scher et al., 2008). The majority of them have chronic migraine (CM) and in more than 70% the headache chronification is associated with excessive intake of analgesics or specific antimigraine drugs, defining so-called medication overuse headache (MOH) (Olesen et al., 2006; Silberstein et al., 2005). The precise mechanisms underlying headache chronification are not fully understood, but central sensitization and dysfunctioning pain control systems are thought to play pivotal roles.

Assuming that the abnormalities of pain-related brain responses, already present in episodic migraine, would be even more pronounced in the chronic forms, electrophysiological studies have been performed in chronic migraine with (Ayzenberg et al., 2006) or without medication overuse (de Tommaso et al., 2003). Not surprisingly, an excessive increase in nociceptive cortical responses was detected in both groups. Interestingly, in patients with MOH, discontinuation of the acute medication overuse (triptans or nonsteroidal anti-inflammatory drugs [NSAIDs]) favored a normalization of the excessive pain-related potential amplitude (Ayzenberg et al., 2006).

In an analysis localizing the source of the most prominent laser-evoked potential peak (P2), de Tommaso et al. found that CM patients were characterized by prevalent activation of the rostral portion of the anterior cingulate

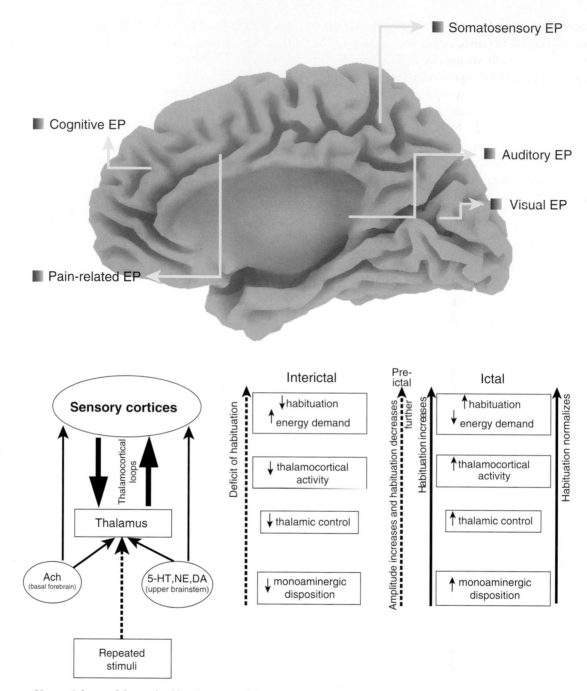

FIGURE 29–2 Upper: *Scheme of the cerebral localizations of the evoked potentials discussed in the chapter.* Lower: *Schematic representation of thalamocortical loops and their normal control by subcortical nuclei in normal conditions* (left) *and the hypothesis of a thalamocortical dysrhythmia in migraine* (right). *The interictal phase in migraine is characterized by a reduced aminergic control of thalamic nuclei leading to thalamocortical dysrhythmia, reduced preactivation, and habituation in sensory cortices. This further worsens preictally, but normalizes during the attack, likely thanks to the activation of brainstem nuclei. EP, evoked potential; ACh, acetylcholine; 5-HT, serotonin; NE, norepinephrine; DA, dopamine.*

cortex respective to episodic migraineurs and normal controls (de Tommaso, Lo Sito, Difruscolo, Libro, et al., 2005). We recently reported excessive cortical activation also in a nonpainful SSEP study, where N20–P25 amplitudes were greater in migraine without aura patients suffering from MOH than in episodic migraineurs recorded

interictally (Coppola, Currà, Di Lorenzo, et al., 2010). The increased SEP amplitude in MOH was proportional to the duration of headache chronification and further increased during stimulus repetition, resulting in a lack of habituation. We interpreted these results as reflecting reinforcement and perpetuation of central sensitization due to the medication overuse and increased headache frequency (Coppola, Currà, Di Lorenzo, et al., 2010). As a further thought-provoking result, we noted that the SSEP changes differed according to the drug overused, since amplitudes were smaller in triptan overusers than in patients overusing NSAIDs or both medications combined.

Siniatchkin et al. studied CNV amplitude and habituation in chronic daily headache (CDH) with analgesic abuse evolving from episodic migraine without aura (also called "transformed migraine") and found that the early CNV component did not habituate in CDH patients and that this occurred at significantly lower amplitudes than in episodic migraine (Siniatchkin et al., 1998). The mean amplitude of the initial block of magnetic visual evoked potentials (P100m) was higher in CM without medication abuse than in interictal episodic migraine. On stimulus repetition, VEP P100m amplitude habituated significantly in CM and in controls, contrasting with the lack of habituation in episodic migraine between attacks (Chen et al., 2011).

Taken together, these findings support the hypothesis that chronic migraine patients with or without medication overuse are locked in a persistent preictal/ictal–like state, probably as a consequence of persistent central sensitization. Medication overuse may promote or reinforce the central sensitization and resulting electrocortical abnormalities.

MEASURES OF CORTICAL EXCITABILITY IN CHILDHOOD MIGRAINE

Electrophysiological studies in pediatric migraine patients, although showing less consistent results than in adults, tend to indicate an impairment of cerebral maturation.

Quantitative EEG analyses yielded controversial results in childhood migraine between attacks. Most reports showed no difference with healthy subjects (Farkas et al., 1987; Polich et al., 1986; Seri et al., 1993), but some found increased theta rhythm in migraineurs (Genco et al., 1994). Delta power increases were observed in the anterior derivations during the aura and posteriorly during the headache phase (Seri et al., 1993) with a higher incidence of parietal alpha asymmetry (Pothmann, 1993; Seri et al., 1993). In a retrospective designed EEG study, it was shown that children with severe or chronic migraine headaches had higher activation of the arousal system compared to those having mild/moderate migraine (Vendrame et al., 2008). Reduction in nocturnal motor activity close to the attack was observed by means of actigraphy and self-report diaries in children with migraine without aura (Bruni et al., 2004). In a recent paper, MEG performed during a finger-tapping task in a small number of children with acute migraine disclosed increased latency and motor area activation compared to healthy subjects (Wang et al., 2010).

An increase in patterned (Lahat et al., 1997, 1999; Unay et al., 2008) and unpatterned (Brinciotti et al., 1986; Genco et al., 1994) VEP amplitudes and a slight delay in latencies (Lahat et al., 1999; Unay et al., 2008) have been described in childhood migraine. BAERs were normal in one study (Unay et al., 2008). A faster recovery curve of the cervical and parietal SSEP components studied by paired-pulse median nerve stimulation has been found in migrainous children (Valeriani et al., 2005). The same authors later observed that prophylactic treatment with topiramate was associated with SSEP recovery curve normalization (Vollono et al., 2010).

It is well known that cortical excitability changes with age. Therefore, the study of habituation in children and adolescents allows a direct assessment of the age-related maturation in sensory information processing.

CNV was used to perform the first detailed study of habituation in a large cohort of child migraineurs. This study showed that the early CNV component decreases and habituation increases with age in healthy controls, while in migraine patients amplitude remains stable and habituation decreases (i.e., habituation deficit) with age (Kropp, Siniatchkin, et al., 1999). In another recent longitudinal study, the reduction of the iCNV amplitude with age was confirmed in healthy subjects, but it occurred in migraine patients only if they had been in remission for at least 8 years after the first recording. Moreover, patients in whom migraine had worsened had the most pronounced loss of iCNV habituation at the first recording and still significantly increased iCNV amplitudes 8 years later (Siniatchkin, Jonas, et al., 2010). In a multielectrode study of CNV, all three CNV components of 6- to 11-year-old migraineurs without aura showed elevated negativity over the supplementary motor area (SMA) and around the vertex, but not at frontal sites; migraine children lacked age-dependent development of late CNV around Cz as previously reported (Bender et al., 2007). The authors interpreted this data as favoring a subcortical dysfunction in migrainous children. The same periodic CNV abnormalities as those found in adult migraineurs (Siniatchkin, Kropp, Gerber, Stephani, 2000) (see above) also occur in childhood migraine (Kropp & Gerber, 1998; Kropp, Kirbach, et al., 1999). Increased CNV negativity and loss of habituation between migraine attacks reflect a higher susceptibility of the brain to the occurrence of an attack.

Self-regulation of CNV with biofeedback (Siniatchkin, Kropp, Gerber, 2000; Siniatchkin, Hierundar, et al., 2000) or special behavioral training of habituation to aversive stimuli (MIPAS-Family [Migraine Patient Seminar for Families]) (Siniatchkin, Gerber-von Müller, et al., 2010) were both associated with a significant increase in iCNV habituation, but only in the MIPAS-treated group was the improvement in habituation paralleled by the favorable outcome in the clinical course of migraine (Siniatchkin, Gerber-von Müller, et al., 2010). Lack of habituation was also found in children and adolescent migraineurs in visual (Evers et al., 1998) and auditory (Valeriani et al., 2009) event-related potentials. By contrast, no abnormalities were found in studies of the auditory P300 (Buodo et al., 2004) and painful or nonpainful sensory P300 (Zohsel et al., 2008), but in the latter study the P300 amplitude was greater in migraineurs.

As for PR-VEPs, some researchers found that in the migraine group, the percentage of subjects showing lack of habituation of the P1–N2 component (Oelkers-Ax et al., 2005) and altered N2 latency (Oelkers-Ax et al., 2004) was higher in older children (12 to 18 years old) than in the early-age group (6 to 11 years old). For the other headache groups and in healthy children, age had no significant effect on the habituation regression slope.

GENETICS AND CORTICAL RESPONSIVITY

Because of the familial and genetic nature of migraine, several studies have attempted to identify with electro-physiological methods abnormalities in cortical or, more broadly, CNS responsivity that could be endophenotypic markers for presymptomatic migraine.

IDAP and VEP habituation slopes, for instance, were more closely correlated in pairs of migrainous parents and their offspring than in unrelated pairs (Sándor et al., 1999). In a later study, Siniatchkin et al. observed that children suffering from migraine had steeper IDAP slopes than age-matched healthy subjects and also steeper slopes than adult migraineurs (Siniatchkin, Kropp, Neumann, et al., 2000). The same authors also observed a considerable familial component in amplitude and habituation of the early CNV component (iCNV) in migraine (Siniatchkin, Kirsch, et al., 2000). For example, they found strong iCNV amplitude and habituation correlations between children with migraine and their parents with migraine, and between young migraineurs and their healthy parents who have a family history of migraine. They subsequently found no iCNV habituation in asymptomatic subjects with a family history of migraine, defined as subjects "at risk," and the iCNV amplitude correlated significantly with the number of migraine sufferers among first- and second-degree relatives (Siniatchkin et al., 2001). The same group has also reported that CNV patterns in

families may be influenced by psychosocial factors (Gerber et al., 2002). Similarly, in a study of a subcortical activity, the nociceptive blink reflex, we found that asymptomatic subjects having a first-degree relative affected by migraine had a lack of habituation comparable to that recorded in migraineurs between attacks (Di Clemente et al., 2007).

Collectively, these findings strongly suggest a link between the underlying genetic load and the interictal abnormal sensory processing in migraineurs. Hence, in subjects with a familial predisposition to migraine, abnormal evoked cortical potential amplitudes and habituation may be neurophysiological markers indicating presymptomatic migraine. Interestingly, familial hemiplegic migraine (FHM) patients, a rare dominant inherited subtype of migraine with aura, are not characterized by a deficient, but rather by an increased habituation in VEP and blink reflex, and by a normal IDAP slope. These results suggest that central neuronal processing differs between FHM and the common forms of migraine (Hansen et al., 2011).

CONCLUSION

To summarize, neurophysiological studies have disclosed abnormalities of cortical responsivity to external stimuli in migraine between attacks:

1. Evidence from electroencephalographic studies tends to indicate *a reduction of cortical arousal in migraine between attacks and reduced cortical activation during sleep*, especially during the night preceding an attack.
2. The majority of evoked potential studies between attacks have shown that, for a number of different sensory modalities, the *migrainous brain is characterized by a deficient habituation during stimulus repetition*. Although the underlying genetic load seems to play an important role, the exact causes are not fully understood, but neuronal hyperexcitability is an oversimplified and ambiguous explanation. On the one hand, based on single-pulse TMS, a tool to interfere briefly with cortical processing, some have proposed that insufficient cortical inhibitory processes might be responsible for the lack of habituation (for a review see Aurora & Wilkinson, 2007; Coppola, Pierelli, et al., 2007). There is, on the other hand, converging evidence from clinical and electrophysiological data that the preactivation level of sensory cortices is reduced because of an inefficient thalamocortical drive. As a matter of

fact, studies of spontaneous EEG and visual or somatosensory evoked high-frequency oscillations clearly indicate that the cortical dysfunction in migraine could be due to abnormal thalamic rhythmic activity, namely, to a "thalamocortical dysrhythmia." This may reconcile the controversy between excessive excitation and deficient inhibition, since a deficient thalamocortical drive (i.e., a low level of cortical preactivation) results in a dysfunction of both inhibitory and excitatory cortical neurons. Lower inhibition and preactivation may thus coexist, since the latter can promote the former via reduction of lateral inhibition. The final common pathway of both dysfunctions is a heightened cortical response to repeated stimuli, that is, hyperresponsivity (Coppola, Pierelli, et al., 2007) (Fig. 29–2).

3. There is some indirect evidence that the *thalamocortical dysrhythmia* and ensuing decreased preactivation levels of sensory cortices might be due to *hypoactivity of the so-called state-setting*, chemically addressed subcortico-cortical projections (Mesulam, 1990). Among the latter, the serotonergic pathway seems to be the most relevant, but other neurotransmitters should be taken into account, since interactions between amines are well documented (Ferrari & Saxena, 1993; Ghelardini et al., 1996; Mascia et al., 1998; Millán-Guerrero, et al. 2007; Sicuteri, 1976; Siniscalchi et al., 1999).

4. It is well established that *cortical responsivity fluctuates over time* in relation to the migraine attack. It grows and leads to increased energy demands during the days immediately preceding the attack when habituation of evoked potentials is minimal and amplitude peaks. By contrast, just before the attack, at a time point when premonitory symptoms may occur, and during the attack, habituation increases and normalizes, which is accompanied by an increased thalamocortical drive (Coppola et al., 2005). We postulate that these electrophysiological changes are due to a further preictal decrease of serotonergic neurotransmission and cortical preactivation level, which flip to increased serotonergic transmission and preactivation levels during the attack. Interestingly, increased serotonin disposition (Evers et al., 1999; Ferrari & Saxena, 1993; Sakai et al., 2008) and activation of brainstem aminergic nuclei (raphe nuclei, locus coeruleus), basal forebrain (nucleus basalis), and the periaqueductal gray matter (Bahra et al., 2001; Farook et al., 2004; Sakai et al., 2008;

Schoenen, 1996; Weiller et al., 1995; Welch, 2009), which seem to play a key role both in attack generation and in the interictal cortical hyperresponsive behavior, were observed during the migraine attack (Fig. 29–2).

5. As hypothesized previously (Schoenen, 1996), the cerebral metabolic homeostasis may be disrupted by the increased energy demands due to the ictal and even more so preictal cortical hyperresponsivity, because the *neuronal energy reserve is reduced in migraineurs* (Barbiroli et al., 1992; Montagna et al., 1994; Welch et al., 1989). This may lead to ignition of the major alarm-signaling system of the brain, the trigeminovascular system, and thus to the migraine attack.

6. *Cortical responsivity fluctuates also in relation to attack frequency*. In fact, electrophysiological findings support the hypothesis that chronic migraine patients are locked in a persistent ictal-like state, since the amplitude of nonnoxious and noxious evoked responses increases probably as a consequence of further brainstem activation (Matharu et al., 2004) that in turn promotes central sensitization. Excessive acute medication intake could further reinforce central sensitization and hence electrocortical abnormalities, since the cortical response patterns in medication overuse headache suggest that the brain is now locked in a preictal state, that is, characterized by an abnormal increase in response amplitude both to a low number of stimuli and during continuous stimulus repetition (deficient habituation).

In conclusion, the methods of clinical neurophysiology seem to be particularly appropriate to provide atraumatically better insight into the nature of the interictal cortical dysfunction in migraine and may allow a better understanding of the cerebral mechanisms subtending headache chronification.

REFERENCES

Áfra, J., Cecchini, A. P., De Pasqua, V., Albert, A., & Schoenen, J. (1998). Visual evoked potentials during long periods of pattern-reversal stimulation in migraine. *Brain, 121*(Pt 2), 233–241.

Áfra, J., Cecchini, A. P., Sándor, P. S., & Schoenen, J. (2000). Comparison of visual and auditory evoked cortical potentials in migraine patients between attacks. *Clinical Neurophysiology, 111*(6), 1124–1129.

Ahmed, I. (1999). Contingent negative variation in migraine: Effect of beta blocker therapy. *Clinical Electroencephalography, 30*(1), 21–23.

Ambrosini, A., Coppola, G., Gérardy, P. Y., Pierelli, F., & Schoenen, J. (2011). Intensity dependence of auditory evoked potentials during light interference in migraine. *Neuroscience Letters, 492*(2), 80–83.

Ambrosini, A., De Pasqua, V., Áfra, J., Sandor, P. S., & Schoenen, J. (2001). Reduced gating of middle-latency auditory evoked potentials (P50) in migraine patients: Another indication of abnormal sensory processing? *Neuroscience Letters, 306*(1–2), 132–134.

Ambrosini, A., Rossi, P., De Pasqua, V., Pierelli, F., & Schoenen, J. (2003). Lack of habituation causes high intensity dependence of auditory evoked cortical potentials in migraine. *Brain, 126*(Pt 9), 2009–2015.

Annovazzi, P., Colombo, B., Bernasconi, L., Schiatti, E., Comi, G., & Leocani, L. (2004). Cortical function abnormalities in migraine: Neurophysiological and neuropsychological evidence from reaction times and event-related potentials to the Stroop test. *Neurological Sciences, 25*(Suppl 3), S285–S287.

Antal, A., Temme, J., Nitsche, M. A., Varga, E. T., Lang, N., & Paulus, W. (2005). Altered motion perception in migraineurs: Evidence for interictal cortical hyperexcitability. *Cephalalgia, 25*(10), 788–794.

Aurora, S. K., Ahmad, B. K., Welch, K. M., Bhardhwaj, P., & Ramadan, N. M. (1998). Transcranial magnetic stimulation confirms hyperexcitability of occipital cortex in migraine. *Neurology, 50*(4), 1111–1114.

Aurora, S. K., & Wilkinson, F. (2007). The brain is hyperexcitable in migraine. *Cephalalgia, 27*(12), 1442–1453.

Ayzenberg, I., Obermann, M., Nyhuis, P., Gastpar, M., Limmroth, V., Diener, H. C., et al. (2006). Central sensitization of the trigeminal and somatic nociceptive systems in medication overuse headache mainly involves cerebral supraspinal structures. *Cephalalgia, 26*(9), 1106–1114.

Bahra, A., Matharu, M. S., Buchel, C., Frackowiak, R. S., & Goadsby, P. J. (2001). Brainstem activation specific to migraine headache. *Lancet, 357*(9261), 1016–1017.

Barbiroli, B., Montagna, P., Cortelli, P., Funicello, R., Iotti, S., Monari, L., et al. (1992). Abnormal brain and muscle energy metabolism shown by 31P magnetic resonance spectroscopy in patients affected by migraine with aura. *Neurology, 42*(6), 1209–1214.

Barkley, G. L., Tepley, N., Nagel-Leiby, S., Moran, J. E., Simkins, R. T., & Welch, K. M. (1990). Magnetoencephalographic studies of migraine. *Headache, 30*(7), 428–434.

Bender, S., Weisbrod, M., Resch, F., & Oelkers-Ax, R. (2007). Stereotyped topography of different elevated contingent negative variation components in children with migraine without aura points towards a subcortical dysfunction. *Pain, 127*(3), 221–233.

Benna, P., Bianco, C., Costa, P., Piazza, D., & Bergamasco, B. (1985). Visual evoked potentials and brainstem auditory evoked potentials in migraine and transient ischemic attacks. *Cephalalgia, 5*(Suppl 2), 53–58.

Birbaumer, N., Elbert, T., Canavan, A. G., & Rockstroh, B. (1990). Slow potentials of the cerebral cortex and behavior. *Physiological Reviews, 70*(1), 1–41.

Bjørk, M., Hagen, K., Stovner, L. J., & Sand, T. (2010). Photic EEG-driving responses related to ictal phases and trigger sensitivity in migraine: A longitudinal, controlled study. *Cephalalgia. 31*(4), 444–455.

Bjørk, M. H., & Sand, T. (2008). Quantitative EEG power and asymmetry increase 36 h before a migraine attack. *Cephalalgia, 28*(9), 960–968.

Bjørk, M. H., Stovner, L. J., Engstrøm, M., Stjern, M., Hagen, K., & Sand, T. (2009). Interictal quantitative EEG in migraine: A blinded controlled study. *Journal of Headache and Pain, 10*(5), 331–339.

Bjørk, M. H., Stovner, L. J., Nilsen, B. M., Stjern, M., Hagen, K., & Sand, T. (2009). The occipital alpha rhythm related to the "migraine cycle" and headache burden: A blinded, controlled longitudinal study. *Clinical Neurophysiology, 120*(3), 464–471.

Böcker, K. B., Timsit-Berthier, M., Schoenen, J., & Brunia, C. H. (1990). Contingent negative variation in migraine. *Headache, 30*(9), 604–609.

Bohotin, V., Fumal, A., Vandenheede, M., Gérard, P., Bohotin, C., Maertens de Noordhout, A., et al. (2002). Effects of repetitive transcranial magnetic stimulation on visual evoked potentials in migraine. *Brain, 125*(Pt 4), 912–922.

Bowyer, S. M., Aurora, K. S., Moran, J. E., Tepley, N., & Welch, K. M. (2001). Magnetoencephalographic fields from patients with spontaneous and induced migraine aura. *Annals of Neurology, 50*(5), 582–587.

Bowyer, S. M., Okada, Y. C., Papuashvili, N., Moran, J. E., Barkley, G. L., Welch, K. M., et al. (1999). Analysis of MEG signals of spreading cortical depression with propagation constrained to a rectangular cortical strip. I. Lissencephalic rabbit model. *Brain Research, 843*(1–2), 71–78.

Bowyer, S. M., Mason, K. M., Moran, J. E., Tepley, N., & Mitsias, P. D. (2005). Cortical hyperexcitability in migraine patients before and after sodium valproate treatment. *Journal of Clinical Neurophysiology, 22*(1), 65–67.

Brinciotti, M., Guidetti, V., Matricardi, M., & Cortesi, F. (1986). Responsivity of the visual system in childhood migraine studied by means of VEPs. *Cephalalgia, 6*(3), 183–185.

Bruni, O., Russo, P. M., Violani, C., & Guidetti, V. (2004). Sleep and migraine: An actigraphic study. *Cephalalgia, 24*(2), 134–139.

Buchgreitz, L., Egsgaard, L. L., Jensen, R., Arendt-Nielsen, L., & Bendtsen, L. (2010). Abnormal brain processing of pain in migraine without aura: A high-density EEG brain mapping study. *Cephalalgia, 30*(2), 191–199.

Buodo, G., Palomba, D., Sarlo, M., Naccarella, C., & Battistella, P. A. (2004). Auditory event-related potentials and reaction times in migraine children. *Cephalalgia, 24*(7), 554–563.

Bussone, G., Sinatra, M. G., Boiardi, A., La Mantia, L., Frediani, F., & Cocchini, F. (1985). Brainstem auditory evoked potentials in migraine patients in basal conditions and after chronic flunarizine treatment. *Cephalalgia, 5*(Suppl 2), 177–180.

Chayasirisobhon, S. (1995). Somatosensory evoked potentials in acute migraine with sensory aura. *Clinical Electroencephalography, 26*(1), 65–69.

Chen, W. T., Wang, S. J., Fuh, J. L., Lin, C. P., Ko, Y. C., & Lin, Y. Y. (2009). Peri-ictal normalization of visual cortex excitability in migraine: An MEG study. *Cephalalgia, 29*(11), 1202–1211.

Chen, W. T., Wang, S. J., Fuh, J. L., Lin, C. P., Ko, Y. C., & Lin, Y. Y. (2011). Persistent ictal-like visual cortical excitability in chronic migraine. *Pain, 152*(2), 254–258.

Chorlton, P., & Kane, N. (2000). Investigation of the cerebral response to flicker stimulation in patients with headache. *Clinical Electroencephalography, 31*(2), 83–87.

Clemens, B., Bánk, J., Piros, P., Bessenyei, M., Veto, S., Tóth, M., et al. (2008). Three-dimensional localization of abnormal EEG activity in migraine: A low resolution electromagnetic tomography (LORETA) study of migraine patients in the pain-free interval. *Brain Topography, 21*(1), 36–42.

Conlon, E., & Hine, T. (2000). The influence of pattern interference on performance in migraine and visual discomfort groups. *Cephalalgia, 20*(8), 708–713.

Connolly, J. F., Gawel, M., & Rose, F. C. (1982). Migraine patients exhibit abnormalities in the visual evoked potential. *Journal of Neurology, Neurosurgery, and Psychiatry, 45*(5), 464–467.

Coppola, G., Ambrosini, A., Di Clemente, L., Magis, D., Fumal, A., Gérard, P., et al. (2007). Interictal abnormalities of gamma band activity in visual evoked responses in migraine: An indication of thalamocortical dysrhythmia? *Cephalalgia, 27*(12), 1360–1367.

Coppola, G., Currà, A., Di Lorenzo, C., Parisi, V., Gorini, M., Sava, S. L., et al. (2010). Abnormal cortical responses to somatosensory stimulation in medication-overuse headache. *BMC Neurology, 10,* 126.

Coppola, G., Currà, A., Sava, S. L., Alibardi, A., Parisi, V., Pierelli, F., et al. (2010). Changes in visual-evoked potential habituation induced by hyperventilation in migraine. *Journal of Headache and Pain, 11*(6), 497–503.

Coppola, G., Currà, A., Serrao, M., Di Lorenzo, C., Gorini, M., Porretta, E., et al. (2010). Lack of cold pressor test-induced effect on visual-evoked potentials in migraine. *Journal of Headache and Pain, 11*(2), 115–121.

Coppola, G., Parisi, V., Fiermonte, G., Restuccia, R., & Pierelli, F. (2007). Asymmetric distribution of visual evoked potentials in patients with migraine with aura during the interictal phase. *European Journal of Ophthalmology, 17*(5), 828–835.

Coppola, G., Pierelli, F., & Schoenen, J. (2007). Is the cerebral cortex hyperexcitable or hyperresponsive in migraine? *Cephalalgia, 27*(12), 1427–1439.

Coppola, G., Serrao, M., Currà, A., Di Lorenzo, C., Vatrika, M., Parisi, V., et al. (2010). Tonic pain abolishes cortical habituation of visual evoked potentials in healthy subjects. *Journal of Pain, 11*(3), 291–296.

Coppola, G., Vandenheede, M., Di Clemente, L., Ambrosini, A., Fumal, A., De Pasqua, V., et al. (2005). Somatosensory evoked high-frequency oscillations reflecting thalamo-cortical activity are decreased in migraine patients between attacks. *Brain, 128*(Pt 1), 98–103.

Coutin-Churchman, P., & Padrón de Freytez, A. (2003). Vector analysis of visual evoked potentials in migraineurs with visual aura. *Clinical Neurophysiology, 114*(11), 2132–2137.

Darabaneanu, S., Kropp, P., Niederberger, U., Strenge, H., & Gerber, W. D. (2008). Effects of pregnancy on slow cortical potentials in migraine patients and healthy controls. *Cephalalgia, 28*(10), 1053–1060.

Dash, A. K., Panda, N., Khandelwal, G., Lal, V., & Mann, S. S. (2008). Migraine and audiovestibular dysfunction: Is there a correlation? *American Journal of Otolaryngology, 29*(5), 295–299.

de Tommaso, M., Baumgartner, U., Sardaro, M., Difruscolo, O., Serpino, C., & Treede, R-D. (2008). Effects of distraction versus spatial discrimination on laser-evoked potentials in migraine. *Headache, 48*(3), 408–416.

de Tommaso, M., Difruscolo, O., Sardaro, M., Libro, G., Pecoraro, C., Serpino, C., et al. (2007). Effects of remote cutaneous pain on trigeminal laser-evoked potentials in migraine patients. *Journal of Headache and Pain, 8*(3), 167–174.

de Tommaso, M., Guido, M., Libro, G., Losito, L., Difruscolo, O., Puca, F., et al. (2004). Topographic and dipolar analysis of laser-evoked potentials during migraine attack. *Headache, 44*(10), 947–960.

de Tommaso, M., Guido, M., Libro, G., Losito, L., Sciruicchio, V., Monetti, C., et al. (2002). Abnormal brain processing of cutaneous pain in migraine patients during the attack. *Neuroscience Letters, 333*(1), 29–32.

de Tommaso, M., Guido, M., Sardaro, M., Serpino, C., Vecchio, E., De, S., et al. (2008). Effects of topiramate and levetiracetam vs placebo on habituation of contingent negative variation in migraine patients. *Neuroscience Letters, 442*(2), 81–85.

de Tommaso, M., Libro, G., Guido, M., Losito, L., Lamberti, P., & Livrea, P. (2005). Habituation of single CO2 laser-evoked responses during interictal phase of migraine. *Journal of Headache and Pain, 6*(4), 195–198.

de Tommaso, M., Losito, L., Di Fruscolo, O., Sardaro, M., Prudenzano, M. P., Lamberti, P., et al. (2005). Lack of habituation of nociceptive evoked responses and pain sensitivity during migraine attack. *Clinical Neurophysiology, 116*(6), 1254–1264.

de Tommaso, M., Losito, L., Difruscolo, O., Libro, G., Guido, M., & Livrea, P. (2005). Changes in cortical processing of pain in chronic migraine. *Headache, 45*(9), 1208–1218.

de Tommaso, M., Marinazzo, D., Guido, M., Libro, G., Stramaglia, S., Nitti, L., et al. (2005). Visually evoked phase synchronization changes of alpha rhythm in migraine: Correlations with clinical features. *International Journal of Psychophysiology, 57*(3), 203–210.

de Tommaso, M., Marinazzo, D., Nitti, L., Pellicoro, M., Guido, M., Serpino, C., et al. (2007). Effects of levetiracetam vs topiramate and placebo on visually evoked phase synchronization changes of alpha rhythm in migraine. *Clinical Neurophysiology, 118*(10), 2297–2304.

de Tommaso, M., Sciruicchio, V., Guido, M., Sasanelli, G., Specchio, L. M., & Puca, F. M. (1998). EEG spectral analysis in migraine without aura attacks. *Cephalalgia, 18*(6), 324–328.

de Tommaso, M., Sciruicchio, V., Tota, P., Megna, M., Guido, M., Genco, S., & Puca, F. (1997). Somatosensory evoked potentials in migraine. *Functional neurology, 12*(2), 77–82.

de Tommaso, M., Stramaglia, S., Brighina, F., Fierro, B., Francesco, V. D., Todarello, O., et al. (2011). Lack of effects of low frequency repetitive transcranial magnetic stimulation on alpha rhythm phase synchronization in migraine patients. *Neuroscience Letters, 488*(2), 143–147.

de Tommaso, M., Valeriani, M., Guido, M., Libro, G., Specchio, L. M., Tonali, P., et al. (2003). Abnormal brain processing of cutaneous pain in patients with chronic migraine. *Pain, 101*(1–2), 25–32.

de Tommaso, M., Valeriani, M., Sardaro, M., Serpino, C., Di Fruscolo, O., Vecchio, E., et al. (2009). Pain perception and laser evoked potentials during menstrual cycle in migraine. *Journal of Headache and Pain, 10*(6), 423–429.

Della Marca, G., Vollono, C., Rubino, M., Di Trapani, G., Mariotti, P., & Tonali, P. A. (2006). Dysfunction of arousal systems in sleep-related migraine without aura. *Cephalalgia, 26*(7), 857–864.

Dexter, J. D. (1979). The relationship between stage III + IV + REM sleep and arousals with migraine. *Headache, 19*(7), 364–369.

Dexter, J. D., & Weitzman, E. D. (1970). The relationship of nocturnal headaches to sleep stage patterns. *Neurology, 20*(5), 513–518.

Di Clemente, L., Coppola, G., Magis, D., Fumal, A., De Pasqua, V., Di Piero, V., et al. (2007). Interictal habituation deficit of the nociceptive blink reflex: An endophenotypic marker for presymptomatic migraine? *Brain, 130*(Pt 3), 765–770.

Di Clemente, L., Coppola, G., Magis, D., Fumal, A., De Pasqua, V., & Schoenen, J. (2005). Nociceptive blink reflex and visual evoked potential habituations are correlated in migraine. *Headache, 45*(10), 1388–1393.

Drake, M. E., Pakalnis, A., Hietter, S. A., & Padamadan, H. (1990). Visual and auditory evoked potentials in migraine. *Electromyography and Clinical Neurophysiology, 30*(2), 77–81.

Evers, S., Bauer, B., Grotemeyer, K. H., Kurlemann, G., & Husstedt, I. W. (1998). Event-related potentials (P300) in primary headache in childhood and adolescence. *Journal of Child Neurology, 13*(7), 322–326.

Evers, S., Bauer, B., Suhr, B., Husstedt, I. W., & Grotemeyer, K. H. (1997). Cognitive processing in primary headache: A study on event-related potentials. *Neurology, 48*(1), 108–113.

Evers, S., Quibeldey, F., Grotemeyer, K. H., Suhr, B., & Husstedt, I. W. (1999). Dynamic changes of cognitive habituation and serotonin metabolism during the migraine interval. *Cephalalgia, 19*(5), 485–491.

Facchetti, D., Marsile, C., Faggi, L., Donati, E., Kokodoko, A., & Poloni, M. (1990). Cerebral mapping in subjects suffering from migraine with aura. *Cephalalgia, 10*(6), 279–284.

Farkas, V., Benninger, C., Matthis, P., Scheffner, D., & Lindeisz, F. (1987). The EEG background activity in children with migraine. *Cephalalgia, 7*(Suppl 6), 59–64.

Farook, J. M., Wang, Q., Moochhala, S. M., Zhu, Z. Y., Lee, L., & Wong, P. T-H. (2004). Distinct regions of periaqueductal gray (PAG) are involved in freezing behavior in hooded PVG rats on the cat-freezing test apparatus. *Neuroscience Letters, 354*(2), 139–142.

Ferrari, M. D., & Saxena, P. R. (1993). On serotonin and migraine: A clinical and pharmacological review. *Cephalalgia, 13*(3), 151–165.

Fierro, B., Ricci, R., Piazza, A., Scalia, S., Giglia, G., Vitello, G., et al. (2003). 1 Hz rTMS enhances extrastriate cortex activity in migraine: Evidence of a reduced inhibition? *Neurology, 61*(10), 1446–1448.

Firenze, C., Del Gatto, F., Mazzotta, G., & Gallai, V. (1988). Somatosensory-evoked potential study in headache patients. *Cephalalgia, 8*(3), 157–162.

Formisano, R., Martucci, N., Fabbrini, G., Cerbo, R., Proietti, R., De Marinis, M., et al. (1988). Spectral EEG analysis and flunarizine treatment in migraine patients. *Cephalalgia, 8*(Suppl 8), 31–33.

Fritzer, G., Strenge, H., Göder, R., Gerber, W-D., & Aldenhoff, J. (2004). Changes in cortical dynamics in the preictal stage of a migraine attack. *Journal of Clinical Neurophysiology, 21*(2), 99–104.

Fumal, A., Coppola, G., Bohotin, V., Gérardy, P-Y., Seidel, L., Donneau, A-F., et al. (2006). Induction of long-lasting changes of visual cortex excitability by five daily sessions of repetitive transcranial magnetic stimulation (rTMS) in healthy volunteers and migraine patients. *Cephalalgia, 26*(2), 143–149.

Genco, S., de Tommaso, M., Prudenzano, A. M., Savarese, M., & Puca, F. M. (1994). EEG features in juvenile migraine: Topographic analysis of spontaneous and visual evoked brain electrical activity: A comparison with adult migraine. *Cephalalgia, 14*(1), 41–46; discussion 4.

Gerber, W-D., Stephani, U., Kirsch, E., Kropp, P., & Siniatchkin, M. (2002). Slow cortical potentials in migraine families are associated with psychosocial factors. *Journal of Psychosomatic Research, 52*(4), 215–222.

Ghelardini, C., Galeotti, N., Figini, M., Imperato, A., Nicolodi, M., Sicuteri, F., et al. (1996). The central cholinergic system has a role in the antinociception induced in rodents and guinea pigs by the antimigraine drug sumatriptan. *Journal of Pharmacology and Experimental Therapeutics, 279*(2), 884–890.

Göder, R., Fritzer, G., Kapsokalyvas, A., Kropp, P., Niederberger, U., Strenge, H., et al. (2001). Polysomnographic findings in nights preceding a migraine attack. *Cephalalgia, 21*(1), 31–37.

Golla, F. L., & Winter, A. L. (1959). Analysis of cerebral responses to flicker in patients complaining of episodic headache. *Electroencephalography and Clinical Neurophysiology, 11*(3), 539–549.

Hall, S. D., Barnes, G. R., Hillebrand, A., Furlong, P. L., Singh, K. D., & Holliday, I. E. (2004). Spatio-temporal imaging of cortical desynchronization in migraine visual aura: A magnetoencephalography case study. *Headache, 44*(3), 204–208.

Hansen, J. M., Bolla, M., Magis, D., de Pasqua, V., Ashina, M., Thomsen, L. L., et al. (2011). Habituation of evoked responses is greater in patients with familial hemiplegic migraine than in controls: A contrast with the common forms of migraine. *European Journal of Neurology, 18*(3), 478–485.

Hebb, D. O. (1955). Drives and the C.N.S. (conceptual nervous system). *Psychological Review, 62*(4), 243–254.

Höffken, O., Stude, P., Lenz, M., Bach, M., Dinse, H. R., & Tegenthoff, M. (2009). Visual paired-pulse stimulation reveals enhanced visual cortex excitability in migraineurs. *European Journal of Neuroscience, 30*(4), 714–720.

Hughes, J. R., & Robbins, L. D. (1990). Brain mapping in migraine. *Clinical Electroencephalography, 21*(1), 14–24.

Jonkman, E. J., & Lelieveld, M. H. (1981). EEG computer analysis in patients with migraine. *Electroencephalography and Clinical Neurophysiology, 52*(6), 652–655.

Judit, A., Sándor, P. S., & Schoenen, J. (2000). Habituation of visual and intensity dependence of auditory evoked cortical potentials tends to normalize just before and during the migraine attack. *Cephalalgia, 20*(8), 714–719.

Kennard, C., Gawel, M., de M Rudolph, N., & Rose, F. C. (1978). Visual evoked potentials in migraine subjects. *Research and Clinical Studies of Headache, 6*, 73–80.

Khalil, N. M., Legg, N. J., & Anderson, D. J. (2000). Long term decline of P100 amplitude in migraine with aura. *Journal of Neurology, Neurosurg, and Psychiatry, 69*(4), 507–511.

Khalil, N. M., Nicotra, A., & Wilkins, A. J. (2011). Asymmetry of visual function in migraine with aura: Correlation with lateralisation of headache and aura. *Cephalalgia, 31*(2), 213–221.

Kropp, P., Kirbach, U., Detlefsen, J. O., Siniatchkin, M., Gerber, W. D., & Stephani, U. (1999). Slow cortical potentials in migraine: A comparison of adults and children. *Cephalalgia, 19*(Suppl 25), 60–64.

Kropp, P., Siniatchkin, M., & Gerber, W. D. (2000). Contingent negative variation as indicator of duration of migraine disease. *Functional Neurology, 15*(Suppl 3), 78–81.

Kropp, P., Siniatchkin, M., Stephani, U., & Gerber, W. D. (1999). Migraine—evidence for a disturbance of cerebral maturation in man? *Neuroscience Letters, 276*(3), 181–184.

Kropp, P., & Gerber, W. D. (1993a). Contingent negative variation—findings and perspectives in migraine. *Cephalalgia, 13*(1), 33–36.

Kropp, P., & Gerber, W. D. (1993b). Is increased amplitude of contingent negative variation in migraine due to cortical hyperactivity or to reduced habituation? *Cephalalgia, 13*(1), 37–41.

Kropp, P., & Gerber, W. D. (1995). Contingent negative variation during migraine attack and interval: Evidence for normalization of slow cortical potentials during the attack. *Cephalalgia, 15*(2), 123–128; discussion 78.

Kropp, P., & Gerber, W. D. (1998). Prediction of migraine attacks using a slow cortical potential, the contingent negative variation. *Neuroscience Letters, 257*(2), 73–76.

Lahat, E., Nadir, E., Barr, J., Eshel, G., Aladjem, M., & Bistritze, T. (1997). Visual evoked potentials: A diagnostic test for migraine headache in children. *Developmental Medicine and Child Neurology, 39*(2), 85–87.

Lahat, E., Barr, J., Barzilai, A., Cohen, H., & Berkovitch, M. (1999). Visual evoked potentials in the diagnosis of headache before 5 years of age. *European Journal of Pediatrics, 158*(11), 892–895.

Lai, C. W., Dean, P., Ziegler, D. K., & Hassanein, R. S. (1989). Clinical and electrophysiological responses to dietary challenge in migraineurs. *Headache, 29*(3), 180–186.

Lang, E., Kaltenhäuser, M., Neundörfer, B., & Seidler, S. (2004). Hyperexcitability of the primary somatosensory cortex in migraine—a magnetoencephalographic study. *Brain, 127*(Pt 11), 2459–2469.

Lehtonen, J. B. (1974). Visual evoked cortical potentials for single flashes and flickering light in migraine. *Headache, 14*(1), 1–12.

Llinás, R. R., Ribary, U., Jeanmonod, D., Kronberg, E., & Mitra, P. P. (1999). Thalamocortical dysrhythmia: A neurological and neuropsychiatric syndrome characterized by magnetoencephalography. *Proceedings of the National Academy of Sciences of the United States of American, 96*(26), 15222–15227.

Logi, F., Bonfiglio, L., Orlandi, G., Bonanni, E., Iudice, A., & Sartucci, F. (2001). Asymmetric scalp distribution of pattern visual evoked potentials during interictal phases in migraine. *Acta Neurologica Scandinavica, 104*(5), 301–307.

Maertens de Noordhout, A., Timsit-Berthier, M., Timsit, M., & Schoenen, J. (1986). Contingent negative variation in headache. *Annals of Neurology, 19*(1), 78–80.

Mariani, E., Moschini, V., Pastorino, G., Rizzi, F., Severgnini, A., & Tiengo, M. (1988). Pattern-reversal visual evoked potentials and EEG correlations in common migraine patients. *Headache, 28*(4), 269–271.

Marlowe, N. (1995). Somatosensory evoked potentials and headache: A further examination of the central theory. *Journal of Psychosomatic Research, 39*(2), 119–131.

Mascia, A., Áfra, J., & Schoenen, J. (1998). Dopamine and migraine: A review of pharmacological, biochemical, neurophysiological, and therapeutic data. *Cephalalgia, 18*(4), 174–182.

Matharu, M. S., Bartsch, T., Ward, N., Frackowiak, R. S. J., Weiner, R., & Goadsby, P. J. (2004). Central neuromodulation in chronic migraine patients with suboccipital stimulators: A PET study. *Brain, 127*(Pt 1), 220–230.

Mazzucchi, A., Sinforiani, E., Zinelli, P., Agostinis, C., Granella, F., Miari, A., et al. (1988). Interhemispheric attentional functioning in classic migraine subjects during paroxysmal and interparoxysmal phases. *Headache, 28*(7), 488–493.

Mesulam, M. M. (1990). Large-scale neurocognitive networks and distributed processing for attention, language, and memory. *Annals of Neurology, 28*(5), 597–613.

Millán-Guerrero, R. O., Isais-Millán, R., Barreto-Vizcaíno, S., Rivera-Castaño, L., Garcia-Solorzano, A., López-Blanca, C., et al. (2007). Subcutaneous histamine versus sodium valproate in migraine prophylaxis: A randomized, controlled, double-blind study. *European Journal of Neurology, 14*(10), 1079–1084.

Montagna, P., Cortelli, P., & Barbiroli, B. (1994). Magnetic resonance spectroscopy studies in migraine. *Cephalalgia, 14*(3), 184–193.

Montagna, P., Zucconi, M., Zappia, M., & Liguori, R. (1985). Somatosensory evoked potentials in migraine and tension headache. *Headache, 25*(2), 115.

Mulder, E. J., Linssen, W. H., Passchier, J., Orlebeke, J. F., & de Geus, E. J. (1999). Interictal and postictal cognitive changes in migraine. *Cephalalgia, 19*(6), 557–65; discussion 541.

Mulder, E. J., Linssen, W. H., & de Geus, E. I. (2002). Reduced sensory anticipation in migraine. *Psychophysiology, 39*(2), 166–174.

Mulleners, W. M., Chronicle, E. P., Palmer, J. E., Koehler, P. J., & Vredeveld, J. W. (2001). Visual cortex excitability in migraine with and without aura. *Headache, 41*(6), 565–572.

Nyrke, T., Kangasniemi, P., & Lang, A. H. (1989). Difference of steady-state visual evoked potentials in classic and common migraine. *Electroencephalography and Clinical Neurophysiology, 73*(4), 285–294.

Nyrke, T., Kangasniemi, P., & Lang, A. H. (1990). Transient asymmetries of steady-state visual evoked potentials in classic migraine. *Headache, 30*(3), 133–137.

Nyrke, T., Kangasniemi, P., Lang, A. H., & Petersen, E. (1984). Steady-state visual evoked potentials during migraine prophylaxis by propranolol and femoxetine. *Acta Neurologica Scandinavica, 69*(1), 9–14.

Nyrke, T., & Lang, A H. (1982). Spectral analysis of visual potentials evoked by sine wave modulated light in migraine. *Electroencephalography and Clinical Neurophysiology, 53*(4), 436–442.

Oelkers-Ax, R., Bender, S., Just, U., Pfüller, U., Parzer, P., Resch, F., et al. (2004). Pattern-reversal visual-evoked potentials in children with migraine and other primary headache: Evidence for maturation disorder? *Pain, 108*(3), 267–275.

Oelkers-Ax, R., Parzer, P., Resch, F., & Weisbrod, M. (2005). Maturation of early visual processing investigated by a pattern-reversal habituation paradigm is altered in migraine. *Cephalalgia, 25*(4), 280–289.

Olesen, J., Bousser, M-G., Diener, H-C., Dodick, D., First, M., Goadsby, P. J., et al. (2006). New appendix criteria open for a broader concept of chronic migraine. *Cephalalgia, 26*(6), 742–746.

Ozkul, Y., & Bozlar, S. (2002). Effects of fluoxetine on habituation of pattern reversal visually evoked potentials in migraine prophylaxis. *Headache, 42*(7), 582–587.

Ozkul, Y., & Uckardes, A. (2002). Median nerve somatosensory evoked potentials in migraine. *European Journal of Neurology, 9*(3), 227–232.

Palmer, J. E., & Chronicle, E. P. (1998). Cognitive processing in migraine: A failure to find facilitation in patients with aura. *Cephalalgia, 18*(3), 125–132.

Péchadre, J. C., & Gibert, J. (1987). [Demonstration, by the cartographic test, of an unusual reaction to intermittent light stimulation in patients with migraine]. *Encephale, 13*(4), 245–247.

Podoshin, L., Ben-David, J., Pratt, H., Fradis, M., Sharf, B., Weller, B., et al. (1987). Auditory brainstem evoked potentials in patients with migraine. *Headache, 27*(1), 27–29.

Polich, J., Ehlers, C. L., & Dalessio, D. J. (1986). Pattern-shift visual evoked responses and EEG in migraine. *Headache, 26*(9), 451–456.

Pothmann, R. (1993). Topographic EEG mapping in childhood headaches. *Cephalalgia, 13*(1), 57–58.

Puca, F. M., de Tommaso, M., Savarese, M. A., Genco, S., & Prudenzano, A. (1992). Topographic analysis of steady-state visual evoked potentials (SVEPs) in the medium frequency range in migraine with and without aura. *Cephalalgia, 12*(4), 244–249; discussion 185.

Puca, F. M., de Tommaso, M., Tota, P., & Sciruicchio, V. (1996). Photic driving in migraine: Correlations with clinical features. *Cephalalgia, 16*(4), 246–250.

Rankin, C. H., Abrams, T., Barry, R. J., Bhatnagar, S., Clayton, D. F., Colombo, J., et al. (2009). Habituation revisited: An updated and revised description of the behavioral characteristics of habituation. *Neurobiology of Learning and Memory, 92*(2), 135–138.

Sakai, Y., Dobson, C., Diksic, M., Aubé, M., & Hamel, E. (2008). Sumatriptan normalizes the migraine attack-related increase in brain serotonin synthesis. *Neurology, 70*(6), 431–439.

Sakuma, K., Takeshima, T., Ishizaki, K., & Nakashima, K. (2004). Somatosensory evoked high-frequency oscillations in migraine patients. *Clinical Neurophysiology, 115*(8), 1857–1862.

Sand, T., & Vingen, J. V. (2000). Visual, long-latency auditory and brainstem auditory evoked potentials in migraine: Relation to pattern size, stimulus intensity, sound and light discomfort thresholds and pre-attack state. *Cephalalgia, 20*(9), 804–820.

Sand, T., White, L. R., Hagen, K., & Stovner, L. J. (2009). Visual evoked potential and spatial frequency in migraine: A longitudinal study. *Acta Neurologica Scandinavica, 120*(suppl. 189), 33–37.

Sand, T., Zhitniy, N., White, L. R., & Stovner, L. J. (2008a). Brainstem auditory-evoked potential habituation and intensity-dependence related to serotonin metabolism in migraine: A longitudinal study. *Clinical Neurophysiology, 119*(5), 1190–1200.

Sand, T., Zhitniy, N., White, L. R., & Stovner, L. J. (2008b). Visual evoked potential latency, amplitude and habituation in migraine: A longitudinal study. *Clinical Neurophysiology, 119*(5), 1020–1027.

Sándor, P. S., Áfra, J., Proietti-Cecchini, A., Albert, A., & Schoenen, J. (1999). Familial influences on cortical evoked potentials in migraine. *Neuroreport, 10*(6), 1235–1238.

Sandrini, G., Friberg, L., Coppola, G., Jänig, W., Jensen, R., Kruit, M., et al. (2011). Neurophysiological tests and neuroimaging procedures in non-acute headache (2nd edition). *European Journal of Neurology, 18*(3), 373–381.

Sauer, S., Schellenberg, R., Hofmann, H. C., & Dimpfel, W. (1997). Functional imaging of headache - first steps in an objective quantitative classification of migraine. *European Journal of Medical Research, 2*(9), 367–376.

Scher, A. I., Midgette, L. A., & Lipton, R. B. (2008). Risk factors for headache chronification. *Headache, 48*(1), 16–25.

Schlake, H. P., Grotemeyer, K. H., Hofferberth, B., Husstedt, I. W., & Wiesner, S. (1990). Brainstem auditory evoked potentials in migraine—evidence of increased side differences during the pain-free interval. *Headache, 30*(3), 129–132.

Schoenen, J. (1986). Beta blockers and the central nervous system. *Cephalalgia, 6*(Suppl 5), 47–54.

Schoenen, J. (1996). Deficient habituation of evoked cortical potentials in migraine: A link between brain biology, behavior and trigeminovascular activation?" *Biomedicine and Pharmacotherapy, 50*(2), 71–78.

Schoenen, J., Jamart, B., & Delwaide, P. J. (1987). Topographic EEG mapping in common and classic migraine during and between attacks. In F. C. Rose (Ed.), *Advances in headache research* (pp. 25–33). London: Smith Gordon.

Schoenen, J., Maertens, A., Timsit-Berthier, M., & Timsit, M. (1985). Contingent negative variation (CNV) as a diagnostic and physiopathologic tool in headache patients. In: F. C. Rose (Ed.), *Migraine: Clinical and research advances* (pp. 17–25). Basel: Karger.

Schoenen, J., Maertens de Noordhout, A., Timsit-Berthier, M., & Timsit, M. (1986). Contingent negative variation and efficacy of beta-blocking agents in migraine. *Cephalalgia, 6*(4), 229–233.

Schoenen, J., & Timsit-Berthier, M. (1993). Contingent negative variation: Methods and potential interest in headache. *Cephalalgia, 13*(1), 28–32.

Schoenen, J., Wang, W., Albert, A., & Delwaide, P. J. (1995). Potentiation instead of habituation characterizes visual evoked potentials in migraine patients between attacks. *European Journal of Neurology, 2*, 115–122.

Sener, H. O., Haktanir, I., & Demirci, S. (1997). Pattern-reversal visual evoked potentials in migraineurs with or without visual aura. *Headache, 37*(7), 449–451.

Seri, S., Cerquiglini, A., & Guidetti, V. (1993). Computerized EEG topography in childhood migraine between and during attacks. *Cephalalgia, 13*(1), 53–56.

Shepherd, A. J., Wyatt, G., & Tibber, M. S. (2011). Visual metacontrast masking in migraine. *Cephalalgia, 31*(3), 346–356.

Shibata, K., Osawa, M., & Iwata, M. (1997a). Pattern reversal visual evoked potentials in classic and common migraine. *Journal of Neurological Sciences, 145*(2), 177–181.

Shibata, K., Osawa, M., & Iwata, M. (1997b). Simultaneous recording of pattern reversal electroretinograms and visual evoked potentials in migraine. *Cephalalgia, 17*(7), 742–747.

Shibata, K., Osawa, M., & Iwata, M. (1998). Pattern reversal visual evoked potentials in migraine with aura and migraine aura without headache. *Cephalalgia, 18*(6), 319–323.

Shibata, K., Yamane, K., Iwata, M., & Ohkawa, S. (2005). Evaluating the effects of spatial frequency on migraines by using pattern-reversal visual evoked potentials. *Clinical Neurophysiology, 116*(9), 2220–2227.

Shibata, K., Yamane, K., Otuka, K., & Iwata, M. (2008). Abnormal visual processing in migraine with aura: A study of steady-state visual evoked potentials. *Journal of Neurological Sciences., 271*(1–2), 119–126.

Sicuteri, F. (1976). Hypothesis: Migraine, a central biochemical dysnociception. *Headache, 16*(4), 145–159.

Silberstein, S. D., Olesen, J., Bousser, M-G., Diener, H-C., Dodick, D., First, M., et al., and International Headache Society. (2005). The international classification of headache disorders, 2nd edition (ICHD-II)—revision of criteria for 8.2 medication-overuse headache. *Cephalalgia, 25*(6), 460–465.

Simon, R. H., Zimmerman, A. W., Sanderson, P., & Tasman, A. (1983). EEG markers of migraine in children and adults. *Headache, 23*(5), 201–205.

Simon, R. H., Zimmerman, A. W., Tasman, A., & Hale, M. S. (1982). Spectral analysis of photic stimulation in migraine. *Electroencephalography and Clinical Neurophysiology, 53*(3), 270–276.

Siniatchkin, M., Andrasik, F., Kropp, P., Niederberger, U., Strenge, H., Averkina, N., et al. (2007). Central mechanisms of controlled-release metoprolol in migraine: A double-blind, placebo-controlled study. *Cephalalgia, 27*(9), 1024–1032.

Siniatchkin, M., Averkina, N., Andrasik, F., Stephani, U., & Gerber, W-D. (2006). Neurophysiological reactivity before a migraine attack. *Neuroscience Letters, 400*(1–2), 121–124.

Siniatchkin, M., Averkina, N., & Gerber, W. D. (2006). Relationship between precipitating agents and neurophysiological abnormalities in migraine. *Cephalalgia, 26*(4), 457–465.

Siniatchkin, M., Gerber, W. D., Kropp, P., Voznesenskaya, T., & Vein, A. M. (2000). Are the periodic changes of neurophysiological parameters during the pain-free interval in migraine related to abnormal orienting activity? *Cephalalgia, 20*(1), 20–29.

Siniatchkin, M., Gerber, W. D., Kropp, P., & Vein, A. (1998). Contingent negative variation in patients with chronic daily headache. *Cephalalgia, 18*(8), 565–569; discussion 531.

Siniatchkin, M., Gerber-von Müller, G., Darabaneanu, S., Petermann, F., Stephani, U., & Gerber, W. D. (2010). Behavioral treatment programme contributes to normalization of contingent negative variation in children with migraine. *Cephalalgia. 31*(5), 562–572.

Siniatchkin, M., Hierundar, A., Kropp, P., Kuhnert, R., Gerber, W. D., & Stephani, U. (2000). Self-regulation of slow cortical potentials in children with migraine: An exploratory study. *Applied Psychophysiology and Biofeedback, 25*(1), 13–32.

Siniatchkin, M., Jonas, A., Baki, H., van Baalen, Gerber, W. D., & Stephani, U. (2010). Developmental changes of the contingent negative variation in migraine and healthy children. *Journal of Headache and Pain, 11*(2), 105–113.

Siniatchkin, M., Kirsch, E., Kropp, P., Stephani, U., & Gerber, W. D. (2000). Slow cortical potentials in migraine families. *Cephalalgia, 20*(10), 881–892.

Siniatchkin, M., Kropp, P., & Gerber, W. D. (2000). Neurofeedback-the significance of reinforcement and the search for an appropriate strategy for the success of self-regulation. *Applied Psychophysiology and Biofeedback, 25*(3), 167–175.

Siniatchkin, M., Kropp, P., & Gerber, W. D. (2001). Contingent negative variation in subjects at risk for migraine without aura. *Pain, 94*(2), 159–167.

Siniatchkin, M., Kropp, P., & Gerber, W-D. (2003). What kind of habituation is impaired in migraine patients? *Cephalalgia, 23*(7), 511–518.

Siniatchkin, M., Kropp, P., Gerber, W. D., & Stephani, U. (2000). Migraine in childhood—are periodically occurring migraine attacks related to dynamic changes of cortical information processing? *Neuroscience Letters, 279*(1), 1–4.

Siniatchkin, M., Kropp, P., Neumann, M., Gerber, W., & Stephani, U. (2000). Intensity dependence of auditory evoked cortical potentials in migraine families. *Pain, 85*(1–2), 247–254.

Siniscalchi, A., Badini, I., Beani, L., & Bianchi, C. (1999). 5-HT4 receptor modulation of acetylcholine outflow in guinea pig brain slices. *Neuroreport, 10*(3), 547–551.

Smyth, V. O., & Winter, A. L. (1964). The EEG in migraine. *Electroencephalography and Clinical Neurophysiology, 16* 194–202.

Strenge, H., Fritzer, G., Göder, R., Niederberger, U., Gerber, W. D., & Aldenhoff, J. (2001). Non-linear electroencephalogram dynamics in patients with spontaneous nocturnal migraine attacks. *Neuroscience Letters, 309*(2), 105–108.

Tagliati, M., Sabbadini, M., Bernardi, G., & Silvestrini, M. (1995). Multichannel visual evoked potentials in migraine. *Electroencephalography and Clinical Neurophysiology, 96*(1), 1–5.

Thompson, R. F., & Spencer, W. A. (1966). Habituation: A model phenomenon for the study of neuronal substrates of behavior. *Psychological Review, 73*(1), 16–43.

Treede, R., Lorenz, J., & Baumgärtner, U. (2003). Clinical usefulness of laser-evoked potentials. *Neurophysiologie Clinique, 33*(6), 303–314.

Tsounis, S., Milonas, J., & Gilliam, F. (1993). Hemi-field pattern reversal visual evoked potentials in migraine. *Cephalalgia, 13*(4), 267–271.

Tsounis, S., & Varfis, G. (1992). Alpha rhythm power and the effect of photic stimulation in migraine with brain mapping. *Clinical Electroencephalography, 23*(1), 1–6.

Unay, B., Ulas, U. H., Karaoglu, B., Eroglu, E., Akin, R., & Gokcay, E. (2008). Visual and brainstem auditory evoked potentials in children with headache. *Pediatrics International, 50*(5), 620–623.

Valdizán, J. R., Andreu, C., Almárcegui, C., & Olivito, A. (1994). Quantitative EEG in children with headache. *Headache, 34*(1), 53–55.

Valeriani, M., de Tommaso, M., Restuccia, D., Le Pera, D., Guido, M., Iannetti, G. D., et al. (2003). Reduced habituation to experimental pain in migraine patients: A CO(2) laser evoked potential study. *Pain, 105*(1–2), 57–64.

Valeriani, M., Galli, F., Tarantino, S., Graceffa, D., Pignata, E., Miliucci, R., et al. (2009). Correlation between abnormal brain excitability and emotional symptomatology in paediatric migraine. *Cephalalgia, 29*(2), 204–213.

Valeriani, M., Rinalduzzi, S., & Vigevano, F. (2005). Multilevel somatosensory system disinhibition in children with migraine. *Pain, 118*(1–2), 137–144.

Vendrame, M., Kaleyias, J., Valencia, I., Legido, A., & Kothare, S. V.. (2008). Polysomnographic findings in children with headaches. *Pediatric Neurology, 39*(1), 6–11.

Vollono, C., Ferraro, D., Miliucci, R., Vigevano, F., & Valeriani, M. (2010). The abnormal recovery cycle of somatosensory evoked potential components in children with migraine can be reversed by topiramate. *Cephalalgia, 30*(1), 17–26.

Walton, K. D., Dubois, M., & Llinás, R. R. (2010). Abnormal thalamocortical activity in patients with complex regional pain syndrome (CRPS) type I. *Pain, 150,* 41–51.

Wang, W., & Schoenen, J. (1998). Interictal potentiation of passive "oddball" auditory event-related potentials in migraine. *Cephalalgia, 18*(5), 261–265; discussion 241.

Wang, W., Schoenen, J., & Timsit-Berthier, M. (1995). Cognitive functions in migraine without aura between attacks: A psychophysiological approach using the "oddball" paradigm. *Clinical Neurophysiology, 25*(1), 3–11.

Wang., W., Timsit-Berthier, M., & Schoenen, J. (1996). Intensity dependence of auditory evoked potentials is pronounced in migraine: An indication of cortical potentiation and low serotonergic neurotransmission? *Neurology, 46*(5), 1404–1409.

Wang, W., Wang, G. P., Ding, X. L., & Wang, Y. H. (1999). Personality and response to repeated visual stimulation in migraine and tension-type headaches. *Cephalalgia, 19*(8), 718–724; discussion 697.

Wang, X., Xiang, J., Wang, Y., Pardos, M., Meng, L., Huo, X., et al. (2010). Identification of abnormal neuromagnetic signatures in the motor cortex of adolescent migraine. *Headache, 50*(6), 1005–1016.

Weckesser, M., Posse, S., Olthoff, U., Kemna, L., Dager, S., & Müller Gärtner, H-W. (1999). Functional imaging of the visual cortex with BOLD-contrast fMRI: Hyperventilation decreases the signal response. *Magnetic Resonance Medicine, 41,* 213–216.

Weiller, C., May, A., Limmroth, V., Jüptner, M., Kaube, H., Schayck, R. V., et al. (1995). Brain stem activation in spontaneous human migraine attacks. *Nature Medicine, 1*(7), 658–660.

Welch, K. M. A. (2009). Iron in the migraine brain; a resilient hypothesis. *Cephalalgia, 29*(3), 283–285.

Welch, K. M., Levine, S. R., D'Andrea, G., Schultz, L. R., & Helpern, J. A. (1989). Preliminary observations on brain energy metabolism in migraine studied by in vivo phosphorus 31 NMR spectroscopy. *Neurology, 39*(4), 538–541.

Woestenburg, J. C., Kramer, C. J., Orlebeke, J. F., & Passchier, J. (1993). Brain potential differences related to spatial attention in migraineurs with and without aura symptoms support supposed differences in activation. *Headache, 33*(8), 413–416.

Wray, S. H., Mijović-Prelec, D., & Kosslyn, S. M. (1995). Visual processing in migraineurs. *Brain, 118*(Pt 1), 25–35.

Zohsel, K., Hohmeister, J., Flor, H., & Hermann, C. (2008). Altered pain processing in children with migraine: An evoked potential study. *European Journal of Pain, 12*(8), 1090–1101.

30 Drug Effects on Cortical Excitability

SUSAN M. BOWYER AND PANAYIOTIS D. MITSIAS

INTRODUCTION

Migraine is associated with a state of increased neuronal excitability. This excitability of the cell membranes appears to be a fundamental factor in the brain's susceptibility to migraine attacks (Aurora & Bowyer, 2006; Welch, 2003; Welch et al., 1990). Understanding the molecular mechanisms underlying the abnormal functioning of hyperactive neuronal circuits has been essential in our effort to develop antimigraine drugs. The neuronal changes that take place with migraine may be thought of as those occurring during the *perimigraine attack phase* (prodrome, ictal events, postictal events) and the *interictal migraine state,* where a hyperexcitable brain state exists.

The neuronal changes that underlie migraine attack are like a well-orchestrated chain of events. Initially, some electrical event takes place that causes the dilation of the blood vessels followed by the painful syndrome. In this initial phase of migraine there is neuronal excitability that reaches a threshold that in turn triggers cortical spreading depression events that cause a depolarization of neuronal activity to spread across the cortex. In the wake of this wave, vessels dilate, leaking substance P, which causes local meningeal inflammation, vascular dilatation, and pain.

A MINI-SUMMARY OF PHARMACOTHERAPY OF MIGRAINE

Migraine drugs fall under two general categories, those addressing the acute attack (acute-phase or abortive medications) and those used for prevention of future attacks (prophylactic medications). There are over 30 types of drugs that are used for migraine treatment: They are divided into the acute-phase or abortive medications and the prophylactic agents. Table 30–1 summarizes these medications and their general mechanism of action.

Acute-phase or abortive migraine treatments usually include nonsteroidal anti-inflammatory drugs (NSAIDs), ergotamines, triptans, or combinations of these. These drugs aim at aborting the acute attack as soon as possible. The *NSAIDs* are effective because of their analgesic actions but also because of more specific effects on the trigeminal and antinociceptive systems in the brainstem and thalamus (Göbel et al., 1992; Jurna & Brune, 1990; Kaube et al., 1993). The *ergotamines* have 5-HT receptor binding, vasoconstrictor, and neuronal properties, especially in the neurons of the trigeminal nucleus caudalis (Hoskin et al., 1996; Müller-Schweinitzer, 1978). The *triptans* were introduced as acute-phase treatment in 1992. They target the 5-HT receptors and they constrict multiple vascular beds. They abort migraine attacks by direct contraction of dilated cranial extracerebral vessels, suppression of neuropeptide release from peripheral nerve endings, and inhibition of impulse transmission centrally in the trigeminal nucleus caudalis (Goadsby & Edvinsson, 1994; Shepherd et al., 1997).

Prophylactic therapies for migraine include, among others, β-blockers, tricyclic antidepressants, calcium channel blockers, and antiepileptic medications. *β-Adrenoceptor blocking agents* that have proven action against migraine include propranolol, nadolol, atenolol, timolol, and metoprolol. They exert their effect by modifying the hyperactivity of the central catecholaminergic system (Schoenen et al., 1986). *Calcium channel blockers* such as verapamil and flunarizine regulate the cellular levels of calcium. Their mechanism of action is most likely through impairing the synthesis and release of nitric oxide from perivascular nerves and, possibly, endothelium (Ayajiki et al., 1997).

In recent years, several *antiepileptic drugs* (AEDs) have been linked to helping reduce the frequency and severity of migraine attacks. This is attributed to the ability of these AEDs to reduce the excitability of the cortical neurons (Rapoport et al., 1989; White, 2005) among other actions. Topiramate has also been shown to inhibit the activation of the trigeminocervical neurons in response to stimulation of the superior sagittal sinus, a plausible mechanism of the action of migraine preventive medications (Storer & Goadsby, 2004). Valproate, on the other hand, increases γ-aminobutyric acid (GABA), but may also increase potassium conductance, producing neuronal hyperpolarization

TABLE 30–1 *Medications Used for Treatment of Migraine*

Drug Category	Drug	Brand Name	Mechanism of Action
Antidepressant Agents			
	Amitriptyline	Elavil	Nonselective biogenic amine reuptake inhibitor
	Duloxetine	Cymbalta	Selective serotonin reuptake inhibitors
	Fluoxetine	Prozac	
	Paroxetine	Paxil	
	Sertraline	Zoloft	
Antiepileptic Agents			
	Gabapentin	Neurontin	Voltage-gated calcium channel antagonists
	Levetiracetam	Keppra	
	Pregabalin	Lyrica	
	Lamotrigine	Lamictal	Voltage-gated sodium channel antagonists
	Valproate	Depakote	
	Zonisamide	Zonegran	
	Topiramate	Topamax	Voltage-gated sodium channel antagonist, AMPA receptor antagonist, $GABA_A$ agonist
Antihypertensive Agents			
	Lisinopril	Zestril, Prinivil	Angiotensin-converting enzyme inhibitor
	Irbesartan	Avapro	Angiotensin II receptor antagonist
	Metoprolol	Lopressor	β-Adrenoceptor antagonists
	Nadolol	Corgard	
	Propranolol	Inderal	
	Timolol	Blocadren	
Nonsteroidal Anti-Inflammatory Drugs (NSAIDs)			
	Diclofenac	Voltaren	Cyclooxygenase inhibitors
	Ibuprofen	Motrin, Advil	
	Indobufen	Lubon	
	Ketorolac	Toradol	
	Ketoprofen	Orudis	
	Naproxen	Anaprox, Aleve	
Triptans			
	Almotriptan	Axert	
	Eletriptan	Relpax	Serotonin receptor agonists, 5-HT receptor agonist that binds with high affinity for $5\text{-}HT_{1B}$ and $5\text{-}HT_{1D}$ receptors
	Frovatriptan	Frova	
	Naratriptan	Amerge	
	Rizatriptan	Maxalt	
	Sumatriptan	Imitrex	
	Zolmitriptan	Zomig	

(Continued)

TABLE 30–1 *Medications Used for Treatment of Migraine (Continued)*

Drug Category	Drug	Brand Name	Mechanism of Action
Ergotamines			
	Ergotamine tartrate	Ergostat, Ergomar	Binds to several receptor populations (α-adrenergic, dopamine, serotonin); can be an agonist or antagonist
Other			
	Acetaminophen	Tylenol	
	Methylprednisolone	Medrol	Glucocorticoid agonist
	Tizanidine	Zanaflex	Adrenergic α_2 agonist
	Metoclopramide	Reglan	Dopamine D_2 receptor antagonists
	Prochlorperazine	Compazine	
	Cyproheptadine	Periactin	Histamine H_1 antagonist

AMPA = α-amino-3-hydroxy-5-methyl-4-isoxazolepropionic acid; $GABA_A$ = γ-aminobutyric acid A.

and turning off the 5-HT neurons of the dorsal raphe nuclei (Cutrer & Moskowitz, 1996; Cutrer et al., 1995).

Studies of topiramate and valproate, but also of propranolol, amitriptyline, and methysergide, have shown that these drugs change the cortical thresholds for the induction of cortical spreading depression (CSD) (Ayata et al., 2006). CSD was first reported by Leão (1944) as a disturbance of the cortical environment that occurs in various pathophysiological conditions such as migraine (Lauritzen, 1994; Milner, 1958), epilepsy (Marshall, 1959), anoxia (Hansen, 1985), cerebral ischemia (Hansen & Zeuthen, 1981), and head trauma (Oka et al., 1977). CSD propagates along the cortex at a rate of a few millimeters per minute. The tissue undergoing CSD exhibits vigorous discharges and then becomes electrically inactive for a few minutes (Grafstein, 1956; Harreras et al., 1994). During CSD, the membrane resistance of the neurons is reduced, and the ionic concentrations across the cell membranes are greatly altered (Bures, 1992; Nicholson & Kraig, 1981).

Several imaging studies provide the basis for detecting neuronal changes that occur in patients before and after migraine treatment. Magnetoencephalography (MEG) was used to study the direct current (DC) MEG shifts that arise in visually stimulated migraine patients (Bowyer et al., 2001). DC MEG shifts provide direct measurement of neuronal excitation and suppression. DC MEG field shifts have previously been demonstrated to arise during spontaneous and visually induced migraine aura (Bowyer et al., 2001). These DC MEG shifts resemble those reported from MEG studies of CSD crossing a sulcus in animal models (Fig. 30–1a), in which electrocorticography was used to confirm the CSD depolarization (Bowyer, Okada, et al., 1999; Bowyer, Tepley, et al. 1999) (Fig. 30–1b).

Migraine patients who received prophylactic treatment with sodium valproate underwent MEG studies before the start of treatment and at follow-up at 1 month (Bowyer et al., 2005). Large-amplitude DC MEG signals, imaged to extended areas of occipital cortex, were seen in patients before drug treatment. After 30 days of prophylactic treatment, reduced DC MEG shifts in the occipital cortex and reduced incidence of migraine attacks were observed (Fig. 30–2). We have also seen similar results from the effect of topiramate in a handful of migraine patients (unpublished). Using visual stimulation, the authors demonstrated the hyperexcitability of widespread regions throughout the occipital cortex in migraine patients, explaining the susceptibility for triggering CSD and migraine aura (Bowyer et al., 2005).

Occipital cortex hyperexcitability has also been demonstrated in migraine using the technique of magnetic suppression of perceptual accuracy (MSPA) (Aurora et al., 2010). The effects of topiramate treatment on patients with migraine have been tested with MSPA and transcranial magnetic stimulation. The interim dose was that at which an improvement in headache frequency was first observed, and the optimal dose was that at which the patient had a $\geq50\%$ reduction in headache frequency, or had reached a 100-mg dose. The dose ranged from 50 to 100 mg of topiramate; the average dose was 75 mg. The interim dose for most patients was 50 mg. In this study there was no significant correlation between mean change in frequency of headache and mean change in inhibition from baseline to

(a)

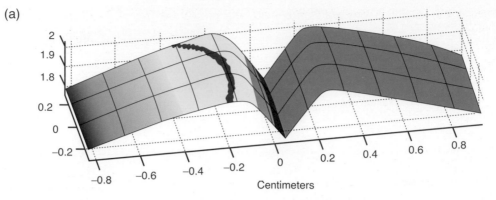

FIGURE 30–1A *Model of cortical spreading depression wave crossing the cortical surface of a lissencephalic brain. From Bowyer, S. M., Okada, Y. C., Papuashvili, N., Moran, J. E., Barkley, G. L., Welch, K. M., et al. (1999). Analysis of MEG signals of spreading cortical depression with propagation constrained to a rectangular cortical strip. I. Lissencephalic rabbit model. Brain Research, 843, 79–86.*

optimal dose (0.04, p = .89). Topiramate modulates occipital cortex excitability in chronic migraine possibly via mechanisms of cortical inhibition. Since there was not a strong correlation between the degree of inhibition and reduction of migraine frequency, it would appear that topiramate did have an independent effect on cortical excitability that was not dependent on reduction in migraine frequency (Aurora et al., 2010).

CONCLUSION

What can the detection of drug effects on cortical excitability mean for the prognosis and treatment of migraine? By understanding the mechanism that underlies the hyperexcitability of the cortex and the mechanism of the drug effects on the cortex, patients may benefit by having treatment therapies individually tailored to their excit-

(b)

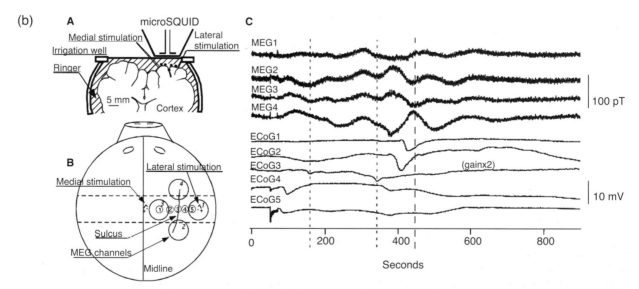

FIGURE 30–1B *Direct current–coupled magnetoencephalography (MEG) and electrocorticography (ECoG) signals associated with cortical spreading depressions (CSD) initiated by stimulation of the lateral portion of the coronal gyrus within the cortical strip. (A) Schematic illustration of the well and the coronal section of the brain at the level of the ECoG electrode array. (B) Top view of experimental setup. Medial and lateral stimulation electrodes are marked. (C) MEG and ECoG traces associated with CSD. Stimulus train was given starting at the time of initial deflection at ECoG5. First two dashed lines correspond to two negative ECoG3 deflections. Third dashed line. represents MEG field due to CSD in the cruciate sulcus_medial to the coronal sulcus indicated in the figure. From Bowyer, S. M., Tepley, N., Papuashvili, N., Kato, S., Barkley, G. L., Welch, K. M. A., et al. (1999). Analysis of MEG signals of spreading cortical depression with propagation constrained to a rectangular cortical strip: II. Gyrencephalic swine model. Brain Research, 843, 71–78.*

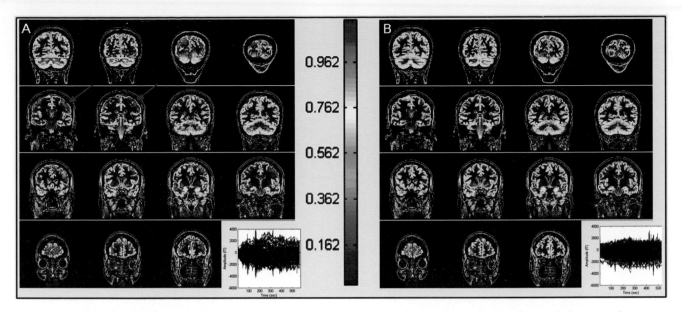

FIGURE 30–2 **(A)** *MR-FOCUSS analysis of the magnetoencephalography (MEG) recordings from a migraine patient before start of treatment with sodium valproate. Averaged MEG image activation results of cortical activity, over the initial 400 seconds, are overlaid onto a standard coronal magnetic resonance imaging (MRI) scan. Scale is in nanoamp meters. Note the extended cortical areas (blue color) of activation in the occipital, parietal (large arrows), and frontal cortex. The 148-channel MEG graph in the lower right-hand corner displays direct current (DC) shifts.* **(B)** *MR-FOCUSS analysis of the MEG recordings from the same migraine patient after 30 days of treatment with sodium valproate. Averaged image activation MEG results of cortical activity are overlaid onto a standard coronal MRI scan. Note the reduced cortical activity in the extended occipital and parietal cortex. The 148-channel MEG graph in the lower right-hand corner displays reduced DC shifts. From Bowyer, S. M., Tepley, N., & Mitsias, P. D. (2005). Cortical hyperexcitability in a migraine patient before and after sodium valproate treatment.* Journal of Clinical Neurophysiology, 22, 65–67.

ability threshold levels or antimigraine drugs may be developed to target specific brain locations of known hyperexcitability.

REFERENCES

Aurora, S. K., Barrodale, P. M., Vermaas, A. R., & Rudra, C. B. (2010). Topiramate modulates excitability of the occipital cortex when measured by transcranial magnetic stimulation. *Cephalalgia, 30*(6), 648–654.

Aurora, S. K., & Bowyer, S. M. (2006). New insights into brain dysfunction in migraine. *Expert Reviews in Neurotherapy, 6*(3), 307–312.

Ayajiki, K., Okamura, T., & Toda, N. (1997). Flunarizine, an antimigraine agent, impairs nitroxidergic nerve function in cerebral arteries. *European Journal of Pharmacology, 329*(1), 49–53.

Ayata, C., Jin, H., Kudo, C., Dalkara, T., & Moskowitz, M. A. (2006). Suppression of cortical spreading depression in migraine prophylaxis. *Annals of Neurology, 59*, 652–661.

Bowyer, S. M., Aurora, K. S., Moran, J. E., Tepley, N., & Welch, K. M. (2001). Magnetoencephalographic fields from patients with spontaneous and induced migraine aura. *Annals of Neurology, 50*(5), 582–587.

Bowyer, S. M., Okada, Y. C., Papuashvili, N., Moran, J. E., Barkley, G. L., Welch, K. M., et al. (1999). Analysis of MEG signals of spreading cortical depression with propagation constrained to a rectangular cortical strip. I. Lissencephalic rabbit model. *Brain Research, 843*, 79–86.

Bowyer, S. M., Tepley, N., & Mitsias, P. D. (2005). Cortical hyperexcitability in a migraine patient before and after sodium valproate treatment. *Journal of Clinical Neurophysiology, 22*, 65–67.

Bowyer, S. M., Tepley, N., Papuashvili, N., Kato, S., Barkley, G. L., Welch, K. M. A., et al. (1999). Analysis of MEG signals of spreading cortical depression with propagation constrained to a rectangular cortical strip: II. Gyrencephalic swine model. *Brain Research, 843*, 71–78.

Bures, J., Korelova, V. I., & Vinogradova, L. V (1992). Synergetics of spreading depression: Reentry waves and reverberation in the rat brain. In: R. J. do Carmo (Ed.), *Spreading depression* (pp. 35–48). Berlin: Springer-Verlag.

Cutrer, F. M., Limmroth, V., Ayata, G., & Moskowitz, M. A. (1995). Attenuation by valproate of c-fos immunoreactivity in trigeminal nucleus caudalis induced by intracisternal capsaicin. *British Journal of Pharmacology, 116*(8), 3199–3204.

Cutrer, F. M., & Moskowitz, M. A. (1996). Wolff Award 1996. The actions of valproate and neurosteroids in a model of trigeminal pain. *Headache, 36*(10), 579–585.

Goadsby, P. J., & Edvinsson, L. (1994). Joint 1994 Wolff Award Presentation. Peripheral and central trigeminovascular activation in cat is blocked by the serotonin (5HT)-1D receptor agonist 311C90. *Headache, 34*(7), 394–399.

Göbel, H., Ernst, M., Jeschke, J., Keil, R., & Weigle, L. (1992). Acetylsalicylic acid activates antinociceptive brain-stem reflex activity in headache patients and in healthy subjects. *Pain, 48*(2), 187–195.

Grafstein, B. (1956). Mechanism of spreading cortical depression. *Journal of Neurophysiology, 19*, 154–171.

Hansen, A. J. (1985). Effect of anoxia on ion distribution in the brain. *Physiological Reviews, 65*, 101–148.

Hansen, A. J., & Zeuthen, T. (1981). Extracellular ion concentration during spreading depression and ischemia in the rat brain cortex. *Acta Physiologica Scandinavica, 113*, 437–445.

Harreras, O., Largo, C., Ibarz, J. M., Somjen, G. G., & Del Rio, R. M. (1994). Role of neuron synchronizing mechanisms in the propagation of spreading depression in the in vivo hippocampus. *Journal of Neuroscience, 14*, 7087–7098.

Hoskin, K. L., Kaube, H., & Goadsby, P. J. (1996). Central activation of the trigeminovascular pathway in the cat is inhibited by dihydroergotamine. A c-Fos and electrophysiological study. *Brain, 119*, 249–256.

Jurna, I., & Brune, K. (1990). Central effect of the non-steroid anti-inflammatory agents, indomethacin, ibuprofen, and diclofenac, determined in C fibre-evoked activity in single neurones of the rat thalamus. *Pain, 41*(1), 71–80.

Kaube, H., Hoskin, K. L., & Goadsby, P. J. (1993). Intravenous acetylsalicylic acid inhibits central trigeminal neurons in the dorsal horn of the upper cervical spinal cord in the cat. *Headache, 33*(10), 541–544.

Lauritzen, M. (1994). Pathophysiology of the migraine aura; the spreading depression theory. *Brain, 117*, 199–210.

Leão, A. (1944). Spreading depression of activity in the cerebral cortex. *Journal of Neurophysiology, 7*, 379–390.

Marshall, W. H. (1959). Spreading cortical depression of Leão. *Physiological Reviews, 39*, 239–279.

Milner, P. M. (1958). Note on possible correspondence between the scotomas of migraine and spreading depression of Leão. *Electroencephalography Clinics and Neurophysiology, 10*, 705.

Müller-Schweinitzer, E. (1978). Basic pharmacological properties. In: B. Berde & H. O. Schild (Eds.), *Ergot alkaloids and related compounds* (pp. 87–232). New York, Berlin, Heidelberg: Springer-Verlag.

Nicholson, C., & Kraig, R. P. (1981). The behavior of extracellular ions during spreading depression. In: T. Zeuther (Ed.), *The application of ion selective microelectrodes* (pp. 217–238). Amsterdam: Elsevier.

Oka, H., Kako, M., Matsushima, M., & Kyozo, A. (1977). Traumatic spreading depression syndrome. Review of a particular type of head injury in 37 patients. *Brain, 100*, 278–298.

Rapoport, A. M., Sheftell, F. D., & Gordon, B. (1989). The successful treatment of migraine with anticonvulsant medication in patients with abnormal EEGs. *Headache, 29*, 309.

Schoenen, J., Maertens de Noordhout, A., Timsit-Berthier, M., & Timsit, M. (1986). Contingent negative variation and efficacy of beta-blocking agents in migraine. *Cephalalgia, 6*(4), 229–233.

Shepherd, S. L., Williamson, D. J., Beer, M. S., Hill, R. G., & Hargreaves, R. J. (1997). Differential effects of 5-HT1B/1D receptor agonists on neurogenic dural plasma extravasation and vasodilation in anaesthetized rats. *Neuropharmacology, 36*(4–5), 525–533.

Storer, R. J., & Goadsby, P. J. (2004). Topiramate inhibits trigeminovascular traffic in the cat. *Cephalalgia, 24*, 1049–1056.

Welch, K. (2003). Contemporary concepts of migraine pathogenesis. *Neurology, 61*(8 Suppl 4), S2–S8.

Welch, K. M. A., D'Andrea, G., Tepley, N., Barkley, G., & Ramadan, N. M. (1990). The concept of migraine as a state of central neuronal hyperexcitability. *Neurological Clinics, 8*, 817–882.

White, H. S. (2005). Molecular pharmacology of topiramate: Managing seizures and preventing migraine. *Headache, 45*(Suppl 1), S48–S56.

Part 5

Conclusions

31 Defining the Migraine Phenotype

TODD J. SCHWEDT AND DAVID W. DODICK

INTRODUCTION

A migraine attack is characterized by headache; hypersensitivities to normal environmental stimuli such as lights, sounds, and odors; and nausea and vomiting. Migraine symptoms are exacerbated by routine physical activities, often leading the migraine patient to seek rest in a dark and quiet room. Neck pain, cutaneous allodynia, and vestibular and cognitive symptoms are also commonly associated with migraine attacks. Approximately one third of people with migraine have aura symptoms associated with at least some of their migraine attacks. Premonitory symptoms, which occur prior to headache onset, and postdromal symptoms, which occur following headache resolution, are common but not universal. Untreated or inadequately treated, migraine attacks last from hours to several days. The different phases of a migraine attack are illustrated in Figure 31–1.

Although the majority of people with migraine have one to four attacks per month, approximately 2% to 3% of the general population has chronic migraine (Bigal, Serrano, Reed, et al., 2008; Castillo et al., 1999; Lipton et al., 2007; Scher et al., 1998). Those with chronic migraine have headaches on at least 15 days per month including at least 8 days on which the patient's symptoms meet diagnostic migraine criteria (Olesen et al., 2006). Although many people with episodic migraine maintain their episodic pattern over time, others transform from episodic to chronic migraine or fluctuate from one pattern to the other. Longitudinal analysis of chronic migraine sufferers over a 3-year period indicates that about one third have persistent chronic migraine, about one quarter remit to having less than 10 headache days per month, and the remainder fluctuate between an episodic and chronic headache pattern (Manack et al., 2011).

Given the episodic nature of full-blown migraine attacks, migraine has typically been considered a chronic disorder with episodic manifestations. However, there is increasing evidence to suggest that people with migraine process and sense painful and environmental stimuli abnormally between individual migraine attacks, even when headache free. Thus, migraine may be more appropriately considered to have persistent manifestations with superimposed paroxysmal episodes of full-blown migraine attacks. Furthermore, migraine is comorbid with or elevates the risk of having several different disorders including psychiatric diseases such as depression and anxiety disorders, myofascial pain, fatigue, epilepsy, sleep disorders, gastrointestinal disorders, cardiac disease, cardiovascular disease, and ischemic stroke.

THE MIGRAINE PATIENT

Migraine has a 1-year prevalence of approximately 12% in the Western population (Lipton et al., 2007; Rasmussen, 1995). This includes 18% of the female population and 6% of the male population (Lipton et al., 2001, 2007). Migraine is equally prevalent in prepubescent boys and girls, with the female predominance becoming apparent with menarche. Prevalence increases in both sexes until reaching a peak in the fourth decade (men 7.4%, women 24.4%), followed by a gradual decline with advancing age (Lipton et al., 2007). In those older than 60 years of age, prevalence is 4% in men and 6.4% in women (Lipton et al., 2007). Lifetime prevalence of migraine is approximately 33% in women and 13% in men (Launer et al., 1999). Migraine is more common in whites than blacks and is more prevalent in those with a lower income (Lipton et al., 2007).

Migraine has a strong genetic component, resulting in many migraineurs having first-degree relatives with migraine (de Vries et al., 2009). First-degree relatives of family members who have migraine without aura are about twice as likely to have migraine without aura compared to the general population (Russell & Olesen, 1995). Migraine with aura may be more heritable, with first-degree relatives of people having migraine with aura being about four times as likely to have migraine with aura compared to the general population (Russell & Olesen, 1995). Genetic and environmental factors are estimated to be equally important in determining the likelihood that a person has migraine (Mulder et al., 2003).

Migraine results in substantial disability. Over 90% of migraine patients report some level of migraine-related

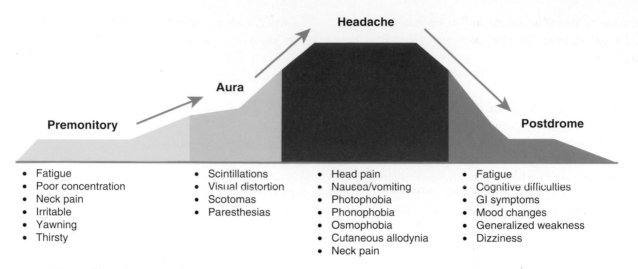

Premonitory	Aura	Headache	Postdrome
• Fatigue • Poor concentration • Neck pain • Irritable • Yawning • Thirsty	• Scintillations • Visual distortion • Scotomas • Paresthesias	• Head pain • Nausea/vomiting • Photophobia • Phonophobia • Osmophobia • Cutaneous allodynia • Neck pain	• Fatigue • Cognitive difficulties • GI symptoms • Mood changes • Generalized weakness • Dizziness

FIGURE 31–1 *Phases of the migraine attack.*

impairment (at least some reduction in functional performance) during attacks, with over 50% reporting severe impairment (inability to function or requiring bed rest) (Lipton et al., 2007). Migraineurs have lower health-related quality of life including physical, social, and emotional domains (Lipton et al., 2000, 2003; Terwindt et al., 2000). One half of migraineurs are substantially disabled on at least 16 days per year (Lipton et al., 2003). As would be expected, patients with more frequent attacks, such as occurs with chronic migraine, have greater migraine-related disability and lower quality of life (Bigal et al., 2003, 2008).

The Migraine Prodrome

The migraine prodrome consists of premonitory symptoms that herald the oncoming migraine attack (Table 31–1). Estimates regarding the prevalence of premonitory symptoms have varied widely, ranging from less than 10% to greater than 90% (Giffin et al., 2003; Kelman, 2004c; Russell et al., 1996). This wide variation is likely due to differing methods of migraine diagnosis/classification (pre–International Classification of Headache Disorders

TABLE 31–1 *Premonitory and Postdromal Symptoms of Migraine*

Fatigue	Thirst
Poor concentration	Yawning
Neck pain/tightness	Dizziness
Hypersensitivity to light	Increased energy
Irritable/emotional	Food cravings
Hypersensitivity to sound	Frequent urination
Blurred vision	

[ICHD] criteria vs. post-ICHD criteria), different populations being investigated (e.g., general population vs. headache clinic), and means by which data were collected (e.g., prospective vs. retrospective). The prevalence of premonitory symptoms is similar in men and women and in patients who have migraine with aura and migraine without aura (Russell et al., 1996). The median duration of premonitory symptoms is about 2 hours, but with almost half of patients reporting premonitory symptoms that endure for less than 1 hour (Kelman, 2004c). According to a prospective analysis of 803 migraine attacks, the most frequent premonitory symptoms included tired/weary, 72.5%; difficulty with concentration, 51.1%; stiff neck, 49.7%; light sensitive, 48.8%; intolerant/irritable, 38.6%; noise sensitive, 38.4%; difficulty with thoughts, 34.6%; blurred vision, 28%; yawning, 27.8%; and thirst, 26% (Giffin et al., 2003). Other reported symptoms included dizziness, increased energy, pale face, sensitive skin, constipation, frequent urination, nausea/vomiting, hunger/food craving, emotional, difficulty reading/writing, and difficulty with speech (Giffin et al., 2003). Of note, all of these symptoms were more common during the migraine headache phase compared to the prodromal phase with the exception of yawning (prodromal phase = 27.8% vs. headache phase = 25.4%) and hunger/food craving (prodromal phase = 18.2% vs. headache phase = 18.1%). Recognition of premonitory symptoms is highly predictive for an impending migraine attack. When premonitory symptoms are observed by the migraine patient, a migraine headache develops within 72 hours, 72% of the time, compared with a 30% random chance of a migraine occurring in the same population (Giffin et al., 2003). Correct predictions more than 24 hours before the start of a migraine headache can be made on 19% of occasions, and more than 6 hours prior to headache onset in 68% of occasions (Giffin et al., 2003).

Migraine Aura

Approximately 4% of the general population and one third of all migraine patients have migraine with aura (Cutrer & Huerter, 2007). Aura may be present with the first migraine attack that a person experiences, the case in about one third of people who have migraine with aura, or may begin later in the course of migraine (Queiroz et al., 1997). Most migraine with aura patients have aura with some attacks interspersed among migraine without aura attacks. Approximately one fifth of migraine with aura patients have aura with every migraine attack (Queiroz et al., 1997).

Aura symptoms develop gradually over several minutes, longer than 5 minutes by definition; endure for less than 60 minutes; and then resolve without sequelae (Committee of the International Classification of Headache Disorders, 2004). Typically, as the aura symptoms resolve, the headache pain begins. Less commonly, aura symptoms can occur after the onset of the migraine headache and sometimes in the absence of headache altogether ("acephalgic migraine"). A study of 163 migraine with aura sufferers in Denmark found that 62 had attacks of both migraine aura with headache and migraine aura without headache (Russell & Olesen, 1996). Considering patients having aura associated with headache, 92.6% had aura preceding headache, 4.7% had aura during headache, and 2.7% had aura following headache. Two main features of the migraine aura help to differentiate migraine aura symptoms from ischemic events and seizures: (a) there is a slow anatomic progression of symptoms over time, often with resolution of symptoms in one location as new symptoms occur in another location (e.g., spread of paresthesias from the hand slowly up to the face); and (b) positive symptoms typically precede negative symptoms (e.g., paresthesias followed by sensory loss). Visual symptoms are the most common during migraine aura, followed by sensory symptoms, aphasic symptoms, and motor symptoms (Eriksen et al., 2004; Manzoni et al., 1985; Russell & Olesen, 1996). Visual auras are reported by well over 80% of people with migraine with aura (reported by 99% of patients with aura in several studies), sensory symptoms by one third to one half, and aphasic symptoms in one fifth to one third (Eriksen et al., 2004; Manzoni et al., 1985; Russell & Olesen, 1996). Motor symptoms are uncommon, occurring in about 5% of aura patients (Russell & Olesen, 1996). Although visual aura commonly occurs in isolation, sensory, aphasic, and motor symptoms are almost always accompanied by visual symptoms (Eriksen et al., 2004; Russell & Olesen, 1996; Ziegler & Hassanein, 1990).

Visual aura may consist of positive visual phenomena (e.g., flickering lights, jagged or waving lines) including perceptive distortions and simple hallucinations (Aleci & Liboni, 2009). Positive visual phenomena are reported by over four fifths of migraine patients with visual aura (Queiroz et al., 1997; Russell & Olesen, 1996). This most commonly includes zigzag lines (fortification), flickering lights, photopsias, and dots. Negative scotomas, which are temporary defects in the binocular visual field, may also be present and may follow the positive symptoms in the parts of the visual field in which the positive phenomena occurred (Aleci & Liboni, 2009). Negative visual phenomena are reported by about half of migraine with aura patients (Queiroz et al., 1997; Russell & Olesen, 1996). Like all aura symptoms, visual aura symptoms develop gradually and progress slowly, moving across the visual field with time. An analysis of visual aura suggested that symptoms develop over 5 to 30 minutes in 82% of patients and total duration of visual symptoms is 60 minutes or less in 89% (30 minutes or less in about two thirds) (Queiroz et al., 1997; Russell & Olesen, 1996). Visual symptoms may begin in the center or the periphery of the visual field (Queiroz et al., 1997; Russell & Olesen, 1996). In a study of 100 migraine with visual aura subjects, 51% reported having visual aura with at least 50% of their migraine attacks, while others had visual auras less frequently (Queiroz et al., 1997). Typical visual auras should be differentiated from symptoms of retinal migraine. Retinal migraine is a rare disorder in which there are recurrent attacks of monocular visual symptoms followed by a migraine headache (Committee of the International Classification of Headache Disorders, 2004). Visual symptoms may include positive phenomena as well as negative phenomena including blindness. It is essential to differentiate retinal migraine from other potential causes of monocular visual symptoms such as transient ischemic attacks, optic nerve pathology, and retinal detachment.

The second most common aura symptoms are sensory in nature. Like other migraine aura symptoms, sensory symptoms are typically predominated by positive sensory symptoms (paresthesias), occasionally followed by negative sensory symptoms (numbness). Sensory symptoms are usually unilateral and began in the hand with a slow spread up the proximal arm, to the ipsilateral face and shoulder. Facial symptoms typically affect the perioral region and tongue (Russell & Olesen, 1996). Although the lower extremity, foot, and body can also be involved, sensory symptoms in these locations are present in less than one quarter of patients with sensory aura (Giffin et al., 2003; Russell & Olesen, 1996). In the majority of patients, symptoms develop over 5 to 30 minutes and resolve within 60 minutes (most within 30 minutes) consistent with ICHD diagnostic criteria for migraine aura (Russell & Olesen, 1996).

Aphasic aura symptoms include difficulties with production of language and impaired comprehension of language. Expressive dysphasias are most common, present in greater than three fourths of patients with aphasic auras, and typically consisting of paraphasic errors (Eriksen et al., 2004; Russell & Olesen, 1996). Receptive dysphasias are reported by approximately one third of patients with aphasic auras (Eriksen et al., 2004; Russell & Olesen, 1996). Approximately half of people with aphasic auras also suffer from dysarthria, possibly associated with sensory phenomena in the mouth and/or tongue (Eriksen et al., 2004; Giffin et al., 2003; Russell & Olesen, 1996).

Motor weakness is most commonly unilateral, affecting one hand and arm (Russell & Olesen, 1996). Like other aura symptoms, motor symptoms typically have a gradual onset. However, unlike other aura symptoms, in about 50% of patients motor symptoms will endure for greater than 60 minutes (Ducros et al., 2001; Russell & Olesen, 1996; Thomsen et al., 2002). Motor symptoms rarely occur in isolation, almost always occurring in conjunction with other aura symptoms (Russell & Olesen, 1996). The presence of motor weakness with visual, sensory, or dysphasic speech symptoms is consistent with a diagnosis of hemiplegic migraine (Committee of the International Classification of Headache Disorders, 2004). Hemiplegic migraine is a rare disorder, estimated to affect 0.01% of the general population (Thomsen et al., 2002). Hemiplegic migraine may be familial or sporadic. Familial hemiplegic migraine is an autosomal dominantly inherited disorder that has been associated with three different mutations in ion channels (CACNA1A, chromosome 19, voltage-gated calcium channel; ATP1A2, chromosome 1, sodium-potassium adenosine triphosphatase pump; SCN1A, chromosome 2, voltage-gated sodium channel) (De Fusco et al., 2003; Dichgans et al., 2005; Ophoff et al., 1996). Sensory aura symptoms occur in about 95% of hemiplegic migraine attacks, visual symptoms in 74% to 91%, and aphasic symptoms in 83% (Black, 2006). Unlike migraine with typical aura, ICHD-II diagnostic criteria for hemiplegic migraine allow for aura symptoms to endure for up to 24 hours (Committee of the International Classification of Headache Disorders, 2004).

THE MIGRAINE HEADACHE AND ASSOCIATED SYMPTOMS

The migraine attack typically consists of head pain; some combination of hypersensitivities to lights, noise, odor, and touch of the skin; and nausea and/or vomiting,

and is often accompanied by neck pain. Migraine symptoms are made worse when the patient participates in routine physical activities. By definition, the migraine attack lasts 4 to 72 hours (Committee of the International Classification of Headache Disorders, 2004). However, the average duration of a migraine attack is from 4 to 24 hours (Kelman, 2006a; Koseoglu et al., 2003; Russell et al., 1996; Wober-Bingol et al., 2004). The typical migraine patient has one to four headache days per month (Koseoglu et al., 2003; Lipton et al., 2007; Wober-Bingol et al., 2004). Table 31–2 shows the ICHD-II diagnostic criteria for migraine (Committee of the International Classification of Headache Disorders, 2004).

TABLE 31–2 *Migraine—International Classification of Headache Disorders Diagnostic Criteria*

A. ≥5 attacks fulfilling criteria B–D
B. Headache attacks lasting 4–72 hours (untreated or unsuccessfully treated)
C. Headache has ≥2 of the following characteristics:
  a. Unilateral location
  b. Pulsating quality
  c. Moderate or severe pain intensity
  d. Aggravation by or causing avoidance of routine physical activity
D. During headache ≥1 of the following:
  a. Nausea and/or vomiting
  b. Photophobia and phonophobia
E. Not attributed to another disorder

HEADACHE

The typical headache of migraine is a unilateral throbbing headache of moderate to severe pain intensity that is aggravated by activity. Although the majority of migraine headaches meet this description, certainly there is variation. In Kelman's investigation of 1,283 migraine patients, approximately 91% of patients described some of their headaches as throbbing, 90% as pressure, 87% as aching, and 71% as stabbing (Kelman, 2006a). Headache aggravated by activity is reported by approximately 90% of patients (Kelman, 2006a; Koseoglu et al., 2003). Median pain intensity is consistent with a moderate to severe rating (Kelman, 2006a; Russell et al., 1996; Wober-Bingol et al., 2004). Migraine headaches do not reach maximal intensity immediately, with a median time to peak intensity of approximately 90 minutes (Kelman, 2006a). This feature helps to differentiate migraine from acute-onset severe headaches (e.g., thunderclap headaches),

headaches that are often secondary in nature. Migraine pain location varies widely among migraineurs. Pain locations in descending order of frequency are eyes (67.1%), temporal (58%), frontal (55.9%), occipital (39.8%), neck (39.7%), vertex (24.1%), and diffusely (17.5%) (Kelman, 2005). When pain is unilateral, the right and left sides of the head are involved with equal frequency, but as many as one quarter to two fifths of migraine patients report that headache pain is felt bilaterally (Kelman, 2005; Russell et al., 1996; Wober-Bingol et al., 2004).

PHOTOPHOBIA

The majority of patients experience an increased sensitivity to light during a migraine attack. Estimates of photophobia prevalence during a migraine range widely, from approximately 48% to 92% (Kececi & Dener, 2002; Koseoglu et al., 2003; Russell et al., 1996; Wober-Bingol et al., 2004). The true frequency of photophobia is probably nearer to the upper end of this range, underestimates likely due to inadequate ascertainment (Choi et al., 2009; Evans et al., 2008). Exposure to light and certain visual patterns may cause generalized discomfort and increase the intensity of the headache pain. Symptoms of photophobia may include an increased sensitivity with exposure to normal lighting conditions, to bright light (e.g., sunlight), and to flickering lights (e.g., fluorescent lights, computer screen) (Friedman & De ver Dye, 2009; Hay et al., 1994; Main et al., 2000). Brighter intensity light causes greater discomfort in migraineurs, a group with lower light discomfort thresholds to begin with (Main et al., 1997, 2000). Migraine patients tend to avoid bright light by laying in dark rooms with lights off and curtains closed and by wearing sunglasses (Choi et al., 2009). Migraineurs are also hypersensitive to certain visual patterns, like alternating light and dark stripes ("gratings"), which may be encountered when viewing road markings and striped wallpaper, an association that may be dependent upon the spatial frequency of the striped pattern (Main et al., 2000; Wilkins et al., 1984).

PHONOPHOBIA

Phonophobia is present in approximately 52% to 82% of patients during a migraine attack (Koseoglu et al., 2003; Russell et al., 1996; Wober-Bingol et al., 2004). Migraine patients have increased sensitivity to normal-volume auditory stimuli (e.g., spoken voice) and to loud noise (e.g., loud music). Exposure to such noises may cause generalized discomfort and increase the pain of the migraine headache. In a study of 51 migraineurs, 98% reported being sensitive to sound during an attack and 94% reported that sound increased their headache intensity (Vingen et al., 1998). Although as many as three fourths of people with migraine report being sensitive to sound between individual migraine attacks, almost all report being even more sound sensitive during an attack (Vingen et al., 1998).

OSMOPHOBIA

Osmophobia occurs with a lower frequency than photophobia and phonophobia. Prevalence estimates for osmophobia during migraine range from about 25% to 43% (De Carlo, 2010; Kelman, 2004a; Zanchin et al., 2007). In the vast majority of migraine patients with osmophobia, this hypersensitivity to odors is present with their first migraine attack and is present with the majority of their migraine attacks (Zanchin et al., 2007). Patients most commonly report osmophobia to scents (e.g., perfumes, deodorants), foods (e.g., coffee, fried foods, onion), and cigarette smoke (De Carlo, 2010; Zanchin et al., 2007). There has been consideration to add osmophobia to the diagnostic criteria for migraine, as evidenced by its inclusion in the ICHD-II appendix criteria. Studies have shown that the presence of osmophobia is highly specific for a migraine diagnosis, but lacks sensitivity. A study investigating the prevalence of osmophobia in 807 migraine patients and 198 tension-type headache patients found osmophobia to be present in 347 of the migraine patients vs. none of the tension-type headache patients, yielding a sensitivity of 43% and a specificity of 100% for the presence of osmophobia in migraine (Zanchin et al., 2007). In a separate study of 1,237 patients, osmophobia was associated with a specificity of 98.4% and a sensitivity of 1.1% for the diagnosis of migraine, while the combination of osmophobia with photophobia had a specificity of 99% and a sensitivity of 1.1%, and the combination of phonophobia and osmophobia was associated with a specificity of 98.6% and a sensitivity of 1.1% (Kelman, 2004b). Thus, investigators found that the addition of osmophobia to diagnostic criteria would result in only a few patients being diagnosed with migraine that would not have been if osmophobia was not included. However, the presence of osmophobia may be helpful to the clinician faced with a patient who does not have nausea or vomiting and has only one of photophobia or phonophobia (probable migraine patient) since its presence is very highly suggestive of a migraine diagnosis.

NAUSEA/VOMITING/GASTRIC STASIS

Nausea is present in greater than three fourths of patients during a migraine attack (estimates ranging from 74.2% to 85.8%) (Kececi & Dener, 2002; Koseoglu et al., 2003; Wober-Bingol et al., 2004). Vomiting is less common, occurring in about one third to two thirds of patients (estimates ranging from 33.5% to 67.3%) (Kececi & Dener,

2002; Koseoglu et al., 2003; Wober-Bingol et al., 2004). Vomiting can add significantly to the discomfort and disability of the migraine attack due to the physical activity of vomiting, worsening of headache pain with vomiting, and subsequent dehydration. Many patients who report the absence of nausea and vomiting during a migraine attack endorse the presence of anorexia.Migraineurs have also been shown to have gastric stasis during and between individual migraine attacks, and to have abnormal absorption of medication during migraine (Aurora et al., 2006, 2007; Thomsen et al., 1996; Volans, 1978). Delayed absorption of migraine medication can result in delayed therapeutic response and the need for additional treatment (Volans, 1978). No direct links between gastric stasis and presence of nausea and/or vomiting have been found, lending support to the theory that nausea and vomiting during migraine is caused by a central (brainstem) process (Aurora et al., 2006, 2007).

WORSENED PAIN WITH NORMAL PHYSICAL ACTIVITIES

Headache pain and malaise associated with the migraine attack are worsened by routine activities. Worsening pain with normal activities is reported by the majority (estimates ranging from 53% to 90%) of migraine patients (Kelman, 2006a; Koseoglu et al., 2003; Wober-Bingol et al., 2004). In Kelman's study in which migraine headache was exacerbated by activity in 90% of subjects, 44.3% very frequently had headache exacerbated by activity, 32.2% frequently, and 13.5% occasionally (Kelman, 2006a). Exacerbating activities are numerous and may differ from patient to patient, but simple activities such as walking stairs, performing household chores, and other routine activities of daily life are common exacerbators. Given this association, the typical migraine patient prefers to lie still in bed during a migraine.

CUTANEOUS ALLODYNIA

The perception of pain to normally nonnoxious stimulation of the skin is referred to as "cutaneous allodynia." Symptoms of cutaneous allodynia occur in approximately 60% to 85% of migraineurs during a migraine attack (Ashkenazi et al., 2007; Bigal, Ashina, et al., 2008; Jakubowski et al., 2005; Lipton et al., 2008; Lovati et al., 2009). The allodynic migraineur may experience pain with activities such as lightly touching the scalp or face; wearing eyeglasses or earrings, contact lenses, or tight collars; shaving one's face; and laying one's head on a pillow. Cutaneous allodynia may develop at body locations beyond the head/face, in such cases typically involving the upper extremity. Symptoms of extracephalic allodynia may be present in up to 26.5% of migraineurs with

allodynia (Mathew et al., 2004). Cutaneous allodynia results in increased pain during the migraine attack and may have implications regarding responsiveness to abortive medication. Some studies have suggested that triptans less effectively abort a migraine attack once allodynia is present, regardless of whether or not the triptan is administered early or later after the migraine attack has started (Burstein et al., 2004; Landy et al., 2007). However, there are substantial difficulties in isolating the potential effects of allodynia development from other features of the prolonged migraine attack. Thus, it is possible that confounding variables (e.g., gastrointestinal absorption of medication) mediate the efficacy of abortive therapies irrespective of allodynia development (Cady et al., 2007; Dahlof, 2006; Lovati et al., 2009).

NECK PAIN

Neck pain is common during a migraine and may occur prior to the development of a full-blown migraine attack, during the attack, or following resolution of other migraine symptoms. Neck pain associated with migraine occurs in 40% or more of migraineurs (Calhoun et al., 2010; Kelman, 2005). A prospective observational study of 113 migraine patients and 786 migraine days has shown that neck pain is more commonly associated with migraine than nausea (Calhoun et al., 2010). In that study, neck pain was more frequently associated with severe migraine attacks (present with 73% of severe attacks) than moderate attacks (61%) and mild attacks (43%) (Calhoun et al., 2010). Furthermore, neck muscular tension has been found predictive of future migraine attacks, associated with a hazard ratio of 1.2 (Wober et al., 2007). Nearly one quarter of migraine attacks may be preceded by neck pain (Kelman, 2006a).

Migraine Postdrome

Approximately two thirds of patients with migraine suffer from nonheadache symptoms following resolution of the migraine headache but prior to feeling completely back to normal, symptoms that are considered to be part of the migraine postdrome (Giffin et al., 2003; Kelman, 2006b) (Table 31–1). The average duration of postdromal symptoms is less than 24 hours, with about 90% of patients with postdromal symptoms reporting a duration of 24 hours or shorter (Blau, 1991; Giffin et al., 2003; Kelman, 2006b). Postdromal symptoms are similar to migraine premonitory symptoms. The most common postdromal symptoms include fatigue, cognitive difficulties, feeling "hung over," gastrointestinal symptoms, mood changes, weakness, and dizziness (Kelman, 2006b). Typically, the migraineur has reduced physical activity until postdromal symptoms resolve (Blau, 1991). Infrequently, the migraine patient feels especially energetic or euphoric following resolution of the migraine attack. In a prospective diary study, the most common symptoms during the migraine postdrome included tired/weary (88.2%), difficulty with concentration (55.5%), neck stiffness (41.9%), sensitivity to light (36%), difficulty with thoughts (33.4%), thirst (32.2%), and noise sensitivity (31.8%) (Giffin et al., 2003). Other frequently occurring symptoms included pale face, frequent urination, irritability, and feeling emotional. The only symptom that occurred more frequently in the postdrome than during the headache phase was tiredness (88.2% vs. 84.3%). The migraineur in the postdromal phase typically has several symptoms in combination, with an average of six symptoms per migraineur (Blau, 1991).

Migraine Triggers

The majority of patients with migraine can identify at least one trigger for their migraine attacks. According to a retrospective study of 1,750 migraine patients, approximately three out of four patients self-identified at least one migraine trigger (Kelman, 2007). Forty percent of these patients reported that their migraine attacks were occasionally triggered, 27% reported frequent triggering, and about 9% reported very frequent triggering. The most commonly identified triggers, in descending order of frequency, included stress, hormones in women, not eating, weather, sleep disturbance, odors, neck pain, light, alcohol, smoke, sleeping late, heat, foods, exercise, and sexual activity. The mean number of triggers per patient was 6.7, with about two thirds of patients identifying between 4 and 9 triggers.

Emotional stress is a very commonly identified migraine trigger. Although this typically refers to times of high stress, stress "let-down," or moving from a time of high stress to lower stress, may also trigger migraine attacks. Thus, it is unfortunately not uncommon for the migraine patient to develop an attack on the weekend or while on vacation. A prospective time-series analysis found that stress accounted for significant variance of migraine headache in 60% of patients, best predicted by the stress level occurring concurrent to the headache (rather than the stress level 1 to 3 days prior to headache onset) (Penzien et al., 2001).

Fluctuations in ovarian hormones are also common migraine triggers. Women with migraine may suffer from menstrual-associated migraines, having migraines triggered by hormonal fluctuation and migraines at other times of the month, or pure menstrual migraine, having migraines only perimenstrually. A migraine is considered perimenstrual if it occurs within 2 days prior to onset of menstruation to 2 days after the onset of menstruation. Risk of migraine is highest on the day of menstruation

onset and the following day (odds ratio = 2), with a slightly lower risk during the 2 days prior to onset of menstruation (odds ratio = 1.8) (Stewart et al., 2000). Approximately one third to one half of women with migraine are thought to have menstrual-related migraines (Granella et al., 1993, 2000; MacGregor et al., 1990). Although the etiology of menstrual migraine has been debated for decades, it is now believed that it is low estrogen levels that are associated with the increased risk of developing a migraine attack. Thus, migraine is more likely just before onset of menstruation when estrogen levels drop, during the menstrual cycle when estrogen levels are low, and during the placebo-pill week in women taking estrogen-containing oral contraceptive pills (MacGregor & Hackshaw, 2004; Martin & Lipton, 2008).

Specific weather conditions are frequently cited as attack triggers by migraine patients, reported by over 50% of migraine patients across several studies (Kelman, 2007; Turner et al., 1995; Wober et al., 2006). Such conditions have included temperature, changes in barometric pressure, humidity, precipitation, wind, and geomagnetic activity. However, self-report of patient-identified weather triggers tend to be inaccurate (Friedman & De ver Dye, 2009). Several studies have not found associations between specific weather conditions and migraine, while other studies have found associations between migraine and barometric pressure, changing weather patterns, and wind patterns (Cooke et al., 2000; Cull, 1981; De Matteis et al., 1994; Prince et al., 2004; Villeneuve et al., 2006; Wilkinson & Woodrow, 1979). Even when specific weather conditions are associated with triggering migraine attacks, patients are often unable to accurately identify the specific weather conditions that trigger their migraines (Prince et al., 2004).

Sleep disturbances and changes in sleep patterns are often reported as migraine triggers. In a study of 1,283 migraineurs, 50% reported sleep disturbance as a migraine trigger (27% reporting this as a frequent or very frequent trigger) and 37% reported oversleeping/sleeping late as a trigger (14% reporting this as a frequent or very frequent trigger) (Kelman & Rains, 2005). A prospective time-series analysis found that the number of hours of sleep per night was significantly associated with headache activity in 60% of migraine patients, headaches best predicted by the sleep on the preceding night (Penzien et al., 2001).

There are numerous potential dietary triggers of migraine. This includes intake of certain foods and beverages as well as skipping meals or fasting, a migraine trigger reported in about 50% of people with migraine (Kelman, 2007; Robbins, 1994; Turner et al., 1995). Identifying dietary triggers can be a daunting task for the migraineur, but when dietary triggers are identified, avoidance can help to reduce attack frequency and can give the migraineur a sense of control over his or her migraines (Martin & Behbehani, 2001; Sun-Edelstein & Mauskop, 2009). More common dietary triggers include skipped meals, foods with monosodium glutamate, foods with nitrates/nitrites (e.g., lunch meats, hot dogs), cheeses, and artificial sweeteners (Henderson & Raskin, 1972; Sun-Edelstein & Mauskop, 2009; Van den Eeden et al., 1994). Alcohol may trigger headaches acutely, within a few hours of ingestion, and may also result in a delayed alcohol hangover headache. Alcoholic beverages that are darker in color, such as red wine, dark beers, and whiskey, might be more likely to trigger headaches than lighter-in-color alcoholic beverages (Peatfield, 1995; Sandler et al., 1995; Sun-Edelstein & Mauskop, 2009). Caffeine can have differing effects on headaches, perhaps dependent upon frequency and magnitude of intake. Caffeine is contained in several prescription and over-the-counter headache treatments due to benefits for acute treatment. However, intake of large amounts of caffeine on a regular basis and withdrawal from caffeine can both lead to headaches. The regular use of caffeine-containing medications to abort migraine is associated with development of medication overuse headache (Mathew et al., 1982, 1987).

A prospective diary study of 327 migraine patients having 8,648 headache days investigated numerous potential migraine triggers. Several factors that occurred prior to headache onset were associated with the risk of developing a migraine headache (Wober et al., 2007). Factors associated with an increased risk included menstruation (days +1 to +3 associated with hazard ratio of 1.96, day +4 hazard ratio 1.43), muscle tension (hazard ratio 1.28), high stress (hazard ratio 1.2), tiredness (hazard ratio 1.1), daily sunshine of 3 hours or longer (hazard ratio 1.1), low pressure over the UK (hazard ratio 1.29), and air advection from the north (hazard ratio 1.22). Factors associated with a reduced risk of migraine included holiday/day off (hazard ratio 0.82), Tuesday (hazard ratio 0.83), and consumption of beer (hazard ratio 0.77).

Episodic Migraine Versus Chronic Migraine

Episodic migraine refers to the migraine patient who has headaches on 14 or fewer days per month. Chronic migraine is a subtype of chronic daily headache and refers to the migraine patient with 15 or more headache days per month with at least 8 days per month with a migraine headache (Table 31–3) (Olesen et al., 2006). Whereas the typical migraineur has one to four attacks per month, the typical chronic migraineur has about 22 days with headache per month (Bigal et al., 2003; Lipton et al., 2007). Each year, approximately 3% of patients in the general population with episodic headache transform to a chronic

daily headache pattern (Scher et al., 1998). Furthermore, 6% of people with infrequent episodic migraine (2 to 104 headache days per year) progress to frequent episodic migraine (105 to 179 headache days per year) annually (Scher et al., 1998). Fortunately, about 57% of those with chronic daily headache transform back to an episodic pattern each year (Scher, Stewart, et al., 2003). Factors associated with transformation to chronic migraine and back to episodic migraine have been identified. The following are associated with an increased risk of transforming to chronic migraine: obesity, high levels of caffeine intake, low socioeconomic status, female, young age, history of head or neck injury, overuse of abortive medications, sleep disorders, snoring, and stress (Bigal & Lipton, 2006; Scher, Stewart, et al., 2003).

Of note, many of these characteristics are modifiable, suggesting that addressing these modifiable risk factors may reduce the risk of converting from episodic to chronic migraine. Reversion back to episodic migraine is positively associated with compliance with prophylactic medication, withdrawal of overused abortive medication, regular exercise (defined as exercising for at least 30 minutes at least four times per week), higher educational level, and nonwhite race (Scher, Stewart, et al., 2003; Seok et al., 2006). A recent prospective longitudinal population-based analysis identified lower baseline headache frequency

TABLE 31–3 *Chronic Migraine—International Classification of Headache Disorders Revised Diagnostic Criteria*

A. Headache on ≥15 days per month for at least 3 months
B. Occurring in a patient who has had ≥5 attacks fulfilling diagnostic criteria for migraine
C. On ≥8 days per month for ≥3 months headache has fulfilled C1 and/or C2 below
　1. ≥2 of a–d:
　　a. Unilateral location
　　b. Pulsating quality
　　c. Moderate or severe pain intensity
　　d. Aggravation by or causing avoidance of routine physical activity
　And ≥1 of a or b:
　　a. Nausea and/or vomiting
　　b. Photophobia and phonophobia
　2. Treated and relieved by triptan(s) or ergot before expected development of C1 above
D. No medication overuse and not attributed to another causative disorder

From Olesen, J., Bousser, M. G., Diener, H. C., Dodick, D., First, M., Goadsby, P. J., et al. (2006). New appendix criteria open for a broader concept of chronic migraine. *Cephalalgia, 26*, 742–746.

(15 to 19 vs. 25 to 31 headache days per month; odds ratio = 0.29; 95% confidence interval [CI]: 0.11–0.75) and absence of allodynia (odds ratio = 0.45; 95% CI: 0.23–0.89) as predictors of remission (Manack et al., 2011).

As would be expected, patients with chronic migraine suffer from more pain and migraine-related disability compared to episodic migraineurs. Chronic migraineurs miss more days of work or school than episodic migraineurs (5.3 days per 3 months vs. 2.3 days per 3 months), have more days with reduced productivity at work or school (5.3 days per 3 months vs. 2.3 days per 3 months), miss more days of housework (16.5 days per 3 months vs. 3.3 days per 3 months), and miss more family and social activities (7 days per 3 months vs. 5.5 days per 3 months) (Bigal et al., 2003). In a large population study, 8.2% of chronic migraineurs reported missing at least 5 days of work or school in the preceding 3 months, 33.8% reported at least 5 days of reduced productivity at work or school, 57.4% reported 5 or more days of missed household work, 58.1% had at least 5 days of reduced productivity in the household, and 36.9% had missed at least 5 days of family activities (Bigal, Serrano, Reed, et al., 2008).

Overuse of Migraine Abortive Medications

It is believed that the frequent use of migraine abortive medications can lead to a worsening and secondary headache pattern termed "medication overuse headache." The general principle is that patients who regularly and frequently use certain abortive medications place themselves at risk of transforming from a pattern of less frequent headaches to a pattern of more frequent headaches. In the general population, the prevalence of chronic migraine with medication overuse is about 1.5% (Castillo et al., 1999; Scher, Stewart, et al., 2003). However, it must be noted that not all patients who meet criteria for medication overuse develop medication overuse headache. Thus, not all patients who stop overusing abortive medications have reductions in headache frequency. Nonetheless, prior to medication withdrawal, it can be very difficult to determine which patients who overuse abortive medications are suffering from medication overuse headache and which are not. Thus, a trial of withdrawal, lasting at least several months, is often required to make this determination.

The definition for medication overuse headache differs according to the medication being used. For all medications, overuse has to be present for at least 3 months, there should be evidence that the headache pattern worsened in some way during the time of overuse, and headaches must be present on at least 15 days per month. According to ICHD-II criteria, overuse is present if a patient uses the following on at least 10 days per month: opiates, combination medications (e.g., medications containing butalbital),

triptans, or ergots. Simple analgesics or a combination of different abortive medications must be used on at least 15 days per month. Although the ICHD-II criteria required improvement in headache frequency following withdrawal of the overused medication, this criterion was excluded from revised ICHD-II diagnostic criteria (Silberstein et al., 2005). The revised criteria allow for the diagnosis of medication overuse headache while it is an active problem, unlike the initial ICHD-II criteria, which allowed for a diagnosis to be made only after resolution of the headache pattern following medication withdrawal.

Several studies have investigated the use of abortive medications in people with episodic and chronic migraine. Treatment with either barbiturates or opioids is consistently shown to be associated with an increased risk for chronic migraine (Bigal et al., 2009; Bigal, Serrano, Buse, et al., 2008; Scher et al., 2010). Compared to those with episodic migraine, people with chronic migraine are more likely to be using opioids (odds ratio = 2.12) or barbiturates (odds ratio = 2.46) (Bigal et al., 2009). The 1-year risk of transforming from episodic migraine to chronic migraine is higher in people taking barbiturates (odds ratio = 1.73) or opioids (odds ratio = 1.44) (Bigal et al., 2009). The critical dose for barbiturate use is administration on about 5 days per month and for opiates is use on about 8 days per month (Bigal & Lipton, 2008). In the American Migraine Prevalence and Prevention Study (AMPP) of 120,000 individuals, 8,219 people had episodic migraine, 209 (2.5%) of which had transformed to chronic migraine at 1 year (Bigal, Serrano, Buse, et al., 2008). The risk of transformation to chronic migraine was increased in episodic migraineurs taking barbiturate-containing medications (odds ratio = 2.06) or opiates (odds ratio = 1.98). The use of triptans did not affect the risk of transformation. Nonsteroidal anti-inflammatory drug use was protective against transition to chronic migraine when episodic migraineurs had low to moderate headache frequency at baseline (fewer than 9 headache days per month), but was associated with increased risk among those with high baseline headache frequency (10 to 14 headache days per month).

The Interictal Migraineur

Although the most obvious migraine features occur during the individual migraine attack, there is less severe phenotypic expression of migraine between migraine attacks (interictal) as well. Defining the interictal period is perhaps the greatest challenge in studying and describing the interictal migraineur. Further understanding of migraine physiology is necessary to specifically define attack onset and offset. Currently, studies have defined the interictal period as a certain number of hours before and after the migraine attack, typically ranging from 24 to 72 hours. Generally, the migraine attack onset and offset is defined according to the presence and disappearance of the headache, since this symptom is more reliably easy to identify. However, the actual duration likely spans from the onset of premonitory symptoms or aura to the resolution of symptoms in the postdromal phase.

The interictal migraineur has persistent hypersensitivities to auditory, visual, and cutaneous stimuli. As many as three quarters of migraine patients report interictal hypersensitivity to sound (Vingen et al., 1998). Quantitative testing shows that the interictal migraineur is more sensitive to sound compared to the nonmigraine control and that the migraine patient is even more sensitive to sound during a migraine attack compared to the interictal period (Ashkenazi et al., 2009; Main et al., 1997; Vingen et al., 1998). A similar phenomenon has been shown for visual sensitivity (Main et al., 1997). Even after being migraine free for 72 hours, migraineurs have significantly lower visual discomfort thresholds compared to nonmigraine controls (Main et al., 1997, 2000). Compared to nonheadache controls and patients with tension-type headache, migraineurs have increased interictal sensitivity to white light (unfiltered light), high-wavelength light (red), and low-wavelength light (blue) (Main et al., 2000). Migraineurs are also more sensitive to stimulation of the skin. Interictal cutaneous pain thresholds have been demonstrated to be lower in episodic and chronic migraine patients compared to nonmigraine controls (Schwedt et al., 2011; Weissman-Fogel et al., 2003). A quantitative sensory testing study showed that both episodic and chronic migraineurs were more sensitive to cold and heat stimuli, even in the absence of overt symptoms of cutaneous allodynia (Schwedt et al., 2011). It is anticipated that migraineurs with low interictal pain thresholds become even more sensitive and develop symptoms of allodynia during a migraine attack (Schwedt et al., 2011).

COMORBID CONDITIONS

Migraine is associated with numerous comorbid conditions including psychiatric disorders, myofascial pain, sleep abnormalities and fatigue, gastrointestinal disorders, and cardiac and vascular disorders (Table 31–4).

Psychiatric comorbidity is common among migraine patients. Major depressive disorder occurs two to four times more commonly in migraine patients than in the general population (Baskin & Smitherman, 2009; Hamelsky & Lipton, 2006). In migraine patients, the lifetime prevalence of major depression is about 34% and the lifetime prevalence of dysthymia is about 8%. Depression is even more common in the chronic migraine population, with major depression reported in over 50% of chronic migraine patients in some studies (Juang et al., 2000; Mathew et al., 1987). Anxiety disorders are also more prevalent in the migraine population compared to the general population. Migraine patients are 4 to 5 times more likely to suffer from generalized anxiety disorder and 3 to 10 times more likely to have panic disorder (Baskin & Smitherman, 2009). Panic disorder may affect as many as 30% of those with transformed migraine (Juang et al., 2000).

Myofascial pain and muscular tension are also commonly reported by migraineurs. Migraineurs tend to have painful craniocervical musculature, abnormal head posture, painful trigger points, and reduced range of motion

TABLE 31–4 *Disorders Comorbid with Migraine*

- Psychiatric disorders
    - Major depressive disorder
    - Dysthymia
    - Generalized anxiety disorder
    - Panic disorder
- Myofascial pain
    - Painful craniocervical musculature
    - Trigger points
    - Fibromyalgia
- Fatigue
- Epilepsy
- Sleep disorders
    - Insomnia
    - Difficulty maintaining sleep
    - Snoring
    - Obstructive sleep apnea
- Gastrointestinal
    - Esophageal reflux
    - Diarrhea
    - Constipation
    - Nausea
    - Irritable bowel syndrome
    - Colitis
    - Celiac disease
- Cardiac
    - Patent foramen ovale
    - Atrial septal defects
    - Mitral valve prolapse
    - Atrial septal aneurysm
    - Pulmonary arteriovenous malformations
- Cardiovascular/cerebrovascular
    - Myocardial infarction
    - Ischemic stroke
    - Cervical artery dissection

at the neck (Bevilaqua-Grossi et al., 2009; Fernandez-de-Las-Penas et al., 2006). As discussed previously, neck pain is commonly associated with the migraine attack and is often persistent between attacks (Calhoun et al., 2010). Neck pain is present during at least 40% of migraine attacks (Calhoun et al., 2010; Kelman, 2005). A study of 15 episodic and 15 chronic migraineurs, over half headache free at the time of evaluation, found migraineurs to have reduced cervical mobility (Bevilaqua-Grossi et al., 2009). A separate study of 20 patients with migraine performed investigations when the migraineurs had been headache free for at least 1 week. Compared to controls, migraineurs had more trigger points in the head and neck muscles (3.6 vs. 1.7), reductions in neck flexion/extension range of motion, and greater head forward position (Fernandez-de-Las-Penas et al., 2006). In addition, approximately 22% to 42% of migraineurs have fibromyalgia (de Tommaso et al., 2009; Ifergane et al., 2006; Peres, 2003). Fibromyalgia is more prevalent in patients with more frequent migraines. Approximately one third of patients with chronic migraine meet American College of Rheumatology diagnostic criteria for fibromyalgia (Peres et al., 2001).

Patients with migraine report fatigue, difficulty falling asleep, difficulty staying asleep, and sleep for fewer hours than people without migraine (Rains & Poceta, 2006). In some studies, over 80% of chronic migraine patients report fatigue (Peres et al., 2002). Furthermore, one half to two thirds of patients with chronic migraine meet diagnostic criteria for chronic fatigue syndrome (Peres et al., 2002). In a study of 1,283 migraine patients, over half reported difficulty falling asleep and maintaining sleep, with 38% sleeping an average of 6 hours or fewer per night (Kelman & Rains, 2005). Those with chronic migraine suffer from greater difficulties with initiating and maintaining sleep and overall sleep fewer hours each night than those with episodic migraine (Kelman & Rains, 2005; Maizels & Burchette, 2004; Rothrock et al., 1996). Habitual snoring and obstructive sleep apnea are also more common in migraine patients (Jennum et al., 1994; Ulfberg et al., 1996). Habitual snoring is more common in those with more frequent headaches, affecting approximately one quarter of chronic daily headache patients (Scher, Lipton, et al., 2003). Sleep-disordered breathing is also associated with migraine, an association that is strongest among those people who wake up with headaches (Alberti et al., 2005; Rains & Poceta, 2006).

Gastrointestinal symptoms and migraine are frequently comorbid. In a large cross-sectional population study, migraine was more commonly reported by people with reflux (odds ratio = 1.8), diarrhea (odds ratio = 1.7), constipation (odds ratio = 1.4), and nausea (odds ratio = 2.2) (Aamodt et al., 2008). There is a positive correlation between increasing headache frequency and presence of gastrointestinal symptoms. Gastrointestinal disorders are reported by 43% of patients with chronic migraine (Ferrari et al., 2007). In migraineurs who have headaches on more than 14 days per month, the odds of reflux symptoms is 2.6, diarrhea is 2.7, constipation is 2.4, and nausea is 6.7 (Aamodt et al., 2008). Furthermore, migraine is positively associated with irritable bowel syndrome, peptic ulcer disease, colitis, and celiac disease (Gabrielli et al., 2003; Gasbarrini et al., 1998; Jones & Lydeard, 1992; Pinessi et al., 2000).

Migraine is positively associated with different cardiac and vascular disorders including right-to-left shunts, cardiovascular disease, and stroke. Compared to the general population, people with migraine are more likely to have patent foramen ovale (PFO). A person with migraine is approximately two times more likely to have a PFO compared to a person without migraine (Schwedt et al., 2008). This increased prevalence of PFO among migraineurs is mostly attributable to patients who have migraine with aura, with just over 50% of migraineurs with aura having a PFO compared to approximately 25% of the general population (Hagen et al., 1984; Schwedt & Dodick, 2006). Atrial septal defects and pulmonary shunts increase the likelihood of having migraine, especially migraine with aura (Azarbal et al., 2005; Mortelmans et al., 2005). Pulmonary arteriovenous malformations (AVMs), as are commonly found in patients with hereditary hemorrhagic telangiectasia (HHT), are associated with increased odds of 2.4 for migraine, about four fifths of which will have migraine with aura (Thenganatt et al., 2006). Migraine is associated with an increased risk of having cardiovascular risk factors and cardiovascular disease. A population study of 5,755 people, including 620 migraineurs, conducted in the Netherlands found migraine to be associated with increased odds of smoking (odds ratio = 1.4) and use of oral contraception (odds ratio = 2.1) and a higher likelihood of having a parent with myocardial infarction at a young age, and decreased odds for alcohol consumption (odds ratio = 0.6) (Scher et al., 2005). Migraineurs are more likely than nonmigraineurs to have diabetes, hypertension, and poor cholesterol profiles (Bigal et al., 2010; Scher et al., 2005). In women, migraine with aura, but not migraine without aura, has been shown to be associated with an increased risk for major cardiovascular disease (e.g., first ischemic stroke or myocardial infarction or death from cardiovascular disease) (hazard ratio = 2.2), ischemic stroke (hazard ratio = 1.9), myocardial infarction (hazard ratio = 2.1), and ischemic cardiovascular death (hazard ratio = 2.3) (Kurth et al., 2006). In men, migraine (with or without aura) is associated with an increased risk of major cardiovascular disease (hazard ratio = 1.2) and myocardial infarction (hazard ratio = 1.4) (Kurth et al., 2007). When men and women with migraine are studied together, migraine with and without aura is associated with increased odds of myocardial infarction (odds ratio = 2.2), stroke (odds ratio = 1.5), and claudication (odds ratio = 2.7), migraine with aura being more highly associated than migraine without aura (Bigal et al., 2010). A meta-analysis investigating the risk of ischemic stroke in people with migraine found a relative risk of 2.16 among all migraineurs, 1.83 among migraineurs without aura, and 2.27 among migraineurs with aura (Etminan et al., 2005). Smoking more than triples this risk and using oral contraceptives quadruples the risk (Chang et al., 1999; Kurth, 2007; Tzourio et al., 1995). A second meta-analysis evaluated studies and reviews published up to January 2009 (Schurks et al., 2009). This meta-analysis included case-control and cohort studies investigating the association between any migraine or specific migraine subtypes and cardiovascular disease. Evaluation of nine studies investigating the association between any migraine and ischemic stroke yielded a pooled relative risk of 1.73 (95% CI: 1.31–2.29). The risk was higher among migraineurs with aura (2.16, 1.53–3.03) compared with people who had migraine without aura (1.23, 0.90–1.69; meta-regression for aura status p = .02). Results also suggested a greater risk among women (2.08, 1.13–3.84) compared with men (1.37, 0.89–2.11). The risk for subjects with migraine aged younger than 45 (2.65, 1.41–4.97) was higher than for the overall group, which was more pronounced among women (3.65, 2.21–6.04). This meta-analysis also confirmed an increased risk of ischemic stroke among smokers (9.03, 4.22–19.34) and women currently using oral contraceptives (7.02, 1.51–32.68). There may be a specific increase in risk for asymptomatic ischemic strokes in cerebellar watershed zones. Migraine is associated with an odds ratio of 7.1 for ischemic cerebellar strokes, with a higher risk in patients who have migraine with aura with at least one attack per month (odds ratio = 15.8) (Kruit et al. 2004).

CONCLUSIONS

Migraine is a very common disorder that preferentially afflicts women in their third to sixth decades of life. Migraine results in substantial pain, hypersensitivities to normal environmental stimuli, workplace and social disability, and costs to individuals and society at large. Most migraineurs have a few attacks or less per month, although 2% to 3% of the general population has 15 or more days per month with headache (chronic migraine). In addition to the headache phase of migraine, the migraine attack may also consist of premonitory symptoms (prodrome), aura, and postdromal symptoms. Although migraine has historically been considered a chronic disorder with episodic manifestations, there is mounting evidence that migraineurs have phenotypic expression of migraine even between individual, full-blown migraine attacks. Furthermore, migraine is associated with numerous comorbid conditions including anxiety, depression, fatigue, myofascial pain, sleep problems, gastrointestinal symptoms, cardiac disease, cardiovascular disease, and stroke.

REFERENCES

Aamodt, A. H., Stovner, L. J., Hagen, K., & Zwart, J. A. (2008). Comorbidity of headache and gastrointestinal complaints. The Head-HUNT Study. *Cephalalgia, 28*, 144–151.

Alberti, A., Mazzotta, G., Gallinella, E., & Sarchielli, P. (2005). Headache characteristics in obstructive sleep apnea syndrome and insomnia. *Acta Neurologica Scandinavica, 111*, 309–316.

Aleci, C., & Liboni, W. (2009). Perceptive aspects of visual aura. *Neurological Sciences, 30*, 447–452.

Ashkenazi, A., Mushtaq, A., Yang, I., & Oshinsky, M. L. (2009). Ictal and interictal phonophobia in migraine-a quantitative controlled study. *Cephalalgia, 29*, 1042–1048.

Ashkenazi, A., Silberstein, S., Jakubowski, M., & Burstein, R. (2007). Improved identification of allodynic migraine patients using a questionnaire. *Cephalalgia, 27*, 325–329.

Aurora, S. K., Kori, S. H., Barrodale, P., McDonald, S. A., & Haseley, D. (2006). Gastric stasis in migraine: More than just a paroxysmal abnormality during a migraine attack. *Headache, 46*, 57–63.

Aurora, S., Kori, S., Barrodale, P., Nelsen, A., & McDonald, S. (2007). Gastric stasis occurs in spontaneous, visually induced, and interictal migraine. *Headache, 47*, 1443–1446.

Azarbal, B., Tobis, J., Suh, W., Chan, V., Dao, C., & Gaster, R. (2005). Association of interatrial shunts and migraine headaches: Impact of transcatheter closure. *Journal of the American College of Cardiology, 45*, 489–492.

Baskin, S. M., & Smitherman, T. A. (2009). Migraine and psychiatric disorders: Comorbidities, mechanisms, and clinical applications. *Neurological Sciences, 30*(Suppl 1), S61–S65.

Bevilaqua-Grossi, D., Pegoretti, K. S., Goncalves, M. C., Speciali, J. G., Bordini, C. A., & Bigal, M. E. (2009). Cervical mobility in women with migraine. *Headache, 49*, 726–731.

Bigal, M. E., Ashina, S., Burstein, R., Reed, M. L., Buse, D., Serrano, D., et al. (2008). Prevalence and characteristics of allodynia in headache sufferers: A population study. *Neurology, 70*, 1525–1533.

Bigal, M. E., Borucho, S., Serrano, D., & Lipton, R. B. (2009). The acute treatment of episodic and chronic migraine in the USA. *Cephalalgia, 29*, 891–897.

Bigal, M. E., Kurth, T., Santanello, N., Buse, D., Golden, W., Robbins, M., et al. (2010) Migraine and cardiovascular disease: A population-based study. *Neurology, 74*, 628–635.

Bigal, M. E., & Lipton, R. B. (2006). Modifiable risk factors for migraine progression. *Headache, 46*, 1334–1343.

Bigal, M. E., & Lipton, R. B. (2008). Excessive acute migraine medication use and migraine progression. *Neurology, 71*, 1821–1828.

Bigal, M. E., Rapoport, A. M., Lipton, R. B., Tepper, S. J., & Sheftell, F. D. (2003). Assessment of migraine disability using the migraine disability assessment (MIDAS) questionnaire: A comparison of chronic migraine with episodic migraine. *Headache, 43,* 336–342.

Bigal, M. E., Serrano, D., Buse, D., Scher, A., Stewart, W. F., & Lipton, R. B. (2008). Acute migraine medications and evolution from episodic to chronic migraine: A longitudinal population-based study. *Headache, 48,* 1157–1168.

Bigal, M. E., Serrano, D., Reed, M., & Lipton, R. B. (2008). Chronic migraine in the population: Burden, diagnosis, and satisfaction with treatment. *Neurology, 71,* 559–566.

Black, D. F. (2006). Sporadic and familial hemiplegic migraine: Diagnosis and treatment. *Seminars in Neurology, 26,* 208–216.

Blau, J. N. (1991). Migraine postdromes: Symptoms after attacks. *Cephalalgia, 11,* 229–231.

Burstein, R., Collins, B., & Jakubowski, M. (2004). Defeating migraine pain with triptans: A race against the development of cutaneous allodynia. *Annals of Neurology, 55,* 19–26.

Cady, R., Martin, V., Mauskop, A., Rodgers, A., Hustad, C. M., Ramsey, K. E., et al. (2007). Symptoms of cutaneous sensitivity pre-treatment and post-treatment: Results from the rizatriptan TAME studies. *Cephalalgia, 27,* 1055–1060.

Calhoun, A. H., Ford, S., Millen, C., Finkel, A. G., Truong, Y., & Nie, Y. (2010) The prevalence of neck pain in migraine. *Headache, 50,* 1273–1277.

Castillo, J., Munoz, P., Guitera, V., & Pascual, J. (1999). Kaplan Award 1998. Epidemiology of chronic daily headache in the general population. *Headache, 39,* 190–196.

Chang, C. L., Donaghy, M., & Poulter, N. (1999). Migraine and stroke in young women: case-control study. The World Health Organisation Collaborative Study of Cardiovascular Disease and Steroid Hormone Contraception. *BMJ, 318,* 13–18.

Choi, J. Y., Oh, K., Kim, B. J., Chung, C. S., Koh, S. B., & Park, K. W. (2009). Usefulness of a photophobia questionnaire in patients with migraine. *Cephalalgia, 29,* 953–959.

Committee of the International Classification of Headache Disorders. (2004). International classification of headache disorders II. *Cephalalgia, 24*(Suppl 1), 1–151.

Cooke, L. J., Rose, M. S., & Becker, W. J. (2000). Chinook winds and migraine headache. *Neurology, 54,* 302–307.

Cull, R. E. (1981). Barometric pressure and other factors in migraine. *Headache, 21,* 102–103.

Cutrer, F. M., & Huerter, K. (2007). Migraine aura. *Neurologist, 13,* 118–125.

Dahlof, C. (2006). Cutaneous allodynia and migraine: Another view. *Current Pain and Headache Reports, 10,* 231–238.

De Carlo, D., Dal Zotto, L., Perissinotto, E., Gallo, L., Gatta, M., Balottin, U., et al. (2010). Osmophobia in migraine classification: A multicentre study in juvenile patients. *Cephalalgia, 30,* 1486–1494.

De Fusco, M., Marconi, R., Silvestri, L., Atorino, L., Rampoldi, L., Morgante, L., et al. (2003). Haploinsufficiency of ATP1A2 encoding the Na+/K+ pump alpha2 subunit associated with familial hemiplegic migraine type 2. *Nature Genetics, 33,* 192–196.

De Matteis, G., Vellante, M., Marrelli, A., Villante, U., Santalucia, P., Tuzi, P., et al. (1994). Geomagnetic activity, humidity, temperature and headache: Is there any correlation? *Headache, 34,* 41–43.

de Tommaso, M., Sardaro, M., Serpino, C., Costantini, F., Vecchio, E., Prudenzano, M. P., et al. (2009). Fibromyalgia comorbidity in primary headaches. *Cephalalgia, 29,* 453–464.

de Vries, B., Frants, R. R., Ferrari, M. D., & van den Maagdenberg, A. M. (2009). Molecular genetics of migraine. *Human Genetics, 126,* 115–132.

Dichgans, M., Freilinger, T., Eckstein, G., Babini, E., Lorenz-Depiereux, B., Biskup, S., et al. (2005). Mutation in the neuronal voltage-gated sodium channel SCN1A in familial hemiplegic migraine. *Lancet, 366,* 371–377.

Ducros, A., Denier, C., Joutel, A., Cecillon, M., Lescoat, C., Vahedi, K., et al. (2001). The clinical spectrum of familial hemiplegic migraine associated with mutations in a neuronal calcium channel. *New England Journal of Medicine, 345,* 17–24.

Eriksen, M. K., Thomsen, L. L., Andersen, I., Nazim, F., & Olesen, J. (2004). Clinical characteristics of 362 patients with familial migraine with aura. *Cephalalgia, 24,* 564–575.

Etminan, M., Takkouche, B., Isorna, F. C., & Samii, A. (2005). Risk of ischaemic stroke in people with migraine: Systematic review and meta-analysis of observational studies. *BMJ, 330,* 63.

Evans, R. W., Seifert, T., Kailasam, J., & Mathew, N. T. (2008). The use of questions to determine the presence of photophobia and phonophobia during migraine. *Headache, 48,* 395–397.

Fernandez-de-Las-Penas, C., Cuadrado, M. L., & Pareja, J. A. (2006). Myofascial trigger points, neck mobility and forward head posture in unilateral migraine. *Cephalalgia, 26,* 1061–1070.

Ferrari, A., Leone, S., Vergoni, A. V., Bertolini, A., Sances, G., Coccia, C. P., et al. (2007). Similarities and differences between chronic migraine and episodic migraine. *Headache, 47,* 65–72.

Friedman, D. I., & De ver Dye, T. (2009). Migraine and the environment. *Headache, 49,* 941–952.

Gabrielli, M., Cremonini, F., Fiore, G., Addolorato, G., Padalino, C., Candelli, M., et al. (2003). Association between migraine and Celiac disease: Results from a preliminary case-control and therapeutic study. *American Journal of Gastroenterology, 98,* 625–629.

Gasbarrini, A., De Luca, A., Fiore, G., Gambrielli, M., Franceschi, F., Ojetti, V., et al. (1998). Beneficial effects of Helicobacter pylori eradication on migraine. *Hepatogastroenterology, 45,* 765–770.

Giffin, N. J., Ruggiero, L., Lipton, R. B., Silberstein, S. D., Tvedskov, J. F., Olesen, J., et al. (2003). Premonitory symptoms in migraine: An electronic diary study. *Neurology, 60,* 935–940.

Granella, F., Sances, G., Pucci, E., Nappi, R. E., Ghiotto, N., & Napp, G. (2000). Migraine with aura and reproductive life events: A case control study. *Cephalalgia, 20,* 701–707.

Granella, F., Sances, G., Zanferrari, C., Costa, A., Martignoni, E., & Manzoni, G. C. (1993). Migraine without aura and reproductive life events: A clinical epidemiological study in 1300 women. *Headache, 33,* 385–389.

Hagen, P. T., Scholz, D. G., & Edwards, W. D. (1984). Incidence and size of patent foramen ovale during the first 10 decades of life: An autopsy study of 965 normal hearts. *Mayo Clinic Proceedings, 59,* 17–20.

Hamelsky, S. W., & Lipton, R. B. (2006). Psychiatric comorbidity of migraine. *Headache, 46,* 1327–1333.

Hay, K. M., Mortimer, M. J., Barker, D. C., Debney, L. M., & Good, P. A. (1994). 1044 women with migraine: The effect of environmental stimuli. *Headache, 34,* 166–168.

Henderson, W. R., & Raskin, N. H. (1972). "Hot-dog" headache: Individual susceptibility to nitrite. *Lancet, 2,* 1162–1163.

Ifergane, G., Buskila, D., Simiseshvely, N., Zeev, K., & Cohen, H. (2006). Prevalence of fibromyalgia syndrome in migraine patients. *Cephalalgia, 26,* 451–456.

Jakubowski, M., Silberstein, S., Ashkenazi, A., & Burstein, R. (2005). Can allodynic migraine patients be identified interictally using a questionnaire? *Neurology, 65,* 1419–1422.

Jennum, P., & Sjol, A. (1994). Self-assessed cognitive function in snorers and sleep apneics. An epidemiological study of 1,504 females and males aged 30–60 years: The Dan-MONICA II Study. *European Neurology, 34,* 204–208.

Jones, R., & Lydeard, S. (1992). Irritable bowel syndrome in the general population. *BMJ, 304,* 87–90.

Juang, K. D., Wang, S. J., Fuh, J. L., Lu, S. R., & Su, T. P. (2000). Comorbidity of depressive and anxiety disorders in chronic daily headache and its subtypes. *Headache, 40,* 818–823.

Kececi, H., & Dener, S. (2002). Epidemiological and clinical characteristics of migraine in Sivas, Turkey. *Headache, 42,* 275–280.

Kelman, L. (2004a). Osmophobia and taste abnormality in migraineurs: A tertiary care study. *Headache, 44,* 1019–1023.

Kelman, L. (2004b). The place of osmophobia and taste abnormalities in migraine classification: A tertiary care study of 1237 patients. *Cephalalgia, 24,* 940–946.

Kelman, L. (2004c). The premonitory symptoms (prodrome): A tertiary care study of 893 migraineurs. *Headache, 44,* 865–872.

Kelman, L. (2005). Migraine pain location: A tertiary care study of 1283 migraineurs. *Headache, 45,* 1038–1047.

Kelman, L. (2006a). Pain characteristics of the acute migraine attack. *Headache, 46,* 942–953.

Kelman, L. (2006b). The postdrome of the acute migraine attack. *Cephalalgia, 26,* 214–220.

Kelman, L. The triggers or precipitants of the acute migraine attack. *Cephalalgia, 27,* 394–402.

Kelman, L., & Rains, J. C. (2005). Headache and sleep: Examination of sleep patterns and complaints in a large clinical sample of migraineurs. *Headache, 45,* 904–910.

Koseoglu, E., Nacar, M., Talaslioglu, A., & Cetinkaya, F. (2003). Epidemiological and clinical characteristics of migraine and tension type headache in 1146 females in Kayseri, Turkey. *Cephalalgia, 23,* 381–388.

Kruit, M. C., van Buchem, M. A., Hofman, P. A., Bakkers, J. T., Terwindt, G. M., Ferrari, M. D., et al. (2004). Migraine as a risk factor for subclinical brain lesions. *Journal of the American Medical Association, 291,* 427–434.

Kurth, T. (2007). Migraine and ischaemic vascular events. *Cephalalgia, 27,* 965–975.

Kurth, T., Gaziano, J. M., Cook, N. R., Bubes, V., Logroscino, G., Diener, H. C., et al. (2007). Migraine and risk of cardiovascular disease in men. *Archives of Internal Medicine, 167,* 795–801.

Kurth, T., Gaziano, J. M., Cook, N. R., Logroscino, G., Diener, H. C., & Buring, J. E. (2006). Migraine and risk of cardiovascular disease in women. *Journal of the American Medical Association, 296,* 283–291.

Landy, S. H., McGinnis, J. E., & McDonald, S. A. (2007). Clarification of developing and established clinical allodynia and pain-free outcomes. *Headache, 47,* 247–252.

Launer, L. J., Terwindt, G. M., & Ferrari, M. D. (1999). The prevalence and characteristics of migraine in a population-based cohort: The GEM study. *Neurology, 53,* 537–542.

Lipton, R. B., Bigal, M. E., Ashina, S., Burstein, R., Silberstein, S., Reed, M. L., et al. (2008). Cutaneous allodynia in the migraine population. *Annals of Neurology, 63,* 148–158.

Lipton, R. B., Bigal, M. E., Diamond, M., Freitag, F., Reed, M. L., & Stewart, W. F. (2007). Migraine prevalence, disease burden, and the need for preventive therapy. *Neurology, 68,* 343–349.

Lipton, R. B., Hamelsky, S. W., Kolodner, K. B., Steiner, T. J., & Stewart, W. F. (2000). Migraine, quality of life, and depression: A population-based case-control study. *Neurology, 55,* 629–635.

Lipton, R. B., Liberman, J. N., Kolodner, K. B., Bigal, M. E., Dowson, A., & Stewart, W. F. (2003). Migraine headache disability and health-related quality-of-life: A population-based case-control study from England. *Cephalalgia, 23,* 441–450.

Lipton, R. B., Stewart, W. F., Diamond, S., Diamond, M. L., & Reed, M. (2001). Prevalence and burden of migraine in the United States: Data from the American Migraine Study II. *Headache, 41,* 646–657.

Lovati, C., D'Amico, D., & Bertora, P. (2009). Allodynia in migraine: Frequent random association or unavoidable consequence? *Expert Reviews in Neurotherapy, 9,* 395–408.

MacGregor, E. A., Chia, H., Vohrah, R. C., & Wilkinson, M. (1990). Migraine and menstruation: A pilot study. *Cephalalgia, 10,* 305–310.

MacGregor, E. A., & Hackshaw, A. (2004). Prevalence of migraine on each day of the natural menstrual cycle. *Neurology, 63,* 351–353.

Main, A., Dowson, A., & Gross, M. (1997). Photophobia and phonophobia in migraineurs between attacks. *Headache, 37,* 492–495.

Main, A., Vlachonikolis, I., & Dowson, A. (2000). The wavelength of light causing photophobia in migraine and tension-type headache between attacks. *Headache, 40,* 194–199.

Maizels, M., & Burchette, R. (2004). Somatic symptoms in headache patients: The influence of headache diagnosis, frequency, and comorbidity. *Headache, 44,* 983–993.

Manack, A., Buse, D. C., Serrano, D., Turkel, C. C., & Lipton, R. B. (2011). Rates, predictors, and consequences of remission from chronic migraine to episodic migraine. *Neurology, 76,* 711–718.

Manzoni, G. C., Farina, S., Lanfranchi, M., & Solari, A. (1985). Classic migraine—clinical findings in 164 patients. *European Neurology, 24,* 163–169.

Martin, V. T., & Behbehani, M. M. (2001). Toward a rational understanding of migraine trigger factors. *Medical Clinics of North America, 85,* 911–941.

Martin, V. T., & Lipton, R. B. (2008). Epidemiology and biology of menstrual migraine. *Headache, 48*(Suppl 3), S124–S130.

Mathew, N. T., Kailasam, J., & Seifert, T. (2004). Clinical recognition of allodynia in migraine. *Neurology, 63,* 848–852.

Mathew, N. T., Reuveni, U., & Perez, F. (1987). Transformed or evolutive migraine. *Headache, 27,* 102–106.

Mathew, N. T., Stubits, E., & Nigam, M. P. (1982). Transformation of episodic migraine into daily headache: Analysis of factors. *Headache, 22,* 66–68.

Mortelmans, K., Post, M., Thijs, V., Herroelen, L., & Budts, W. (2005). The influence of percutaneous atrial septal defect closure on the occurrence of migraine. *European Heart Journal, 26,* 1533–1537.

Mulder, E. J., Van Baal, C., Gaist, D., Kallela, M., Kaprio, J., Svensson, D. A., et al. (2003). Genetic and environmental influences on migraine: A twin study across six countries. *Twin Research, 6,* 422–431.

Olesen, J., Bousser, M. G., Diener, H. C., Dodick, D., First, M., Goadsby, P. J., et al. (2006). New appendix criteria open for a broader concept of chronic migraine. *Cephalalgia, 26,* 742–746.

Ophoff, R. A., Terwindt, G. M., Vergouwe, M. N., van Eijk, R., Oefner, P. J., Hoffman, S. M., et al. (1996). Familial hemiplegic migraine and episodic ataxia type-2 are caused by mutations in the Ca2+ channel gene CACNL1A4. *Cell, 87,* 543–552.

Peatfield, R. C. (1995). Relationships between food, wine, and beer-precipitated migrainous headaches. *Headache, 35,* 355–357.

Penzien, D. B., Rains, J. C., Andrew, M. E., Galovski, T. E., Mohammad, Y., & Mosley, T. H. (2001). Relationships of daily stress, sleep, and headache: A time-series analysis. *Cephalalgia, 21,* 262–263.

Peres, M. F. (2003). Fibromyalgia, fatigue, and headache disorders. *Current Neurology and Neuroscience Reports, 3,* 97–103.

Peres, M. F., Young, W. B., Kaup, A. O., Zukerman, E., & Silberstein, S. D. (2001). Fibromyalgia is common in patients with trans-formed migraine. *Neurology, 57,* 1326–1328.

Peres, M. F., Zukerman, E., Young, W. B., & Silberstein, S. D. (2002). Fatigue in chronic migraine patients. *Cephalalgia, 22,* 720–724.

Pinessi, L., Savi, L., Pellicano, R., Rainero, I., Valfre, W., Gentile, S., et al. (2000). Chronic Helicobacter pylori infection and migraine: A case-control study. *Headache, 40,* 836–839.

Prince, P. B., Rapoport, A. M., Sheftell, F. D., Tepper, S. J., & Bigal, M. E. (2004). The effect of weather on headache. *Headache, 44,* 596–602.

Queiroz, L. P., Rapoport, A. M., Weeks, R. E., Sheftell, F. D., Siegel, S. E., & Baskin, S. M. (1997). Characteristics of migraine visual aura. *Headache, 37,* 137–141.

Rains, J. C., & Poceta, J. S. (2006). Headache and sleep disorders: Review and clinical implications for headache management. *Headache, 46,* 1344–1363.

Rasmussen, B. K. (1995). Epidemiology of headache. *Cephalalgia, 15,* 45–68.

Robbins, L. (1994). Precipitating factors in migraine: A retrospective review of 494 patients. *Headache, 34,* 214–216.

Rothrock, J., Patel, M., Lyden, P., & Jackson, C. (1996). Demographic and clinical characteristics of patients with episodic migraine versus chronic daily headache. *Cephalalgia, 16,* 44–49; discussion 4.

Russell, M. B., & Olesen, J. (1995). Increased familial risk and evidence of genetic factor in migraine. *BMJ, 311,* 541–544.

Russell, M. B., & Olesen, J. (1996). A nosographic analysis of the migraine aura in a general population. *Brain, 119*(Pt 2), 355–361.

Russell, M. B., Rasmussen, B. K., Fenger, K., & Olesen, J. (1996). Migraine without aura and migraine with aura are distinct clinical entities: A study of four hundred and eighty-four male and female migraineurs from the general population. *Cephalalgia, 16,* 239–245.

Sandler, M., Li, N. Y., Jarrett, N., & Glover, V. (1995). Dietary migraine: Recent progress in the red (and white) wine story. *Cephalalgia, 15,* 101–103.

Scher, A. I., Lipton, R. B., & Stewart, W. F. (2003). Habitual snoring as a risk factor for chronic daily headache. *Neurology, 60,* 1366–1368.

Scher, A. I., Lipton, R. B., Stewart, W. F., & Bigal, M. (2010) Patterns of medication use by chronic and episodic headache sufferers in the general population: Results from the frequent headache epidemiology study. *Cephalalgia, 30,* 321–328.

Scher, A. I., Stewart, W. F., Liberman, J., & Lipton, R. B. (1998). Prevalence of frequent headache in a population sample. *Headache, 38,* 497–506.

Scher, A. I., Stewart, W. F., Ricci, J. A., & Lipton, R. B. (2003). Factors associated with the onset and remission of chronic daily head-ache in a population-based study. *Pain, 106,* 81–89.

Scher, A. I., Terwindt, G. M., Picavet, H. S., Verschuren, W. M., Ferrari, M. D., & Launer, L. J. (2005). Cardiovascular risk factors and migraine: The GEM population-based study. *Neurology, 64,* 614–620.

Schurks, M., Rist, P. M., Bigal, M. E., Buring, J. E., Lipton, R. B., & Kurth, T. (2009). Migraine and cardiovascular disease: Systematic review and meta-analysis. *BMJ, 339,* b3914.

Schwedt, T. J., Demaerschalk, B. M., & Dodick, D. W. (2008). Patent foramen ovale and migraine: A quantitative systematic review. *Cephalalgia, 28,* 531–540.

Schwedt, T. J., & Dodick, D. W. (2006). Patent foramen ovale and migraine—bringing closure to the subject. *Headache, 46,* 663–671.

Schwedt, T. J., Krauss, M. J., Frey, K., & Gereau, R. W. (2011). Episodic and chronic migraineurs are hypersensitive to thermal stimuli between migraine attacks. *Cephalalgia, 31,* 6–12.

Seok, J. I., Cho, H. I., & Chung, C. S. (2006). From transformed migraine to episodic migraine: Reversion factors. *Headache, 46,* 1186–1190.

Silberstein, S. D., Olesen, J., Bousser, M. G., Diener, H. C., Dodick, D., First, M., et al. (2005). The international classification of headache disorders, 2nd edition (ICHD-II)—revision of criteria for 8.2 medication-overuse headache. *Cephalalgia, 25,* 460–465.

Stewart, W. F., Lipton, R. B., Chee, E., Sawyer, J., & Silberstein, S. D. (2000). Menstrual cycle and headache in a population sample of migraineurs. *Neurology, 55,* 1517–1523.

Sun-Edelstein, C., & Mauskop, A. (2009). Foods and supplements in the management of migraine headaches. *Clinical Journal of Pain, 25,* 446–452.

Terwindt, G. M., Ferrari, M. D., Tijhuis, M., Groenen, S. M., Picavet, H. S., & Launer, L. J. (2000). The impact of migraine on quality of life in the general population: The GEM study. *Neurology, 55,* 624–629.

Thenganatt, J., Schneiderman, J., Hyland, R. H., Edmeads, J., Mandzia, J. L., & Faughnan, M. E. (2006). Migraines linked to intrapulmonary right-to-left shunt. *Headache, 46,* 439–443.

Thomsen, L. L., Dixon, R., Lassen, L. H., Gibbens, M., Langemark, M., Bendtsen, L., et al. (1996). 311C90 (Zolmitriptan), a novel centrally and peripheral acting oral 5-hydroxytryptamine-1D agonist: A comparison of its absorption during a migraine attack and in a migraine-free period. *Cephalalgia, 16,* 270–275.

Thomsen, L. L., Eriksen, M. K., Roemer, S. F., Andersen, I., Olesen, J., & Russell, M. B. (2002). A population-based study of familial hemiplegic migraine suggests revised diagnostic criteria. *Brain, 125,* 1379–1391.

Turner, L. C., Molgaard, C. A., Gardner, C. H., Rothrock, J. F., & Stang, P. E. (1995). Migraine trigger factors in non-clinical Mexican-American population in San Diego county: Implications for etiology. *Cephalalgia, 15,* 523–530.

Tzourio, C., Tehindrazanarivelo, A., Iglesias, S., Alperovitch, A., Chedru, F., d'Anglejan-Chatillon, J., et al. (1995). Case-control study of migraine and risk of ischaemic stroke in young women. *BMJ, 310,* 830–833.

Ulfberg, J., Carter, N., Talback, M., & Edling, C. (1996). Headache, snoring and sleep apnoea. *Journal of Neurology, 243,* 621–625.

Van den Eeden, S. K., Koepsell, T. D., Longstreth, W. T., Jr., van Belle, G., Daling, J. R., & McKnight, B. (1994). Aspartame inges-tion and headaches: A randomized crossover trial. *Neurology, 44,* 1787–1793.

Villeneuve, P. J., Szyszkowicz, M., Stieb, D., & Bourque, D. A. (2006). Weather and emergency room visits for migraine headaches in Ottawa, Canada. *Headache, 46,* 64–72.

Vingen, J. V., Pareja, J. A., Storen, O., White, L. R., & Stovner, L. J. (1998). Phonophobia in migraine. *Cephalalgia, 18,* 243–249.

Volans, G. N. (1978). Migraine and drug absorption. *Clinical Pharmacokinetics, 3,* 313–318.

Weissman-Fogel, I., Sprecher, E., Granovsky, Y., & Yarnitsky, D. (2003). Repeated noxious stimulation of the skin enhances cutaneous pain perception of migraine patients in-between attacks: Clinical evidence for continuous sub-threshold increase in membrane excitability of central trigeminovascular neurons. *Pain, 104,* 693–700.

Wilkins, A., Nimmo-Smith, I., Tait, A., McManus, C., Della Sala, S., Tilley, A., et al. (1984). A neurological basis for visual discomfort. *Brain, 107*(Pt 4), 989–1017.

Wilkinson, M., & Woodrow, J. (1979). Migraine and weather. *Headache, 19,* 375–378.

Wober, C., Brannath, W., Schmidt, K., Kapitan, M., Rudel, E., Wessely, P., et al. (2007). Prospective analysis of factors related to migraine attacks: The PAMINA study. *Cephalalgia, 27,* 304–314.

Wober, C., Holzhammer, J., Zeitlhofer, J., Wessely, P., & Wober-Bingol, C. (2006). Trigger factors of migraine and tension-type headache: Experience and knowledge of the patients. *Journal of Headache and Pain, 7,* 188–195.

Wober-Bingol, C., Wober, C., Karwautz, A., Auterith, A., Serim, M., Zebenholzer, K., et al. (2004). Clinical features of migraine: A cross-sectional study in patients aged three to sixty-nine. *Cephalalgia, 24,* 12–17.

Zanchin, G., Dainese, F., Trucco, M., Mainardi, F., Mampreso, E., & Maggioni, F. (2007). Osmophobia in migraine and tension-type headache and its clinical features in patients with migraine. *Cephalalgia, 27,* 1061–1068.

Ziegler, D. K., & Hassanein, R. S. (1990). Specific headache phenomena: Their frequency and coincidence. *Headache, 30,* 152–156.

32 The Future of Imaging in Migraine Diagnosis and Treatment

DAVID BORSOOK AND LINO BECERRA

INTRODUCTION

Migraine is the most common neurological disease that profoundly affects the brain (Sprenger & Goadsby, 2009). The disease does so in terms of how it affects the brain (e.g., with and without aura), gender distribution (affecting women during their reproductive years more frequently than men), has a relatively abrupt onset and offset (most individuals will eventually have a remission) (Bigal & Lipton, 2011; Bigal et al., 2005; Manack et al., 2011; Robbins & Lipton, 2010). However, these relatively easily defined measures do not provide indices for how the brain is affected by migraine and how the brain may respond to different therapies. With respect to the latter, objective measures of a drug's effect are critical in the clinic and in the development of new pharmacotherapies (see Borsook et al., 2011a, 2011b).

There have been enormous strides in imaging from brain structural measures (magnetic resonance imaging [MRI]) capturing changes such as white matter and small infarcts associated with migraine (see Chapter 11). More recent advanced high-magnetic-field imaging that can measure functional, morphometric, and chemical changes has reported significant differences in the brains of those suffering from the disorder compared with healthy controls (May, 2009; Moulton et al., 2011; Prescot et al., 2009; Stankewitz et al., 2011). Treating migraine, as with many disorders affecting the central nervous system, is fraught with difficulties related to specific diagnoses and measures of treatment efficacy (Cole & Marmura, 2010; D'Amico et al., 2008; Silberstein, 2010). Given the recent advances in brain imaging techniques that have contributed to our understanding of how chronic pain affects multiple aspects of brain function, including sensory, emotional, cognitive, and modulatory, opportunities to adopt these approaches in the clinic are now becoming possible (Borsook & Hargreaves, 2010). The routine application of brain imaging as a clinical marker of disease state or therapeutic (drug) efficacy would significantly enhance the clinical process by providing objective markers for clinicians and patients (see Borsook et al., 2011a, 2011b).

Here we offer our insights into (a) how new techniques in functional imaging may change how we diagnose patients with migraine, (b) how imaging could contribute to evaluating disease state and risk of future changes such as progression of disease, (c) how imaging may evaluate treatment effects including potential deleterious effects of drugs used to treat the disorder, and (d) how imaging may influence the development of novel migraine medications and accelerate future treatments through innovative clinical trials. One of the unique features of migraine is that it is a disease involving the trigeminal system, and thus for most imaging techniques, the whole system can be captured—from trigeminal ganglion to brainstem, subcortical to cortical regions (Borsook et al., 2004; Borsook, Burstein, et al., 2006). Given the nature of peripheral and central nervous system involvement and the central or peripheral pathophysiology of migraine, fundamental hypotheses can be tested and applied to imaging with the potential for clinical applications (i.e., clinical functional imaging).

THE USE OF FUNCTIONAL IMAGING TO DIAGNOSE MIGRAINE IN PATIENTS: DEVELOPMENT OF BRAIN MIGRAINE BIOMARKERS

Critical to future use of functional imaging in the clinical setting is the development of validated biomarkers (see Borsook et al., 2011a, 2011b). Although migraine is a relatively easy disease to diagnose (see International Headache Society [IHS] guidelines on disease definition—http://ihs-classification.org/en/), the specific brain alterations are not known. As we come to understand the effects on brain systems, specific metrics may be helpful in evaluating migraine patients. Episodic migraine is a unique pain disorder with explosive periods of headache (ictal phase) separated by periods of no pain (interictal phase). Many patients experience more pain-free days per month than painful days. However, migraine may progress from a few episodic attacks to many per month (14 headache days per month) (http://ihs-classification.org/en/). Some patients further progress to chronic daily headache (Bigal, 2009; Bigal & Lipton, 2008). Identifying those patients who are prone to progression may provide an opportunity for a different treatment approach than for patients who do not progress. Already some insights from imaging into this aspect of migraine have been made possible. The search for and adopting of specific biomarkers in migraine may indeed become possible in a way that may even allow us to renew our definitions of episodic and chronic migraine "substates". Examples of such states include patients who have predominantly sensory systems altered compared with those who have more complex effects, such as alterations in temporal lobe processing (Moulton et al., 2011), that confer differences in behavioral manifestations of the disease.

Subtyping migraine patients based on brain state provides a potential opportunity to improve treatments by offering specific opportunities for interictal therapeutic choices. Specific measures include those discussed elsewhere in this book—functional measures, anatomical or morphometric measures, and chemical measures. Since all utilize high-field 3-Tesla MRI scanners, which are becoming the standard in radiological practice, the implementation of acquisition paradigms that are relatively simple, reproducible, and sensitive is clearly possible in the near future. Radiological reports of functional changes (e.g., increased brain sensitivity), morphological changes (e.g., increased or decreased volume in specific structures

defined in the disease state), or chemical changes (e.g., diminished cortical inhibitory neurotransmitters such as γ-aminobutyric acid [GABA]) are being honed and tuned (simplification, standardized imaging sequences, standardized protocols, etc.) for adaptation in the clinic.

Comorbidity in migraine (e.g., depression, anxiety) is clearly a component of subtyping the disease state (Casucci et al., 2010; Finocchi et al., 2010). Other migraine subtypes may depend on the chronicity and frequency of the disease (discussed below).

HOW IMAGING MAY CONTRIBUTE TO EVALUATING DISEASE STATE

Brain Measures in the Interictal State

The interictal state (see Chapter 5) is a more convenient time for imaging patients since they do not have pain, but their brains have changed as a consequence of their disease state. Imaging approaches are summarized in Figure 32–1. As noted in the figure, specific brain measures may be obtained. Some features are already well defined in migraine patients (e.g., increased cortical excitability). However, efforts to validate such findings and develop clinical protocols/paradigms are still required. Opportunities for the use of imaging are noted for each imaging domain below (functional magnetic resonance imaging [fMRI], magnetic resonance spectroscopy [MRS], voxel-based morphometry [VBM]).

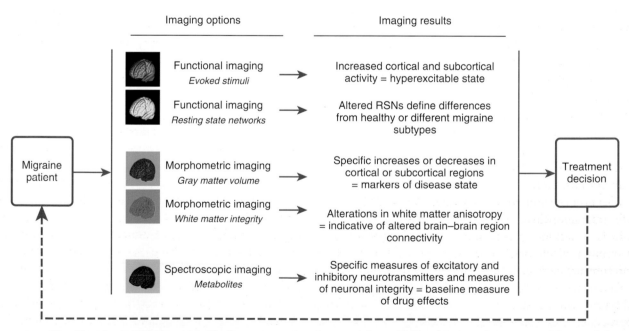

FIGURE 32–1 *Use of imaging in clinical practice. The figure summarizes the potential use of different functional imaging modalities in defining alterations in the brains of migraine patients (see text for details).*

Functional Measures of Brain Activity

Functional—circuit specific: Current data indicate that significant alterations in general circuits may be observed in migraine. These include changes in trigeminal systems (Borsook, Burstein, et al., 2006; Moulton et al., 2008; Stankewitz et al., 2011; Weissman-Fogel et al., 2003). Such circuits represent sensory systems in migraine, but more likely than not, other circuits will be shown to be altered in the disease (e.g., thalamo-cortico-basal ganglia).

Functional—region specific: Relatively little has been evaluated in this domain. Regions evaluated include the posterior thalamus (Burstein et al., 2010) which may serve as a marker of general sensitivity, since this is observed not only in the migraine state with generalized allodynia but also in patients with increased frequency (Maleki et al., 2010). Changes are also observed in other brain regions such as the cingulate and temporal pole (Moulton et al., 2011). More recent data suggest that the basal ganglia (Maleki et al., 2010) and hippocampus (Maleki et al., 2011) may be specific markers for migraine frequency.

Functional changes—resting state networks: Resting state networks have the advantage of evaluating a brain state without stimuli (Deco et al., 2011). Few studies have been reported in the migraine field, but numerous reports have been published in different disease states including pain. The current hurdles are in objective evaluation of these networks (Ferrarini et al., 2009).

Morphometric Measures of Gray and White Matter Changes

Gray matter (voxel-based morphometry or cortical thickness)—region specific: Ever since the groundbreaking observations of alterations in cortical thickness (dorsolateral prefrontal) in chronic pain, (Apkarian et al., 2004), numerous studies have supported the idea that changes in specific morphometric regions are observed in migraine (see Chapter 18). Of great interest is that these regions may "normalize" with treatment. As such, this approach is not experimenter determined as with functional changes.

Chemical Changes as Correlates of Abnormal Brain Function

Chemical—neurotransmitter specific: A few MRS studies in the migraine field have been reported (Prescot et al., 2009). MRS is an advancing field and the technologies are now becoming available for clinical magnets (3 Tesla) that together with software packages can be deployed in the clinic.

Classification of the above results to identify migraine subtypes will result in better-designed treatment approaches. For some conditions, such as migraineurs who experience high recurrence of migraines or have evolved to having daily headaches, collection of imaging data in a large number of patients longitudinally may be required to potentially specify those changes predicting evolution of low-incidence migraine into a more severe condition.

BRAIN MEASURE IN THE ICTAL STATE

All of the above studies may be performed in the ictal state. However, evaluating migraine patients using imaging in their ictal state is extremely difficult in routine medical practice. Provocative tests may also be used to activate a migraine. Nitroglycerine has been used successfully to induce migraine (Bank, 2001; Juhasz et al., 2003). Advantages of measures during the ictal state are evaluation of brain features including the severity of the attack on neural networks (sensory, emotional, cognitive) as well as the opportunity to evaluate specificity of drug effects on the ictal event.

HOW IMAGING MAY EVALUATE TREATMENT EFFECTS INCLUDING POTENTIAL DELETERIOUS EFFECTS OF DRUGS USED TO TREAT THE DISORDER

Figure 32–2 depicts possible uses of imaging in evaluating drug effects in the clinic and in clinical trials. Some drugs such as opioids alter the brain state in migraine patients so as to render them less responsive to treatments. Opioids alter brain systems in a profound manner (Upadhyay et al., 2010), and triptan overuse has been implicated in migraine chronification (Bigal & Lipton, 2009). Specific markers for such changes may now be available (Maleki et al., 2010).

Direct central nervous system (CNS) effects of triptans are still a matter of debate (Tfelt-Hansen, 2010), although several lines of evidence support the presence of direct CNS effects: (a) triptans, such as zolmitriptan, do cross the blood-brain barrier (Boshuisen & den Boer, 2000), although the degree to which they do so may vary according to their lipid solubility; (b) patients display CNS symptoms related to triptans that can be differentiated from placebo (Dodick & Martin, 2004); (c) 3-H-labeled sumatriptan-binding studies of human brain show increased binding in a number of regions of the brain including the basal ganglia, with the highest binding in the caudate (Lopez-Alemany et al., 1997); and (d) there are some reports of triptan-induced motor changes (dystonia, akathisia) suggestive of actions of these drugs on the basal ganglia (Lopez-Alemany et al., 1997; Oterino & Pascual, 1998), supporting the postmortem binding studies. The

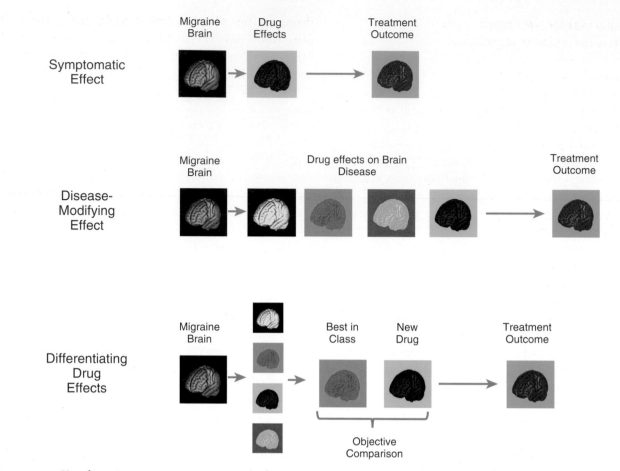

Symptomatic Effect

Migraine Brain → Drug Effects → Treatment Outcome

Disease-Modifying Effect

Migraine Brain → Drug effects on Brain Disease → Treatment Outcome

Differentiating Drug Effects

Migraine Brain → Best in Class | New Drug → Treatment Outcome

Objective Comparison

FIGURE 32–2 *Use of imaging in migraine treatments. The figure shows three main processes in utilizing imaging for evaluating treatments. As such, these approaches may be used in clinical trials or potentially in individual patients. From Borsook et al., 2011b, Discovery Medicine, with permission.*

only differences between the groups that we studied were migraine frequency and concomitant use of triptans (increased in the high frequency migraineurs). Thus, our observations may be a result of direct triptan-mediated effects on these structures (Cupini & Calabresi, 2005). Placebo-controlled, longitudinal studies are needed. However, the results of such approaches could be transformative in potentially defining those drugs that cross the blood-brain barrier as potentially harmful to individuals.

HOW IMAGING MAY INFLUENCE THE DEVELOPMENT OF NOVEL MIGRAINE MEDICATIONS AND ACCELERATE FUTURE TREATMENTS THROUGH INNOVATIVE CLINICAL TRIALS

The use of imaging in drug development has been reviewed in a number of recent papers (Borsook, Becerra,

et al., 2006). The field of migraine imaging has some interesting opportunities to contribute to the evaluation of new drugs (see Borsook & Hargreaves, 2010). Some drugs approved for migraine preventive treatments have relatively low efficacy profiles (e.g., botulinum toxin A and topiramate). No data exist on how these drugs affect brain systems, and the marginal effects in clinical trials may relate to a number of issues including lack of segregation of responders and nonresponders or false-positive results. In addition to efficacy, measures of CNS side effects can also be defined using imaging. Thus, in the future, the addition of imaging in early clinical trials for drug effects on symptom management and in later trials on disease modification will provide useful additional information. Imaging combined with other metrics clearly diminishes the variance of measures of drug effects, allowing for fewer patients to be enrolled when comparing drug versus placebo or best-in-class medication.

THE PATIENT, IMAGING, AND INDIVIDUALIZED MEDICINE

How could imaging be integrated into clinical practice? Genetic markers may define certain aspects of disease vulnerability of migraine subtype (Anttila et al., 2010) or drug metabolism. Markers of pharmacogenomics evaluating sensitivity or drug metabolism may be useful in choosing specific drugs (Gentile et al., 2011; Van Den Maagdenberg et al., 2010). However, brain markers can provide insights into the dynamic disease state until effective therapies (symptomatic and disease modifying) essentially "cure" the disease. In the days of personalized medicine, when data-driven approaches to treatments are driving the new era in medicine, specific diagnoses of disease state and drug effects for migraine patients are now possible with imaging.

Imaging migraine in individualized medicine will tailor specific treatments to specific patients (Ma & Lu, 2011). The focus has been on genetic and other information on patients, but imaging has the opportunity to be a leader in this field, particularly in the domain of drug use related to treatment response and disease modification (Gerretsen et al., 2009).

Technical issues including validation, clinical standards, and rapid methods for acquiring, analyzing, and interpreting data from individual patients need to be implemented. Given the current standing in the field of vendor products, technical know-how, and radiology entrepreneurship, these issues are not seen as hurdles to accomplishing "radiological readouts." The issues relate more to the reproducibility and specificity of brain targets for disease diagnosis and treatment effects. Access to normative and patient data will be critical to the evolution of application in the clinic. An example includes datasets/databanks from centers such as the Laboratory of Neuroimaging at UCLA (LONI; http://www.loni.ucla.edu/).

CONCLUSIONS: A NEW HORIZON

Any objective assay of a disease state is a major contribution to improving clinical care. The development of deployable neuroimaging measures of function, morphology, and chemistry will contribute to personalized medicine. In recent years, significant progress has been made in the use of functional brain imaging to complement observational studies of migraine phenotypes by highlighting pathways within the brain that may be involved in predisposition to migraine or modulation of migraine pain, or that could be sensitive to pharmacological or behavioral therapeutic intervention. Improvements in diagnosis may offer new opportunities for more specific therapies, for adaptive clinical trials, and perhaps for drug development (see Borsook & Hargreaves, 2010). Many of the medications used in migraine treatments are not specifically indicated for the disease, particularly in the domain of high-frequency episodic and chronic daily headache. The arbitrary nature of these classifications (based on symptomatology) will probably be modified as functional imaging makes its impact in the clinic.

Symptomatic measures/effects: Imaging may define the effects of acute or chronic medications on symptoms associated with the ictal event. Such targeted effects relate to control of pain and associated symptoms (e.g., photophobia) and signs (e.g., nausea and vomiting) present during the ictal event.

Disease-modifying measures/effects: How current medications affect the brain is unclear. Medications used as preventive treatments could act on brain systems to modify them over time. Such changes presumably involve neural adaptive changes. Understanding specific brain dysfunction in migraine may allow for new targets for preemptive medications. Using specific imaging modalities (e.g., MRS for chemical changes or VBM for anatomical changes) can allow measurement of the effects of a drug over time.

Differentiating new drugs: Antimigraine drugs may have different effects in individuals or within specific classes of drugs (e.g., triptans may have different brain penetration based on their ability to cross the blood-brain barrier). Differentiating new drugs within the same class or in different classes can be accomplished using pharmacological imaging as well as those modalities noted in Figure 32–1.

REFERENCES

Anttila, V., Stefansson H., Kallela M., Todt U., Terwindt G. M., Calafato M. S., et al. (2010). Genome-wide association study of migraine implicates a common susceptibility variant on 8q22.1. *Nature Genetics, 42,* 869–873.

Apkarian, A. V., Sosa, Y., Sonty, S., Levy, R. M., Harden, R. N., Parrish, T. B., et al. (2004). Chronic back pain is associated with decreased prefrontal and thalamic gray matter density. *Journal of Neuroscience, 24,* 10410–10415.

Bank, J. (2001). Migraine with aura after administration of sublingual nitroglycerin tablets. *Headache, 41,* 84–87.

Bigal, M. (2009). Migraine chronification—concept and risk factors. *Discovery Medicine, 8,* 145–150.

Bigal, M. E., & Lipton, R. B. (2008). Clinical course in migraine: Conceptualizing migraine transformation. *Neurology, 71,* 848–855.

Bigal, M. E., & Lipton, R. B. (2009). Overuse of acute migraine medications and migraine chronification. *Current Pain and Headache Reports, 13,* 301–307.

Bigal, M. E., & Lipton, R. B. (2011). Migraine chronification. *Current Neurology and Neuroscience Reports, 11*, 139–148.

Bigal, M. E., Sheftell, F. D., Tepper, S. J., Rapoport, A. M., & Lipton, R. B. (2005). Migraine days decline with duration of illness in adolescents with transformed migraine. *Cephalalgia, 25*, 482–487.

Borsook, D., Becerra, L., & Hargreaves, R. (2006). A role for fMRI in optimizing CNS drug development. *Nature Reviews Drug Discovery, 5*, 411–424.

Borsook, D., Becerra, L., & Hargreaves, R. (2011a). Biomarkers of chronic pain and analgesia part 1: The need, reality, challenges and solutions. *Discovery Medicine, 11*(58), 197–207.

Borsook, D., Becerra, L., & Hargreaves, R. (2011b). Biomarkers of chronic pain and analgesics part 2: How, where and what to look for using functional imaging. *Discovery Medicine, 11*(58), 209–19.

Borsook, D., Burstein, R., & Becerra, L. (2004). Functional imaging of the human trigeminal system: Opportunities for new insights into pain processing in health and disease. *Journal of Neurobiology, 61*, 107–125.

Borsook, D., Burstein, R., Moulton, E., & Becerra, L. (2006). Functional imaging of the trigeminal system: Applications to migraine pathophysiology. *Headache, 46*(Suppl 1), S32–S38.

Borsook, D., & Hargreaves, R. (2010). Brain imaging in migraine research. *Headache, 50*, 1523–1527.

Boshuisen, M. L., & den Boer, J. A. (2000). Zolmitriptan (a 5-HT1B/1D receptor agonist with central action) does not increase symptoms in obsessive compulsive disorder. *Psychopharmacology (Berlin), 152*, 74–79.

Burstein, R., Jakubowski, M., Garcia-Nicas, E., Kainz, V., Bajwa, Z., Hargreaves, R., et al. (2010). Thalamic sensitization transforms localized pain into widespread allodynia. *Annals of Neurology, 68*, 81–91.

Casucci, G., Villani, V., & Finocchi, C. (2010). Therapeutic strategies in migraine patients with mood and anxiety disorders: Physiopathological basis. *Neurological Sciences, 31*(Suppl 1), S99–S101.

Cole, A. K., & Marmura, M. J. (2010). Triptans: Where things stand. *Current Treatment Options in Neurology, 12*, 454–463.

Cupini, L. M., & Calabresi, P. (2005). Medication-overuse headache: Pathophysiological insights. *Journal of Headache and Pain, 6*, 199–202.

D'Amico, D., Leone, M., Grazzi, L., & Bussone, G. (2008). When should "chronic migraine" patients be considered "refractory" to pharmacological prophylaxis? *Neurological Sciences, 29*(Suppl 1), S55–S58.

Deco, G., Jirsa, V. K., & McIntosh, A. R. (2011). Emerging concepts for the dynamical organization of resting-state activity in the brain. *Nature Reviews Neuroscience, 12*, 43–56.

Dodick, D. W., & Martin, V. (2004). Triptans and CNS side-effects: Pharmacokinetic and metabolic mechanisms. *Cephalalgia, 24*, 417–424.

Ferrarini, L., Veer, I. M., Baerends, E., van Tol, M. J., Renken, R. J., van der Wee, N. J., et al. (2009). Hierarchical functional modularity in the resting-state human brain. *Human Brain Mapping, 30*, 2220–2231.

Finocchi, C., Villani, V., & Casucci, G. (2010) Therapeutic strategies in migraine patients with mood and anxiety disorders: clinical evidence. *Neurological Sciences, 31*(Suppl 1), S95–S98.

Gentile, G., Borro, M., Simmaco, M., Missori, S., Lala, N., & Martelletti, P. (2011). Gene polymorphisms involved in triptans pharmacokinetics and pharmacodynamics in migraine therapy. *Expert Opinions in Drug Metabolism and Toxicology, 7*, 39–47.

Gerretsen, P., Muller, D. J., Tiwari, A., Mamo, D., & Pollock, B. G. (2009). The intersection of pharmacology, imaging, and genetics in the development of personalized medicine. *Dialogues in Clinical Neuroscience, 11*, 363–376.

Juhasz, G., Zsombok, T., Modos, E. A., Olajos, S., Jakab, B., Nemeth, J., et al. (2003). NO-induced migraine attack: Strong increase in plasma calcitonin gene-related peptide (CGRP) concentration and negative correlation with platelet serotonin release. *Pain, 106*, 461–470.

Lopez-Alemany, M., Ferrer-Tuset, C., & Bernacer-Alpera, B. (1997). Akathisia and acute dystonia induced by sumatriptan. *Journal of Neurology, 244*, 131–132.

Ma, Q., & Lu, A. Y. (2011). Pharmacogenetics, pharmacogenomics, and individualized medicine. *Pharmacological Reviews, 63*, 437–59.

Maleki, N., Becerra, L., Nutile, L., Burstein, R., & Borsook, D. (2010). Structural differences in migraine brain are related to the attack frequency [Abstract]. *The Society of Neuroscience.*

Maleki, N., Becerra, L., Nutile, L., Pendse, G., Bigal, M., Burstein, R., et al. (2011). Hippocampal changes in episodic migraine patients: Morphometric and functional evidence [Abstract]. *Human Brain Mapping.* Quebec City, Canada, 2011.

Manack, A. N., Buse, D. C., & Lipton, R. B. (2011). Chronic migraine: Epidemiology and disease burden. *Current Pain and Headache Reports, 15*, 70–78.

May, A. (2009). Morphing voxels: The hype around structural imaging of headache patients. *Brain, 132*, 1419–1425.

Moulton, F. A., Becerra, L., Maleki, N., Pendse, G., Tully, S., Hargreaves, R., et al. (2011). Painful heat reveals hyperexcitability of the temporal pole in interictal and ictal migraine states. *Cerebral Cortex, 21*, 435–448.

Moulton, E. A., Burstein, R., Tully, S., Hargreaves, R., Becerra, L., & Borsook, D. (2008). Interictal dysfunction of a brainstem descending modulatory center in migraine patients. *PLoS One, 3*, e3799.

Oterino, A., & Pascual, J. (1998). Sumatriptan-induced axial dystonia in a patient with cluster headache. *Cephalalgia, 18*, 360–361.

Prescot, A., Becerra, L., Pendse, G., Tully, S., Jensen, E., Hargreaves, R., et al. (2009). Excitatory neurotransmitters in brain regions in interictal migraine patients. *Molecular Pain, 5*, 34.

Robbins, M. S., & Lipton, R. B. (2010). The epidemiology of primary headache disorders. *Seminars in Neurology, 30*, 107–119.

Silberstein, S. D. (2010). Migraine preventive treatment. *Handbooks of Clinical Neurology, 97*, 337–354.

Sprenger, T., & Goadsby, P. J. (2009). Migraine pathogenesis and state of pharmacological treatment options. *BMC Medicine, 7*, 71.

Stankewitz, A., Aderjan, D., Eippert, F., & May, A. (2011). Trigeminal nociceptive transmission in migraineurs predicts migraine attacks. *Journal of Neuroscience, 31*, 1937–1943.

Tfelt-Hansen, P. C. (2010). Does sumatriptan cross the blood-brain barrier in animals and man? *Journal of Headache and Pain, 11*, 5–12.

Upadhyay, J., Maleki, N., Potter, J., Elman, I., Rudrauf, D., Knudsen, J., et al. (2010). Alterations in brain structure and functional connectivity in prescription opioid-dependent patients. *Brain, 133,* 2098–2114.

Van Den Maagdenberg, A. M., Terwindt, G. M., Haan, J., Frants, R. R., & Ferrari, M. D. (2010). Genetics of headaches. *Handbook of Clinical Neurology, 97,* 85–97.

Weissman-Fogel, I., Sprecher, E., Granovsky, Y., & Yarnitsky, D. (2003). Repeated noxious stimulation of the skin enhances cutaneous pain perception of migraine patients in-between attacks: Clinical evidence for continuous sub-threshold increase in membrane excitability of central trigeminovascular neurons. *Pain, 104,* 693–700.

33 Can Imaging Change Migraine Treatment Paradigms?

DAVID BORSOOK, ARNE MAY, PETER J. GOADSBY, AND

RICHARD HARGREAVES

INTRODUCTION

Optimal treatment for migraine is still elusive. We do not fully understand the disease state (e.g., differences in the episodic and chronic migraine brain or neural circuits involved in transformation), nor how drugs used in the treatment of acute and chronic migraine affect the migraine condition in either the short or long term. Clearly, understanding the pathophysiology and pharmacology of migraine has been driven by clinical contributions and clinical studies and through research on agents highly effective against migraine in the laboratory and clinic.

How can we optimize migraine treatments? Significant progress has been made in the use of functional brain imaging to complement observational studies of migraine phenotypes by highlighting pathways within the brain that may be involved in predisposition to migraine or modulating migraine pain, or that could be sensitive to therapeutic interventions (e.g., pharmacological or behavioral). Imaging will not be a panacea, but can define the disease state and drug effects in human subjects. Clearly, the ideal is to evaluate and treat the individual patient—that is, *individualized medicine.*

Migraine may in some cases progress. Developing our knowledge of where drugs act in the brain and of how the brain is altered in both episodic migraine (interictal state and ictal state) and chronic migraine is an important step to understanding why there is such differential responsiveness to therapeutics among migraine patients, and to improving how they are evaluated and treated. Functional (functional magnetic resonance imaging [fMRI], resting state networks, arterial spin labeling) and molecular neuroimaging (positron emission tomography) research can help understand the neural systems biology of acute and chronic migraine. Neuroimaging tools can visualize the interaction of promising antimigraine therapeutics with their brain targets and so guide clinical trials, patient selection, and therapy. Chemical imaging (magnetic resonance spectroscopy) can define normal and abnormal levels of brain chemicals (including excitatory and inhibitory neurotransmitters) in the migraine state and in response to treatments. Imaging research can reveal the neural circuits that predispose to migraine, the consequences of trigeminovascular activation, and altered pain-related brain processes (including affect modulation), all of which may impact the comorbid symptoms of migraine. Neuroimaging-based observations will impact our understanding of migraine pathophysiology and provide a rich framework within which to design and test future migraine treatment strategies.

MAKING IMAGING USEFUL IN MIGRAINE—DEFINING DISEASE STATE AND DRUG EFFECTS

Imaging has already confirmed old ideas and provided new insights into the disease state—both in the ictal and interictal times (May, 2009). Advances in understanding how acute migraine attacks or chronic migraine alters brain function (neuronal circuit activation), structure (morphometrically), or neurochemistry (neurotransmitters and their metabolites) has the potential to transform our understanding of the migraine brain and its progression to chronic disease (Bigal, 2009; Bigal & Lipton, 2008; Raskin et al., 1987), thereby providing a foundation for new therapeutic approaches. Defining *biomarkers* for migraine would be an enormous contribution to defining a disease state and drug effects in individual patients (Borsook et al., 2011a, 2011b).

Functional imaging has entered into a phase where the effects of drugs on brain systems can now be measured. Though the mechanisms of action for acute agents such as triptans and calcitonin gene–related peptide antagonists are somewhat well defined, many drugs that are used in the prophylaxis of migraine (anticonvulsants, antidepressants) do not have focused, specific mechanisms. What is now possible is that measures of drug effects on brain circuits can be made independently of knowing all the effects of a drug (see Becerra et al., 2006; Borras et al., 2004). fMRI "signatures" of known active and inactive antimigraine drug classes after either acute or chronic drug administration can provide fingerprints of drug activity that can be used to assess and discover new migraine drug approaches.

Molecular imaging merges neuroanatomy, neuropharmacology, and imaging technologies. Molecular imaging techniques such as positron emission tomography enable the visualization, characterization, and measurement of biological processes with exquisite, spatial, temporal, and biochemical resolution at molecular and cellular levels in living subjects. The value of molecular imaging is that it is translational between the laboratory and the clinic, allowing one to probe, noninvasively or minimally invasively, physiological, pathophysiological, and disease processes in a relevant tissue context.

CONCLUSIONS

Significant progress has been made in the use of imaging to study activity within the brain during pain, suffering, and therapy. Functional brain imaging has been successfully interwoven into fundamental studies of pain and analgesia. Specifically, brain patterns of activation can be evaluated alongside responses to nociceptive stimuli, which can then be simply evaluated and communicated by healthy individuals and patient populations. fMRI has helped define the sensory and emotional neural circuits that are involved in pain processing and its psychophysical modulation in diverse acute and chronic pain syndromes, including migraine. It can highlight the pathways that may be sensitive to pharmacological or behavioral therapeutic intervention.

Future imaging studies will continue to provide insights into disease state. Translating this information into therapeutic opportunities is clearly a challenge. Having objective markers of disease state should, however, help transform development and deployment of new therapeutic opportunities. The use of imaging should provide useful aids in evaluating treatments for *disease symptoms* or for *disease modification*. At the end of the day, the principles of evidence-based datasets need to be applied to the individual. Imaging is very close to being able to do this, that is, to provide objective measures of anatomical and chemical changes in brain systems where disease state and drug effects can be monitored.

REFERENCES

Becerra, L., Harter, K., Gonzalez, R. G., & Borsook, D. (2006). Functional magnetic resonance imaging measures of the effects of morphine on central nervous system circuitry in opioid-naive healthy volunteers. *Anesthesia and Analgesia, 103,* 208–216, table of contents.

Bigal, M. (2009). Migraine chronification—concept and risk factors. *Discovery Medicine, 8,* 145–150.

Bigal, M. E., & Lipton, R. B. (2008). Clinical course in migraine: Conceptualizing migraine transformation. *Neurology, 71,* 848–855.

Borras, M. C., Becerra, L., Ploghaus, A., Gostic, J. M., DaSilva, A., Gonzalez, R. G., et al. (2004). fMRI measurement of CNS responses to naloxone infusion and subsequent mild noxious thermal stimuli in healthy volunteers. *Journal of Neurophysiology, 91,* 2723–2733.

Borsook, D., Becerra, L., & Hargreaves, R. (2011a). Biomarkers for chronic pain and analgesia. Part 1: The need, reality, challenges, and solutions. *Discovery Medicine, 11,* 197–207.

Borsook, D., Becerra, L., & Hargreaves, R. (2011b). Biomarkers for chronic pain and analgesia. Part 2: How, where, and what to look for using functional imaging. *Discovery Medicine, 11,* 209–219.

May, A. (2009). New insights into headache: an update on functional and structural imaging findings. *Nature* Reviews Neurology, 5, 199–209.

Raskin, N. H., Hosobuchi, Y., & Lamb, S. (1987). Headache may arise from perturbation of brain. *Headache, 27,* 416–420.

INDEX

Note: Page numbers followed by *f* or *n* refer to figures or tables, respectively.

gastrointestinal disturbances
    comorbid disorders, 98t, 356t, 357
    migraine, 36, 351–352
gender, chronic and episodic
    migraine, 64, 65t
gene association studies, migraine, 154
genetic factors, chronic migraine
    (CM), 64, 66
genetics. *See also* migraine genes
    cortical responsivity, 330
    epidemiology of migraine, 145–146
    markers and disease vulnerability, 367
    migraine, 14, 58
    migraine and comorbid bipolar
        disorder, 156
    migraine and comorbid depression,
        155–156
    monogenic disorders associated
        with migraine, 150, 151t
genome-wide association (GWA),
    common migraine, 155, 159
glutamate receptors, migraine, 219–220
glyceryl trinitrate (GTN), model of
    migraine, 304
Gowers, William, 12, 14, 275
gray matter changes
    altered brain, 52f
    diffusion tensor MRI, 191
    migraine indicator, 196–197
    morphometric measures, 364f, 365
Greco-Roman medicine, 4
Greek medical authors, 4

habituation
    contingent negative variation
        (CNV), 326
    evoked potentials, 138, 323, 324f
    laser-evoked potential (LEP), 327
    migraine cycle, 321, 325
    migrainous brain, 330–331
Hall, Marshall, 9
Harris, Wilfred, 12
headache
    botulinum toxin in treatment, 109t
    daily incidence of, with nausea, 37f
    mechanism of botulinum toxin for, 107
    mechanisms, 31–32
    migraine, 350–351
    migraine mimics, 91–92
    morphometric studies of, syndromes,
        195–197
    morphometric study of chronic tension-
        type, 196
    morphometric study of cluster, 195–196
    neural system changes, 30–33
    neuroimaging, 137–138
    pain arising within brain, 32–33
    progression, 67–68
    source of pain in migraine, 30
    structural changes, 199
    temporomandibular disorder, 69, 70t

trigeminovascular system, 30–31
    vascular disturbances, 32
head pain, vicious circle of migraine
    symptoms, 36f
Heberden, William, 8
hemicrania
    definition, 9
    word, 3, 6–7
hemiplegic migraine, headache, 5
hemodynamics, cerebrovascular, of
    migraine patients, 56
high-frequency oscillations (HFOs),
    evoked potentials, 324f, 326
HIHRATL (hereditary infantile
    hemiparesis, retinal arteriolar
    tortuosity, and leukoencephalopathy),
    disorder with migraine, 151t, 152
Hildegard of Bingen, 5
Hippocratic school, medical writing, 3, 8
history of migraine
    17th century, 5–7
    18th century, 7–8
    20th century, 12–14
    antiquity, 3–4
    Arabic and medieval European
        medicine, 5
    early Christian era Greco-Roman
        medicine, 4
    imaging, 169–174
    natural, 63–64
    nineteenth century, 8–12
homeostatis, iron, 117
hormones, migraine trigger, 353
household income, chronic and
    episodic migraine, 64, 65t
human cerebral cortex
    cortical thickness, 205–206, 209–210
    structure, 203
    visualization and quantification of,
        203–204
Huntington disease
    cortical thickness, 205
    iron, 118
hyperexcitability
    functional imaging demonstrating,
        298–299
    occipital cortex, 341–342
    repetitive transcranial magnetic
        stimulation, 298
hyperexcitable trigeminovascular
    system, vicious circle of migraine
    symptoms, 36f
hypersensitivity
    computed tomography vs. magnetic
        resonance imaging, 86
    interictal olfactory, 224, 225f
    sensory input, 75
hyperventilation, visual evoked
    responses, 323, 325
hypocretins, hypothalamus and, 23
hypoperfusion

cortical spreading depression (CSD),
    237–238
    migraine without aura, 234, 236f, 248
    neurovascular event, 238
    posterior, and migraine, 234, 236
hypothalamus
    activation during spontaneous
        migraine attacks, 179f
    antinociceptive effect, 22
    autonomic symptoms in migraine,
        22–23
    circadian rhythm, 23
    cluster headache, 199
    migraine and, 21–24
    neuroimaging studies, 24
    obesity, and migraine, 23–24
    orexins, 23

ictal phase
    blood flow, 279–280
    diffusivity abnormalities, 189–190
individualized medicine, patient and
    imaging, 367, 371
infarction
    migrainous, 123, 137
    risk of silent, 124–125
infarcts
    cerebellar, 129f
    infratentorial posterior circulation,
        in cerebellum, 128f
    magnetic resonance imaging (MRI),
        126–127
    migraine with aura, 89
    silent, 124–125
intensity dependence of auditory evoked
    potentials (IDAP)
    evoked potentials, 324f, 325
    migraine, 138
interictal migraine brain state (IMBS)
    alterations, 287, 288–291
    cerebrovascular hemodynamics, 56
    chemical alterations, 55–56
    definition, 51
    electroencephalography (EEG), 287
    functional alterations, 53–54
    neuroimaging techniques and, 52f
    neuronal changes, 339
    pathophysiology of interictal brain,
        56–58
    structural alterations, 51–53
    white matter alterations, 54–55
interictal phase
    alterations, 287
    altered cortical processing, 289–291
    brain activation by noxious heat
        stimulation, 247, 248f
    brain measures in, 364
    brainstem and modulatory
        circuitry, 288
    caveats in neuroimaging, 291–292
    cerebral cortex, 288–289

synaptic activity, correlation with regional cerebral blood flow, 233
synthetic analgesics, migraine treatment, 12
systemic lupus erythematosus (SLE), white matter abnormalities, 89

Tanacetum parthenium (feverfew), migraine prevention, 111
teichopsia, term, 10
temporal lobe, altered cortical processing, 289–291
temporal pole, interictal migraine, 289–291
temporomandibular disorders (TMDs), chronic migraine, 69, 70t
TGFR2 gene (transforming growth factor-b receptor 2), mutation in, 151t, 152
thalamocortical dysrhythmia, sensory cortices, 331
thioctic acid, migraine treatment, 269
Thomas, Louis Hyacinthe, 12
thromboxanes, receptor, 220
timolol, migraine preventive agent, 98, 99t
Tissot, Samuel, 7–8
tobacco exposure, pregnancy, 66, 67t
tonic pain, visual evoked responses, 323
topiramate, migraine prevention, 102t, 103–104, 340t, 341
town-wall vision, migraine, 10
trait component analysis (TCA), linkage analysis for migraine, 153t
transcranial direct current stimulation (tDCS), migraine, 312–313, 316–317
transcranial Doppler
  cardiac shunts, 140
  imaging technique, 303
transcranial magnetic stimulation (TMS)
  acute therapy and abortive intervention in migraine, 315–316
  basic principles, 309–310
  clinical tool and intervention, 317
  cortical silent period in migraine, 297
  functional imaging demonstrating hyperexcitability, 298–299
  magnetic suppression of perceptual accuracy (MSPA), 298
  migraine assessment, 208, 313–317
  motor cortex in migraine, 295–297
  motor cortex studies of migraineurs, 297t
  occipital cortex in migraine, 297–298
  paired-pulse TMS, 311
  picture of TMS application, 310f
  prevention of attacks, 316
  rationale for TMS in migraine, 315
  repetitive, 316
  repetitive TMS, 298, 311–312, 312f, 313–315
  safety, 317
  single-pulse TMS, 310–311, 315–316

transcranial direct current stimulation (tDCS), 312–313, 316–317
visual evoked potentials (VEPs), 140, 141t
transient ischemic attack (TIA), risk of silent infarction, 124–125
transient receptor potential vanilloid receptors, migraine, 219
trauma
  head and neck, 71
  producing migraine, 57–58
treatment. *See also* preventive therapy for migraine
  migraine prevention, 111–112, 339–342
tricyclic antidepressants, migraine prevention, 100–101
trigeminal ganglion, sensitized neurons, 45, 46f
trigeminal nucleus caudalis (TNC)
  hypothalamus, 22
  migraine, 31
  neural systems, 37, 38f
trigeminal-vestibular interaction, neural system, 35–36
trigeminocervical complex, dopamine, 218
trigeminovascular neurons
  hypothalamus, 22
  sensitization of first-order, 45, 46f
  sensitization of second-order, 45–46, 47f
  sensitization of third-order, 46–47, 48f
trigeminovascular system
  headache, 30–31, 32
  migraine, 37–38
triptans
  direct central nervous system effects, 365
  migraine, 24, 25, 339, 340t
tryptophan, migraine, 38
Turenne, Auzias, 8–9
twentieth century, migraines, 12–14

ultrasound, cranial arteries, 140–141

valproate, migraine prevention, 102t, 103, 339, 340t, 341
valproic acid, migraine prevention, 102t, 103
Van der Linden, J. A., 6
vascular changes, migraine, 32
vascular hypothesis
  imaging techniques, 303
  migraine, 303–306
  provoked migraine attacks, 304–306
  spontaneous migraine attacks, 303–304
vascular theory, migraine, 19, 169
vasodilation, migraine and, 169
vasodilators, blood-brain barrier, 24–25
vasospastic theory, cerebral blood flow, 169, 170

venlafaxine, migraine prevention, 99t, 101
verapamil, migraine prevention, 102, 339
vestibular nuclei, neural systems, 37, 38f
vestibular symptoms, migraine, 35–36
vicious circle, migraine symptoms, 36f
visual aura (VA). *See also* migraine with aura
  Alice in Wonderland syndrome, 275–276
  blood flow, 279–280
  cortical spreading depression and role in, imaging, 277–278
  drawing by girl, 276f
  functional magnetic resonance imaging (fMRI), 280–282
  functional somatotopy, 275
  migraine, 275, 349–350
  neuroimaging, 278–279
  scintillations in visual field, 283, 284f
  teichopsia, 275
  variations, 275–276
  visual agnosias, 276
  visual cortex, 276
visual cortex
  activations by light, 76, 77f, 276
  activations by luminous stimulation, 240f
  functional magnetic resonance imaging (fMRI), 30
  photophobia, 239–241
  retinotopic organization, 276–277
  three-dimensional form of primary, 278f
visual evoked potentials (VEPs)
  cortical excitability in childhood migraine, 329
  migraine patients, 138–140
  transcranial magnetic stimulation (TMS), 140
vitamin B₂, riboflavin, 267–268
vitamins, migraine prevention, 111, 267–268
vomiting center
  migraine attack, 351–352
  nausea, 36
voxel-based morphometry (VBM). *See also* surface-based morphometry (SBM)
  chronic pain, 197–198
  chronic tension–type headache, 196
  cluster headache, 195–196
  gray matter change, 365
  limitation, 199–200
  migraine, 196–197
  structural alterations in brain, 195
  structural change specific for headache, 199
  structural data for chronic pain, 197, 198f
  white matter of migraine patients, 191